ADVANCED PRACTICE NURSING

Essentials for Role Development

FOURTH EDITION

ADVANCED PRACTICE NURSING

Essentials for Role Development

FOURTH EDITION

Lucille A. Joel, EdD, APN, FAAN

Distinguished Professor
Rutgers, The State University of New Jersey
School of Nursing, New Brunswick–Newark, New Jersey

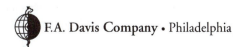

F.A. Davis Company • Philadelphia

F.A. Davis Company
1915 Arch Street
Philadelphia, PA 19103
www.fadavis.com

Printed in the United States of America

Last digit indicates print number: 10 9 8 7 6 5 4 3 2 1

Sponsoring Editor: Jacalyn Sharp
Content Project Manager II: Amy M. Romano
Design and Illustration Manager: Carolyn O'Brien

As new scientific information becomes available through basic and clinical research, recommended treatments and drug therapies undergo changes. The author(s) and publisher have done everything possible to make this book accurate, up-to-date, and in accord with accepted standards at the time of publication. The author(s), editors, and publisher are not responsible for errors or omissions or for consequences from application of the book, and make no warranty, expressed or implied, in regard to the contents of the book. Any practice described in this book should be applied by the reader in accordance with professional standards of care used in regard to the unique circumstances that may apply in each situation. The reader is advised always to check product information (package inserts) for changes and new information regarding dose and contraindications before administering any drug. Caution is especially urged when using new or infrequently ordered drugs.

Library of Congress Cataloging-in-Publication Data

Names: Joel, Lucille A., editor.
Title: Advanced practice nursing : essentials for role development / [edited
  by] Lucille A. Joel, EdD, APN, FAAN, Distinguished Professor, Rutgers, The
  State University of New Jersey, School of Nursing, New Brunswick-Newark,
  New Jersey.
Description: Fourth edition. | Philadelphia, PA : F.A. Davis Company, [2018]
  | Includes bibliographical references and index.
Identifiers: LCCN 2017023590 | ISBN 9780803660441
Classification: LCC RT82.8 .J64 2018 | DDC 610.7306/92--dc23 LC record available at https://lccn.loc.
gov/2017023590

Preface

The content of this text was identified only after a careful review of the documents that shape both the advanced practice nursing role and the educational programs that prepare these individuals for practice. That review allowed some decisions about topics that were essential to all advanced practice nurses (APNs)*, whereas others were excluded because they are traditionally introduced during baccalaureate studies. This text is written for the graduate-level student in advanced practice and is intended to address the nonclinical aspects of the role.

Unit 1 explores *The Evolution of Advanced Practice* from the historical perspective of each of the specialties: the clinical nurse-midwife (CNM), nurse anesthetist (NA), clinical nurse specialist (CNS), and nurse practitioner (NP). This historical background moves to a contemporary focus with the introduction of the many and varied hybrids of these roles that have appeared over time. These dramatic changes in practice have been a response to societal need. Adjustment to these changes is possible only from the kaleidoscopic view that theory allows. Skill acquisition, socialization, and adjustment to stress and strain are theoretical constructs and processes that will challenge the occupants of these roles many times over the course of a career, but coping can be taught and learned. Our accommodation to change is further challenged as we realize that advanced practice is neither unique to North America nor new on the global stage. Advanced practice roles, although accompanied by varied educational requirements and practice opportunities, are well embedded and highly respected in international culture. In the United States, education for advanced practice had become well stabilized at the master's degree level. This is no longer true. The story of our recent transition to doctoral preparation is laid before us with the subsequent issues this creates.

The Practice Environment, the topic of Unit 2, dramatically affects the care we give. With the addition of medical diagnosis and prescribing to the advanced practice repertoire, we became competitive with other disciplines, deserving the rights of reimbursement, prescriptive authority, clinical privileges, and participation as members on health plan panels. There is the further responsibility to understand budgeting and material resource management, as well as the nature of different collaborative, responding, and reporting relationships. The APN often provides care within a mediated role, working through other professionals, including nurses, to improve the human condition.

Competency in Advanced Practice, the topic of Unit 3, demands an incisive mind capable of the highest order of critical thinking. This cognitive skill becomes refined as the subroles for practice emerge. The APN is ultimately a direct caregiver, client advocate, teacher, consultant, researcher, and case manager. The APN's forte is to coach individuals and populations so that they may take control of their own health in their own way, ideally even seeing chronic disease as a new trajectory of wellness. The APN's clients are as diverse as the many ethnicities of the U.S. public, and the challenge is often to learn from them, taking care to do no harm. The APN's therapeutic modalities go beyond traditional Western medicine, reaching into the realm of complementary therapies and integrative health-care practices that have become expected by many consumers. Any or all of these role competencies are potential areas for conflict, needing to be understood, managed, and resolved in the best interests of the client. Some of the most pressing issues confronting APNs today are how to mobilize informational technology in the service of the client, securing visibility for their work, and thinking

---

*Please note that the terms advanced practice nurse (APN) and advanced practice registered nurse (APRN) are used interchangeably in this text according to the author's choice.

through publication. The chapters in this section aim to introduce these competencies, not to provide closure on any one topic; the art of direct care in specialty practice is not broached.

When you have completed your course of studies, you will have many choices to make. There are opportunities to pursue your practice as an employee, an employer, or an independent contractor. Each holds different rights and responsibilities. Each demands *Ethical, Legal, and Business Acumen,* which is covered in Unit 4. Each requires you to prove the value you hold for your clients and for the systems in which you work. Cost efficiency and therapeutic effectiveness cannot be dismissed lightly today. The nuts and bolts of establishing a practice are detailed, and although these particulars apply directly to independent practice, they can be easily extrapolated to employee status. Finally, experts in the field discuss the legal and ethical dimensions of practice and how they uniquely apply to the role of the APN to ensure protection for ourselves and our clients.

This text has been carefully crafted based on over 40 years of experience in practice and teaching APNs. It substantially includes the nonclinical knowledge necessary to perform successfully in the APN role and raises the issues that still have to be resolved to leave this practice area better than we found it.

LUCILLE A. JOEL

Contributors

Cindy Aiena, MBA
Executive Director of Finance
Partners HealthCare/MGH
Boston, Massachusetts

Judith Barberio, PhD, APNC
Associate Clinical Professor
Rutgers-The State University of New Jersey
School of Nursing
New Brunswick-Newark, New Jersey

Deborah Becker, PhD, ACNP, BC, CCNS
Director, Adult Gerontology Acute Care Program
University of Pennsylvania
School of Nursing
Philadelphia, Pennsylvania

Andrea Brassard, PhD, FNP-BC, FAANP
Senior Strategic Policy Advisor
Center to Champion Nursing in America at AARP
Washington, District of Columbia

Edna Cadmus, RN, PhD, NEA-BC
Clinical Professor and Speciality Director-Nursing
    Leadership Program
Executive Director NJCCN
Rutgers-The State University of New Jersey
School of Nursing
New Brunswick-Newark, New Jersey

Ann H. Cary, PhD, MPH, FN, FNAP, FAAN
Dean and Professor
University of Missouri
Kansas City, School of Nursing and Health Studies
Kansas City, Missouri

Patricia DiFusco, MS, NP-C, FNP-BC, AAHIVS
Nurse Practitioner
SUNY Downstate Medical Center
Brooklyn, New York

Caroline Doherty, AGACNP, AACC
Advanced Senior Lecturer
University of Pennsylvania
School of Nursing
Philadelphia, Pennsylvania

Carole Ann Drick, PhD, RN, AHN-BC
President
American Holistic Nurses Association
Topeka, Kansas

Lynne M. Dunphy, PhD, APRN, FNP-BC, FAAN, FAANP
Professor and Associate Dean for Practice
    and Community Engagement
Florida Atlantic University
Christine E. Lynn College of Nursing
Boca Raton, Florida

Denise Fessler, RN, MSN, CMAC
Principal/CEO
Fessler and Associates
Healthcare Management Consulting, LLC
Lancaster, Pennsylvania

Eileen Flaherty, RN, MBA, MPH
Staff Specialist
Massachusetts General Hospital
Boston, Massachusetts

Jane M. Flanagan, PhD, ANP-BC

Associate Professor and Program Director
Adult Gerontology
Boston College
Connell School of Nursing
Chestnut Hill, Massachusetts

Rita Munley Gallagher, RN, PhD

Nursing and Healthcare Consultant
Washington, District of Columbia

Mary Masterson Germain, EdD, ANP-BC, FNAP, D.S. (Hon)

Professor Emeritus
State University of New York–Downstate
    Medical Center College of Nursing
Brooklyn, New York

Kathleen M. Gialanella, JD, LLM, RN

Law Offices
Westfield, New Jersey
Associate Adjunct Professor
Teachers College, Columbia University
New York, New York

Shirley Girouard, RN, PhD, FAAN

Professor and Associate Dean
State University of New York-Downstate
    Medical Center
College of Nursing
Brooklyn, New York

Antigone Grasso, MBA

Director
Patient Care Services Management Systems
    and Financial Performance
Massachusetts General Hospital
Boston, Massachusetts

Anna Green, RN, Crit Care Cert, MNP

Project Manager
Australian Red Cross Blood Service
Melbourne, Australia

Phyllis Shanley Hansell, EdD, RN, FNAP, FAAN

Professor
Seton Hall University
College of Nursing
South Orange, New Jersey

Allyssa Harris, RN, PhD, WHNP-BC

Assistant Professor
William F. Connell School of Nursing
Boston College
Boston, Massachusetts

Gladys L. Husted, RN, PhD

Professor Emeritus
Duquesne University
Pittsburgh, Pennsylvania

James H. Husted

Independent Scholar
Pittsburgh, Pennsylvania

Joseph Jennas, CRNA, MS

Program Director
Clinical Assistant Professor
SUNY Downstate Medical Center
Brooklyn, New York

Lucille A. Joel, EdD, APN, FAAN

Distinguished Professor
Rutgers-The State University of New Jersey
School of Nursing
New Brunswick-Newark
New Jersey

Dorothy A. Jones, EdD, RNC-ANP, FAAN

Professor, Boston College
Connell School of Nursing
Senior Nurse, Massachusetts General Hospital
Boston, Massachusetts

David M. Keepnews, PhD, JD, RN, NEA-BC, FAAN

Dean and Professor
Long Island University (LIU) Brooklyn
Harriet Rothkopf Heilbrunn School of Nursing
Brooklyn, New York

Alice F. Kuehn, RN, PhD, BC-FNP/GNP

Associate Professor Emeritus
University of Missouri-Columbia
School of Nursing
Columbia, Missouri
Parish Nurse
St. Peter Catholic Church
Jefferson City, Missouri

Irene McEachen, RN, MSN, EdD

Associate Professor
Saint Peter's University
Division of Nursing
Jersey City, New Jersey

Deborah C. Messecar, PhD, MPH, AGCNS-BC, RN

Associate Professor
Oregon Health and Science University
School of Nursing
Portland, Oregon

Patricia A. Murphy, PhD, APRN, FAAN

Associate Professor
Rutgers-The State University of New Jersey
New Jersey Medical School
Newark, New Jersey

Marilyn H. Oermann, RN, PhD, FAAN, ANEF

Thelma Ingles Professor of Nursing
Director of Evaluation and Educational Research
Duke University
School of Nursing
Durham, North Carolina

Marie-Eileen Onieal, PhD, MMHS, RN, CPNP, FAANP

Faculty, Doctor of Nursing Practice
Rocky Mountain University of Health Professions
Provo, Utah

David M. Price, MD, PhD

Founding Faculty
Center for Personalized Education of Physicians
    (CDEP)
Denver, Colorado

Beth Quatrara, DNP, RN, CMSRN, ACNS-BC

Advanced Practice Nurse–CNS
University of Virginia Health System
Charlottesville, Virginia

Kelly Reilly, MSN, RN, BC

Director of Nursing
Maimonides Medical Center
Brooklyn, New York

Valerie Sabol, PhD, ACNP-BC, GNP-BC, ANEF, FAANP

Professor and Division Chair
Healthcare in Adult Population
Duke University
School of Nursing
Durham, North Carolina

Mary E. Samost, RN, MSN, DNP, CENP

System Director Surgical Services
Hallmark Health System
Medford, Massachusetts

Madrean Schober, PhD, MSN, ANP, FAANP

President
Schober Global Healthcare Consulting International
Indianapolis, Indiana

Robert Scoloveno, PhD, RN

Director–Simulation Laboratories
Assistant Professor
Rutgers-The State University of New Jersey
School of Nursing
Camden, New Jersey

Carrie Scotto, RN, PhD

Associate Professor
The University of Akron
College of Nursing
Akron, Ohio

Dale Shaw, RN, DNP, ACNP-BC

ACNP–Acute Care Neurosurgery
University of Virginia Health System
Charlottesville, Virginia

Benjamin A. Smallheer, PhD, RN, ACNP-BC, FNP-BC, CCRN, CNE

Assistant Professor of Nursing
Duke University
School of Nursing
Durham, North Carolina

Thomas D. Smith, DNP, RN, NEA-BC, FAAN

Chief Nursing Officer
Maimonides Medical Center
Brooklyn, New York

Mary C. Smolenski, MS, EdD, FNP, FAANP

Independent Consultant
Washington, District of Columbia

Shirley A. Smoyak, RN, PhD, FAAN

Distinguished Professor
Rutgers-The State University of New Jersey
School of Nursing
New Brunswick-Newark, New Jersey

Christine A. Tanner, RN, PhD, ANEF

Professor Emerita
Oregon Health and Science University
Portland, Oregon

Caroline T. Torre, RN, MA, APN, FAANP

Nursing Policy Consultant
Princeton, New Jersey
Formerly, Director, Regulatory Affairs
New Jersey State Nurses Association
Trenton, New Jersey

Jan Towers, PhD, NP-C, CRNP (FNP), FAANP

Director of Health Policy
Federal Government and Professional Affairs
American Academy of Nurse Practitioners
Washington, District of Columbia

Maria L. Vezina, RN, EdD, NEA-BC

Chief Nursing Officer/Vice President, Nursing
The Mount Sinai Hospital
New York, New York

Reviewers

Nancy Bittner, RN, PhD

Associate Dean
School of Nursing Science and Health Professions
Regis College
Weston, Massachusetts

Cynthia Bostick, PMHCNS-BC, PhD

Lecturer
California State University
Carson, California

Susan S. Fairchild, EdD, APRN

Dean, School of Nursing
Grantham University
Kansas City, Missouri

Cris Finn, RN, PhD, FNP

Assistant Professor
Regis University
Denver, Colorado

Susan C. Fox, RN, PhD, CNS-BC

Associate Professor
College of Nursing
University of New Mexico
Albuquerque, New Mexico

Eileen P. Geraci, PhD candidate, MA, ANP-BC

Professor of Nursing
Western Connecticut State University
Danbury, Connecticut

Sheila Grossman, PhD, APRN, FNP-BC, FAAN

Professor and Coordinator
Family Nurse Practitioner Program
Fairfield University
Fairfield, Connecticut

Elisabeth Jensen, RN, PhD

Associate Professor
School of Nursing
York University
Toronto, Ontario
Canada

Linda E. Jensen, PhD, MN, RN

Professor Graduate Nursing
Clarkson College
Omaha, Nebraska

Julie Ann Koch, DNP, RN, FNP-BC, FAANP

Assistant Dean of Graduate Nursing
DNP Program Coordinator
Valparaiso University College of Nursing & Health
    Professions
Valparaiso, Indiana

Linda U. Krebs, RN, PhD, AOCN, FAAN

Associate Professor
University of Colorado
Anschutz Medical Campus, College of Nursing
Aurora, Colorado

Joy Lewis, CRNA, MSN

Interim Assistant Program Director Nurse
Anesthesia
Lincoln Memorial University
Harrogate, Tennessee

Laurie Kennedy-Malone, PhD, GNP-BC, FAANP, FGSA

Professor of Nursing
University of North Carolina at Greensboro School
of Nursing
Greensboro, North Carolina

Susan McCrone, PhD, PMHCNS-BC

Professor
West Virginia University
Morgantown, West Virginia

Sandra Nadelson, RN, MS Ed, PhD

Associate Professor
Boise State University
Boise, Idaho

Geri B. Neuberger, RN, MN, EdD, ARNP-CS

Professor
University of Kansas School of Nursing
Kansas City, Kansas

Crystal Odle, DNAP, CRNA

Director, Assistant Professor Nurse Anesthesia
Program
Lincoln Memorial University
Harrogate, Tennessee

Julie Ponto, RN, PhD, ACNS-BC, AOCN

Professor
Winona State University–Rochester
Rochester, Minnesota

Susan D. Schaffer, PhD, ARNP, FNP-BC

Chair, Department of Women's, Children's
and Family Nursing
FNP Track Coordinator
University of Florida College of Nursing
Gainesville, Florida

Beth R. Steinfeld, DNP, WHNP-BC

Assistant Professor
SUNY Downstate Medical Center
Brooklyn, New York

Lynn Wimett, EdD, APRN-C

Professor
Regis University
Denver, Colorado

Jennifer Klimek Yingling, PhD, RN, ANP-BC, FNP-BC

Advanced Practice Nurse
Faxton-St. Luke's Healthcare
SUNY Institute of Technology
Utica, New York

Acknowledgments

This book belongs to its authors. I am proud to be one among them. Beyond that, I have been the instrument to make these written contributions accessible to today's students and faculty. I thank each author for the products of his or her intellect, experience, and commitment to advanced practice.

Contents

1

The Evolution of Advanced Practice

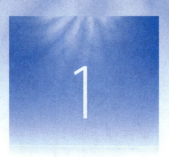

Advanced Practice Nursing
Doing What Has to Be Done

Lynne M. Dunphy

Learning Outcomes
Learning outcomes expected as a result of this chapter:

- Recognize the historical role of women as healers.
- Identify the roots of professional nursing in the United States including the public health movement and turn-of-the-century settlement houses.
- Describe early innovative care models created by nurses in the first half of the 20th century such as the Frontier Nursing Service (FNS).
- Trace the trajectory of the role of the *nurse midwife* across the 20th century as well as the present status of this role.
- Recognize the emergence of *nurse anesthetists* as highly autonomous practitioners and their contributions to the advancement of surgical techniques and developments in anesthesia.
- Describe the development of the *clinical nurse specialist* (*CNS*) role in the context of 20th-century nursing education and professional development with particular attention to the current challenges of this role.
- Describe the historical and social forces that led to emergence of the nurse practitioner (NP) role and understand key events in the evolution of this role.
- Describe the development of the doctor of nursing practice (DNP) and distinguish this role from the others described in this chapter.
- Describe the current challenges to *all* advanced roles and formulate ways to meet these challenges going forward.

Advanced practice is a contemporary term that has evolved to label an old phenomenon: nurses or women providing care to those in need in their surrounding communities. As Barbara Ehrenreich and Deidre English (1973) note, "Women have always been healers. They were the unlicensed doctors and anatomists of western history . . . they were pharmacists, cultivating herbs and exchanging the secrets of their uses. They were midwives, travelling from home to home and village to village" (p. 3). Today, with health care dominated by a male-oriented medical profession, advanced practice nurses (APNs) (especially those cheeky enough to call themselves "doctor" even while clarifying their nursing role and background) are viewed as nurses "pushing the envelope"—the envelope of regulated, standardized nursing practice. The reality is that the boundaries of professional nursing practice have always been fluid, with changes in the practice setting speeding ahead of the educational and regulatory environments. It has always been those nurses caring for persons and families who see a need and respond—at times in concert with the medical profession and at times at odds—who are the true trailblazers of contemporary advanced practice nursing.

This chapter makes the case that, far from being a new creation, APNs actually predate the founding of modern professional nursing. A look back into our past reveals legendary figures always responding to the challenges of human need, changing the landscape of health care, and improving the health of the populace. The titles may change—such as a doctor of nursing practice (DNP)—but the essence remains the same.

PRECURSORS AND ANTECEDENTS

There is a long and rich history of female lay healing with roots in both European and African cultures. Well into the 19th century, the female lay healer was the primary health-care provider for most of the population. The sharing of skills and knowledge was seen as one's obligation as a member of a community. These skills were broad based and might have included midwifery, the use of herbal remedies, and even bone setting (Ehrenreich, 2000, p. xxxiii). Laurel Ulrich, in *A Midwife's Tale* (1990), notes that when the diary of the midwife Martha Ballard opens in 1785, ". . . she knew how to manufacture salves, syrups, pills, teas, ointments, how to prepare an oil emulsion, how to poultice

wounds, dress burns, treat dysentery, sore throat, frost bite, measles, colic, 'whooping cough,' 'chin cough,' . . . and 'the itch,' how to cut an infant's tongue, administer a 'clister' (enema), lance an abscessed breast . . . induce vomiting, assuage bleeding, reduce swelling and relieve a toothache, as well as deliver babies" (p. 11).

Ulrich notes the tiny headstones marking the graves of midwife Ballard's deceased babies and children as further evidence of her ability to provide compassionate, knowledgeable care; she was able to understand the pain and suffering of others. The emergence of a male medical establishment in the 19th century marked the beginning of the end of the era of female lay healers, including midwives. The lay healers saw their role as intertwined with one's obligations to the community, whereas the emerging medical class saw healing as a commodity to be bought and sold (Ehrenreich & English, 1978). Has this really changed? Are not our current struggles still bound up with issues of gender, class, social position, and money? Have we not entered a phase of more radical than ever splits between the haves and have-nots, with grave consequences to our social fabric?

Nursing histories (O'Brien, 1987) have documented the emergence of professional nursing in the 19th century from women's domestic duties and roles, extensions of the things that women and servants had always done for their families. Modern nursing is usually pinpointed as beginning in 1873, the year of the opening of the first three U.S. training schools for nurses, "as an effort on the part of women reformers to help clean up the mess the male doctors were making" (Ehrenreich, 2000, p. xxxiv). The incoming nurses, for example, are credited with introducing the first bar of soap into Bellevue Hospital in the dark days when the medical profession was still resisting the germ theory of disease and aseptic techniques.

The emergence of a strong public health movement in the 19th century, coupled with the Settlement House Movement, created a new vista for independent and autonomous nursing practice. The Henry Street Settlement, a brainchild of a recently graduated trained nurse named Lillian Wald, was a unique community-based nursing practice on the lower east side of New York City. Wald described these nurses who flocked to work with her at Henry Street Settlement as women of above average "intellectual equipment," of "exceptional character, mentality and scholarship" (Daniels, 1989, p. 24). These nurses, as has been well documented, enjoyed an exceptional degree of independence and autonomy in their nursing practice caring for the poor, often recent immigrants.

In 1893, Wald described a typical day. First, she visited the Goldberg baby and then Hattie Isaacs, a patient with consumption to whom she brought flowers. Wald spent 2 hours bathing her ("the poor girl had been without this attention for so long that it took me nearly two hours to get her skin clean"). Next, she inspected some houses on Hester Street where she found water closets that needed "chloride of lime" and notified the appropriate authorities. In the next house, she found a child with "running ears," which she "syringed," showing the mother how to do it at the same time. In another room, there was a child with a "summer complaint"; Wald gave the child bismuth and tickets for a seaside excursion. After lunch she saw the O'Briens and took the "little one, with whooping cough" to play in the back of the Settlement House yard. On the next floor of that tenement, she found the Costria baby who had a sore mouth. Wald "gave the mother honey and borax and little cloths to keep it clean" (Coss, 1989, pp. 43–44). This was all before 2 p.m.! Far from being some new invention, midwives, nurse anesthetists, clinical nurse specialists (CNSs), and nurse practitioners (NPs) are merely new permutations of these long-standing nursing commitments and roles.

NURSE-MIDWIVES

Throughout the 20th century, nurse-midwifery remained an anomaly in the U.S. health-care system. Nurse-midwives attend only a small percentage of all U.S. births. Since the early decades of the 20th century, physicians laid claim to being the sole legitimate birth attendants in the United States (Dye, 1984). This is in contrast to Great Britain and many other European countries where trained midwives attend a significant percentage of births. In Europe, homes remain an accepted place to give birth, whereas hospital births reign supreme in the United States. In contrast to Europe, the United States has little in the way of a tradition of professional midwifery.

As late as 1910, 50% of all births in the United States were reportedly attended by midwives, and the percentage in large cities was often higher. However, the health status of the U.S. population, particularly in regard to perinatal health indicators, was poor (Bigbee & Amidi-Nouri, 2000). Midwives—unregulated and by most accounts unprofessional—were easy scapegoats on which to blame the problem of poor maternal and infant outcomes. New York City's Department of Health commissioned a study that claimed that the New York midwife was essentially "medieval." According to this report, fully 90% were "hopelessly dirty, ignorant, and incompetent" (Edgar, 1911, p. 882). There was a concerted movement away from home births. This was all part of a mass assault on midwifery by an increasingly powerful medical elite of obstetricians determined to control the birthing process.

These revelations resulted in the tightening of existing laws and the creation of new legislation for the licensing and supervision of midwives (Kobrin, 1984). Several states passed laws granting legal recognition and regulation of midwives, resulting in the establishment of schools of midwifery. One example, the Bellevue School for Midwives in New York City, lasted until 1935, when the diminishing need for midwives made it difficult to justify its existence (Komnenich, 1998). Obstetrical care continued the move into hospitals in urban areas that did not provide midwifery. For the most part, the advance of nurse-midwifery has been a slow and arduous struggle often at odds with mainstream nursing. For example, Lavinia Dock (1901) wrote that all births must be attended by physicians. Public health nurses, committed to the professionalizing of nursing and adherence to scientific standards, chose to distance themselves from lay midwives. The heritage of the unprofessional image of the lay midwife would linger for many years.

A more successful example of midwifery was the founding of the Frontier Nursing Service (FNS) in 1925 by Myra Breckinridge in Kentucky. Breckinridge, having been educated as a public health nurse and traveling to Great Britain to become a certified nurse-midwife (CNM), pursued a vision of autonomous nurse-midwifery practice. She aimed to implement the British system in the United States (always a daunting enterprise on any front). In rural settings, where doctors were scarce and hospitals virtually nonexistent, midwifery found more fertile soil. However, even in these settings, professional nurse-midwifery had to struggle to bloom.

Breckinridge founded the FNS at a time when the national maternal death rate stood at 6.7 per 1,000 live births, one of the highest rates in the Western world. More than 250,000 infants, nearly 1 in 10, died before they reached their first birthday (U.S. Department of Labor, 1920). The Sheppard-Towner Maternity and Infancy Act, enacted to provide public funds for maternal and child health programs, was the first federal legislation passed for specifically this purpose. Part of the intention of this act was to provide money to the states to train public health nurses in midwifery; however, this proved short-lived. By 1929, the bill lapsed; this was attributed by some to major opposition by the American Medical Association (AMA), which advocated the establishment of a "single standard" of obstetrical care, care that is provided by doctors in hospital settings (Kobrin, 1984).

Breckinridge saw nurse-midwives working as independent practitioners and continued to advocate home births. And even more radically, the FNS saw nurse-midwives as offering complete care to women with normal pregnancies and deliveries. However, even Breckinridge and her supporters did not advocate the FNS model for cities where doctors were plentiful and middle-class women could afford medical care. She stressed that the FNS was designed for impoverished "remotely rural areas" without physicians (Dye, 1984).

The American Association of Nurse-Midwives (AANM) was founded in 1928, originally as the Kentucky State Association of Midwives, which was an outgrowth of the FNS. First organized as a section of the National Organization of Public Health Nurses (NOPHN), the American College of Nurse-Midwives (ACNM) was incorporated as an independent specialty nursing organization in 1955 when the NOPHN was subsumed within the National League for Nursing (NLN). In 1956, the AANM merged with the college, forming the ACNM as it continues today. The ACNM sponsored the *Journal of Nurse-Midwifery*, implemented an accreditation process of programs in 1962, and established a certification examination and process in 1971. This body also currently certifies non-nurses as midwives and maintains alliances with professional midwives who are not nurses. As noted by Bigbee and Amidi-Nouri (2000), CNMs are distinct from other APNs in that "they conceptualize their role as the combination of two disciplines, nursing and midwifery" (p. 12).

At their core, midwives as a group remain focused on their primary commitment: care of mothers and babies regardless of setting and ability to pay. Rooted in holistic care and the most natural approaches possible, in 2015 there were 11,194 CNMs and 97 certified midwives. In 2014, CNMs or CMs attended 332,107 births, accounting for 12.1% of all vaginal births and 8.3% of total U.S. births (National Center for Health Statistics, 2014).

CNMs are licensed, independent health-care providers with prescriptive authority in all 50 states, the District of Columbia, American Samoa, Guam, and Puerto Rico. CNMs are defined as primary care providers under federal law. CMs are also licensed, independent health-care providers who have completed the same midwifery education as CNMs. CMs are authorized to practice in Delaware, Missouri, New Jersey, New York, and Rhode Island and have prescriptive authority in New York and Rhode Island. The first accredited CM education program began in 1996. The CM credential is not yet recognized in all states.

Although midwives are well-known for attending births, 53.3% of CNMs and CMs identify reproductive care and 33.1% identify primary care as main responsibilities in their full-time positions. Examples include annual examinations, writing prescriptions, basic nutrition counseling, parenting education, patient education, and reproductive health visits.

NURSE ANESTHETISTS

Nursing made medicine look good.   —Baer, 1982

Surgical anesthesia was born in the United States in the mid 19th century. Immediately there were rival claimants to its "discovery" (Bankert, 1989). In 1846 at Massachusetts General Hospital, William T. G. Morton first successfully demonstrated surgical anesthesia. Nitrous oxide was the first agent used and adopted by U.S. dentists. Ether and chloroform followed shortly as agents for use in anesthetizing a patient. One barrier to surgery had been removed. However, it would take infection control and consistent, careful techniques in the administration of the various anesthetic agents for surgery to enter its "Golden Age." It was only then that "surgery was transformed from an act of desperation to a scientific method of dealing with illness" (Rothstein, 1958, p. 258).

For surgeons to advance their specialty, they needed someone to administer anesthesia with care. However, anesthesiology lacked medical status; the surgeon collected the fee. No incentive existed for anyone with a medical degree to take up the work. Who would administer the anesthesia? And who would do so reliably and carefully? There was only one answer: nurses.

In her landmark book *Watchful Care: A History of America's Nurse Anesthetists* (1989), Marianne Bankert explains how economics changed anesthesia practice. Physician-anesthetists "needed to establish their 'claim' to a field of practice they had earlier rejected" (p. 16), and to do this it became necessary to deny, ignore, or denigrate the achievements of their nurse colleagues. The most intriguing part of her study, she says, was "the process by which a rival—and less moneyed—group (in this case, nurses) is rendered historically 'invisible'" (p. 16).

St. Mary's Hospital, later to become known as the Mayo Clinic, played an important role in the development of anesthesia. It was here that Alice Magaw, sometimes referred to as the "Mother of Anesthesia," practiced from 1860 to 1928. In 1899, she published a paper titled "Observations in Anesthesia" in *Northwestern Lancet* in which she reported giving anesthesia in more than 3,000 cases (Magaw, 1899). In 1906, she published another review of more than 14,000 successful anesthesia cases (Magaw, 1906). Bigbee and Amidi-Nouri (2000) note, "She stressed individual attention for all patients and identified the experience of anesthetists as critical elements in quickly responding to the patient" (p. 21). She also paid special attention to her patients' psyches: She believed that "suggestion" was a great help "in producing a comfortable narcosis" (Bankert, 1989, p. 32). She noted that the anesthetist "must be able to inspire confidence in the patient" and that much of this depends on the approach (Bankert, 1989, p. 32). She stressed preparing the patient for each phase of the experience and of the need to "'talk him to sleep' with the addition of as little ether as possible" (p. 33). Magaw contended that hospital-based anesthesia services, as a specialized field, should remain separate from nursing service administrative structures (Bigbee & Amidi-Nouri, 2000). This presaged the estrangement that has historically existed between nurse anesthetists and "regular" nursing; we see a nursing specialty with expanded clinical responsibilities developing outside of mainstream nursing.

The medical specialty of anesthesiology began to gain a foothold around the turn of the 20th century, led largely by women physicians. However, these physicians were unsympathetic to the role of the nurse anesthetists; they wanted to replace them to establish their own controls. Different variants of this old power struggle echo today in legislative battles over the need for on-site oversight by an anesthesiologist.

The American Association of Nurse Anesthetists (AANA) was founded in 1931 by Hodgins and originally named the National Association for Nurse Anesthetists. This group voted to affiliate with the American Nurses Association (ANA), only to be turned away. As early as 1909, Florence Henderson, a successor of Magaw's, was invited to present a paper at the ANA convention, with no subsequent extension of an invitation to become a member of the organization (Komnenich, 1998). Thatcher (1953) speculates that organized nursing was fearful that nurse anesthetists could be charged with practicing medicine, a theme we will see repeated when we examine the history of the development of the NP role. This rejection led the AANA to affiliate with the American Hospital Association (AHA).

The relationship between nurse anesthetists and anesthesiologists has always been, and continues to be, contentious. Consistent with health-care workforce data in general, there is a maldistribution of MDs, including anesthesiologists, who frequently choose to practice in areas where patients can afford to pay or in desirable areas to live. Rural areas continue to be underserved as well as indigent areas in general. CRNAs pick up the slack, "doing what has to be done" to meet the needs of underserved patients. Complicating this picture is that there is an uneven supply of CRNAs in different geographic areas. As CRNAs retire later, unwilling to give up lucrative positions, some regions experience intergenerational hostility as well.

Despite a brief period of relative harmony from 1972 to 1976, when the AANA and the American Society of Anesthesiologists (ASA) issued the "Joint Statement on Anesthesia Practice," their partnership ended when the board of directors of the ASA withdrew its support of this statement, returning to a model that maintained physician control (Bankert, 1989, pp. 140–150).

The Certified Registered Nurse Anesthetist (CRNA) credential came into existence in 1956. At present, there are approximately more than 50,000 CRNAs (AANA, 2016),* 41% of whom are males (compared with the approximately 13% male population in nursing overall, a figure that has held steady for some time). CRNAs safely

---

*In some states, the title CRNA has been changed to APN-Anesthesia.

administer *approximately 43 million anesthetics* to patients each year in the United States according to the AANA 2016 Practice Profile Survey.

Interestingly, the inclusion of large numbers of males in its ranks has not eased the advance of this venerable nursing specialty; turf wars between practicing anesthesiologists and nurse anesthetists remain intense as of this writing, further aggravated by the incursion of "doctor-nurses" or "nurse-doctors." Nonetheless, nurse anesthetists continue to thrive and have situated themselves in the mainstream of graduate-level nursing education, including a large portion of programs adapting curriculums leading to the DNP. Their inclusion in the spectrum of advanced practice nursing continues to be invigorating for us.

THE CLINICAL NURSE SPECIALIST

The role of the CNS is the one strand of advanced practice nursing that arose and was nurtured by mainstream nursing education and nursing organizations. Indeed, one could say it arose from the very bosom of traditional nursing practice. As early as 1900, in the *American Journal of Nursing*, Katherine DeWitt wrote that the development of nursing specialties, in her view, responded to a "need for perfection within a limited domain" (Sparacino, 1986, p. 1). According to DeWitt, nursing specialties were a response to "present civilization and modern science [that] demand a perfection along each line of work formerly unknown" (Sparacino, 1986, p. 1). She argued that "the new nurse is more useful, at least to the patient himself, and ultimately to the family and community. Her sphere is more limited, but her patient receives better care" (Sparacino, 1986, p. 1).

Historically, nurses were trained and worked in hospitals that were structured for the convenience of the doctors around specific populations of patients. Early on, nurses initiated guidelines for the care of unique populations and often garnered a hands-on kind of intimacy, an expertise in the care of certain patients that was not to be denied. Caring day in and day out for patients suffering from similar conditions enabled nurses to develop specialized and advanced skills not practiced by other nurses. Think of the nurses who cared exclusively for patients with tuberculosis, syphilis, and polio. Because these conditions are no longer common, any nursing expertise that might have been developed has been lost.

In a 1943 speech, Frances Reiter first used the term *nurse-clinician*. She believed that "practice is the absolute primary function of our profession" and "that means the direct care of patients" (Reiter, 1966). The nurse-clinician, as Reiter conceived the role, consisted of three spheres. The first sphere, clinical competence, included three additional dimensions of function, which she termed *care, cure,* and *counseling.* The nurse-clinician was labeled "the Mother Role," in which the nurse protects, teaches, comforts, and encourages the patient. The second sphere, as envisioned by Reiter, involved clinical expertise in the coordination and continuity of the patient's care. In the final sphere, she believed in what she called "professional maturity," wherein the physician and nurse "share a mutual responsibility for the welfare of patients" (Reiter, 1966, p. 277). It was only through such working together that the patient could best be served and nursing achieve "its greatest potential" (Reiter, 1966). Although Reiter believed that the nurse-clinician should have advanced clinical competence, she did not specify that the nurse-clinician should be prepared at the master's level.

In 1943, the National League for Nursing Education advocated a plan to develop these *nurse-clinicians,* enlisting universities to educate them (Menard, 1987). Traditionally, advanced education in nursing had focused on "functional" areas, that is, nursing education and nursing administration. Esther Lucile Brown, in her 1948 report *Nursing for the Future,* promoted developing clinical specialties in nursing as a way of strengthening and advancing the profession. The GI Bill was also available. Nurses in the Armed Services were eligible to receive funds for their education.

It took the entrance of another strong nurse leader, Hildegard Peplau, to move these ideas forward to fruition. In 1953, she had both a vision and a plan: She wanted to prepare psychiatric nurse clinicians at the graduate level who could offer direct care to psychiatric patients, thus helping to close the gap between psychiatric theory and nursing practice (Callaway, 2002). In addition, as always there was a great need for health-care providers of all stripes in psychiatric settings. In her first 2 years at Rutgers University in New Jersey, Peplau developed a 19-month master's program that prepared only CNSs in psychiatric nursing. In contrast, existing programs, such as that at Teachers College in New York City, attempted to prepare nurses for teaching and supervision in a 10-month program.

The field of psychiatric nursing was in the process of inventing itself. Before the passage of the National Mental Health Act in 1946, there was no such field as psychiatric nursing. It was the availability of National Institute of Mental Health funds to "seed" such programs as Peplau's that allowed psychiatric nursing to begin and eventually to flourish.

In retrospect, Peplau would note that no encouragement was received from the two major nursing organizations of the day, the NLN and the ANA. She stated, "We were highly stigmatized. Any nurse who worked in [the field of mental health] was considered almost certifiable. . . . We were thoroughly unpopular, we were considered queer enough to be avoided" (Callaway, 2002, p. 229).

It should be emphasized that at this point in nursing history it was inconceivable that any nurse, under any circumstances, could become a specialist. The "received wisdom" of the day was the axiom, followed by the vast majority of nurses, that "a nurse is a nurse is a nurse," opposing any differentiation between who was doing what among them. Peplau's rigorous curriculum and clinical and academic program requirements expected that faculty would continue their own clinical practice, do clinical research, and publish the results (Callaway, 2002). This was a radical model for nursing faculty, few of whom were doctorally prepared in the 1950s. In 1956, only 2 years following the initiation of the first clinically focused graduate program, a national working conference on graduate education in psychiatric nursing formally developed the role of the psychiatric clinical specialist.

Most hospital training schools remained embedded in a functional method of nursing well into the 1960s. As originally conceptualized by Isabel Stewart in the 1930s, "nurses were trained and much of nursing practice was rule-based and activity-oriented" (Fairman, 1999, p. 42), relying heavily on repetition of skills and procedures. There was little, if any, scientific understanding of the principles underlying care. There was little, if any, intellectual content to be found in the nursing curriculum.

With the advent of antibiotics in the 1940s and the resulting decline of infectious diseases, nurses' practice shifted to caring for patients with acute, often rapidly changing exacerbations of chronic conditions. Leaders such as Peplau, along with others such as Virginia Henderson, Frances Reiter, and later Dorothy Smith, began developing a theoretical orientation for practice. Students were being taught to assess patient responses to their illnesses and to make analytical decisions. Smith experimented with the idea of a nurse-clinician who

had 24-hour responsibility for a patient area and who was on call. Laura Simms at Cornell University–New York Hospital School of Nursing developed a CNS role to provide consultation to more generalist nurses. As opposed to the nurse who might have been expert in procedures, these new clinicians were experts in clinical care for a certain population of patients. This development occurred across specialties and was seen in oncology, nephrology, psychiatry, and intensive care units (Sills, 1983).

Role expansion of the CNS grew rapidly during the 1960s because of several factors. Advances in medical technology and medical specialization increased the need for nurses who were competent to care for patients with complex health needs. Nurses returning from the battlefields of Vietnam sought to increase their knowledge and skills and continued to practice in advanced roles and nontraditional areas (such as trauma or anesthesia). Role definitions for women loosened and expanded. There was a shortage of physicians. The Nurse Training Act of 1964 allocated necessary federal funds for additional graduate nursing education programs in several different clinical specialties (Mirr & Snyder, 1995).

The terms *nurse-clinician, CNS,* and *nurse specialist,* among others, were used extensively by nurses with experience or advanced knowledge who had developed an expertise within a given area of patient care. There were no standards regarding educational requirements or experience. In 1965, the ANA developed a position statement declaring that only those nurses with a master's degree or higher in nursing should claim the role of CNS (ANA, 1965). These trends continued into the 1970s. The number of academic programs providing master's preparation in a variety of practice areas increased. Federal grants, including those from the Department of Health, Education, and Welfare, continued to provide funding for nursing education at the master's and doctoral levels.

In 1976, during the ANA's Congress on Nursing Practice, a position statement on the role of the CNS was issued. The ANA position statement read as follows (ANA Congress for Nursing Practice, 1976):

> The clinical nurse specialist (CNS) is a practitioner holding a master's degree with a concentration in specific areas of clinical nursing. The role of the CNS is defined by the needs of a select client population, the expectation of the larger society and the clinical expertise of the nurse.

The statement went on to elaborate that "by exercising leadership ability and judgment," the CNS is able to affect client care on the individual, direct-care provider level as well as affect change within the broader health-care system (ANA Congress for Nursing Practice, 1976).

The 1970s were a time of growth in academic CNS programs; the 1980s were years in which refinements occurred. In 1980, the ANA revised its earlier policy statement of 1976 to define the CNS as "a registered nurse who, through study and supervised clinical practice at the graduate level (master's or doctorate) has become an expert in a defined area of knowledge and practice in a selected clinical area of nursing" (ANA, 1980, p. 23). This statement was significant because it was the first time that education at the master's level had been dictated as a mandatory criterion for entry into expert practice.

The CNS role more than any other advanced nursing role was situated in the mainstream of graduate nursing education, with the first master's degree in psychiatric and mental health nursing conferred by Rutgers University in 1955. The inclusion of clinical content in master's degree education was an essential step forward for nursing's advancement. But the implementation and use of the CNS avoided easy categorization and their efficacy was elusive.

In February 1983, the ANA Council of Clinical Nurse Specialists met for the first time (Sparacino, 1990). The Council grew rapidly throughout the subsequent years, supporting and providing educational conferences for the increasing numbers of CNSs. In 1986, the Council published the CNS's role statement. This statement identified the roles of the CNS as specialist in clinical practice and as educator, consultant, researcher, and administrator. This role statement by the Council depicted the changing role of the CNS, notably delegating and overseeing practice as its primary focus (Fulton, 2002). The year 1986 was also notable for the publication of the journal *Clinical Nurse Specialist: The Journal for Advanced Nursing*.

In 1986, the ANA's Council of Clinical Nurse Specialists and the Council of Primary Health Care Providers published an editorial outlining the similarities of the CNS and NP roles. Discussion surrounding the commonalities of both specialties occurred throughout the decade. In 1989, during the annual meeting of the National Organization of Nurse Practitioner Faculty (NONPF), the 10-year-old debate regarding the merger of the two roles reached a crescendo without resolution (Lincoln, 2000). It remains an issue of contention to the present day. Despite this, the two ANA councils did merge in 1990, becoming the Council of Nurses in Advanced Practice (Busen & Engleman, 1996; Lincoln, 2000). Following the merger of the councils, several studies were published comparing CNS and NP roles, finding the education for practice generally comparable (Joel, 2011).

The 1990s was an era of health-care "reform." Health-care costs were skyrocketing; hospital stays were shorter, with acutely ill patients being discharged quicker and sicker. Because of fiscal mandates, hospitals were decreasing the number of beds and personnel and the focus of health care shifted from hospital to ambulatory care within the community and home. The historically hospital-based CNS was considered too expensive and unproven. Thus, CNSs all over were losing positions.

In 1993, the American Association of Colleges of Nursing (AACN) met to discuss educational needs and requirements for the 21st century. At the AACN's annual conference in December 1994, members voted to support the merging of the CNS and NP roles in the curricula of graduate education in nursing. Although the structure of the curricula suggested in the "Essentials of Graduate Education" (AACN, 1995) has been widely adopted, the lived reality of role adaptation and its implementation in the marketplace has been less uniform and more divisive. Sparacino (1990) defined the scope of the CNS as "client-centered practice, utilizing an in-depth assessment, practiced within the domain of secondary and tertiary care settings" (p. 8). The NP role is defined by Sparacino (1986) as being responsible for providing a full range of primary health-care services, using the appropriate knowledge base and practicing in multiple settings outside of secondary and tertiary settings. To some degree this has been the nature of these roles, though many exceptions can be observed today.

Scope of practice barriers continue in this area of advanced practice nursing. The latest setback occurred when the Standard Occupational Classification Policy Committee (SOCPC) announced its recommendations to the Office of Management and Budget for the 2018 Standard Occupational Classification on July 22, 2016. The SOCPC declined to include the CNS in a separate broad occupation and detailed occupation category, stating:

> Multiple dockets requested a new detailed occupation for Clinical Nurse Specialists. The SOCPC did not accept this recommendation based on Classification Principle 2 which states that occupations are classified based on work performed and on Classification Principle 9 on collectability.

In July 2014, the National Association of Clinical Nurse Specialists (NACNS) submitted an extensive filing on why the CNS should be included in the Standard Occupational Classification (SOC) as a "broad category." This is the second time that the SOCPC did not accept the request to make the CNS a new detailed occupation in the SOC. Retaining CNSs in the RNs 2010 classifications is inconsistent with federal agencies, with nursing practice in the states, and with the larger nursing community, all of which distinguish CNSs as APRNs. Congress has accepted CNSs as APRNs for nearly two decades. The *Balanced Budget Act of 1997* allowed CNSs to directly bill their services through the Centers for Medicare and Medicaid Services under Part B participation in Medicare. CNSs were recognized as eligible for Medicare's Primary Care Incentive Program in the *Patient Protection and Affordable Care Act* (PPACA, 2010).

CNSs prescribe medications, durable medical equipment, and medical supplies as well as order, perform, and interpret diagnostic tests including laboratory work and x-rays. Two unequivocal differences exist between CNSs and RNs: diagnosing patients and prescribing pharmaceuticals. CNSs can perform both; RNs are not authorized to perform either. The SOCPC's recommendation to not recognize the CNS as a broad occupation and detailed occupation, similar to how other APRNs are categorized, skews the quality and utility of federal health-care policy data. Linking the CNS workforce data with the RN workforce does not allow CNS contributions to be differentiated from or compared with any other APRN data. Simply put, a database set up by any federal, state, regional, local, research, or private entity using the 2010 SOC categories has no data on the more than 72,000 CNSs in the United States (NACNS, 2016).

The "other side" of this story of advanced practice nursing—NP evolution—is addressed in the next section of this chapter. The futures of these various roles remain on some level intertwined and are further complicated by the emergence of a new model of educational preparation: the DNP.

THE EVOLUTION OF THE NURSE PRACTITIONER ROLE: "A DISRUPTIVE INNOVATION"

The history of the NP "movement" has been well documented (Brush & Capezuti, 1996; Fairman, 1999, 2008;

Jacox, 2002). A lesser known story involves Dr. Eugene A. Stead, Jr., of Duke University, who in 1957 conceived of an advanced role for nurses somewhere between the role of the nurse and the doctor. Thelma Ingles, a nursing faculty member on a sabbatical, worked with Stead, accompanying the interns and residents on rounds, seeing patients, and managing increasingly ill patients with acumen and sensitivity. Ingles shared Stead's ideas and returned to the Duke Nursing School to create a master of science in nursing program modeled on her experience with Stead. Stead was gratified and anxious to impart this expanded role to other nursing faculty, envisioning a new role for nurses, with, in his view, expanded autonomy. He was shocked at the "lukewarm" response of the dean of nursing at Duke and the unsupportive stance of several prominent nurses at the university. On top of that, the NLN, the school's accrediting body, did not approve of Ingles's new program for nurse clinical specialization and withheld the program's accreditation. They found the program "unstructured" and criticized the use of physicians as instructors to teach courses for nurses in a nursing program. They disavowed the study of the esteemed discipline of medicine that Stead was so anxious to impart (Holt, 1998). Instead, they wanted the students to study "nursing." Stead could not understand this. What was there in nursing to study? Rejected and disheartened, Stead eventually turned to military corpsmen to actualize this new role, which he named *physician assistant*. He insisted that they be male. In his view, nurse leaders were very antagonistic to innovation and change (Christman, 1998). In the view of some, this was a missed opportunity for organized nursing but one governed by historical circumstances when viewed on the broader stage of history. Fairman (2008), in an extensive study of Stead's papers, offers the appraisement that "Stead's difficulties went beyond his experiences with organized and academic nursing. They reflected his perceptions of the kind of help his physician colleagues needed" (Fairman, 2008, p. 98).

Stead's original proposal was quite prescient. Gender roles were loosening as were hierarchical structures in general; nurses were better educated and well able to assume the role responsibilities that Stead envisioned. Yet it came at a time when nursing was merely a fledgling discipline, new to the university, new to development as an academic discipline, and new to doctoral education. Academic nursing was fixated on defining its own knowledge base and developing its own unique science. Along with expanded opportunities for women came ideas of an autonomous nursing role separate and distinct from medicine. Stead's deeply rooted gender-role stereotyping no doubt further inflamed nursing resistance to "his" new role. Other settings—such as the University of Colorado, where Henry Silver, a pediatrician, and Loretta Ford, a master's-prepared public health nurse, founded a partnership rooted in collaboration—provided more fruitful results. All these factors were in play when the first NPs emerged in the 1960s.

However, the NP was not really a new role for nurses. Examining our history, it is apparent that nurses functioned independently and autonomously before the rise of organized medicine. If medicine was ambivalent about the emergence of this new role, nursing itself was no less conflicted.

In 1978, the following statement appeared in the *American Journal of Nursing* (Roy & Obloy, 1978, p. 1698):

> The nurse practitioner movement has become an issue in nursing, a topic on which there is no consensus. One question about the movement is whether the development of the nurse practitioner role adds to, or detracts from, the development of nursing as a distinct scientific discipline.

This statement was issued more than 13 years after the initiation of the first NP program at the University of Colorado. If, as Sparacino (1990) spells out, the domain of the CNS is situated in the secondary and tertiary setting, the domain of the NP originally arose as a role situated in primary care.

Loretta Ford and Dr. Henry Silver designed a graduate curriculum for pediatric nurses to provide ambulatory care to poor rural Colorado children. The goal of this program was to bridge the gap between the health-care needs of children and the family's ability to access and afford primary health care (Ford & Silver, 1967; Silver, Ford, & Stearly, 1967). This program was situated in graduate education and included courses such as pathophysiology, health promotion, and growth and development, with the intent of the student understanding the principles of healthy child care and patient education. Nurses would then be able to provide preventive nursing services outside of the hospital setting in collaboration with physicians. Students had to have a baccalaureate degree and public health nursing experience to be admitted to the program.

Ford states the following in an interview: "We looked at the nurse practitioner preparation not as a separate program but as integrated into a role that had already been designed at the graduate level" (Jacox, 2002, p. 155). Ford notes that the lack of organizational leadership in the profession coupled with a lack of responsiveness in academic settings caused a "bastardization of the model" (Jacox, 2002, p. 157). She had envisioned that our professional organization, as in other professions, would identify, credential, and make public advanced NPs. However, Ford was to discover that the "ANA in those early years was reluctant to stick its neck out and give some leadership to the NP groups that were growing rapidly" and that the lack of leadership in nursing education created "a patchwork quilt" of differently prepared NPs (Jacox, 2002, p. 157). Although clinically based programs were growing, there remained resistance to the NP model. Ford (Jacox, 2002, p. 155) says,

> I understood that faculty members were supposed to be doing just that—push the borders of knowledge and publish their work. In my naiveté of faculty politics, I expected that since the NP model grew out of professional nursing and public health nursing—including primary, secondary, and tertiary prevention and community-based services—it was a perfectly legitimate investigation. Instead, it became a battleground, and even recently was labeled in the Harvard Business Review as a "Disruptive Innovation." What a compliment!

The collaboration between NP and physician has been analyzed and debated since the advent of the NP role, including the relationship between Ford and Silver (Fairman, 2002, 2008). The sticking point of collaboration is that it has included the heavy implication of supervision and thus control. In truth, in the early 1970s both NPs and physicians had to give up their traditional roles, tasks, and knowledge to establish this new provider role, often in the face of organizational and societal opposition. Jan Towers describes the growth of her own NP practice as follows: "The area that I perhaps most feared turned out to be the least troublesome, after some initial adjustments between the physician with whom I was working and me were made" (Towers, 1995, p. 269). What would often be impossible on an organizational level was more easily resolvable among professionals with a shared interest and commitment: the good of the patient.

Prescriptive authority was a major issue, and it was either delegated from the medical practice act and carried out under physicians' standing orders or protocols or it came directly from the nursing practice acts. Nurse historian Arlene Keeling has argued that far from being a new realm of nursing practice, the "prescribing"—or use—of a variety of techniques and substances for therapeutic effect has always been a dimension of nursing practice (Keeling, 2007). The states of Oregon and Washington allowed nurses the freedom to prescribe independently in 1983 (Kalisch & Kalisch, 1986). Some of the fiercest turf battles have heated up over prescriptive privileges. By 1984, nurses were accused of practicing medicine, although they were practicing well within the scope of their expanded role. Physicians remained ambivalent. They pushed NPs to function broadly but did not usually support legislation that authorized an increased scope of practice, especially in the area of prescriptive privileges. Joan Lynaugh, nurse historian, describes NPs as looking for an "exam room of their own"—essentially a clinical space in which to provide nursing care (Fairman, 2008, p. 7). This space is indeed a crowded one (Fairman, 2008, p. 200, note 9). Prescriptive authority is discussed in greater detail in Chapter 6.

The Great Society entitlement programs significantly influenced the need for NPs to care for people who were covered under Medicare and Medicaid. Predominant social movements—women's rights, civil rights, antiwar protest, consumerism—had a profound impact on the need for groups to assert their place in the society of the 1960s and early 1970s. Nurses were not immune to the forces unleashed in these years and took advantage of the opportunities to work with physicians "in relationships that were entrepreneurial and groundbreaking, and to engage in a kind of dialogue that supported new models of care" (Fairman, 2002, p. 165). These nurses were pioneers, rebels, and renegades treading on uncertain ground.

The National Advisory Commission on Health Manpower supported the NP movement (Moxley, 1968). The Committee to Study Extended Roles for Nurses in the early 1970s recommended that the expanded role for nurses was necessary to provide the consumer with access to health care and proposed the inclusion of highly developed health assessment skills (Kalisch & Kalisch, 1986; Leininger, Little, & Carnevali, 1972; Marchione & Garland, 1997). Although the Committee did stop short of providing a definitive scope of practice statement, it recommended support for licensure and certification for advanced practice, recognition in the nursing practice act, further cost-benefit research, and surveys on role impact.

Government and private groups rapidly developed funding support for educational programs (Hamric, Spross, & Hanson, 2013). According to Marchione and Garland (1997), "The traditional role of humanistic caring, comforting, nurturing and supporting was to be maintained and improved by the addition" of new primary care functions that the Department of Health, Education, and Welfare approved: total patient assessment, monitoring, health promotion, and a focus that encompassed not only disease prevention but health promotion and maintenance, treatment, and continuity of care.

The Division of Nursing of the Department of Health, Education, and Welfare tracked the development of the NP role from 1974 to 1977. During that time, the number of NP programs rose from 86 to 178 across the country, with significant governmental support through the Nurse Training Act to advanced practice nursing education programs of all types. Although nurse educators by this time wanted NP education standardized, in 1977 most NP programs awarded a certificate with some still using continuing education models and accepting less than a baccalaureate degree for entry. However, the number of NP graduates of master's programs did increase from 20% in 1975 to 26% in 1977, again largely encouraged by the availability of federal funds for support. The education of NPs was the rallying cry for the formation of the NONPF in 1980, dedicated to defining curriculum and evaluation standards as well as pioneering research and development related to NP practice and teaching-learning methodologies. The political voice for NPs was enhanced with the formation of the American Academy of Nurse Practitioners (AANP) in 1985 and the American College of Nurse Practitioners (ACNP) in 2003.

The Nurse Training Acts of 1971 and 1975 were critical in providing federal funding to support NP programs. By 1979, more than 133 programs and tracks existed, and approximately 15,000 NPs were in practice. By 1983 and 1984, NP graduates numbered approximately 20,000 to 24,000; they were primarily employed in sites that served those in greatest need: public health departments, community health centers, outpatient and rural clinics, health maintenance organizations, school-based clinics, and occupational health clinics (Hamric et al, 2013; Kalisch & Kalisch, 1986; Pulcini & Wagner, 2001). NPs were typically providing care for health promotion, disease prevention, minor acute problems, chronic stabilized illness, and the full range of teaching and coaching that nurses have always provided for patients and families.

A hindrance to practice in rural areas was finding appropriate physician backup. By 1987, the federal government had spent $100 million to promote NP education, primarily through the U.S. Public Health Service Division of Nursing (Pulcini & Wagner, 2001). By the 1980s, the master's degree was viewed broadly as the educational standard for advanced practice (Geolot, 1987; Sultz et al, 1983), and by 1989, 90% of programs were master's and post-master's level (Pulcini & Wagner, 2001). NONPF thrived in the 1980s, developing curriculum guidelines and competencies, surveying faculties, and studying role components.

An interorganizational task force to identify criteria for quality NP educational programs occurred as an outgrowth of the work to unify certification. This work, begun in 1995 by NONPF and the NLN, was the beginning of the development of a model curriculum for NP education that would be used nationally and provide the basis for certification eligibility (Hamric et al, 2013). At that time, the NLN was the only accrediting body for nursing graduate programs, and program standards, curriculum guides, and domains and competencies for NP education from NONPF were often used by the NLN in the accreditation process. In 1998, the Commission on Collegiate Nursing Education, an accreditation arm of the AACN, was formed to provide an alternative to the NLN as a source of accreditation to schools offering baccalaureate and higher degrees in nursing. The thrust of the 2001 meeting of the NP task force when it reconvened was for accrediting bodies to move toward the approval of NONPF guidelines and standards as the reigning accepted standards for accreditation of programs preparing NPs (Edwards et al, 2003). In addition, the APRN Consensus Model (see later section) spells out specific criteria for preapproval and accreditation of APRN education.

There is a cautionary note to this perception of progress. Despite clear statutes in some states, credentialing by insurers for NPs may still lag, providing additional barriers to care. Scope of practice, a primary focus of the 2011 Institute of Medicine (IOM) *Future of Nursing* recommendations, remains a contested battleground for control of professional practice and reimbursement.

In 2008, the adoption of the Consensus Model for Advanced Practice Registered Nurse (APRN) Regulation by the National Council of State Boards of Nursing (NCSBN) gave direction for gains in legal authority, prescriptive privilege, and reimbursement mechanisms across the 50 states and the District of Columbia. Current NPs have achieved a higher degree of autonomy in practice and associated prestige (Phillips, 2011) with the mandate for continued advancement contained in the IOM report, *The Future of Nursing* (2011). More victories than failures provide evidence of success, but, as in the late 1970s, today's NP is still battling for autonomy and consumer recognition in practice, especially in states with many physicians. Veterans' Health Affairs (VHA) Advanced Practice Registered Nurses Proposed Rule (81 Fed.Reg.33155, May 25, 2016) to the Federal Register is under siege. Opponents, as noted earlier, are still trying to block implementation of this policy and are reaching out to members of Congress to delay the proposal through legislation that extends expiring benefits for our nation's veterans. New legislation was introduced late in 2016, the *Veterans Affairs Expiring Authorities Act* (HR 5985).

As early as 1985, Hayes stated, "No role in nursing, or for that matter, in any field has been so debated in the literature, and possibly no other nursing function has ever been so obsessed about by those performing it as has been the NP role" (Hayes, 1985, p. 145). Yet, as Hayes asserts, there has been an avalanche of support from satisfied consumers of NP services.

THE CONSENSUS MODEL

In an effort to bring some clarity to and standardization of advanced practice nursing roles, in 2008 the APRN Consensus Model, also referred to as a regulatory model, was published by the APRN Consensus Work Group and the NCSBN APRN Advisory Committee with extensive input from a larger APRN stakeholder community. The nomenclature *APRN* was adopted, and four APRN roles were defined in the document: CNMs, CRNAs, CNSs, and certified nurse practitioners (CNPs). An APRN is further defined as an RN who has completed a graduate degree or postgraduate program that has prepared him or her to practice in one of these four roles. The acronym LACE—standing for "licensure, accreditation, certification, and education"—demonstrates alliances across these spheres for implementation of the APRN Consensus

Model, thus promoting uniformity and standardization of the APRN role for the safety of the consumer of health care. The target date for model implementation was 2015, with an alignment of current certifying examinations with educational program offerings and subsequent licensure. By December 2016, according to the NCSBN, 15 states were in full compliance with the LACE model and most others were in some stage of change. This is amazing given the continued strength of states' rights and the opposition of organized medicine.

YET ANOTHER "DISRUPTIVE INNOVATION": THE DOCTOR OF NURSING PRACTICE

The future contains clouds on the horizon as well as sunshine. Fairman (1999) cautions that although local negotiations between individual physicians and nurses may have been, in some cases, easily traversed in the interest of the good of the patient, on the professional level hierarchical relationships and power are at stake. As noted at the start of this chapter, within this hotly competitive health-care environment, with the still controversial implementation of the PPACA (2010), the entire health-care sector continues to face hurdles, challenges, and assaults.

In October 2004, the members of the AACN endorsed the *Position Statement on the Practice Doctorate in Nursing,* which called for the movement of educational preparation for advanced practice nursing roles from the master's degree to the doctoral level by 2015. Though this target date has not been achieved, there has been much movement in this direction. This "new" doctorate is a "practice" doctorate in contrast to the doctor of philosophy (PhD)—the traditional research degree—and is not intended to "replace" the PhD. There are many reasons for this development. Some master's programs for APNs had become very lengthy, without any change in the credential awarded at the completion of studies. The number of credits, in many cases, approaches what is required for a doctoral degree. And many educators believe this is necessary to ensure clinical competency. Furthermore, other practice disciplines such as pharmacy, physiotherapy, and occupational therapy have moved on to doctoral-level preparation. The debate continues.

The case can also be made that APNs across the country have been expanding their skills, both formally and informally. One example is the role of "intensivist" in the hospital, which is being assumed by many NPs and CNSs (Mundinger, 2005). This is consistent with nursing's lengthy history of moving where the need in health care surfaces—always "doing what had to be done." The aging of the population, the increased acuity of patients with multiple comorbidities, the complexity of care, the continuation of a dwindling number of primary care physicians, and the decreased hours for residents in the hospital because of legislative and accreditation criteria have fostered the need for these nurses to move well beyond the primary care arena. For example, when Columbia University School of Nursing was asked by Presbyterian Hospital to establish two new ambulatory care clinics to meet the growing demand for primary care among the underserved immigrant populations, the faculty accepted. They also proposed conducting a randomized trial comparing independent NPs and primary care physicians. To reduce the variability among roles and strengthen the study, the faculty requested that the hospital's medical board grant the faculty NPs admitting privileges. Mundinger (2005) describes this evolution at Columbia: "Several physician(s) . . . provided additional training for our faculty nurse practitioners in dermatology, radiology, and cardiology and helped mentor them through the process of admitting, and co-managing patients and conducting emergency room evaluation" (p. 175).

The results of the randomized trials, with excellent patient care outcomes achieved by NPs on a par with primary care physicians, were published in the *Journal of the American Medical Association* (Mundinger et al, 2000). This contributed to a change in hospital bylaws and granted faculty NPs hospital admitting privileges. Mundinger sees the level of service delivered by these faculty NPs as beyond that achieved by colleagues with the traditional master's degree preparation for practice. Based on these observations comes the call for a formal and standardized curriculum leading to a doctoral degree consistent with the practice needs for advanced competencies and increased knowledge. Mundinger (2005) states, "We know that thousands of nurses aspire to this level of education and schools are responding by developing the new degree. We know that the research degree is asynchronous with these goals, and we know from every other profession that when you reach the competency associated with doctoral achievement, one should receive a doctorate not another MS degree" (p. 175).

As part of the APRN Consensus Model, 2015 was targeted as the year anyone seeking to sit for certification as an APRN would need a DNP. Although the DNP degree has spread and prospered since 2008, there have always been vocal detractors. Recently, opposition to this mandate was voiced by a significant cohort of national nursing leaders in a paper titled "The Doctor of Nursing Practice: A National Workforce Perspective" (Cronenwett et al, 2011), making the case that the need for care providers should take precedence over a professionalizing agenda. Significant retrenchment of the 2015 mandate has occurred, with moves to preserve existing master's programs producing APRNs. See Chapter 4 for more discussion on this issue.

THE INSTITUTE OF MEDICINE ISSUES ITS 2010 REPORT: *THE FUTURE OF NURSING: LEADING CHANGE, ADVANCING HEALTH*

This dramatic, evidence-based report presents the results of 2 years of study by the Committee on the Robert Wood Johnson Foundation Initiative on the Future of Nursing at the IOM. This committee was chaired by Donna Shalala, PhD, FAAN, long-time nurse advocate, former head of the U.S. Department of Health and Human Services (1992–2000), and now University of Miami president, in concert with Nursing Vice Chair Linda Burnes Bolton,

RN, DrPH, FAAN. This report was presented in November 2010. The far-reaching impact of the report's recommendations are just now beginning to be fully absorbed. Key recommendations begin with the assumption that "nursing can fill . . . new and expanded roles in a redesigned healthcare system" (IOM, 2011, p. xi). We will need our renegades, rebels, and trailblazers more than ever.

CONCLUSION

The boundaries of practice are always malleable. They are always subject to myriad external forces—political, economic, social, and cultural—and are interpreted in different ways by different practitioners. APNs are a mixed breed; each trajectory under the umbrella of advanced nursing practice has evolved differently and under variable circumstances. This leads to vigor, strength, and diversity. The struggles documented within this chapter have aimed to strengthen each variant of the nursing advanced practice role. The struggles are not over; in many ways, they are just beginning. It is our hope that nursing will continue to produce rebels, renegades, and trailblazers motivated by concern for patients, concern for community, and concern for humanity. We have no doubt that we will continue to take on new and challenging roles using creative and diverse strategies. Nursing continues to lurch forward; progress is sometimes slow, sometimes variable, sometimes unsteady—but, as always, continuing to find opportunity in chaos, motivated, as ever, by commitment to patients, families, and communities, to human need and suffering.

2

Emerging Roles of the Advanced Practice Nurse

Deborah Becker and Caroline Doherty

Learning Outcomes

Learning outcomes expected as a result of this chapter:

- Describe the advanced practice registered nurses (APRN) Scope of Practice and the Consensus Model.
- Describe the clinical nurse specialist (CNS) role and discuss how their contributions contribute to cost savings and implementation of evidence-based practice.
- Identify role highlights of the nurse practitioner (NP) in primary care with adult and pediatric populations, in various community settings, in psychiatric and mental health care, in women's health/gender-related care and transitional care, and in acute care with neonatal, pediatric adult, and elderly populations.
- Discuss nurse-midwifery with an emphasis on primary care and first-assistant services.
- Summarize the new certification requirements for nurse anesthetists.
- Distinguish palliative care as an emerging practice area for all APRNs.
- Propose diverse practice opportunities for APRNs.

INTRODUCTION

Advanced practice nursing continues to evolve to meet the changing and increasing needs of patients, communities, and society as a whole. Advanced practice registered nurses (APRNs)* have successfully adapted their roles to meet these ever-changing needs and the expectations that go along with them. The growth occurring now can be attributed to several elements, such as health-care reform and fuller implementation of the Affordable Care Act (ACA), a national emphasis on the provision of safe and high-quality care, pay-for-performance initiatives, and the call by the Institute of Medicine (IOM)'s *Future of Nursing* (2011) report for APRNs to work to the fullest extent of their scopes of practice without restrictions or barriers. These initiatives foster new opportunities for the development of advanced practice nursing roles.

Several factors have influenced the emergence and acceptability of advanced practice roles. These factors include the growing numbers of elderly patients as baby boomers reach retirement age, increased complexity and severity of illness in hospitalized patients, further reductions in medical residents' clinical work hours, a call for greater access to care for all citizens, and a varying degree of nursing and primary care physician shortages, depending on geographical region. These and other factors will continue to influence the emergence of the APRN role in the coming decades.

The four major groups of APRNs currently in the United States are certified registered nurse anesthetists (CRNAs), certified nurse-midwives (CNMs), clinical nurse specialists (CNSs), and nurse practitioners (NPs). The range of current advanced practice roles and the numbers of nurses in these roles demonstrate the continued success and acceptance of APRNs. See **Table 2.1.** Studies evaluating clinical outcomes of care delivered by APRNs are overwhelmingly positive as are surveys of patient satisfaction with the delivery of care by APRNs.

---

*APRN is the title preferred by the American Nurses Association (ANA) and used in most state practice acts. Throughout this chapter, various acronyms will be presented to distinguish between specialty preparations, but the generic title for all these practice roles is APRN. Please note that not all of the four specialty preparations are recognized in their state as APRNs.

TABLE 2.1	
Numbers of Advanced Practice Nurses	
Clinical nurse specialists	8,395
Certified registered nurse anesthetists	49,113
Certified nurse-midwives	8,332
Nurse practitioners	186,656

Source: Adapted from Phillips, S. J. (2016). 28th annual legislative update. *Nurse Practitioner, 41*(1), 21–52.

A systematic review of outcomes studies conducted between 1990 and 2008 was performed to compare patient outcomes between physician- and APRN-directed teams (Newhouse et al, 2011). The review found that patient outcomes of care provided by NPs and CNMs (in collaboration with physicians as required by state regulations) were similar to—and in some ways better than—care provided by physicians alone for the populations and in the settings included (Newhouse et al, 2011). The review found that CNSs working in acute care settings can reduce length of stay and cost of care for hospitalized patients. Although no specific conclusions regarding CRNA patient outcomes were provided by this review, a few studies show CRNA patient outcomes to be comparable with those of anesthesiologists (Newhouse et al, 2011). A recent Cochrane Review of studies comparing outcomes of anesthesiologists and CRNAs found that, although the quality of studies available to review was poor, there is no available study demonstrating any difference between the quality of care provided by CRNAs or anesthesiologists (Lewis, Nicholson, Smith, & Alderson, 2014).

By accepting the responsibilities of the advanced practice role, APRNs have understood the need to expand legislative recognition of their professional status, including prescriptive authority and reimbursement for care delivered. Recognition of APRNs in the United States varies, with most states providing some level of legal recognition and prescriptive authority.

SCOPE OF PRACTICE

Professional nursing organizations and state boards of nursing understand the need to describe and interpret the responsibilities of advanced practitioners in their areas of specialization. Underlying the recognition of this need is the obligation to ensure public safety, to identify the essential characteristics of advanced practice, and to interpret for the practitioner the components of competent care (American Association of Critical Care Nurses and American Nurses Association, 1995). The scope of practice may be described by the functions performed by the APRN and the minimal competencies needed to perform those functions. These descriptions and guidelines direct APRNs in the implementation and conceptualization of their roles and responsibilities.

In addition, each state has a legislative and regulatory stance on issues affecting advanced practice within its jurisdiction (Phillips, 2016). The legal scope of practice, including prerogatives for diagnosing, prescriptive authority, and reimbursement, is described within these regulations. Scope and standards of practice are defined by the professional organization and enacted into law at the state level. The actual role is further delineated through credentialing of practice responsibilities and activities at the institutional or employment level. Hospitals and other health-care organizations typically define role responsibilities and prerogatives through a review by other practitioners, and this is generally expressed through a contract identifying responsibilities, prerogatives, and limitations of the role. This review results in the granting of institutional- or organizational-based practice privileges for the APRN.

Although scope of practice guidelines are important philosophically and may even have the weight of law, they do not imply that the roles of APRNs are unchanging. When knowledge evolves and different care delivery models emerge, roles also evolve. More commonly, roles change as different practice settings become available and opportunities for improved patient access to care appear. The nature of advanced practice is broader than individual roles or functions.

Regulation of the Advanced Practice Registered Nurse

Regulation of APRNs occurs at the state level, but there are both educational and certification prerequisites.

Graduate-level educational preparation of APRNs is guided by educators and members of professional organizations who identify essential curricular goals, content, and competencies expected of APRN graduates. In 2004, the American Association of Colleges of Nursing (AACN) called for doctoral-level preparation as entry level for APRNs, with a proposed implementation date of 2015. However, several barriers to moving entry-level practice preparation to the doctoral level have been identified. These barriers include financial costs, limited faculty resources, the need to obtain permissions from numerous levels of leadership, boards and regulatory bodies, finding clinical sites, and more (Rand Corporation, 2010). Many schools of nursing moved their APRN education to the doctoral level, with most offering the doctorate of nursing practice (DNP) degree; however, only the American Association of Nurse Anesthetists (AANA) has mandated that as of 2022, all graduates of educational programs must be prepared at the doctoral level for entry into practice (AANA, 2010). The remaining APRN groups have not embraced mandating doctoral education for entry into practice.

Content and competencies core to all APRNs and those specific to a particular role must be provided in all APRN educational programs. **Table 2.2** lists major APRN organizations that develop the educational and certification prerequisites and the APRN essential content and competency documents that direct the preparation of APRNs for entry into practice. On completion of an accredited master's or doctoral-level program, graduates generally must pass a national certification examination in the area of intended practice before applying for licensure at the state level.

APRNs may be recognized and licensed at the state level in one of the four aforementioned roles. However, many issues have been identified with the current regulatory process, particularly eligibility for reciprocity of licensure between states. In response to this need to develop more consistent standards for APRN recognition across states, the APRN Consensus Work Group and the National Council of State Boards of Nursing have developed the Consensus Model for APRN Regulation: Licensure, Accreditation, Certification and Education (Consensus Model, 2008). This document has been accepted by numerous nursing organizations and stakeholder groups. The regulatory model acknowledges the four APRN roles and recommends that advanced practice registered nursing must be

TABLE 2.2

Professional Organizations and Essential Educational Content

Organization	Landmark Publications
American Association of Colleges of Nursing	*The essentials of master's education in nursing.* Washington, DC: Author, 2011. *The essentials of doctoral education for advanced nursing practice.* Washington, DC: Author, 2006.
American College of Nurse-Midwives	*Core competencies for basic midwifery practice.* Silver Spring, MD: Author, 2012. *Competencies for master's level midwifery education.* Silver Spring, MD: Author, 2014. *The practice doctorate in midwifery.* Silver Spring, MD: Author, 2011.
American Association of Women's Health, Obstetric and Neonatal Nurses, and National Association of Nurse Practitioners Women's Health	*The women's health nurse practitioner: Guidelines for practice and education* (7th ed.). Washington, DC: Author, 2014.
Council on Accreditation of Nurse Anesthesia Educational Programs	*Standards for accreditation of nurse anesthesia educational programs.* Chicago, IL: Author, 2016.
National Association of Clinical Nurse Specialists	*Criteria for the evaluation of clinical nurse specialist master's, practice doctorate, and post-graduate certificate educational programs.* Philadelphia, PA: Author, 2012. *Organizing framework and CNS core competencies.* Philadelphia, PA: Author, 2008.
National Organization of Nurse Practitioner Faculties	*NP core competencies with curriculum content.* Washington, DC: Author, 2014. *Adult-gerontological acute care nurse practitioner competencies.* Washington, DC: Author, 2012. *Adult-gerontological primary care nurse practitioner competencies.* Washington, DC: Author, 2010. *Population-focused nurse practitioner competencies: Family/Across the lifespan, neonatal, pediatric acute care, pediatric primary care, psychiatric-mental health, women's health/gender-related.* Washington, DC: Author, 2013.

regulated in one of the four roles and in at least one of six population foci: psychiatric or mental health, women's health/gender-related, adult-gerontology, pediatrics, neonatal, and individual families across the life span. The adult-gerontology and pediatrics populations are further distinguished by either an acute care or a primary care focus. Of note, the CNS practice is described to occur across primary and acute care settings and as such must be reflected in their education.

Requirements for consistent educational preparation across all APRN roles have provided greater uniformity. Content for all APRNs must include graduate-level courses in advanced pathophysiology, advanced physical assessment, and advanced pharmacology, called the *APRN core* (Consensus Model, 2008). In addition, content related

to the population served, role development, and clinical experience in the specific role is required. The recommendations of the Consensus Model have and will continue to influence the licensure, accreditation, certification, and educational preparation of all future APRNs, and can be found in **Table 2.3.**

Clinical Nurse Specialist

CNSs are nurses with masters- or doctorate-level education in a defined area of knowledge and practice. They typically work in unit- or population-based settings; in hospitals, offices, or outpatient clinic settings; and in community practice. In an analysis of acute care advanced practice nurses performed by the American Association of Critical

TABLE 2.3
Essential Characteristics of the Advanced Practice Registered Nurse*
1. Completion of an accredited graduate-level program in one of four areas: nurse-midwifery, nurse anesthesia, NP, or CNS
2. Successful completion of a national certification examination measuring APRN role and population of focus competencies and maintains competence through recertification
3. Possession of advanced clinical knowledge and skills needed for direct patient care, and a significant component of education and practice focuses on direct care of individuals
4. Practice builds on RN competencies and demonstrates depth and breadth of knowledge, data synthesis, complex skills, intervention, and role autonomy
5. Educational preparation for health promotion and maintenance, assessment, diagnosis, and management of patient problems including use and prescription of pharmacological and nonpharmacological interventions
6. Possesses depth and breadth of clinical experience reflecting intended area of practice
7. Possesses license to practice as an RN, and then further as a CRNA, CNM, CNS, or CNP

APRN, advanced practice registered nurse; *CNM,* certified nurse-midwife; *CNP,* certified nurse practitioner; *CNS,* clinical nurse specialist; *CRNA,* certified registered nurse anesthetist; *RN,* registered nurse.

*Adapted from Consensus Model for APRN Regulation: Licensure, Accreditation, Certification and Education. (2008). Completed through the work of the APRN Consensus Work Group and the National Council of State Boards of Nursing APRN Advisory Committee.

Care Nurses (Becker et al, 2006), CNSs were asked to rate activities they perform that are most critical to their practices. Activities selected included the following:

- Synthesizing, interpreting, making decisions and recommendations, and evaluating responses on the basis of complex, sometimes conflicting, sources of data
- Identifying and prioritizing clinical problems on the basis of education, research, and experiential knowledge
- Facilitating development of clinical judgment in health-care team members (e.g., nursing staff, medical staff, other health-care providers) through serving as a role model, teaching, coaching, and/or mentoring
- Promoting a caring and supportive environment
- Promoting the value of lifelong learning and evidence-based practice while continually acquiring knowledge and skills needed to address questions arising in practice to improve patients' care
- Evaluating current and innovative practices in patients' care on the basis of evidence-based practice, research, and experiential knowledge
- Incorporating evidence-based practice guidelines, research, and experiential knowledge to formulate, evaluate, and/or revise policies, procedures, and protocols.

These results demonstrated the performance of activities that at one time were performed solely by physicians and currently also overlap with those performed by acute care nurse practitioners (ACNPs).

The CNS shifts functions depending on the needs of the situation and participates in a mix of direct and indirect patient care activities. Still, the traditional roles of CNS practice remain, including those of expert practitioner, educator, consultant, manager, and researcher. See **Boxes 2.1** and **2.2**.

The Clinical Nurse Specialist and Cost Savings

Multiple studies have demonstrated the positive contributions of CNSs to patient care outcomes and patient satisfaction, but fewer studies have evaluated their economic impact and their ability to generate income and save costs. A recent study by Richardson and Tjoelker (2012) demonstrated a CNS-led initiative to decrease central line associated bloodstream infections (CLABSI), saving the organization $214,712 in terms of cost avoidance and 1.4 lives saved out of 8 patients with CLABSI. Similarly, Maze and Riggins (2011) demonstrated a CNS-led initiative resulting in the CLABSI rate to be consistently below the National Healthcare Safety Network (NHSN) benchmark. These savings are real, but they may not be returned to the CNS's home (usually nursing) department. Because of this, the immediate supervisors of CNSs may not appreciate the benefits of expert CNS practice. This reality is compounded by the inability of CNSs to bill directly for services if they are hospital-based, salaried employees. Skilled advanced practice nursing care is not directly reimbursed and remains bundled in the hospital's

---

Box 2.1

The Unit-Based Clinical Nurse Specialist Profile

Margo is an adult critical care CNS who is master's prepared and has been working in a large academic health system for more than 6 years. Margo works on a neurosurgery step-down unit where her clientele ranges from patients with seizure disorders, those recovering from major strokes or traumatic brain injuries, and a host of neurosurgical conditions. She is a key member of the health-care team, especially because of her wealth of knowledge and experience with neurologically impaired patients. Margo leads interdisciplinary rounds that include attending physicians, fellows and residents in training, nurses, APRNs, pharmacists, dietitians, and physiatrists. She empowers her nursing staff to actively participate in rounds and provides them the resources and encouragement they need to have their voices heard. Margo is instrumental in assuring that the patients on her unit are receiving high-quality and safe care. Recently her unit was recognized for having met or exceeded quality metrics for 6 months in a row. Margo currently leads the CNS Leadership Group in her hospital. This group meets monthly to network with the 30+ CNSs that work throughout the system. This group sets internal standards for clinical and professional activities, reviews initiatives, and provides support to CNSs who often work in silos caring for their specific patient populations.

Box 2.2

Corporate Clinical Nurse Specialist Profile

Sue is a nurse who has doctoral-level training and has been a CNS for the past 20 years. She began her CNS career in a major teaching hospital during which she worked on the writing group to help the organization to achieve Magnet status. She also developed a postcardiothoracic surgery glycemic protocol, an orientation for BSN-prepared nurses and CNSs, along with many other significant initiatives. Subsequently, she was hired by a corporation as a consultant for all their ICUs. In this role, she helped to establish standards of care, has served as chair of numerous committees, developed protocols for safe handoffs, and worked with the interdisciplinary team to address quality and core measures. The significant travel requirement is a challenge, but she is pleased to know that her expertise has had such a significant impact across many organizations, resulting in a positive impact on the interdisciplinary team and the patients that they serve.

---

room, food, laundry, and supplies bill. More creative and appropriate financial models that could remedy the situation are needed. This limitation on role functioning is usually not faced by self-employed or practice-based CNSs, who likely are not institutional employees and generally work in outpatient or community settings.

One recent randomized controlled trial identified that cost savings were achieved, without loss of quality, by substituting physicians with diabetes nurse specialists in caring for patients with diabetes (Arts, Landewe-Cleuren, Schaper, & Vrijhoef, 2012). Few studies comparing CNS care to physicians exist primarily because of most CNSs working in hospitals. However, the CNS can play a key role in providing care to underserved populations and should be considered instrumental in achieving the goals of the ACA.

The Clinical Nurse Specialist and Evidence-Based Practice (EBP)

CNSs have long been considered change agents; recently, the implementation of EBP is where many CNSs spend their time. However, several barriers to implementing change exist in clinical settings such as reluctance to change approaches when the "old way still works." A recent study by Campbell and Profetto-McGrath (2013) identified five challenges to implementing EBP by CNSs: time constraints for the CNS, time constraints for the bedside nurses, multiple roles of the CNS reducing dedicated time to focus on EBP implementation, heavy workload and lack of resources, and both individual and organization support (Campbell & Profetto-McGrath, 2013).

However, when CNSs are provided the time and resources to perform their role, positive outcomes occur. Recently, CNS involvement in quality initiatives and their contributions to improved patient outcomes has been recognized as agencies apply for Magnet Recognition. The Magnet Recognition Program® offered by the American Nurses Credentialing Center (ANCC) recognizes health-care organizations for quality patient care, nursing excellence, and innovations in professional nursing practice (ANCC, 2011). The CNS role is essential to implementing innovation and sustaining improved patient outcomes, which are integral components of the Magnet Recognition Program (Muller, Hujcs, Dubendorf, & Harrington, 2010). The CNS role broadly and specifically supports the process by which care is delineated, changes are made, and improvements are noted. CNS participation in the attainment of these goals and the movement of organizations toward achieving Magnet status likely will provide new and expanded opportunities for the CNS.

Ambiguity and the Clinical Nurse Specialist Role

The observation that CNS practice reflects role ambiguity undoubtedly grows out of the ability of the CNS to adapt to changing patient, family, and nursing staff needs, supported by a broad clinical repertoire of skills and knowledge. This adaptability provides role confusion not only for those implementing the role, but also for those observing it. There have been several responses to the problem of role ambiguity with in-hospital CNS roles. One has been the development of AACN's Scope and Standards for Acute and Critical Care Clinical Nurse Specialist Practice (Bell & McNamara, 2010). This document provides guidelines for competent and professional care for acutely and critically ill patients. It also reflects the three spheres of CNS influence: patient and family, nursing personnel and other health-care providers, and the organizational system for care delivery in different settings (Bell & McNamara, 2010). Within this framework, the CNS is expected to provide continuous and comprehensive care to improve outcomes for acutely and critically ill patients. This is done in a collaborative model that includes patients, families, significant others, nurses, and other providers and administrators (Bell & McNamara, 2010).

A contribution of this document is that it sets goals and standards for CNS practice and contributes to further role clarification for hospital-based CNSs. The values identified in this document for continuous and comprehensive care for acutely and critically ill patients suggest that the scope of the critical care CNS's responsibilities are not limited to acute or special care units. Seriously ill patients are found in most hospital units, and their continuing specialized care needs are now frequently required in nonhospital or outpatient settings. It is likely that postdischarge role functions will become more common for the acute or critical care CNS.

The publishing of CNS Core Competencies by the National CNS Competency Task Force (Clinical Nurse Specialist Core Competencies, 2010) also attempts to reduce role ambiguity for the CNS. This task force identified the various roles and activities of CNSs in numerous practice settings and validated them by surveying more than 2,000 CNSs. The range of agreement was 90% to 98%. These competencies will aid educators, employers, and new CNSs in understanding their role and responsibilities as well as their contributions to patient care outcomes.

However, CNSs have not obtained the clarity they are seeking. Recently, the Office of Management and Budget's Standard Occupational Classification (SOC) Policy Committee inaccurately designated CNSs as general registered nurses instead of APRNs. This miscategorization will result in the inability of researchers to capture accurate data and statistics as they relate to the CNS workforce, further reducing the importance of the CNS role to the health care of U.S. citizens (NACNS news release, 2016).

Nurse Practitioner

NPs are frontline health-care providers essential to developing and maintaining successful communication and collaboration among providers across health-care settings. In both primary and urgent care settings, NPs can ensure continuity of care, decrease health-care costs, and optimize health outcomes for patients (Villasenor & Krouse, 2016).

The educational preparation of NPs has moved from continuing education programs offering certification on completion to university-based graduate programs granting a master's or doctorate degree in nursing. Today, NPs are the largest group of APRNs and have prescriptive authority in all 50 states and the District of Columbia (Phillips, 2016). APRNs assess and manage both medical and nursing problems and serve as both primary and acute care providers.

Changing Roles for the Primary Care Nurse Practitioner

Initially, patient populations cared for by NPs were often uninsured immigrants or low-income individuals who were Medicaid recipients. However, NPs since have sought to meet the needs of larger groups of patients and have expanded their practices to include clients from suburban and urban outpatient settings and clinics. This shift to highly populated, high-income areas where physicians are also readily available shows the increased acceptance of NPs.

Retail and Urgent Care Clinics

The development of walk-in, retail, and urgent care clinics has changed the landscape for accessing primary care services. These clinics are major employers of NPs and thus provide an opportunity to showcase to the public some of the care that NPs can provide. According to the National Conference of State Legislatures (NCSL) website, as of 2015, 2,000 retail clinics operate in 41 states and Washington, DC (NCSL, 2015). Recognizing the potential impact of these clinics on the APRNs, the American Academy of Nurse Practitioners (AANP) published *Standards for Nurse Practitioner Practice in Retail-Based Clinics* (AANP, 2007).

Nurse Practitioners in the Community

Primary care NPs have established unique community-centered practice models. In an effort to develop an independent NP service model and to study the ways health care is delivered to various populations in the United States, many schools of nursing opened Academic Community Nursing Centers (Naylor & Kurtzman, 2010; Oros, Johantgen, Antol, Heller, & Ravella, 2001). These centers are used as settings in which to study how health care is provided to vulnerable populations with limited access to care, who face inefficiencies and a lack of coordination in health-care delivery; to determine the specific needs of the community

in which the center is located; and to provide a means of improving the quality of the care delivered (Zachariah & Lundeen, 1997).

Building on the concept of nurse-run clinics, the National Committee for Quality Assurance (NCQA), a prominent health-care quality organization, reports that it will recognize "nurse-led" primary care practices as patient-centered medical homes under the Physician Practice Connections®–Patient-Centered Medical Home recognition program (Schram, 2010). In this program, practices are encouraged to add names of eligible NPs to their practice information. The "medical home" concept was developed to reward providers for the coordination and management of patient-centered care of individuals with complex and multiple chronic illnesses, activities that NPs can easily perform. What is uncertain is whether NPs were actually included in the staffing of Medical Homes. In a study conducted in New York (NY) State, Park (2015) compared the number of NPs and physician assistants (PAs) to primary care physicians in both designated and undesignated PCMHs. She found a significant increase in the number of NPs and PAs relative to Primary Care Physicians in designated PCMHs. This is a promising result, but only reflects the current condition in NY State.

Pediatric Nurse Practitioners

Societal changes also affect the care of children. Child abuse continues to be one of the nation's most serious concerns. During 2012, 3.4 million referrals for child abuse were made in the United States, involving 6.3 million children and resulting in 1,640 deaths (CDC, 2014c). Childhood immunization is also a top health priority in the United States. More than 600 cases of measles were reported in 2014, a disease thought to have been eradicated in the United States in 2000 (CDC, 2014b).

Recent reports show serious issues with childhood obesity, bullying, and increases in suicide attempts in adolescents aged 10 to 14 years (CDC, 2014a). The need for appropriately prepared pediatric NPs is urgent. However, few U.S. nurses gravitate toward pediatrics or the NP role. So, although the role is not new, the opportunities for nurses to care for our nation's children are abundant.

Nurse Practitioners in Transitional Care Settings

Hospital-based nurses have traditionally focused their interventions on preparing patients for discharge from the hospital. However, the time for providing discharge teaching and answering patient and family questions is limited and often results in patients returning to the hospital because they did not completely understand their discharge instructions.

If patients were lucky enough to have a home health nurse visit them when they were discharged, these nurses often identified problems and concerns regarding the health of their patients and have had to contact the patient's physician to determine the next course of action, a step that often caused a delay in treatment. Therefore, the need for APRNs who can provide transitional care from hospital to community became particularly evident.

Several viable models of APRNs in transitional roles have been demonstrated through research efforts (Blewett et al, 2010; Hirschman & Bixby, 2014; Naylor et al, 2000). The clearly demonstrated, favorable patient-centered outcomes of Naylor's Transitional Care Model (2000) have gained significant recognition to the point of being named in the ACA as an example of a program showing substantial contributions to reducing health-care costs. However, there is still a need to further develop reimbursement systems for the services of APRNs.

Nurse Practitioners as Consultants in the Community

The NP as consultant in community health settings is another emerging advanced practice role. Long-term care facilities, nursing homes, and rehabilitation centers are settings that have few APRNs or professional nurses. However, residents in these settings often have chronic health needs that go untreated or unnoticed until they become serious. In response, some administrators have developed roles for APRNs to address health issues more quickly (Neal-Boylan, Mager, & Wallace-Kazer, 2012). More APRNs can be found in rehabilitation centers, inpatient hospice, skilled nursing facilities, and other nontraditional health-care settings. These community-based APRNs assess problems and develop plans of care in an attempt to prevent further progression of symptoms or needless suffering. Restrictions on APRNs' ability to function independently may limit the range of services they can provide. In addition, there are restrictions on the type of services for which APRNs can bill directly. However, as changes in health-care reimbursement policies continue to occur, the consultant role in the community will grow more popular.

The Psychiatric and Mental Health Nurse Practitioner

In the 1950s, the APRN role of the psychiatric and mental health nurse was conceptualized as a CNS role. With developments in the science underpinning mental health and psychiatric illnesses, emphasis shifted from a traditional psychosocial approach to care to a biopsychosocial paradigm. In the latter model, psychopharmacology assumed a prominent place in the treatment inventory. Acceptance of this movement was demonstrated by the development of national certification examinations for the psychiatric and mental health NP. Initially, there were two examinations available—adult and family (American Nurses Credentialing Center [ANCC], 2016). With the adoption of the Consensus Model (2008), the psychiatric and mental health APRN shifted to a focus on the individual across the life span. Prescriptive authority is available in 40 states for both CNSs and NPs (NACNS, 2015). However, NPs have prescriptive authority in all 50 states. For this reason, the psychiatric and mental health NP has become the only educational preparation for this APRN role. See **Box 2.3**.

A newly designed role for the psychiatric mental health NP is being developed through the University of Nebraska Medical Center College of Nursing (UNMC CON). Recognizing the needs of our citizens for both primary care and mental health services, UNMC CON has proposed a new program for an integrated family nurse practitioner/psychiatric–mental health nurse practitioner (Hulme, Houfek, Fiandt, Barron, & Mulhbauer, 2015). It is anticipated that this provider will care for patients across the mind–body spectrum in integrated mental health–primary care positions. Opportunities for APRN educational innovations will continue to emerge as nurses continue to respond to societal needs.

Women's Health/Gender-Related Nurse Practitioners

The women's health/gender-related NP role grew out of identification of the unique needs of women and initially focused on family planning, infertility, sexual dysfunction, gynecological care, perimenopausal issues, and the diagnosis and treatment of sexually transmitted infections (STIs) throughout the life span. Because of low income and the lack of resources available to many women, the role expanded to include well-woman health with a focus

Box 2.3

Adult Acute Care Nurse Practitioner in Palliative Care Profile

Rochelle is an adult ACNP working in palliative care in a university hospital. In her role, she is a member of the multidisciplinary team that includes several NPs, a pharmacist, collaborating physicians, fellows, a chaplain, a social worker, and an art and music therapist. Her role is solely inpatient, Monday through Friday, during daytime hours. She serves as a consultant for patients facing serious and often life-threatening illness to provide support in making care decisions and managing diverse symptoms with a significant focus on pain management. Billing is done under her NPI or the collaborating physician's.

Rochelle enjoys being able to tap into the expertise of her diverse team. Because she is in a university hospital, she has the opportunity to participate in daily huddles, a weekly conference including expert guest lecturers, team member presentations, journal club, and case presentations. She also feels her patients benefit from

the strong collaboration of the palliative team with nursing, attending physicians, hospital social workers, and case managers.

This role is a great fit for her; however, it is very different than her former colleague's role in a rural setting across the country. Amelia joined a private practice in which she has the dual role of both palliative care and hospice NP and is the only provider of these services for the entire community. Her role includes seeing patients in the office, rounding in the hospital, making home hospice visits, and handling on-call responsibilities for evenings and weekends. Although she sometimes feels isolated and often misses the daily peer collaboration, educational, and other benefits of working in a university environment, she enjoys the intensive continuity of care that she can provide her patients in multiple settings. In her practice, she bills for all her services.

on holistic care, prevention and healthy lifestyles, mental health issues, and identification of issues such as partner violence. The women's health NP also focuses on common urological problems such as incontinence and cystitis, and performs procedures such as cystoscopy, circumcision, intrauterine device (IUD) insertion, endometrial biopsy, and obstetrical ultrasonography.

Over the years, these experts recognized a lack of providers to address men's sexual and reproductive health needs. Thus, the education and role of the women's health NP expanded to include the diagnosis of, screening for, and evaluation and management of men's issues such as STIs and fertility issues. In recognition of the effectiveness of these women's health practitioners, the Consensus Model (2008) calls for women's health practitioners to expand their population focus. The formal recognition of care to men will undoubtedly provide for future expansion of the role. Additionally, women's health NPs have increased their focus on the need of the aging woman. AACN has developed specific competencies to address the special needs of this population; these include issues such as assessing falls risk, recognizing the impact of sensory deficits, assisting

with transitions of care, and advocating for the special needs of the older adult (AACN, 2010).

The National Association of Nurse Practitioners in Women's Health (NPWH) has demonstrated its leadership and commitment to health policy by partnering with the American Academy of Family Physicians (AAFP), the American College of Physicians (ACP), and the American College of Obstetricians and Gynecologists (ACOG) to update the Women's Preventive Service Guidelines (HRSA, 2016).

Women's health NPs have recently expanded into general primary care practices that need a clinician to focus on women's health issues. They have also expanded their role in specialty problem areas such as incontinence care, sexuality, and caregivers support as most often women in the family assume the role of transitioning parents into elder care after or sometimes during the time they are raising their families (Wysocki, 2014).

Acute Care Nurse Practitioner

NPs are found not only in primary care but also in specialized areas such as neonatal, pediatric, geriatric, and acute and critical care settings. The term *acute* has always been associated with the type of facility in which patient care is provided, but it is also used to describe the patient who is experiencing either a new onset or an exacerbation between an existing illness and those patients who have complex chronic illnesses that teeter on the edge of wellness and illness (Bell, 2012). Thus, ACNPs are no longer defined by the geographical setting in which they provide care but by the patient population they serve. ACNPs provide care in a variety of settings such as hospitals, intensive care units (ICUs), long-term acute care hospitals, outpatient and inpatient hospices, specialty offices, and operating rooms. They may be practice based, such as those working on a cardiothoracic service, or unit based, such as those working in a medical ICU or cardiac step-down unit. They may also be on teams that provide care across settings such as those in hospitalist positions or on consultative teams such as acute diabetes management services (see **Box 2.4**).

A new leadership role that has emerged is director of NPs or advanced practice providers. This role has improved the work environment for NPs who had previously reported to office managers or physicians. The director of NPs is familiar with issues regarding scope of practice, licensure, and certification. He or she can serve as an advocate as well as a mentor for professional development projects such as publications and presentations (D'Agostino & Halpern, 2010). These new practice areas demonstrate the diversity of practice opportunities available to meet the needs of acutely ill patients.

Neonatal Nurse Practitioner

The neonatal NP (NNP) role is a collaborative one. Several studies have examined the quality of outcomes of care delivered by neonatal NPs compared with that delivered by medical house staff. Results demonstrated that care delivered by NPs was as good as or better than that delivered by house staff on measures of cost-effectiveness and quality. In addition, care delivered by neonatal NPs had greater continuity and consistency (Bissinger, Allred, Arford, & Bellig, 1997; Mitchell-DiCenso et al, 1996).

The supply of NNPs has rarely met the national demand for services. Consistent shortages of NNPs leave a significant gap in the team approach to care (Kaminski, Meier, & Staebler, 2015). However, the care NNPs provide is often viewed to be so specialized that few nurses seek to fulfill this role (Bellini, 2014). This shortage of NNPs is anticipated to worsen. In addition, the Accreditation Council for Graduate Medical Education (ACGME) proposes to reduce the required number of neonatal intensive care unit (NICU) hours pediatric residents must complete. This is especially concerning with an inherent shortage of providers, as it is thought that individuals who become neonatal providers are those who have trained and worked in the collaborative environment of the NICU. However, this does provide opportunities for NNPs to fill the gap.

The Pediatric Acute Care Nurse Practitioner

The pediatric ACNP was a relatively late arriver to the NP workforce. This was due in part to the strong role held

---

Box 2.4

Psychiatric Mental Health Nurse Practitioner Profile

Anya is a psychiatric mental health NP who is prepared at the master's level and for the past 5 years has worked with a private oncology practice supporting clients with multiple psychological problems. Her clients include late adolescents and adults undergoing cancer treatment. She is a critical member of the team, especially because she manages psychological issues that can get in the way of treatment decisions, disease management, and patient follow-through. She is also recognized by the palliative care team as a consultant

and expert clinician in managing psychological issues in those facing life-threatening diseases. Although she sees clients of her own, she has helped the oncology and palliative care MD and NP providers manage issues such as depression and identify when they should consult a psychiatric mental health professional for particularly challenging cases. Although she is very satisfied with her work, she is frustrated by state requirements such as the need for a collaborating physician and limitations on her ability to prescribe certain medications.

by CNSs in pediatric settings. When the role of ACNP first started, it was a blended role of the CNS and NP in an attempt to provide comprehensive services and direct patient care to pediatric patients and their families. Now the APRN roles in pediatric acute care are distinctly separate.

With implementation of the Consensus Model (2008), CNSs and NPs must be certified distinctly in one of these roles based on their educational preparation and eligibility for licensure in the state they practice. The many responsibilities of the APRN in pediatrics include such activities as performing health histories and physical examinations; evaluating clinical data; prescribing treatments; performing invasive procedures, such as tracheal intubation and insertion of arterial lines; educating and supporting patients and families; facilitating patient discharge; participating in interdisciplinary rounds; and providing consultative services regarding such issues as wound care and infant feeding problems (Reuter-Rice, Madden, Gutknecht, & Foerster, 2016).

The pediatric ACNP can be found on specific patient care units such as the medical-surgical floor or the ICU; function in the hospitalist role; or be a member of a specialty service such as cardiology, pulmonary, oncology, transplantation, gastrointestinal, and general surgery (Reuter-Rice, Madden, Gutknecht, & Foerster, 2016). Pediatric ACNPs may also work outside the hospital setting in other areas in which acutely ill pediatric patients are found. Such areas include long-term acute care centers, centers for the management of mechanically ventilated patients, transport services, and home settings (Reuter-Rice, Madden, Gutknecht, & Foerster, 2016).

The role that each NP assumes depends largely on the specific needs of the patients cared for. The focus of the role, regardless of the geographical location in which the pediatric ACNP works, is to provide cost-effective and high-quality patient care.

Adult Gerontology Acute Care Nurse Practitioners

Acknowledging the aging of the American public and the need to properly train providers who can meet the multifaceted needs of older adults, the crafters of the Consensus Model (2008) explicitly changed the population focus of adult care NPs to adult gerontology. With this significant emphasis on the needs of older adults, educational programs had to revise their curricula to clearly address the competency requirements of the adult gerontology patient across the adult age continuum and certifying bodies

had to change their examinations to cover the breadth of knowledge required to implement the role.

Similar to the roles of their pediatric counterparts, the roles of adult-gerontology ACNPs (AGACNPs) are evolving and expanding throughout the acute care setting. AGACNPs are found in traditional care settings such as emergency rooms, ICUs, step-down or progressive care units, and medical-surgical floors. Adult gerontology ACNPs also deliver care to patients outside the tertiary or quaternary care institutions in settings such as outpatient surgical centers, centers for the management of mechanically ventilated patients, long-term acute care hospitals, psychiatric evaluation centers, dialysis units, heart failure centers, and correctional facilities.

In the Kleinpell and Goolsby (2012) study of ACNP practice as part of the larger 2009–2010 National NP Sample Survey, ACNP respondents continued to develop new roles to fulfill identified needs for APRNs to manage aspects of patient care in a variety of settings. NPs were found to be practicing in specialty care areas such as the cardiology, pulmonary, and specialized neurology settings; hematology and oncology; specialty ear-nose-throat (ENT) services; a variety of surgery services; palliative care; pain management services; and others. New areas of practice for ACNPs were hospitalist roles, palliative care, and roles in physician private practices (Kleinpell & Goolsby, 2012).

Adult Gerontology Acute Care Nurse Practitioners in Specialty Practices

In tertiary health-care centers, further reductions in medical resident work hours have contributed to fragmented care and a shortage of providers. The AGACNP can provide much-needed stability and continuity, which is known to produce positive patient outcomes. Complex settings, where continuous follow-up of patients is necessary, are ideal practice areas for AGACNPs. AGACNPs can make a positive impact on the health-care delivery system by providing a continuous and comprehensive approach to the management of their patients' needs.

Acute Care Nurse Practitioners in Oncology

Oncology is one specialty area in which NP expertise for continuous and comprehensive care is crucial. Oncology settings span the cancer trajectory from high-risk cancer clinics to hospice and palliative care (Vogel, 2010; Volker & Limerick, 2007). NPs in oncology bring a unique holistic perspective that enables them to provide expert care with issues such as pain management, symptom palliation, and sensitivity to the psychological aspects of a cancer diagnosis. NP roles in oncology are varied and can include outpatient roles in radiation therapy, chemotherapy, surgical clinics (preoperative and postoperative global care), palliative care, survivorship and prevention, and genetic counseling related to cancer risk. These NPs can also be found in ICUs as well as medical or surgical oncology units. Because of the Consensus Model, there are no longer stand-alone oncology NP programs. NPs must be prepared as either primary care or ACNPs and then can complete additional training and obtain specialty certification in oncology. See Box 2.4.

In 2007, the American Society of Clinical Oncology (ASCO) Workforce Study predicted a 48% increase in the demand for medical oncology services by the year 2020. This need far exceeds the number of medicine trainees that will be available (Erikson et al, 2009).

Nurse-Midwifery

Nurse-midwives are registered nurses who are primary health-care providers to women throughout the life span. They perform physical examinations; prescribe medications, including contraceptive methods; order laboratory tests as needed; and provide prenatal care, gynecological care, and labor and birth care, as well as health education and counseling to women of all ages. Per the American College of Nurse-Midwives (ACNM) position statement, *Mandatory Degree Requirements for Entry Into Midwifery Practice,* a graduate degree is required for entry into midwifery practice (ACNM, 2012b). All midwifery education programs provide the necessary education for graduates to be eligible to take the examination offered by the American Midwifery Certification Board (AMCB) and become CNMs. The Accreditation Commission for Midwifery Education (ACME) (formerly the ACNM Division of Accreditation [DOA]) assesses the quality and content of midwifery education programs and ensures that they reflect the ACNM core competencies.

The ACNM has mandated graduate-level education for entry into midwifery clinical practice since 2010. In the past master's programs predominated in nurse-midwifery preparation, however, many programs have discontinued their master's degree option and only offer a DNP (ACNM, 2012a).

Nurse-midwifery is recognized in all 50 states, although it is regulated by various agencies in the different states and has varying scopes of practice from state to state. The main scope of practice issue has to do with independent versus collaborative practice with physicians. Physician practices (21.7%) and hospitals (29.5%) continue to be identified as the primary employers of nurse-midwives (Schuiling, Sipe, & Fullerton, 2013). For nurse-midwives practicing in hospital settings, clinical privileges may be granted through membership in the medical staff or through other privileging routes. The purpose of requiring institutional credentialing and practice privileges is to ensure that nurse-midwives provide patient care within the parameters of professional practice that are consistent with national standards and state regulations (ACNM, 2006).

Although nurse-midwives practice predominantly in hospitals and physician-owned practices, they also practice in educational institutions, midwife-owned practices, community health centers, nonprofit health agencies, military or federal government agencies, and birthing centers (Schuiling et al, 2013). Nurse-midwives have advocated for women for years. An exciting initiative started by the American College of Nurse-Midwives in 2015 is the *Healthy Birth Initiative: Reducing Primary Cesareans Project* (http://birthtools.org/HBI-Reducing-Primary-Cesareans). The goal of this project is to set up care bundles in birthing centers and hospitals that proactively work with the laboring woman in such a way that the experience does not require the delivery of the baby via Cesarean section.

A recent consequence of nurse-midwives expanding their practices and becoming entrepreneurial is the expansion of their duties into more administrative areas such as budgeting, setting up and interpreting quality metrics, taking on human resource responsibilities, scheduling, and developing policies and procedures (Slager, 2016). As these activities become more commonplace, the educational preparation for nurse-midwives may have to include these content areas. See **Box 2.5.**

Primary Care Focus in Nurse-Midwifery

As nurse-midwives provided obstetrical care to women throughout their childbearing years, they realized that many women did not have access to primary care services. It became a natural progression for women to seek their primary health-care needs from the health-care provider they had trusted during their childbirths; thus,

---

BOX 2.5

Certified Nurse-Midwife Clinical Profile

Siji is the practice director of a busy obstetrical, gyne-cological, and midwifery care program that includes nine midwives and five physicians. She is responsible for the recruitment and evaluation of staff members and serves as liaison to hospital administrators and to the professional and lay community.

As she has progressed in her role, she has assumed more administrative responsibilities including managing the practice budget, overseeing productivity, and creating a vision for the future of the practice. She has had to learn the intricacies of reimbursement because her practice accepts numerous health insurance plans, and she acknowledges a steep learning curve. Because this practice is new, she also oversees the development of marketing strategies, new practice policies and procedures, and the collection of quality measures. She finds it hard to balance this with her clinical responsibilities, but she enjoys having the opportunity to develop her administrative skills.

---

nurse-midwives began to provide care to perimenopausal and postmenopausal women, a natural expansion of their scope of practice. As the aging of U.S. Americans evolves in the 21st century, the number of women approaching menopause is growing. Large numbers of women are ex-pected to seek menopausal and postmenopausal care from nurse-midwives. In response to this change in demographics and the need for greater access to primary care providers, CNMs have expanded their scope of practice to include provision of primary care to women across the life span from adolescence to beyond menopause, with a special emphasis on pregnancy, childbirth, and gynecological and reproductive health.

The scope of practice for CNMs also includes treatment of male partners for sexually transmitted infections and reproductive health and care of the normal newborn during the first 28 days of life (ACNM, 2012c). Interestingly, this scope of practice reflects the changes in the Consensus Model: the population focus of midwives from women's health to women's health/gender-related care. CNMs con-tinue to focus on midwifery so as to not lose the essence of nurse-midwifery practice, while acknowledging those aspects of primary care that are part of the services offered to patients and their families.

Issues Related to Primary Care Practice

CNMs provide primary and preventive care in clinics and other outpatient settings. The ACNM calls for care delivered by CNMs to include all essential factors of primary care and case management. This focus on the ambulatory care of women and newborns emphasizes health promotion, education, and disease prevention and identifies women as central in providing this care (ACNM, 2012c). CNMs have also focused on the care of adolescent women, noting that they are largely a medically underserved group. They are recognized as a key component of the Patient Centered Medical Home, also referred to as the Maternity Care Home (ACNM, 2012b).

Nurse-Midwife as First Assistant for Cesarean Section

Another role of the CNM that has grown is that of the sur-gical first assistant. Because of obstetrical residency programs across the nation closing and cost containment resulting in fewer physicians available to serve as first assistants, CNMs have expanded their roles to fill the gap (Tharpe, 2015). Additionally, because in many cases the CNM is already present at the time of an emergency Cesarean section, a delivery can progress without interruption, resulting in better outcomes for both the mother and the newborn, when the CNM is prepared as a surgical first assistant.

Not unexpectedly, there is opposition to this expan-sion of the CNM role. The Association for Perioperative Registered Nurses (AORN) and some surgeons are not convinced that CNMs possess adequate knowledge to perform the first assistant role safely. In response to this criticism, the ACNM (2016) has set guidelines for those CNMs who wish to serve as a first assistant and defined the role of the first assistant in Cesarean sections as a frequently performed advanced midwifery skill requiring training and supervision in patient assessment, anatomy and physiology, principles of wound repair, and the development of basic surgical skills such as aseptic technique and suturing. At present, each state is addressing the requirements for CNMs who practice as first assistants. Although the number of CNM–first assistants has grown substantially, this skill is not part of the Core Competencies for CNMs, and therefore requires additional education.

More recently, midwives have added the use of obstetrical and gynecological ultrasound examinations to their repertoire of skills (ACNM, 2012d). Ultrasound examinations may be performed in all trimesters of pregnancy to obtain specific information: determining gestational age, assessing fetal well-being, monitoring interval fetal growth, and measuring maternal cervical length. ACNM (2012d) recognizes the need for additional educational content, credentialing, and privileging for midwives who choose to incorporate this into their practices. ACNM is not mandating this as a required skill for all midwives but recognizes that ultrasound examinations may be a necessary tool in meeting the needs of one's patients.

As the needs of childbearing women have changed over the years, the practice and skills of the nurse-midwife have expanded to meet them. This trend will continue as additional needs are identified.

Nurse Anesthetist

CRNAs are anesthesia specialists with authority to practice in all 50 states and the District of Columbia. They administer all types of anesthesia and provide anesthesia-related care in the following categories: preanesthetic preparations and evaluation; anesthesia induction, maintenance, and emergence; postanesthesia care; and perianesthetic and clinical support functions (Department of Health and Human Services [DHHS], Public Health Service [PHS] Division of Acquisition Management, 1995). Chronic pain is a major issue in the United States. Unfortunately, access to care can be limited as pain management procedures, such as epidural steroid injections, are regulated at the state level and thus cannot be performed by all CRNAs (AANA, 2014).

Nurse anesthetists provide a significant amount of the anesthesia given for surgical procedures in the United States. These APRNs work in urban and rural settings, and provide more than 50% of the anesthesia administered in rural areas (RAND Corporation, 2010). In contrast to the high numbers of women in the other APRN categories, 41% of CRNAs are men (Rand Corporation, 2010).

The AANA serves as the guiding professional organization for CRNAs, setting the educational and certification standards and promulgating a code of ethics for CRNAs (AANA, 2005b), along with the scope of nurse anesthesia practice (AANA, 2013a), standards of nurse anesthesia practice (AANA, 2013b), and standards for office-based anesthesia practice (AANA, 2015). Nurse anesthetist students must enroll in schools accredited by the AANA, and upon graduation they must successfully complete a certification examination. As of August 2016, they must also participate in mandatory Continued Professional Certification (CPC) every 4 years (with a 2-year check-in) through the National Board on Certification and Recertification of Nurse Anesthetists (NBCRNA) that includes 100 hours of accredited continuing education and core modules. They must also take a recertification examination every 8 years (NBCRNA, 2016).

In 1998, master's degree preparation was required for beginning nurse anesthesia practice. Although the required master's degree does not have to be in nursing, about 50% of graduate CRNA programs are located within schools of nursing (AANA, 2010). By 2022 the entry-into-practice educational requirement will be at the doctoral level.

CRNAs face significant ongoing difficulties in establishing their practice prerogatives. They face considerable pressures from anesthesiologists who have attempted to limit their scope of practice by conceptualizing the administration of anesthesia as the practice of medicine (Shumway & Del Risco, 2000). In 1982, the American Society of Anesthesiologists (ASA) introduced the concept of an anesthesia care team (ACT), a practice model requiring that all anesthetics be given under the direction of an anesthesiologist (Shumway & Del Risco, 2000).

These restrictive efforts were inadvertently fostered with the introduction of an insurance reimbursement regulation policy by Medicare in 1982. This policy attempted to reduce charges of fraud for anesthesia care by establishing specific conditions that held anesthesiologists accountable for services they claimed to perform when working with or employing CRNAs (Shumway & Del Risco, 2000). The Tax Equity and Fiscal Responsibility Act (TEFRA) regulations set specific conditions for reimbursable services that seemed to require physician leadership for the delivery of anesthesia as a standard of care. Later attempts to eliminate the necessity for anesthesiologist supervision for Medicare reimbursement of CRNA services resulted in an "opt out" option for states (AANA, 2005a). This effort has given way to the current movement for APRN independent practice. CRNAs' quest for independent practice is a result of the Consensus Model (2008). According to NCSBN.org, CRNAs currently have the ability to provide anesthesia without physician supervision in 27 states (NCSBN, 2016).

One result of the struggle for CRNA practice prerogatives and leadership has been the establishment of the ACT as the predominant practice model. To clarify whether differences exist between CRNAs who work in ACTs and those who do not, Shumway and Del Risco (2000) evaluated personal and professional characteristics, scope of practice, work load, income, and employment arrangements in a sample of more than 400 CRNAs. They found that CRNAs who practiced in ACTs were more likely to be women, have less experience, be younger, have a master's degree, and practice in larger cities. ACT-based CRNAs also had a broader scope of practice and used more airways, regional anesthesia, and monitoring techniques, and performed more varied cases and services. They used more laryngeal mask airways and arterial catheters, and provided more anesthesia for cardiopulmonary bypass, pediatric, intracranial, and trauma cases than non-ACT anesthetists. However, they were less likely to be involved with the placement of epidural and central venous catheters and to participate in pain management and critical care services (Shumway & Del Risco, 2000).

Non–ACT-based anesthetists worked more hours per week and were reimbursed $40,000 more per year.

Finally, 91% of ACT-based anesthetists in this sample were employees compared with 4% who were self-employed, whereas 49% of non–ACT-based anesthetists were employees compared with 43% who were self-employed (Shumway & Del Risco, 2000). See **Box 2.6.**

AN EMERGING PRACTICE AREA FOR ALL ADVANCED PRACTICE REGISTERED NURSES: HOSPICE AND PALLIATIVE CARE

As the number of individuals in the United States with life-limiting and serious illnesses increases, there is a need to increase palliative care services that can help to improve access and quality of life, increase patient and family satisfaction, and contain costs. In 2014, the authors of the IOM's report, *Dying in America: Improving Quality and Honoring Individual Preferences Near the End of Life,* made recommendations that included an increase in access to care for our aging population (Meghani & Hinds, 2015). In 2010, the American Academy of Hospice and Palliative Medicine published a workforce study that demonstrated the need for up to 18,000 physicians in hospice and palliative care (Lupu, 2016).

APRNs have stepped up to try to fill the need in this growing area. Palliative care APRNs can be found across settings including inpatient, outpatient, skilled nursing and rehabilitation facilities, and in the home. Although one typically thinks of these specialists working in Primary

---

Box 2.6

Certified Registered Nurse Anesthetist Clinical Profile

Josh has been a CRNA for 20 years. He began his career in a large university-based medical center focusing on cardiac cases. He subsequently developed the skills and expertise to rotate through different cases including craniotomies. As outpatient surgical centers began to open in his area, he thought about transitioning to a position in the community. However, he had a friend who had been doing this for several years, and although the hours were better and the stress level lower, she missed the challenge of working with acutely ill and medically complex

patients and felt unprepared to return to a high-acuity environment.

Josh ultimately decided to leave his hospital-based job and work per diem as an independent contractor. Because he is a seasoned clinician with a broad skill set and a great local reputation, he found work in many settings including a community hospital, university-based medical center, and surgicenter. He has the best of both worlds in that he can make his own schedule, experience the challenges of managing high-acuity patients, and work more independently in the outpatient arena.

Care and Oncology, there has been a shift to increase access to patients with other life-limiting illnesses such as neurological and cardiopulmonary disease. All APRNs have a role in palliative care. As nurses first, APRNs have always focused and excelled with symptom management, assessing patients' responses to treatments and ascertaining patients' goals. CNSs and NPs are the roles many people think of as being the "typical" palliative care provider; however, the palliative care APRN can also be a nurse-midwife, as these professionals are skilled in managing individuals through life transitions, pain, and anxiety, or a nurse anesthetist, who may participate in palliative sedation (Van Hoover & Holt, 2016; Wolf, 2013). Certification as an advanced practice hospice and palliative nurse (ACHPN), often a job requirement for this specialty area, is available for the CNS and the NP through the Hospice and Palliative Nurses Association (http://hpcc.advancingexpertcare.org/competence/aprn-achpn/).

FUTURE DIRECTIONS FOR ADVANCED PRACTICE NURSES

APRNs are thriving, as shown in the increased numbers of practitioners; in the expansion of practice roles and settings; in the opportunity for independent practice without physician collaboration or supervision; and with the support of major health-care organizations; for example, the Veterans Healthcare Association endorses their use throughout their health-care network (U.S. Department of Veterans Affairs, 2016).

The future for APRNs is promising but will continue to be affected by knowledge development in the biological and social sciences and in the evolving political and social climate. What effect this will have on APRN practice is yet to be seen.

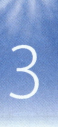

3

Role Development
A Theoretical Perspective

Lucille A. Joel

Learning Outcomes

Learning outcomes expected as a result of this chapter:

- Explain structural-functionalist and symbolic-interactionist theories and how they influence role adjustment.
- Define reference groups and distinguish between normative, comparison, and audience groups.
- Evaluate role-taking and role-making in the workplace and explain the role of socialization in these processes.
- Explain the nature of second-order change and how it leads to the development of new behaviors.
- Apply the skill acquisition model to nursing (Benner, Dreyfus, & Dreyfus).
- Describe setbacks experienced by new role expectations.
- Justify the need for anticipatory socialization during the educational process.
- Discuss challenges to socialization in the advanced practice nurse (APN) role.
- Distinguish stress and strain.

A nurse's role is constantly changing. There is no role that a nurse will serve exclusively for the entire life of a career. Role modifications depend on a theoretical body of knowledge, more of it hypothetical than empirical research. These concepts and relationships allow a comfortable paradigm shift as necessary, with an awareness of the elements of continuity from here to there.

A THEORETICAL PERSPECTIVE ON ROLE: AN OVERVIEW

There are two diametrically opposed theoretical perspectives in the behavioral sciences that provide a context for the study of role performance: structural-functionalist theory and symbolic-interactionist theory. Structural-functionalist theory is based on the assumption that roles are more or less fixed within the society to which they are attached and that opportunities for individuals to alter patterns of social interaction are limited. In contrast, symbolic interactionist theory proposes the more individualistic perspective, that people do not merely learn responses but organize and interpret cues in the environment and choose those to which they wish to react (Conway, 1988).

Structural-functionalist theory subordinates the individual to the society; it is deductive in its analysis of role. All situations that arise within a society do so because they fill a social need. One such example is the division of labor. The more complex a society, the more differentiated its labor source will become, readjusting and reconstructing over time. Specialization becomes guaranteed, and associates and assistants are created to share in a domain of the work. This concept is dramatically displayed by the division of labor and reordered roles within the health-care delivery system, each role creating its own cadre of technologists, technicians, associates, and assistants. Why should nursing be different?

Altruism also plays a major part here because individuals subordinate their will to the social order. The social forces in a given society validate the roles and the associated behaviors of the individual. Consensual validation is the vehicle for both the maintenance and change of these norms. In many instances, norms are codified by government; in others, they continue to exist in veritable limbo, changing or resisting change according to time and place. A continuing debate exists about the relationship between the fixed norms of a society and the individual's perception of those norms. Often there is no route to interpretation of the social norm except cues offered by others in the situation, and often those cues may be misleading. From another perspective, where may nonconformity be tolerated, to what degree, and in what areas of social participation? Examples abound both professionally and in life. Consider for a moment the immigrant family whose children are schooled in the United States and socialized to the prevailing culture in this country. Are their new ways accepted at home and to what extent? Must they change the way a chameleon does from place to place or jeopardize belonging or perhaps even sustenance? To what extent can advanced practice nurses (APNs) feel confident in establishing their personally preferred values, attitudes, and behaviors in a new role or employment situation? See **Box 3.1** for cues that may predict limits on flexibility in defining role behaviors.

In contrast, the symbolic-interactionist view emphasizes the meaning that symbols hold for actors in the process of

---

Box 3.1

Cues That May Predict Limits on Flexibility in Defining Role Behaviors

Highly precise and detailed job descriptions

Management by memorandum in situations in which personal communication would have sufficed

Guarded interdisciplinary boundaries that hamper smooth operation

A hierarchy that is an obstacle to work rather than a facilitator

Policies, procedures, and documentation systems that are cumbersome and even inconsistent with current practice

Absence of staff nurse autonomy in caring for patients

Organizational relationships designed for supervision, as opposed to reporting

Absence of inventiveness and creativity

Verbalized discontent from staff, but no evidence of any attempt to change things

High turnover rate among employees

Maintenance of a "screen" for attitudes, values, and behaviors not supported by historic antecedents role development, rather than the constraints presumed to be exerted by the social structure. The interactionist sees the formation of role identity as inductive and complex. The role is a creative adaptation to the social environment and the result of the reciprocal interaction of individuals. It is the product of self-conception and the perspective of generalized others. To facilitate communication toward these ends, symbols are essential, and they must be social and hold the same meaning for each actor in the process. In other words, self-identity is shaped by the reflected appraisals of others, and it is desirable that individuals' self-perception should be highly congruent with the way they are perceived by others and the way they see themselves as being perceived by others. Should these pieces show a poor fit, an individual could waste a lifetime of effort creating evidence that justifies his or her personal view of self.

Many have rejected the structuralist approach because it seems limited in accounting for the wide variation in roles and behaviors that we see today. Yet, it is impossible to ignore the effect that the culture and the "collective conscience" have on our development of identity and role behaviors. There is recent interest in building conceptual frameworks that are inclusive of both the interactionist and structural perspectives, and promise a greatly enlarged understanding of role development. This eclecticism characterizes this chapter's discussion.

ROLE DEVELOPMENT

The concept of reference groups and the process of socialization are central to role development. Reference groups are the frame of reference for the process of socialization. Through socialization, individual behavior is shaped to conform to the standard of the group in which one chooses to seek membership.

Reference Groups

Reference groups convey a standard of normative behavior in terms of values, attitudes, knowledge, and skills. For an individual, this may be a group to which he or she belongs or aspires to belong. In moving toward a standard that is either consciously or unconsciously desired, discussion of several reference groups is in order, including normative

groups, comparison groups, and audience groups. The normative group sets explicit standards and expects compliance, and it rewards or punishes relative to that degree of compliance. The church, community, and family are good examples of normative groups. The behaviors that are expected may have wide or narrow latitude, but somewhere there is a "bottom line."

The comparison group sets its own standards and becomes a comparison group only when an individual accepts it as such (Lum, 1988). The nursing staff of a Magnet facility may be a comparison group, demonstrating longevity in employment and satisfaction with work, seeking upward mobility through education, and so on. The nursing staff and their leadership in other facilities may aspire to these qualities, making it a comparison group for them.

The audience group is a collective group whose attention an individual wishes to attract. The audience group holds certain values but does not demand compliance from the person for whom they serve as a referent (Lum, 1988). In fact, the audience group may not even be aware of this individual. To be recognized, the individual takes note of the group's values and plays to that audience for attention. Staff nurses may observe that physicians value being able to proceed with the treatment of their patients unencumbered by the bureaucratic constraints of health care. Administrators are overwhelmed by the cost factors in health care. Nurses are best positioned if they are aware of these values and attitudes, and try to minimize the obstacles they represent to these groups. In other words, they play to the audience through either word or deed.

Socialization

Socialization refers to the learning of the values, attitudes, knowledge, and skills that enable the behavior prescribed for a specific social position or role. The fact that these components are society-specific indicates that there are social norms involved. Values are ideas held in common by members of a social structure that prioritizes goals and objectives (Scott, 1970). Values are generally the abstract but relatively stable aspects of a person's belief system. Attitude is the tendency to respond to social objects or events in a favorable or unfavorable way. Opinion is defined as expressed attitude. Behaviors are observable social acts performed by an individual. Attitudes guide judgment and subsequently behavior, but this assumption of a relationship between attitude and behavior is controversial.

Operationally, the concept of socialization refers to individuals acquiring the necessary knowledge and skills, as well as internalizing and shaping the values and attitudes of a particular social system, in preparation for fulfilling a specific role in that system (Lum, 1988). This process is no less true for the roles of nurse and APN than it is for the role of mother, father, husband, or wife. Further, whereas some roles or statuses have highly specific role prescriptions, others are extremely vague and open to wide variation of interpretation. This latitude may be observed in the setting in which the role is played out, the society in which it is placed, or both. Harmony among these systems enhances role execution. There is often significant discrepancy between the public, professional, legal, and institutional definitions of the role of the nurse. Even if the society and role occupant are bound by the legal role as defined, discrepancies among the other definitions cause problems in recruitment, retention, job satisfaction, and more (Harley-Wilson, 1988).

Socialization is a continuous and cumulative process that evolves over time through role-taking and role-making, both of which are techniques of role bargaining. Social behavior is not simply a learned response. It depends on the processes of interaction and communication. To be successful, role-taking requires skill in empathic communication. The individual must project him- or herself into the circumstances of another and then step back to imagine how he or she would feel in the other's situation. If there is accurate determination of the motives and feelings of the other, the actor can modify his or her own behavior to sustain or alter the other's response (Hardy & Hardy, 1988a). The process here is unidirectional. For example, the APN "reads" his or her peers and supervisor as seeing staff development as the major focus of the APN role, although she or he may have preferred to carry a significant personal caseload of the most complex patients. Staff development is accepted as the priority, but the APN takes on cases as vehicles for teaching at every opportunity.

Put in another way, the less desirable activities are accommodated (first-order change) and even eventually assimilated (second-order change), becoming an integral part of the role. First-order changes are *behavioral shifts* that do not permanently achieve a desired result. Old preferences keep returning the way antagonists do because we shift our behaviors, but not the core values or attitudes causing the behaviors. Second-order changes are *permanent attitude shifts that cause new behaviors* (Watzlawick, Weakland, & Fisch, 2011). The "old ways" stay gone and are not replaced by a new version (such as giving up alcohol and starting a nicotine or work addiction).

In contrast, role-making is bidirectional and interactive, with both actors presenting behaviors that are interpreted reciprocally for the purpose of creating and modifying their own roles. This process is analogous to a dance, with each partner seeking to complement the other while maintaining his or her own uniqueness. For example, the APN notices surprise from the physician when suggesting a modification in treatment for a patient. The APN supplies cogent and sophisticated reasoning, and the physician agrees, although skeptical of this behavior. Over time, the physician becomes comfortable with the APN's prescriptions and actually looks for the clinical input. Both role-taking and role-making depend on success in reading role partners correctly. This skill is enhanced by broad social experience, rehearsal of the role anticipated, the recentness of those experiences, attentiveness to role behaviors, and good memory skills. These skills can be developed and honed during the educational experience (Ter Maten-Speksnijder, Grypdonck, Pool, Meurs, & Van Staa, 2015).

Equally challenging as internalizing role behaviors is the movement from one role or subrole to another. This process is described in **Box 3.2.** Not only must one learn new behaviors, but one must break from old ones. Inadequate socialization predicts marginalization or the inability to either remain in a previous role or move on to another. A case in point is the nurse who hangs on to the periphery of a system, never quite becoming part of it or bothering to know the personalities involved and refusing to assimilate nursing with the other aspects of life. This is particularly common in people who try to juggle multiple aspects of life, keeping each separate—obligations everywhere, multiple lists of things to do, each with a first-place priority, a comprehensive plan nowhere. The wiser strategy is to integrate the dimensions of life, with professional colleagues becoming personal friends, family participating in workplace and professional events, and so on (one list with one rank ordering of priorities).

Box 3.2

Socialization as a Continuous Process

Break From Previous Roles

Minimize previous advantage.

Break previous peer relationships.

Convert previous peer relationships into friendship relationships.

Maintain a portfolio or clinical log reflecting on your evolving practice, values, and attitudes.

Establish a New Peer Group

Clarify new responsibilities that accompany changed status.

Consider the values, attitudes, knowledge, and skills that will contribute to success.

Develop new peer group associations.

Move to the New Role Prescription (Accommodation)

Provide role rehearsal opportunities.

Review benefits of mastery.

Consider a mentor.

Identify support systems among role partners.*

Assimilate Role Behaviors

Be aware of change of self-concept.

Recognize the rites of passage as more than symbolic.

Create opportunities for success.

Treat failure as a learning experience.

Move on to process and outcome evaluation once the role is established, although not matured.

*A role partner may hold the same role or a role that is reciprocal but definitely has role expectations of the primary role occupant.

Role Acquisition

Knowledge and skill acquisition are important aspects of role implementation in nursing, both for the entry-level registered nurse and for the APN. This is not to ignore the essential part played by attitudes and values (the belief system), but to acknowledge that knowledge and skill are expected of professionals by the public (audience group), leadership in the field (comparative group), and peers (normative group). The skill acquisition model, developed by Dreyfus and Dreyfus (1977) and later applied to nursing by Benner (1984), tells us that even experts perform as novices when they enter new roles or subroles, although they proceed to acquisition at a quicker pace. This pattern is verified by several authorities, including Brykczynski (2000) and Roberts, Tabloski, and Bova (1997). In observing APN students, they report periods of regression, anxiety, and conflict before the incorporation of new role behaviors. This is not unexpected, and an analogy can be drawn from work with groups. It is common that in the beginning of a group or when a new member is introduced into an established group, there is a loss of confidence among individual members. The introduction of a person into a milieu with new role expectations is a temporary setback, even when some of the behaviors have been well established in a previous role. The regression and loss of confidence are often followed by anger directed toward faculty and preceptors whom they see as guilty of not giving them enough knowledge or skill. In many ways, they are grieving the role they had previously mastered and responding to the anxiety over moving on.

Anticipatory socialization should be a planned goal during the student period and not left to chance. Ample opportunity should be provided for students to get to know APNs who may just be beginning their careers (peer group) and to participate in discussions with seasoned APNs regarding practice issues (accommodation). Both of these goals may be accomplished through the state nurses association, especially if there is a forum or division on advanced practice. Other experiences should be incorporated in the educational program, such as the opportunity to dialogue with employers and practicing APNs about their expectations of the role. **Box 3.3** contains a format for the participation of APNs on a panel describing their practice and role development for students. These anticipatory experiences should facilitate the period of resocialization as a graduate.

It would be remiss not to mention the clinical competency of faculty. Clinically competent faculty are necessary to give credibility to the program and to narrow the gap "between education and practice" (Brykczynski, 2000, p. 121). The best of all worlds would be for faculty to teach using their own panel of patients. Although this is often impossible, it is still necessary for faculty to maintain their clinical skills to be able to critique practice and provide the proper oversight for preceptors (Moore & Watters, 2013).

Box 3.3

Questions to Guide Advanced Practice Nurse Participation in a Panel on Advanced Practice

How did you find your first position after graduation?

What job-seeking strategies would you advise new graduates to use in today's market?

How do any or all of the following fit into your specific position?

What is your prescriptive authority?

What kind of practice privileges (i.e., admitting, treating, consulting, and discharging) do you have?

What system do you have for reimbursement?

Do you participate in a managed-care panel?

How have your functions or role changed over the years, and were those changes the result of the evolution of the profession, your choices, your advocacy, or the expectations of an employer?

Have you been an active participant in developing your role? How so?

What are the major stresses and strains in your practice? How do you handle them?

Describe your collaborative arrangement with a physician.

How do you show outcomes or document the value of your contribution to the practice (or to your employer)?

How do you maintain your practice credibility?

Do you plan to further develop your own role or skill set? If so, how?

What were the most valuable aspects of your graduate educational preparation for advanced practice? The least valuable?

What do you know now that you wish you had known earlier in your career?

What is your experience with mentoring, either as mentor or protégé?

How important to your professional development was this mentor(ed) experience?

Benner (2001) describes five levels of skill acquisition: novice, advanced beginner, competent, proficient, and expert. As one proceeds along this continuum, one becomes more involved in the process of caring, until at the expert stage, situations are recognized in terms of their holistic patterns rather than a cluster of component parts, and the context becomes somewhat irrelevant. In the early stages, new behaviors are accommodated, and they later become assimilated in the practice repertoire, until at the highest level they appear intuitive. Movement from accommodation to assimilation or from novice to expert with its intermediate steps is best accomplished through accruing experience with the opportunity to apply both practical and theoretical knowledge, and providing situations in which failure is allowed and treated as a learning experience (Roberts et al, 1997). It should be noted that Benner's model is experiential and does not consider education as a variable in distinguishing these skill levels. However, you cannot apply what you do not know. It would be interesting to use Benner's model to compare an APN and a non–master's-prepared registered nurse, both with similar experience.

It is helpful for APN students to consciously approach the socialization process knowing their normative, comparative, and audience groups, and being aware of the changes that are expected to take place in their own behaviors, values, and attitudes. Socializing experiences, provided during the course of studies, are presented in **Box 3.4.**

Socialization Deficits

One of the most compelling challenges in professional education is to provide adequate socialization. Socialization deficits are guaranteed to inhibit role performance, introducing additional stress into roles that are already by nature stressful.

APNs are increasingly prepared in programs of part-time study. In addition, the movement into the community college and university settings for entry-level education has, to some degree, diluted the intensity of the socialization experience for nursing. Off-campus living arrangements, a cohort of students who depend on full-time or part-time employment or who have family obligations, courses of study that may be protracted over many years, and so on,

Box 3.4

Role-Enhancing Experiences Planned During Your Education (Applicable to Either Entry-Level or Graduate Education)

A synthesis semester at the end of the educational program that incorporates, as far as legally possible, all the ingredients of full-time employment

Work-study programs that alternate semesters with work placements in your anticipated field

A curriculum that progresses toward more independence and personal accountability, with students and faculty moving to a collegial relationship as opposed to superiors and subordinates

Service-education partnerships, with faculty teaching students as they practice with their own patients

Opportunity for students to work with faculty on their personal research or in their practice

Summer externships and new graduate internships or residencies

Patient clinical areas with a primary commitment to the clinical learning needs of students (the designated teaching unit)

Participation in activities suited to APNs (e.g., conferences, meetings, and peer review sessions)

Preceptor or "buddy" system involving agency staff

An experience with interdisciplinary (or at the least multidisciplinary) education (Joel, 2011)

---

all reduce the strength of the primary socialization into the profession. What is the result of an incomplete or weak primary socialization into nursing when moving on to the next role transition to advanced practice (Chen, Chen, Tsai, & Lo, 2007)? This remains a serious question yet to be answered. Further, even if the primary socialization is solid, what does incomplete anticipatory socialization as an APN mean for role acquisition? This could create a situation of "marginal man," in which a person is a member of one or more cultures but belongs to none. It also presents a strong case for externships and residency programs through which a concentrated exposure to the role is guaranteed (Santucci, 2004; Starr, 2006). Certification also promises to help role acquisition and role progression with its expectation of additional education and investment in practice.

STRESS AND STRAIN

Stress and strain are natural companions of advanced practice, given the chaotic health-care environment and the fact that these roles are evolving and growing in prominence. Hardy and Hardy (1988b) tell us that role stress is primarily located in the social structure, external to the individual, and owing to incompatible normative expectations. It may or may not generate role strain, the feeling of frustration and anxiety internal to the individual.

Antecedents of Stress and Strain

Many situations can create stress and strain for the APN. These include the educational preparation in which we may overlook opportunities for anticipatory socialization and in a rapidly restructuring health-care delivery system that demands continuous minor or major modification in roles. Specialization and advances in technology make roles that have become well established over time obsolete and require the role occupants to face a new cycle of ambiguity and transition (Creakbaum, 2011). Beyond this, there is also the growing emphasis on cost efficiency, consumerism, and the demedicalization of health care. None of these trends are surprising to the reader, but the effect they have on roles is often unexpected and unintended. The traditional hierarchy of the system is radically changed, and the primary care provider is as likely to be an APN or physician assistant as a physician. Consumer is "king," and health-care organizations are competing to corner their market share of clients. Consumer satisfaction is a major outcome measure against which everyone is measured. Given the availability of information, consumers often enter the system with as much information about their condition as the professional who attends them. At the same time, we see the slow but decisive movement toward complementary therapies that have not been part of our nursing repertoire in the past, but that are demanded by the public.

To further complicate the situation, reality finds most nurses as employees in health-care systems. One should never lose sight of the fact that systems (whether large or small, simple or complex) exist to secure their goals and preserve their values. They accomplish this by responding to changing conditions, achieving solidarity among their parts, using a division of labor to accomplish work, controlling the environment, maintaining order, and using resources efficiently. Efficiency has caused a move to accomplish many things through "adhocracy"—systems established for a limited goal and then disbanded. Subcontracting in addition to internal departments allow greater flexibility to adjust to change. In a similar manner, the nursing role has been forced to readjust or jeopardize organizational stability (Ball, 2011), so resocialization becomes a continuing process, and stress and strain a constant by-product of this process.

Classifying Role Stress

After an exhaustive analysis of research on role stress as it existed in 1988, Hardy and Hardy (1988) developed the classification system presented in **Box 3.5** that was subsequently expanded by the work of Schumacher and Meleis (1994).

Stress and strain are predictable in situations that include ambiguity, ambivalence, incongruity, conflict, and underload and overload, and in situations in which the role occupants see themselves as underqualified or

---

Box 3.5

Classification of Role Stress

Role ambiguity—There is vagueness and lack of clarity of the role expectations.

Role conflict—Role expectations are incompatible.

Role incongruity—There is a poor fit between the persons' abilities and their expectations or the expectations of the systems with which they interface.

Role overload—There is too much expected in the time available.

Role underload—Role expectations are minimal and underuse the abilities of the role occupant.

Role overqualification—Role occupant's motivation, skills, and knowledge far exceed those required.

Role underqualification (role incompetence)—Role occupant lacks the necessary resources (Hardy & Hardy, 1988b).

Role transition—Person moves to a new role.

Role supplementation—There is anticipatory socialization (Schumacher & Meleis, 1994).

---

overqualified or are moving into a new role or are engaged in anticipatory socialization. An example of ambiguity is the new APN who accepts a position without an adequate job description in a setting where there has been little experience with advanced practice, and so there are no seasoned peers to provide direction or support. An example of incongruity is the nurse who has been prepared exclusively for primary care practice and accepts a position that requires extensive coaching and teaching of nursing staff in a specialty area. Role conflict may result when the staff nurse feels an obligation to provide quality care but then finds it impossible to achieve satisfactory outcomes within the limits of a predetermined length of stay or in a situation in which the nurse believes that his or her clinical judgment is superior to the client's own choices, but the client refuses to comply. Overload and underload often require a more objective opinion as well as the self-assurance to revisit goals and objectives to make them more realistic. Being overqualified or underqualified moves into areas of competence. Some individuals may consider themselves overqualified because they never strain to see or are untrained to see the complexities of a situation. The same circumstances may give rise to feelings of underload. Peer discussion of such clinical situations is helpful to verify your opinion of yourself. Feelings of being underqualified must be talked through and validated, or they result in living the life of an "impostor" (Arena & Page, 1992).

The stress and strain that come with most of the service occupations are labeled *codependency* or *burnout* in the literature. These two terms are related but different. In codependency, a person controls a situation through the assurance that he or she is needed and works to keep things that way, whereas in burnout there is difficulty determining who owns a problem. The result is anger stemming from the moral imperative to make a difference, yet the inability to succeed. The natural impulse of nurses to feel for their patients and occasionally bring home their frustrations is played out with exaggeration and eventually rejected. With time, where once they felt too much, they now feel too little in defense of their ego. The result is poor judgment, insensitivity, and intolerance (Joel, 1994). This is the end result of burnout. The codependent personality is at particularly high risk for burnout, which eventually results in negativism and the severe loss of self-esteem as one's clinical competence is questioned.

Responding to Role Strain

Kramer (1974), in an extensive longitudinal study that is still relevant after 40 years, identified the problems of new graduates in establishing their roles in the midst of bureaucratic-professional conflict and termed it *reality shock*. Kramer speaks of "the specific shock-like reactions of new workers when they find themselves in a work situation for which they have spent several years preparing and for which they thought they were going to be prepared, and then suddenly find that they are not" (p. vi). When the new nurse, who has been *in* the work setting but not *of* it, embarks on a first professional work experience, there is not an easy adaptation of previously learned values, attitudes, and behaviors, but the necessity of an entirely new socialization to practice and simultaneous resolution of conflict with the bureaucracy. This process of resocialization from student to graduate can be easily applied to the APN. Kramer (1974) describes the steps as follows:

Skills and routine mastery: The expectations are those of the employment setting. A major value is competent, efficient delivery of procedures and techniques to clients. New graduates immediately concentrate on skill and routine mastery.

Social integration: [Social integration is] getting along with the group; being taught by them how to work and behave; the "backstage" reality behaviors. If individuals stay at stage one, they may not be perceived as competent peers; if they try to incorporate some of the professional concepts brought over from the educational setting and adhere to those values, the group may be alienated.

Moral outrage: With the incongruence identified and labeled, new graduates feel angry and betrayed by both their teachers and employers. They weren't told how it would be and they aren't allowed to practice as they were taught.

Conflict resolution: The graduates may and do change their behavior, but maintain their values, or change both values and behaviors to match the work setting; or change neither values nor behavior; or work out a relationship that allows them to keep their values, but begin to integrate them into the new setting (pp. 155–162).

The individuals who make the first choice have selected what is called *behavioral capitulation*. They may be the group with potential for making change, but they simply slide into the bureaucratic mold, or more likely, they withdraw from nursing practice altogether. Those who choose bureaucracy (*value capitulation*) may either become "rutters" (staying in a rut), with an "it's a job" attitude, or they may eventually reject the values of both themselves and the system. Others become organization men and women, who move rapidly into the administrative ranks and totally absorb the bureaucratic values. Those who will change neither values nor behavior, what might be called "going it alone," either seek to practice where professional values are accepted or try the "academic lateral arabesque" (also used by the first group), going on to advanced education with the hope of new horizons or escape. The most desirable choice, says Kramer (1974, p. 162), is biculturalism:

In this approach the nurse has learned that she possesses a value orientation that is perhaps different from the dominant one in the work organization, but that she has the responsibility to listen to and seek out the ideas of others as resource material in effecting a viable integration of both value systems. She has learned that she is not just a target of influence and pressure from others, but that she is in a reciprocal relationship with others and has the right and responsibility to attempt to influence them and to direct their influence attempts . . . she has learned a basic posture of interdependence with respect to the conflicting value systems.

Even though complicated by the bureaucratic-professional conflict, our original paradigm for socialization is visible in biculturalism.

New graduates do indeed go through variations of this experience, including role-taking, role-making, and bargaining. That there was little change in the adjustment process for decades can be seen by reviewing journals in the interim and by the nomadic workplace patterns of nurses, which must reflect deep-seated job dissatisfaction. Turnover may be a response to boredom, lack of involvement, and apathy, and may trace its origin to incomplete or ineffective socialization, or more correctly, ignorance of the socialization process. Hardy and Hardy (1988a) propose that strain may be handled by redefining the role or its expectations, by bargaining among role partners to reestablish priorities, or by decreasing or increasing the degree of interaction.

Managing Role Strain

There is no one prescription for coming to terms with an unmanageable personal or professional life. The problems are relative to the personality of the afflicted, and solutions must be individualized. The ultimate goal is to establish control and identity that is driven by internal strength, rather than being captive to the volatility of the environment. Given that your best investment is in self-care, consider the following (Joel, 2011, p. 584):

Learn to use distance therapeutically. Allow people to fail and learn from their own mistakes.

Find a comfortable and private place to which you can retreat when you are stressed. If you cannot physically distance yourself, try meditation techniques.

Decide who owns a problem. If you don't own it, you have no obligation to fix it, especially if it requires self-sacrifice.

Examine the quality of the peer support you give and get, and correct the situation if needed. Sometimes support systems become habits as opposed to helps.

Invest in upgrading yourself. Expose yourself to new experiences; learn new skills. Plan your self-care as seriously as you plan your patient care.

Consciously schedule routine tasks and those requiring physical exertion as a break from complex and stressful activities.

Learn to trust your instincts. Every problem does not have a rational and logical solution.

Sometimes think in terms of what could be the worst consequence, then anything short of that is a bonus.

Identify one person willing to serve as your objective sounding board. This may be one way to find out how you come across to people.

Make contact with your feelings about situations. Feelings are neither good nor bad; they just are.

Create options for yourself. Identify those circumstances that you need to personally control, those that are just as well controlled for you, and those that you choose to wait out.

CONCLUSION

Socialization into role is a major responsibility of the nursing profession, whether at the point of immersion into the student role and anticipatory socialization to the profession or later with transition to registered nurse and for some on to advanced practice. Socialization requires personalizing a role to your preferences while complying with norms established by the government, the profession, the public, and the employing institution. These are your normative, comparative, and audience groups, your major referents; there may be others. The norms held by these groups may be broadly or narrowly interpreted and are revealed through the process of role-taking or empathic communication. There is an opportunity to modify these expectations once you are sensitive to the degree of flexibility allowed by each referent system. This process involves skill in reading our role partners and the environment and reciprocally working to make the role to our liking. This skill can be learned.

Stress and strain are natural companions to nurses, given the environment in which we work and the work we do. Role stress is located in the social structure, and role strain in the person. Not all stressful circumstances produce strain; this depends on the individual and his or her ability to cope, problem solve, and search for meaning in difficult situations. Success in dealing with stress and strain may be related to complete and effective socialization. This observation reinforces the obligation to both provide socialization experiences and to equip nurses with the resources for self-care.

4

Educational Preparation of Advanced Practice Nurses

Looking to the Future

Phyllis Shanley Hansell

Learning Outcomes

Learning outcomes expected as a result of this chapter:

- Understand the historical background of education for advanced practice.
- Describe external factors that drive demand and influence education for advanced practice.
- Distinguish the advanced practice nurse (APN) role and educational requirements for the nurse practitioner (NP), nurse-anesthetist (NA), clinical nurse-midwife (CNM), and clinical nurse specialist.
- Determine the factors that initiated interest in the doctorate of nursing practice (DNP).
- Identify distinctions in scholarship between the DNP and the PhD.
- Explain the process of transition from MSN to DNP for the APN.
- Compare the doctoral dissertation to the DNP project.
- Propose potential synergy between the DNP and PhD.
- Demonstrate a faculty role for the DNP graduate.
- Anticipate the future for the DNP and PhD.

BACKGROUND

The education of advanced practice nurses (APNs) has increased in complexity as curricula have evolved in response to societal needs. These curricular changes are primarily in response to health-care reform and the transformation of health-care delivery brought about by the Patient Protection and Affordable Care Act (PPACA) (Public Law 111-148). Henry Silver and Loretta Ford created the first certificate program for nurse practitioners (NPs) at the University of Colorado in 1965; since that time, the NP role and educational preparation for the role has been met with some degree of controversy from both inside and outside of the nursing profession. This dissonance has extended beyond NP education and also includes nurse-midwives, nurse anesthetists, and clinical nurse specialists.

The PPACA (2010) has resulted in improved access to health care, particularly for underserved populations in rural and inner city areas, and subsequently increased demand for primary health care. Many of the provisions included in the PPACA acknowledge the important contributions that nurses, especially APNs, have to offer. The PPACA has therefore provided funded support that includes (a) the establishment of nurse managed health centers, (b) funding for school-based health centers, (c) funding to support collaboration between nursing schools and health-care facilities, (d) loan forgiveness for individuals willing to practice in a pediatric subspecialty (including mental health) in an underserved area, (e) funding to support Independence at Home Demonstration for chronically ill Medicare beneficiaries that uses both NPs and physicians and is aimed at reducing expenditures and improving health outcomes, and (f) an increase in the reimbursement rate for certified nurse-midwives (CNMs) for covered services from 65% to 100%.

These PPACA-funded initiatives will serve to support and further deploy the professional expertise of APNs, enabling them to make a difference in the delivery of health care, especially to those who are underserved. A recent study by the Rand Corporation (Auerbach, Martsolf, Pearson et al, sponsored by Rand Corporation, 2015), commissioned by the AACN Board of Directors, found that there is now universal agreement within the nursing community on the value of doctor of nursing practice (DNP) education that is preparing nurses to meet the future health-care needs (Auerbach, 2014). Because of this study the AACN Board

of Directors convened a task force to review the state of DNP programs in order to better clarify both curricular and practice expectations as outlined in the *Essentials of Doctoral Education for Advanced Nursing Practice* (AACN, 2006) and to highlight practice scholarship and academic partnership opportunities.

The 21st century has been a significant time for nursing, first with recognition by the Carnegie Foundation that nursing has met the criteria for professional status, and second, that APNs are being recognized for their important contributions to health care. A major factor in this newfound recognition has much to do with the exponential growth of nursing science and translational nursing research that has enlarged the foundation of scientific evidence supporting nursing practice (AACN, 2010b).

One of the lingering controversies for APNs has to do with the preferred academic credential for entry into advanced practice. At the semiannual meeting of the American Association of Colleges of Nursing in 2004 (AACN, 2004), the member deans present voted to endorse and support the DNP degree as the entry-level educational credential for APNs, effective as of 2015. The discussion that ensued in response to the resolution was very heated. When the members' secret ballot votes were tallied, the results were 162 in affirmative, 101 in opposition, and 13 in abstention. Voices in opposition came from two divergent factions of the assembly: deans that viewed the DNP as beyond the resources of their institutions, and deans of schools with highly developed and well-funded PhD programs. I voted in the affirmative, as I believed that the APN curriculum fell short in both depth and breadth, had become increasingly narrow, and needed to be broadened. In addition, for APNs to achieve parity with other major health professionals, a terminal clinical practice degree would both reinforce the status of nursing as a major autonomous health-care provider and enable the achievement of better patient care outcomes. Other major considerations were the proposed requirement of 1,000 supervised hours of clinical practice along with the focus on clinical scholarship and analytical methods for evidence-based practice.

The movement to advance doctoral education for nurses in the United States is strong and has gained significant momentum. According to AACN (2016) data, there are currently 403 doctoral level nursing programs in the United States: 134 PhD programs and 269 DNP programs. Interestingly, most schools that offer the PhD nursing degree also offer the DNP. There are few exceptions to this pattern with only 16 schools offering only the research doctorate. At this time, there are DNP programs in 49 states with online access delivering DNP education to all 50 states.

According to the AACN's 2015 *Annual Report: Leading Excellence and Innovation in Academic Nursing* (2016), 113,788 students are currently enrolled in master's programs (including master's entry students), 5,290 students are enrolled in research focused doctoral programs, and 18,352 students are enrolled in practice focused doctoral programs. Although the master of science in nursing (MSN) continues to be the predominant route to certification for APNs, the trend is moving in the direction of the bachelor of science of nursing (BSN) to DNP with MSN advanced practice programs coexisting in 75% of schools that offer the DNP. BSN to DNP programs currently comprise more than half of existing DNP programs (with an additional 60 BSN to DNP programs reported to be in the planning stage). Although the postbaccalaureate DNP is taking hold, most nurses often seek the more expeditious option, which is the MSN. At this time, the MSN still meets the requirement for APN certification.

When one takes a retrospective look at the credentialing of NPs, it is noteworthy that in 1965, the certificate became the first advanced educational postbaccalaureate credential for the first generation of pediatric NPs (the first NP role). Two years later in 1967, Boston College introduced the first MSN with an NP track. Similar to the certificate program at the University of Colorado, the program at Boston College (Historical Timeline AANP. org) included efforts that were collaboratively led by nursing and medicine. As the educational requirements for NPs uniformly advanced to the master's level, there were many concerns arising over grandfathering NPs with certificates when MSN degree preparation became the standard requirement for certification (Ford, 1975). Although there once was a defined period of grandfathering for certificate NP graduates, there is currently no grandfathering clause remaining in any state that would allow any APN (nurse-midwife, nurse anesthetist, clinical nurse specialist [CNS], or NP) to enter into practice without an advanced degree. It is important to note that because advanced practice nursing is regulated by state statute, older nurses with an advanced practice certificate have been able to continue to practice so long as the state and their specialty-certifying bodies recognize their status. In the United States there are 50 different state nurse practice acts (NPAs) under which the advanced practice roles are regulated. For this reason, in 2008 the State Boards of Nursing (NCSBN) introduced the *Consensus Model for APRN Regulation: Licensure, Accreditation, Certification and Education,* designed to provide some common structural guidance for the preparation and practice of APNs.

APNs are prepared through a variety of educational programs with oversight carried out by specialty certification boards; hence, there are different requirements for different advanced practice roles. The American Midwifery Certification Board (AMCB) and the American College of Nurse-Midwives (ACNM) have eliminated recognition of all postbaccalaureate certificate programs, and in July of 2009 required a graduate degree for entry into practice, which went into effect in 2010 (ACNM, 2009). Moreover, in 2009 the ACNM also moved to require recertification for CNMs who were certified before 1996 to ensure the highest quality of nurse-midwifery care. In 1990, the Council on Accreditation of Nurse Anesthesia Educational Programs (2003, 2004) moved to require the master's degree requirement for entry into nurse anesthesia practice. It is important to note that the master's degree is not mandated to be in nursing, as many nurse anesthesia programs do not reside in schools of nursing. The Council included a grandfather clause that allowed current certified registered nurse anesthetists (CRNAs) to continue to practice without obtaining a master's degree (Kinslow, 2005). In September 2007 the American Association of Nurse Anesthetists (AANA) announced support for doctoral level entry into nurse anesthesia practice by 2025 (AANA, 2007). The DNP degree was not specifically endorsed, allowing for other types of doctoral education to meet these criteria. In states where the status of CNS is recognized, the master's degree in nursing is required as the educational requirement for practice. In June 2015 the National Association of Clinical Nurse Specialists (NACNS, 2016) endorsed the DNP degree as the entry requirement for CNSs by 2030.

The typical MSN curriculum for APNs has become highly focused on the specialty area of practice, leaving minimal opportunity for students to select elective areas of study. When one peruses the eight *Essentials of Doctoral Education for Advanced Practice Nursing* (AACN, 2006), the DNP offers much to round out the knowledge, skills, and expertise of the graduate with the inclusion of (a) interprofessional collaboration, (b) health policy advocacy, (c) clinical scholarship and analytical methods for evidence-based practice, and (d) organizational and systems leadership and the scientific underpinnings of practice. The AACN *Essentials* (2006) clearly augments the 2015 MSN curriculum in needed ways by equipping the APN of the future to create and advance patient care as never before envisioned.

The American Association of Nurse Practitioners (AANP) has been proactive, and although a master's degree is required for certification of NPs, the board of directors of the National Organization of Nurse Practitioner Faculties (NONPF) reaffirmed its allegiance (NONPF, September 2015) to advancing the DNP degree as the entry-level academic preparation for NPs. Their statement on the matter is as follows "Now—2015—is our time to make a commitment collectively on behalf of our students, the profession and our patients to making NP education doctoral-level preparation." The sooner the educational standards for NPs advance to the DNP, the better it will be for APNs and their patients.

It is clear that the coursework required in NP MSN programs is rigorous and comparable with the coursework required of typical clinical doctoral programs such as those involving pharmacy and physical therapy. However, it is tantamount that the transition to the practice doctorate preparation continue to be conducted so that NPs collectively advance together in unity.

THE DOCTOR OF NURSING PRACTICE

According to the AANP there are more than 359,194 NPs licensed in the United States (AANP, 2016). The other APN roles comprise a relatively small proportion of APNs as follows: 77,000 CNSs, 49,000 nurse anesthetists, and 11,194 CNMs, among which 82% are prepared with the minimum of a master's degree (American Nurses Association [ANA], 2011).

The goal to migrate all these APNs to the doctorate (excluding those who already have the degree) is a highly ambitious undertaking. Some question whether this is a realistic goal when, in reality, the movement to require the entry-level doctorate for advanced nursing practice will be a complex process. Although the AACN has a role in contributing to the development of standards, it lacks the legal authority to enforce this on the various

state nursing regulatory bodies and with the respective advanced practice specialty organizations. Furthermore, the two chief accrediting bodies in nursing, the Commission on Collegiate Nursing Education (CCNE) and the Commission for Nursing Education Accreditation (CNEA, formerly The National League for Nursing Accreditation Commission [NLNAC]), have elected to accredit DNP programs. The CCNE has elected to accredit only practice doctorate programs with the initials "DNP," whereas the CNEA believes as advanced practice doctorates move in this new direction, they will accredit whatever title suits the program, believing that nursing is best served by focusing on competencies, learning outcomes, and curriculum (CNEA, 2016) (NLN-CNEA, 2016).

In the past, APNs who pursued doctoral education were limited to research-focused doctorates such as the PhD, DNSc, DNS, DSN, and EdD, as well as doctorates in other disciplines. By 2008 most of the various nursing doctoral degrees had converted to the PhD (Dreher, Fasolka, & Clark, 2008), leaving the PhD in Nursing as the professional standard for research doctoral degrees in the field. APNs enter a new conundrum with the emergence of the practice doctorate, which is best suited to those who are dedicated practitioners. Those who instead opt for the PhD degree have the advancement of nursing science as their goal. Prospectively, as one looks to the future when the DNP becomes the standard for entry into advanced practice, the PhD will eventually become the step beyond the practice doctorate, similar to what exists in medicine where the MD/PhD is the degree of choice for those with a research focus.

Transition From the MSN to the DNP

When experienced APNs continue their education at the DNP level, what is the gain? I interviewed four recent DNP students/graduates to find out what they gained from the DNP program and how it changed them. Here are the responses that I received:

1. "The Doctor of Nursing Practice offers the highest level of quality and safety to the patients in their care, the nurses on their team and the system within which they practice. Let us welcome this new recognition of Nursing Practice excellence! Changed attitudes = changed outcomes!"

2. "The DNP has provided the essential knowledge necessary to translate evidence into practice in order to improve health quality, cost efficiency and sustainability of effective processes."
3. "Coming from such a strong clinical background, the DNP program has helped me integrate my collaborative clinical practice and research with current trends in the evolution of health care issues."
4. "The DNP enabled me to recognize health delivery system problems and conduct evidence-based scholarly projects toward rectifying those issues."

Based on these quotes, it is evident that even for the most experienced APNs there is much to be gained from the DNP curriculum that will shape the APN's practice and ultimately benefit the patient.

The Tipping Point for the DNP

The DNP is still a relatively new degree; it was first offered by the College of Nursing at the University of Kentucky in 2001, with nine students initially graduating with the degree in 2005. (In contrast, the first EdD in Nursing Education was first offered in 1932 at Teachers College, Columbia University, and the first PhD in 1934 at New York University.) The genesis of today's DNP practitioner-focused model can be traced to Mary Mundinger of Columbia University's School of Nursing. In 2000, Mundinger and her colleagues published a clinical trial in the *Journal of the American Medical Association* titled "Primary Care Outcomes in Patients Treated by Nurse Practitioners or Physicians: A Randomized Trial." This innovative project at Columbia University on the NP model ultimately led to development of the clinical doctorate or DrNP degree. Columbia's DrNP was finally approved in 2005. Nevertheless, even the Columbia DrNP model went through an evolution during which the faculty first described the degree as a "DrNP in Primary Care," later simply the "first clinical doctorate" (instead of a "practice doctorate" as it is commonly called). In 2008, the degree was changed to the DNP to comply with CCNE standards.

Before the presentation of the proposal for the DNP degree, the AACN sponsored speakers from the American Association of Colleges of Pharmacy at their semiannual meeting. They presented their 10-year transition from the bachelor of pharmacy to doctor of pharmacy degree, the first professional degree that is a nonresearch doctorate. An AACN task force was subsequently constituted in 2002 to explore the DNP. The report of this task force provided the impetus for the 2004 vote by the AACN membership, which then was followed by the development and approval of the *Essentials for the Practice Doctorate in Nursing* published in 2006. Other degrees considered analogous to the DNP by AACN include doctorates in medicine (MD), dentistry (DDS and DMD), pharmacy (PharmD), psychology (PsyD), physical therapy (DPT), and audiology (AudD) (AACN, 2011b).

Rationale for the DNP Degree

Despite the plethora of DNP programs, the numbers of MSN students far outnumber those enrolled in BSN/DNP programs. There are convincing reasons in support of an entry-level doctorate for nursing. These include reform in health profession education mainly because of rising health-care errors, patient safety issues, and the changing roles of providers; failure of the health disciplines to work collaboratively and deliver optimal health outcomes; and the rising cost of health-care services. The central arguments for why the AACN advocated that entry into advanced practice nursing should require the doctorate instead of the master's degree are as follows: (a) master's in nursing degrees, especially those preparing the NP, nurse anesthetist, or CNM, often required as many credit hours as some clinical doctorate programs in other disciplines; (b) other disciplines such as physical therapy (DPT) and pharmacy (PharmD) had begun offering a clinical doctorate; and (c) contemporary knowledge is growing exponentially and the master's degree can no longer fully encompass the breadth of coursework necessary for advanced practice (Apold, 2008).

As compelling as these arguments are, they are not all data based. Although the statement about the total number of credits could be considered a salient one, the attainment of credits alone is not sufficient to merit the attainment of a doctoral degree. One could argue that the decades of strong outcome data supporting the excellence of the APN, particularly in comparison to primary medical care (Horrocks, Anderson, & Salisbury, 2002; Mundinger et al, 2000), is reason enough to maintain the status quo. Such reasoning is not without flaws, however, as it totally ignores the changes that have evolved through health-care reform, the growing aging population, and the implementation of the PPACA. In our changed, complex world of health care, ANPs must stay on top of their patients' needs; more education about health systems, evidence-based practice, and health systems is in order.

The DNP degree has gained wide acceptance by the academic nursing community, and it is highly probable that candidates with a practice doctorate will have an advantage in a highly competitive changing job market. The nursing community is challenged to substantiate that the added cost, time, and resources needed to educate the DNP graduate will improve health care, as well as the status and expertise of the practitioner.

The "tipping point" has been reached and the DNP is well along on its way to acceptance especially within the clinical practice arena. Within academia, the DNP credential is accepted and well suited for clinical track appointments. However, most major universities do not accept the DNP for tenure track positions and require a research doctorate for those appointments.

The DNP has existed for slightly more than a decade with some of the early programs developed before the AACN's *Essentials of Doctoral Education for Advanced Practice Nurses* (2006). This has resulted in some degree of irregularity from program to program, particularly concerning the final capstone project. Fink (2006) indicates that the professional (or practice) doctorate "should not be a watered down version of the PhD, but offer a valid alternative in doctoral education" (p. 38). The AACN *Essentials* (2006) state scholarship and research represent the hallmark of doctoral level education. Although original research is paramount in the advancement of science, a much broader view has emerged that enlarges that perspective through alternative paradigms (Boyer, 1990). This perspective acknowledges the following: (a) The scholarship of integration and discovery more specifically "reflects the investigative and synthesizing traditions of academic life" (Boyer, p. 21); (b) Scholars give meaning to isolated facts and make connections across disciplines through the scholarship of integration; and (c) The scholar applies knowledge to solve problems via the scholarship of application (in nursing this is practice).

Essential III of the *Essentials of Doctoral Education for Advanced Nursing Practice* (AACN, 2006) specifies that Clinical Scholarship and Analytical Methods for Evidence-Based Practice is an important component of the DNP curriculum. In contrast to the PhD curriculum, the DNP graduate engages as an APN, thus providing the leadership for evidence-based practice, whereas the PhD graduate acquires the research skills needed for discovering new knowledge in the discipline. The DNP graduate requires competence in knowledge application activities including translation of research into practice, practice evaluation of the improvement of the reliability of health-care practices and outcomes, and participation in collaborative research (De Palma & McGuire, 2005). The graduates of research and practice doctorates are both critical to the advancement of the profession and are optimally complementary to each other in the advancement of nursing science. The DNP is not intended to be a watered down version of the PhD or, as some may say, a "PhD light"; rather, it is a rigorous professional practice terminal degree. If nursing science is to advance practice, graduates of both degrees are needed to achieve this important goal.

FORK IN THE ROAD: THE DNP OR THE PHD

The Dissertation Versus the DNP Project

The hallmark of doctoral education is scholarship, and the research doctorate in nursing is designed to prepare the graduate with the research skills needed to discover new knowledge to advance the discipline. In contrast, the DNP prepares graduates to be experts in the practice of nursing and to lead in the formulation and appropriate application of evidence-based practice. De Palma and McGuire (2005) state that in order to provide leadership in translational research, the graduate needs to be competent in the translation of research in practice, the evaluation of practice, the improvement of the reliability of health-care practice and outcomes, and participation in collaborative research. Accordingly, the DNP curriculum needs to focus on the translation of new nursing science and its application and evaluation.

For the research doctorate in nursing, the doctoral dissertation is the culminating requirement through which the PhD student is required to create new research. The steps associated with the dissertation process across programs in the United States is relatively standard. The typical steps of the dissertation process include proposal development and approval, data collection, data analysis, synthesis of findings, completion of a five to six chapter dissertation, and oral defense of the dissertation. All this occurs under the guidance and supervision of a dissertation chairperson and committee.

The rapid growth of DNP programs has resulted in significant variability in the final project or capstone requirement. Some DNP programs have required students to complete a dissertation-type project that includes a committee and oral defense; others have focused on the generation of original practice research, whereas still others require a systematic review of the literature on a clinical topic with no actual involvement in the clinical practice setting. In contrast to the dissertation process, there is typically a mentor without a committee structure and the final presentation of the capstone project is less of an oral defense than a presentation of results of the project to faculty and students.

Consistent with the AACN *Essentials of Doctoral Education for Advanced Nursing Practice* (2006), Waldrop, Caruso, Fuchs, and Hypes (2014) have defined five criteria for executing a successful DNP final project. In order for the DNP project to be consistent with the standards articulated by the AACN (2006) and NONPF (2007), they have stated that the project should address a complex practice, process, or systems problem in the particular setting. Evidence should then be used to improve practice, process, or outcomes; this makes it clear that the DNP graduate must actually have completed a project in the practice setting and must evaluate what was implemented to determine the outcomes (p. 302). This is in accordance with Waldrop et al (2014), who represent the criteria with the acronym "EC as PIE" where E = Enhance, C = Culmination, P = Partnerships, I = Implements, and E = Evaluates.

In 2015 the AACN convened a task force on the current state of implementation of the DNP to clarify curricular and practice expectations as outlined in the DNP *Essentials* (AACN, 2006). An important outcome of the task force was the articulation of the distinction between research and practice-focused doctorates. According to their statement, "Graduates of both research and practice based doctorates are prepared to generate new knowledge. However, research focused graduates are prepared to generate knowledge through rigorous research and statistical methodologies that may be broadly applicable or generalizable; whereas, practice focused graduates are prepared to generate new

knowledge through innovation of practice change, the translation of evidence, and the implementation of quality improvement processes in specific practice settings, systems, or with specific populations to improve health or health outcomes" (AACN, 2015).

The AACN task force (2015) has clarified the scope of the final scholarly project regarding the DNP. The title of the project should be the DNP project to avoid confusion with the dissertation. Because the DNP project is not a research dissertation the term *dissertation* should not be used. The scholarly DNP project may take on various forms as stipulated by an institution's requirement along with the students' area of advanced practice, but should remain standard for all students and include planning, implementation, and evaluation components. Contrary to the DNP *Essentials* (AACN, 2006), the task force "believes that an integrative and systematic review alone is not considered a DNP project, and does not provide opportunities for students to develop and integrate scholarship into practice" (AACN, 2015b, p. 4). Additional recommendations from the task force include (a) there is no committee, but rather a project team; (b) the dissemination of the project should describe its purpose, planning, implementation, and evaluation components; and (c) evaluation of the final project is the responsibility of the faculty and should include academic, peer, and stakeholder review. As a programmatic outcome of the DNP curriculum, all students must have the opportunity to integrate all eight of the DNP *Essentials* (AACN, 2006, 2015a). They do not have to be demonstrated in the DNP project, but rather through the completion of the curriculum. As DNP programs mature into a unique identity of their own and become more standardized and consistent with the DNP *Essentials* (AACN, 2006) and DNP task force recommendations (AACN, 2015a) there will be increased congruence across DNP programs.

The Potential for Synergy Between the PhD and DNP

In an article in *Nursing Outlook* entitled "Strategic Innovation Between PhD and DNP Programs: Collaboration, Collegiality and Shared Resources" (Edwards, Rayman, Diffenderfer, & Stidham, 2016), the authors share the results of a collaborative DNP and PhD project within the context of the East Tennessee State University's Academic

TABLE 4.1

Complementary Residency Experiences in the DNP and PhD Programs

PhD Research Residency Activities	DNP Practice Residency Activities
Literature review in area of nursing science	Literature review of evidence in nursing
Pilot research projects for dissertation	Participation in quality improvement
Participation in full scope of research	Development in capstone with mentors
Presentation at research conferences	Presentation at practice conferences
IPE (interprofessional education) collaborative experiences	IPE collaborative experiences
Submission of research grant proposals	Submission of practice or leadership grant proposals
Participation to influence health policy	Participation to influence health policy

Health Science Center along with medicine, pharmacy, clinical, and rehabilitative health sciences and public health, who each have a longstanding commitment to interprofessional education (p. 313). Their project provides an excellent example of the catalytic synergy that can take place when the strengths of DNP and PhD education are brought together. **Table 4.1** contains examples of complementary residency experiences in the DNP and PhD programs (p. 317).

As these common and complementary areas illustrate, there is much to be gained from the strategic collaboration between PhD and DNP students. Within the right context, this collaboration will continue to develop beyond graduation to advance nursing science and evidence-based practice in innovative ways. Combining PhD and DNP resources will translate and deliver best practices to the patient as never before envisioned. Partnerships between DNP and PhD students selected for the natural synergy of their dissertations and DNP projects would greatly speed the educational process, generate publications, and produce other outcomes that are both useful and fundable.

As to whether the DNP or PhD degree is the best option or fit for an individual APN, it is more about an individual's professional goals. The APN who is focused and immersed in clinical practice is probably best advised to seek the DNP degree, whereas the APN who is passionate about research and testing innovative interventions and models of care probably has goals that are more in alignment with the PhD. There is also the option of completing both the PhD and DNP, either as a dual degree or separately as one's focus evolves and different methodologies are needed. Each can be completed as a separate complementary degree that further builds on the practice or research foundation of the other degree. The important conclusion is that APNs have choices in the selection of a terminal degree that best fits with their goals as they advance their careers. In the long view, there will probably come a time when all APNs complete the DNP, which then will form the foundation for all PhD students in nursing. Joint DNP/PhD degree programs analogous to the MD/PhD now exist at Barnes/Jewish College of Nursing in St. Louis, University of Tennessee Health Sciences Center, and Case Western Reserve University in Cleveland. Looking forward, the PhD as a sequel to the DNP may in fact become a reality for the profession in the long view.

Moving forward, there are important strategic implications for the nursing profession with the rise of the DNP. PhD programs optimally will attract those who are serious about their interest and passion for research, which will ultimately have the outcome of a more highly engaged scientific cadre of nursing scholars. Clearly complementary scholarship that includes PhD and DNP students on the same team will serve to advance nursing science and practice to the next level.

The PhD in Nursing: The Future Is Bright

AACN data from 2004–2014 (AACN, 2016, p. 7) reveal that there has been an increase in research doctoral program enrollment from 3,715 in 2005 to 5,290 in 2014 with steady incremental increases in enrollment each year. In contrast, DNP enrollment has increased from 269 students in 2005 to 18,352 in 2014. These strong numbers bode well for the nursing profession with a clear focus on the future of health care and how we can achieve the greatest difference. These numbers also clearly indicate that the DNP is not diverting applicants from PhD programs, which are continuing to grow in enrollment to almost nearly double what they were in 2005 before the DNP took hold.

The DNP and the Faculty Role

In 2006, the AACN stated that DNP graduates are not prepared for the full scope of the faculty role without additional education and supervision (McKenna, 2005; Wittmann-Price, Waite, & Woda, 2011). Lack of preparation for the faculty role is a problem that is also evident for recent PhD graduates, especially if they have had little or no previous teaching experience. The exception involves recent graduates of PhD programs in Nursing Education such as those at Villanova University and the EdD program at Teachers College, Columbia University. For new graduates of DNP and PhD programs alike, deans need to provide support systems that include senior faculty mentors with the understanding that the new DNP or PhD graduates are novices in need of support to succeed in all the dimensions of the demands of the faculty role.

Although there has been an increase in the number of new PhD in Nursing programs during the past decade, there has been limited support to properly socialize and mentor doctoral students in the nurse scientist role, leaving many unprepared for the rigors of conducting postdissertation research (Dreher & Smith Glasgow, 2011; Potempa, Redman, & Anderson, 2008). This is a criticism widely proffered by the University of Washington's project on *Re-envisioning the PhD* (Nyquist & Wulff, 2000). Similar commentary is found in "How Business Schools Lost Their Way" from the *Harvard Business Review* (Bennis & O'Toole, 2005). The parallels between business education and nursing are striking. For almost a decade, professional business schools have come under intense criticism for failing to impart useful skills and instill norms for ethical business behavior. Similar to business, in academia nursing finds itself trying to replicate the academic and scientific traditions of fields such as chemistry and history. This is especially common when PhD faculty have left clinical nursing practice perhaps even decades earlier. The mission to educate the doctoral-prepared practitioner or scholar seems to have been lost to create the proper nurse scientist.

Nursing science that contributes critical, high-impact translational health research can distinguish the profession of nursing, raise credibility, better position the discipline within the community of science, and move the science from "bench to bedside." At present, nursing research lacks wide recognition and receives limited grant-funded support. In 2015 the National Institute for Nursing Research received $145,912,000 in funding; although at first glance this number appears to be a robust allocation, it represents the lowest level of funding of any institute within the National Institutes of Health (NIH). In 2015 the NIH received a total budget of $4,300,145,614; that leaves nursing with less than 1% of the NIH budget. In 2014 575 applications were received by the National Institute for Nursing Research but only 46 were awarded funding. In 2014 nursing achieved an overall success rate of 8%, which is the lowest of any institute or center within the NIH (NIH Research Portfolio Online Reporting Tools, 2015). Nurse researchers conduct studies that are key to the management of chronic disease, health promotion, and end of life care. In order to increase the funding allocation for the NINR, nursing research needs to be better understood by the public with translational research projects conducted in tandem to demonstrate the importance of our work. I believe that in concert the DNP and PhD graduate can make this happen.

Given the move by the government to fund more interdisciplinary translational research, the need for well-trained nurse scientists is more apparent than ever (National Academy of Sciences, 2005). Nurse scientists and researchers should not confine their research efforts to those funded solely by the NIH and other government agencies; rather, they should also seek private sector foundation funding. The bar is very high, however; with the growing enrollment in PhD programs and the extremely robust enrollment in DNP programs, a critical mass of expertise is being created that will have a measurable impact on the advancement of nursing science.

Settling the Dust Between the DNP and the PhD

New doctoral programs in any discipline are not created without in-depth analysis. Additional resources or the reallocation of resources from other academic programs often will be needed. At this time, the majority of universities that offer the PhD in Nursing also offer the DNP. Over the past decade, substantial enrollment increases have occurred in both DNP and PhD programs.

With the advent of the DNP, it is risky for the profession to rely solely on nursing PhD graduates to advance the science. There is much to be accomplished through the collaborative efforts between the DNP and PhD graduates who will work together to advance translational research projects, bringing the best evidence-based practice to patient care. O'Sullivan and colleagues (2005) rightly raise the argument that because many PhD graduates never conduct research past their dissertation, these students might have been better served by a practice doctorate option. The DNP option now enables those who are clinically immersed in their passion for practice to improve practice through evidence-based projects.

The Advanced Practice Nurse With an MSN, DNP, or PhD

Luther Christman, a leader and visionary in nursing (1915–2011), proposed through the Rush Unification Model for nursing that all nurses have advanced education to practice. His Unification Model incorporated interprofessional teams composed of physicians, nurses, and other health professionals practicing together for the benefit of patients. Christman (Pittman, 2005) was the dean and vice president of nursing at Rush-Presbyterian University Medical Center in Chicago. Education, practice, and research were evident on every nursing unit (Pittman, 2005). Christman believed that nursing was poised to achieve parity with medicine and other health professionals if all possessed terminal degree credentials. Although health-care delivery has changed dramatically since Christman articulated his vision of a Unification Model, certain elements remain constant. It is now well understood that no one profession can provide holistic comprehensive interprofessional care where health professionals work collaboratively to ensure the best patient outcomes.

Health-care reform within the context of the PPACA (2017) has enabled many previously uninsured individuals to gain access to health care, increasing the demand for primary and tertiary care services that will ultimately increase the demand for NPs and primary care physicians. This creates a strategic opportunity for APNs to step up to the needs of society and practice to the full extent of their educational preparation. Attainment of the DNP as the new standard will serve to bring APNs to their rightful position as an equal partner on the interprofessional health-care team. In order to achieve this goal of parity with the major health professions, APNs need to unify and strategize to advance to the next level. APNs have the potential to be leaders in the delivery of primary care because physicians are more typically attracted to specialty practice. Using the DNP as entry for advanced practice is a reasonable expectation and goal, which will support excellence in patient care with vastly improved clinical outcomes.

SUMMARY: A NEW VISION FOR THE FUTURE OF THE EDUCATION OF APNS

As APNs, specialty organizations, and other stakeholders consider the implications of the AACN 2015 goal, some suggestions for the future of nursing education for advanced practice are offered. Although the 2015 goal for transition to the DNP for entry into advanced practice has passed, there is mounting dynamic movement within the profession to move to the next level. With more than 18,000 currently enrolled DNP students, change is occurring within the profession at a fast pace never before experienced. With NONPF endorsing the movement to the DNP for NPs, we are at the crossroads, beginning transformation in the education of APNs.

In order to achieve parity with other major health professionals, the education of APNs must equip them with competencies that hold some level of "extra value" *in addition to* the MD and the other major health professions. Quite evident is the clinical research skill of the DNP graduate, which focuses on translational evidence-based projects along with those that focus on patient safety issues that will clearly place the DNP-prepared APN in key leadership positions. Beyond that, the DNP-educated nurse possesses skills in the understanding and advancement of health-care system issues, which with the PPACA are on the forefront and cutting edge of health-care problems to be solved.

In 2005, Broome identified two serious issues that nursing still faces today: an urgent need for more BSN-prepared nurses and a severe nursing faculty shortage that is only going to escalate in the decade to come. Discussion of the DNP for advanced practice students cannot be separated from a discussion about what type of academic preparation is best to teach them. Mundinger (2005) of Columbia University has described the ways in which the doctoral role of advanced practice differs from MS-level practice. She emphasized that the DNP graduate shows "a greater depth and breadth of knowledge and practice with significant additional science education provided by courses in genetics, advanced pathophysiology, pharmacology, differential diagnoses, chronic illness, bioinformatics, research methods, and identification and use of medical evidence" (p. 173). How do new DNP programs *really effect change* because of their curricula beyond the scope of the MSN? One of the challenges with the wide array of DNP programs has to do with its unevenness with regard to skills, knowledge, and competencies beyond the MSN. As more and more DNP programs become accredited by either CCNE or CNEA, these differences should become somewhat diminished with firmer standards emerging. As the number of DNP graduates increases, programmatic evaluation data will be generated to identify how these graduates are making a difference. It is likely that MSN preparation will continue for a time; however, as outcome data are generated we will be able to measure the difference that the DNP makes, which will hopefully fuel the transition to full acceptance of the DNP as the new standard of education for APNs. As we look to the future, and hold on, the best is yet to come for the nursing profession and patients alike.

5

Global Perspectives on Advanced Nursing Practice

Madrean Schober and Anna Green

Learning Outcomes

Learning outcomes expected as a result of this chapter:

- Identify the growth of advanced nursing practice (ANP) worldwide.
- Demonstrate issues influencing the development of advanced practice nursing globally.
- Illustrate the impact of the International Council of Nurses (ICN) in setting international standards.
- Compare country illustrations of growth and progress of advanced practice nursing.
- Detail controversial practice issues and challenges faced with emerging roles.
- Distinguish the diversity of international health-care systems.
- Contrast the lack of role clarity and international consensus on the meaning of ANP.

INTRODUCTION

There is growing international recognition that advanced nursing practice (ANP)* should be developed, acknowledged,

and legitimized. Factors contributing to a greater willingness to explore ANP options are multifaceted. Physician shortages, increased demand for highly specialized nurses, a greater emphasis on primary health care (PHC) and home-based services, and the increased acuity and complexity of hospitalized patients are among the issues motivating decision makers to rethink provision of health-care services (Buchan et al, 2013; Delamaire & LaFortune, 2010; DiCenso et al, 2010; Sastre-Fullana et al, 2014; Schober,

---

Advanced nursing practice (ANP) is used as a comprehensive "umbrella" term for the discipline or function of APNs. The term *advanced practice nurse (APN)* is used in reference to APN roles, APN practice, APN curriculum, APN positions, or individuals who are APNs.

2016). Professional factors for nursing are also influencing developments in this field. The acquisition of more highly developed qualifications as nursing education moves into the academic education sector is matched by a demand for clinical career ladders or pathways that acknowledge professional advancement and give nurses an incentive to remain in clinical practice (De Geest et al, 2008; ICN, 2007; Schober, 2013, 2016; Zurn, Dolea, & Stilwell, 2005).

The predicted global deficit of 12.9 million physicians, nurses, and midwives by 2035 has stimulated a renewed examination of skill mix including options for introducing new types of health-care workers; these options include task shifting, task reallocation, and the expansion of current roles of all health-care professionals (WHO, 2014). Historically, Buchan and Calman (2005) identified several drivers in health systems in countries belonging to the Organization for Economic Co-operation and Development (OECD) contributing to a heightened interest in the advanced practice nurse (APN) role. In addition to staff shortages faced by these countries, these authors suggested that health sector reform and new initiatives have stimulated serious consideration of the appropriateness of current role definitions for health-care workers and skill mix. Aspects affecting these deliberations include cost containment measures, actions to improve service quality, the introduction of technological innovations and new therapeutic interventions, and alterations in the legislative and regulatory environment. The growing body of literature continues to confirm this diversity in motivation globally when countries consider the option of advanced nursing roles (De Geest et al, 2008; Delamaire & LaFortune, 2010; Schober, 2016). See **Box 5.1** for a summary of factors contributing to ANP growth.

However, enthusiasm and motivation when redefining roles for health-care professionals is not enough to support a strong climate of advocacy for these changes (Buchan et al, 2013). Continuing clarity on who the advanced nurse is and the place of an advanced nursing role in the health-care workforce are themes that take center stage in the evolving international drama of development. The World Health Organization (WHO) in its continued efforts to maximize the capacities and potential of nurses and midwives emphasizes the need to mobilize political will to build effective workforce development (WHO, 2016). The maturing nature of the discipline calls leaders and decision makers to assess models of governance specific

---

Box 5.1

Factors Contributing to International Growth in Advanced Nursing Practice

Escalating disease burden worldwide: communicable and noncommunicable diseases

Increased inpatient acuity and complexity of treatment

Impact of technological innovations and new therapeutic approaches

Increased emphasis on PHC and community-based services

Increasing requests for and complexity of home-based care

General global shortage of health-care workers stimulating consideration of skill mix, task-shifting, and task reallocation options

Physician shortages

Increased demand for specialized nurses

Nursing's desire for a clinical career ladder and professional advancement

Better-informed health-care consumers

Intensified demand for options to address out-of-control health-care costs

Search to improve quality of and access to health-care services

---

to country context that could be effective in influencing optimal practice for ANP (Maier, 2015).

This chapter examines some of the issues influencing the development of ANP globally. The emergence of the role in different regions of the world, the role of the International Council of Nurses (ICN) in setting international guidelines, and some of the controversial practice issues affecting the nature of ANP are explored. Country illustrations provide examples of growth, progress, governance, and challenges experienced worldwide.

THE ROLE OF THE INTERNATIONAL COUNCIL OF NURSES

The International Nurse Practitioner/Advanced Practice Nursing Network (INP/APNN) was launched in 2000 under the auspices of ICN to follow trends and act as a resource for ANP. Following the initiation of the

TABLE 5.1		
International Council of Nurses Characteristics for the Advanced Practice Nurse		
Educational Preparation	**Nature of Practice**	**Regulatory Mechanisms (Country-Specific Regulations That Underpin Advanced Practice Nursing Practice)**
Educational preparation at an advanced level	The ability to integrate research, education, and clinical management	Right to diagnose Authority to prescribe medications and treatments
Formal recognition of educational programs	High degree of autonomy and independent practice Case management Advanced assessment and decision-making skills	Authority to refer to other professionals
A formal system of licensure, registration, certification, or credentialing	Recognized advanced clinical competencies The ability to provide consultant services to other health professionals Recognized first point of entry for services	Authority to admit to hospital Title protection Legislation specific to advanced practice

International Council of Nurses. (2008b). *The scope of practice, standards and competencies of the advanced practice nurse.* Geneva: Author.

INP/APNN ICN consulted extensively with members of the network to reach a consensus on the definition, characteristics, and scope of practice for an APN. Because of this consultation ICN provided the following definition (ICN, 2008b):

> a registered nurse who has acquired the expert knowledge base, complex decision-making skills and clinical competencies for expanded practice, the characteristics of which are shaped by the context and/or country in which s/he is credentialed to practice. A master's degree is recommended for entry level.

See **Table 5.1** for ICN-recommended role characteristics.

Although ICN does not specifically define the scope of practice, it draws on the definition and characteristics described in Table 5.1 in recommending that countries should keep the following points in mind when developing a scope of practice for the APN:

- Requires cognitive, integrative, and technical abilities to put into practice ethical and culturally safe acts, procedures, protocols, and practice guidelines.
- Has the capacity for delivery of evidence-based care in primary, secondary, and tertiary settings in urban and rural communities.

- Practices a high level of autonomy in direct patient care and management of health problems, including case management competencies.
- Accepts accountability for providing health promotion, patient and peer education, mentorship, leadership, and management of the practice environment.
- Maintains current nursing practice and seeks improvement through the translation, use, and implementation of meaningful research.
- Engages in partnerships with patients and health team members for determining resources needed for continuous care and partnering with stakeholders in influencing policies that direct the health-care environment (adapted from ICN, 2008b, p. 13).

Core competencies have been identified and published in the following ICN documents: *The Scope of Practice, Standards and Competencies of the Advanced Practice Nurse* (ICN, 2008b) and *Nursing Care Continuum—Framework and Competencies* (ICN, 2008a). Since the time that ICN developed these guidelines, additional competencies have emerged as prominent aspects of the role. As the field of ANP has matured, the nurse in an APN role is often seen as a clinical expert with characteristics of the role crosscutting over numerous themes that include increased understanding of issues of governance, policy development, leadership, and research (Schober, 2016). This developmental issue along with the varying nature of the discipline globally suggests that a review and revision of international competency guidelines defining the APN is needed.

Progress in this direction has been initiated by Bird and Schumann (2016) in their 2014 survey of 16 countries that identified competencies for APNs. This survey provides a comparison of the Strong Model of Advanced Practice Nursing (Ackerman et al, 1996) and the ICN APN competencies (ICN, 2008b) with APN competencies provided from respondent countries. As of July 2016 the data are being analyzed with publication of findings expected in 2017 (B. Bird & L. Schumann, personal communication, June 30, 2016).

Following 16 years acting as an international resource for ANP presence globally and a change in ICN administration, the ICN in July 2016 reviewed the functionality of their nine networks including the INP/APNN. Further, at the ICN 2017 Congress in Barcelona, Spain the formation of a Global Alliance was announced with the intent of broadening ICN access to international resources. The ICN NP/APN Network will be the prototype for this concept leading with the development of a resource cluster for APNs. It is expected that ICN will continue to follow ANP trends and development with the introduction of a new organizational model.

ADVANCED NURSING PRACTICE: A GROWING GLOBAL PRESENCE

Since the 1990s the ICN has monitored the progress of ANP globally. In 1999, in response to an ICN survey sent to 125 nation members, 33 countries reported having nursing roles with advanced practice elements (Schober & Affara, 2006). In a follow-up survey, Roodbol (2004) reported that 60 countries indicated an interest in ANP or were in the process of developing advanced practice roles.

Information on the state of ANP globally and associated developmental issues was obtained from a Strength/Weakness/Opportunities/Threats (SWOT) analysis carried out with participants attending the 2006 ICN APNN Conference in the Republic of South Africa. This analysis highlighted important areas of concern affecting the evolution of ANP in many of the participating countries attending the conference (Affara, 2006). Issues surfacing were similar to those uncovered by Schober and Affara (2006) from their survey of key informants and the literature, published and unpublished, on the status of ANP internationally.

An ICN survey of 32 countries conducted in 2008 provided additional confirmation of the expansion of NP and APN roles internationally while also highlighting some of the challenges encountered (Pulcini et al, 2010). At the 2011 ICN Congress in Malta, Roodbol (2011) reported that membership in the ICN International NP/APNN represented 78 countries with an interest in ANP. As of June 2016 ICN reported that membership in the INP/APNN included representation from 94 countries (A. Canedo, personal communication, June 9, 2016). The numbers based on INP/APNN membership as of 2011 and 2016 suggest an interest in exploring the concept of advanced nursing roles but do not necessarily represent an active presence of APN roles.

CHALLENGES AND CONTROVERSY

Development and implementation of APN roles is fraught with difficulties even when there is enthusiasm to integrate this new category of nurses into the health-care workforce. The following section identifies some of the key challenges in role development and realization of the ANP concept.

Role Ambiguity and Lack of Role Clarity

Role ambiguity and lack of role clarity is related to an inability to define a scope of practice for the APN and what this nurse will do in the health-care workforce (Donald et al, 2010; Gardner et al, 2007; Schober, 2016). In the absence of a clearly defined scope of practice, it is difficult to delineate accountability and responsibility. In addition, the lack of a defined identity affects the ability of APNs to communicate clear messages about the nature of their role to clients, policy makers, other health-care professionals, regulators, and educators, among others.

Findings from the Canadian Decision Support Synthesis on Clinical Nurse Specialists and Nurse Practitioners in Canada further indicate that regulators, educators, government officials, and administrators consistently raised concerns regarding the lack of clarity surrounding APN roles and the potential of losing the role during economic downturns or when other roles are introduced if the contributions of the APN role were not clear (DiCenso et al, 2010).

Proliferation of Titles

Identification of ANP globally is plagued by a proliferation of titles. This diversity leads to confusion and lack of understanding as researchers attempt definitive research and regulators look for guidance when developing professional regulation. In addition, functions and responsibility vary considerably from one setting to another even when one title is used within the same country (Pulcini et al, 2010; Schober, 2016). This lack of consensus adds to the mystery as to what title should be applied as distinctive roles emerge in countries in the early stages of role development. Titles currently being used throughout the world include nurse practitioner (NP), family NP (FNP), adult NP, advanced NP, primary care practitioner (PCP), clinical nurse-midwife (CNM), clinical nurse specialist (CNS), nurse anesthetist (NA), community health NP (CHNP), and women's health NP (WHNP). Pediatric NP, gerontological NP, emergency room NP, and acute care NP are also titles applied to APN roles. Some titles indicate the specialty of the APN; other titles have been developed to fit the context of the systems or the situations in which the APN role exists. The ICN survey of 32 countries discovered 14 different titles being used to designate ANP (Pulcini et al, 2010). The variety of titles being used reveals the explorative nature and diverse perspectives of advanced practice internationally with respect to the parameters of the role and where it sits in relation to other nursing and professional roles in the health-care system (Schober, 2016).

Lack of Recognition by Other Professionals in the Health-Care System

Medical dominance and control over the provision of health-care services, especially in more developed countries, are cited as major obstacles to implementing APN roles. In addition, scope of practice conflicts and overlap with other health professionals' scope of practice, especially medicine, contributes to APNs feeling unwelcome within the health-care team. Interestingly, one of the particular problem areas revealed by research conducted in Singapore by Schober (2013) was a mistrust that may exist between APNs and other nurses. Schober and Affara (2006) had uncovered a similar sentiment in information obtained from key informants who reported obstacles to the role arising from other nurses. In the Netherlands, Roodbol

(2005) found that even though physicians believed that the APN presence had a positive effect on the social identity of nurses in general, nurses as a whole did not share this view and were not prepared to accept them into their professional group.

Varying Levels of Autonomy

The degree of autonomy afforded to APNs varies from country to country and even within the same country. This appears to be related to the degree of recognition and acceptance of the role and to the type of regulatory mechanisms in place (Schober, 2016).

Variable Standards and Quality of Education Programs

Historically and up to the present time, educational qualifications for the APN role have varied from the awarding of certificates for postbasic or baccalaureate courses of various lengths to undertaking a formal university program and obtaining a master's degree. Information from an ICN INP/APNN survey indicated that among 31 responding countries, 50% replied that the most prevalent credential was the master's degree (Pulcini et al, 2010). Education and preparation beyond the level of the generalist nurse is a critical component in the development of the APN role. The ICN guidelines suggest that entry-level education at the master's level should be a recommended goal (ICN, 2008b). See **Box 5.2** for the ICN-recommended education standards.

Professional Regulation, Credentialing, and Standard Setting

Standards, supportive legislation, and professional regulation ultimately provide the underpinnings for successful ANP implementation and sustainability. Development of appropriate policies, although essential, can contribute to intense discussions and lengthy debate. The lag between actual APN practice and supportive legislation can be attributed to uneven starts in initiating new roles and the diversity of health issues challenging the communities and countries where these roles seek to grow. Also, restrictive regulations that unnecessarily limit the expertise and scope of practice for APN roles can considerably affect to what extent advanced practice will be embraced by a health-care system and permit

---

Box 5.2

International Council of Nurses Standards for Education of the Advanced Practice Nurse

Programs prepare the student, a registered/licensed nurse, for practice beyond that of the generalist nurse by including opportunities to access knowledge and skills, as well as demonstrate their integration in clinical practice as a safe, competent, and autonomous practitioner.

Programs prepare the authorized nurse to practice within the nation's health-care system to the full extent of the role as set out in the scope of practice.

Programs are staffed by faculty who are qualified and prepared at or beyond the level of the student undertaking the program of study.

Programs are accredited or approved by the authorized national or international credentialing body.

Programs facilitate lifelong learning and maintenance of competencies.

Programs provide student access to a sufficient range of clinical experience to apply and consolidate under supervision the theoretical course content.

International Council of Nurses. (2008b). *The scope of practice, standards and competencies of the advanced practice nurse.* Geneva: Author.

Box 5.3

International Council of Nurses Minimal Standards for Regulating the Advanced Practice Nurse

Develop and maintain sound credentialing mechanisms that enable the authorized nurse to practice in the advanced role within the established scope of practice.

Establish relevant civil legislation or rules to acknowledge the authorized role, monitor the competence, and protect the public through issuance of guidance,

assessment processes, and, when necessary, fitness to practice procedures and processes.

Periodically revise regulatory language to maintain currency with nursing practice and scientific advancement.

Establish title protection through rule making or civil legislation.

International Council of Nurses. (2008a). *Nursing care continuum—framework and competencies.* Geneva: Author.

APNs to contribute to their fullest capacity. A process of evaluation and revision of professional regulation may be the only option to follow when regulations are found to hinder optimal professional practice. This, in turn, poses another set of challenges as to who has the authority to initiate and the power to supply leverage in provision of solutions in the credentialing and regulatory arena.

National nursing associations and nursing leadership would seem to provide the likely foundation for development and exploration of educational requirements and standards, especially because the core of ANP is grounded in nursing theory and nursing science. However, there appears to be a lack of consensus among nursing academics and leaders as to what ANP really means, and at times overt

support by nursing bodies is lacking as the roles develop. Key decision makers and advisors have begun to provide regulatory and credentialing guidance and make policy decisions. International organizations, such as the ICN, are taking official organizational positions regarding ANP and offer publications (ICN, 2008a, 2008b) to facilitate a better understanding of ANP. **Box 5.3** identifies the minimal regulatory standards recommended by ICN (2008b).

Flexible regulatory language has been encouraged to ensure quality health-care services that are protective of the populations receiving those services. However, especially in countries that are newly developing standards, restrictive regulatory legislation affecting APNs is promulgated to protect the practice of other health-care professionals.

Clarity and consistency in defining the process and structure of credentialing for APNs and accreditation of educational programs is essential as the APN investigates intercountry choices for employment and educational opportunities. Professional mobility may potentially shape a move toward consensus for credentialing among countries as APNs relocate, immigrate, or accept temporary assignment. The capability of agencies and organizations in addressing legislative issues, standards, and professional regulation will increasingly come under scrutiny as the international nursing community looks for authoritative guidance.

In ANP development and implementation, professional regulation often needs to catch up with innovation if understanding and confidence in the role is to be established for the benefit of key decision makers, the profession, and the public. However, the setting up of suitable regulatory mechanisms needs to be approached in such a manner that new problems are not created, health-care systems are not made less efficient, or access is reduced to those who benefit by APN services.

Authority to Prescribe Medicines and Therapeutics

Nurse prescribing of medicines or therapeutics describes various types of nursing practice currently undertaken in different countries or regions of the world. In general, discussion of this issue focuses on the suitability of prescriptive authority for nurses and the appropriateness of nurse prescribing as it relates to defined characteristics and expected competencies for APN roles. Nevertheless, discourse and comment reveal that nurses have been prescribing medicines, treatments, and other therapies in certain health-care settings, but the reality of carrying out these activities within a legal framework and in a supportive health-care environment, such as one that has enabling workplace policies in place, lags behind the requisites of actual practice. However, as more countries implement APN roles in a variety of settings, the issue of nurse prescribing is becoming less of a controversial issue.

It appears that advancement for APN and NP roles necessitates prescriptive authority, but it is worth noting that health-care services in some areas of the world have for some time included nurse prescribing of a range of essential drugs at the first level of practice in primary health-care systems (Ball, 2009). Ball (2009, p. 67) suggests that the

question underlying the topic of nurse prescribing is not "Can nurses prescribe?" in a particular country, but "To what extent is nurse prescribing established?" How nurse prescribing evolves and becomes an integral part of the health-care system is as important as whether or not nurses have the legal authority to prescribe.

Nurse prescribing prototypes internationally provide models by which nurses may potentially be involved in prescribing (Ball, 2009). Nurse prescribing is not always associated with ANP as evidenced by countries or regions with authority for nurses to prescribe. Sweden, Australia, Canada, New Zealand, and countries of the United Kingdom (UK) have well-established community nursing or general nursing roles supportive of this capability.

In appraisal of the key global issues associated with nurses' prescribing, Ball (2009) indicates that there is little uniformity as to what role nurses should have with regard to prescriptive authority. Educational programs to prepare nurses for prescribing range from master's degree preparation to a designated program of a few study days. Although these issues are varied, there are common approaches when considering nurses' prescriptive authority. These include the acceptability of nurse prescribing within the health-care setting, designation of which nurses will prescribe, and strategies for implementation and feasibility from an administrative and health policy perspective. The differences between countries reflect differences in health-care systems, the population demographics of the country, and the status of nursing (Ball, 2009).

GLOBAL PERSPECTIVE— COUNTRY ILLUSTRATIONS

The development of ANP internationally has progressed significantly in numerous regions of the world. To review this global growth, examples are presented from diverse experiences of countries introducing, developing, and implementing APN roles. To grasp perspectives of emerging development, country illustrations are arranged according to WHO-designated regions. Descriptions of country progress and interpretation of ANP are intended to provide representative examples of a region but are not meant to portray all activity in any one area of the world. The authors acknowledge that wherever the concept or level of ANP arises the occurrence of this phenomenon is subject to specific health-care, nursing, and political cultures. The dynamic authority of leaders within local, national, and institutional settings ultimately drive policy that impacts the APN role and the manner in which the APN practices.

Africa: WHO-AFRO

The WHO Regional Office for Africa is located in Brazzaville, Republic of Congo. Personnel in the office include the WHO regional committee for Africa, a secretariat for the African region, three intercountry support teams, and country and liaison staff located in 47 member states.

Botswana

In Botswana, a poorly developed health-care system and a severe shortage of physicians following independence in 1966 triggered the need for nurses with advanced skills and decision making to provide services usually associated with physician practice. Nurses accepted these increased responsibilities but demanded further education to enhance their ability to meet the health-care needs of the country.

The Ministry of Health, through the Institute of Health Sciences (IHS), responded by establishing the first FNP diploma program in 1981 with the aim to educate nurses in advanced skills in diagnosis and management of PHC problems common in Botswana. The program evolved to 18 months of postbasic education in 1991, followed by a revision and update in curriculum in 2001 with increased emphasis on comprehensive family health services (National Health Insurance [NHI], 2002). In 2007, a four-semester format was introduced (Pilane et al, 2007). Currently, the diploma programs at IHS are at an advanced stage of curricula revision and upgrading to degree levels. At the same time the master's program at the University of Botswana is being revised and is likely going to address articulation and recognition of prior learning issues from the IHS diploma program.

The University of Botswana offers a master of nursing science degree that includes specialization as a FNP (University of Botswana, 2016). Although the University of Botswana has begun to graduate FNP students, the diploma program at the IHS simultaneously continues to offer a FNP program at IHS Gabarone and Kanye SDA College of Nursing (Institute of Health Sciences, Botswanna, 2017). Candidates for the IHS program must

have a diploma in general nursing (G.N.) with a minimum of 2 years' service as a general nurse, be registered as a general nurse with the Nursing and Advance Diploma in Midwifery Council of Botswana, and be in possession of a Botswana General Certificate of Secondary Education (BGCSE) or its equivalent.

Because the University of Botswana now offers a master's degree in nursing science with the option for FNP study, a comparative analysis of the master's degree and FNP curricula at IHS is underway to identify how the two programs could combine common coursework and remove redundant or repetitious study while still supporting educational advancement for the FNP educated in the IHS program. Possibilities for credit transfer and opportunities for challenge examinations or applying for exemption from retaking courses when seeking further study at the University of Botswana are being considered (C. Pilane, personal communication, August 14, 2014).

NPs in Botswana provide primary care in outpatient departments, clinics, industry, schools, and private practice throughout the country. The health-care environment in Botswana supports autonomy in provision of PHC services as evidenced in nurse-managed facilities and prescribing privileges. Challenges are lack of specific regulations, the absence of clear qualifications, no designated career advancement for FNPs, and lack of availability of qualified faculty for the educational programs. Study findings by Seitio-Kgokgwe et al (2015) confirm issues associated with lack of central coordination, weak leadership, weak policy and regulatory frameworks, and inadequate resources with a focus on the lack of attention to organizational structure. The conclusion from this study is that there is an opportunity for the Ministry of Health in Botswana to reorganize and enhance the associated health-care infrastructure in hopes that this would solidify support for FNPs and nursing.

Republic of South Africa

The "key challenges for NPs in South Africa lie in lobbying for enabling legislation, obtaining access to education and training opportunities, and managing risks within the rapidly changing environment" (Geyer et al, 2002, p. 11). Even though this statement was made in 2002, the commentary remains true today (N. Geyer, personal communication, July 2, 2016).

The move since 1994 from a mainly hospital-based health-care service to increased emphasis on PHC and community-based services increased the visibility of the NP. The creation of a more unified health-care system, while dealing with rapid change in the health-care environment, posed challenges and opportunities for the primary clinical practitioner (PCP). PCP has been used as a title for NPs in the Republic of South Africa (RSA); however, with the development and introduction of new qualifications post 2016, the title will become FNP.

The 2005 Nursing Act and its regulations call for NPs to possess required competencies. Standards for the education and training of nurses and midwives have also been established. Basic preparation for FNPs follows either acquisition of a 4-year diploma or 4-year degree for general nursing, midwifery, psychiatry, or community health nursing followed by a specialization program in diagnosis, treatment, and care. However, the rapid acceleration in use of nurses in PHC services has resulted in FNPs that have not received specialist education. Therefore, one of the challenges is providing sufficient access to education to ensure nurses in the FNP role have the required competence to provide high-quality care.

The scope-of-practice regulations provided by the South African Nursing Council in 1984 provided practice principles that support nurses and midwives to "perform any acts for which they have been trained" (Geyer et al, 2002, p. 13). The FNP scope of practice will be written in such a way that it emphasizes the provision of comprehensive clinical services such as the following:

• Comprehensive assessment
• Diagnosis of health and disease, especially diseases common in the RSA
• Treatment and management (pharmacological and nonpharmacological)
• Referral to other professionals
• Counseling
• Leadership and management
• Health promotion and disease prevention

However, the legal framework for the FNP has not evolved as rapidly as practice. As of July 2016 a new scope of practice for nursing was approved and is awaiting promulgation by the Ministry of Health. See the first numbered item in Box 5.4. This scope will make a clear distinction between the roles for professional nurses,

staff nurses, and auxiliary nurses while also providing the basis for progression to specialist nurse and FNP scopes of practice. The South African Nursing Council has revised the qualifications framework for nurses in alignment with changes in education legislation in the country that transfers all nursing programs to the higher education band. The specialist nurse has been described in legislation, but not the FNP.

The FNP scope of practice overlaps with aspects of scopes of practice for other health practitioners, such as physicians and, in the case of medicines, pharmacists. Dispensing of drugs falls under the pharmacist's function, whereas the control of drugs as associated with prescribing is exclusive to the physician, unless the practitioner or professional, such as a nurse, has been authorized to prescribe by his or her respective councils or regulatory bodies. Nurses are listed as one of these professions (see numbered items 3 and 4 in **Box 5.4**). A nurse who wishes to dispense medicines must undergo a course accredited with the pharmacy council. Application for a license to dispense medication is made through the national department of health. The license is valid for 3 years, after which reapplication is required.

NPs in RSA are mainly employed in the public health sector at the provincial and local authority level. Nurses and midwives provide the majority of health services, with nurses identified as the first point of contact for preventive health and minor ailments. With the growing need for home-based care, resulting mainly from the epidemic proportions of HIV and AIDS, nurses and NPs are increasingly holding leadership and supervisory responsibilities for other workers and volunteers in health-care systems. The publication of the White Paper on NHI for the country includes roles for NPs as well as contracting for private practitioners that is said to include nurses. This is where the NP can make a significant contribution.

Establishing collaborative practice in the RSA context is fraught with difficulty because language contained in separate practice acts and regulations governing practice of each category of health-care professional poses a significant barrier. Health-care practitioners can employ each other, but stipulations within regulations prohibit group practice. Such limitations either discourage formation of multiprofessional groups or require development of involved legal contracts to bypass the rules. Conflict arises when existing scopes of practice are seen to overlap with other professions, thus contributing to lack of agreement

---

Box 5.4

Developments for Nurse Practitioners in the Republic of South Africa

1. The scope of practice has been structured for three categories of nurses within a framework of professional-ethical practice, clinical practice, and quality of practice. This lends itself to developing a structured scope that progresses to the next levels of specialist nurses and NPs.

2. Educational programs linked to this scope will prepare staff nurses who will be independent/autonomous practitioners able to plan and execute comprehensive care for stable and uncomplicated patients. Professional nurses can specialize in a variety of areas, including family nurse practice. A criterion has been built in that no nurse can specialize until he or she has a 2-year clinical experience (this includes 1 year of community service after completion of basic training plus 1 additional year of clinical practice).

3. Although there is a new Nursing Act, the profession has not managed to get rid of government control regarding the authorization of nurses to prescribe. Section 56 of the Nursing Act of 2005 places more controls into the system; nurses will now be licensed to prescribe and reapply for licensing.

4. Work is currently in process on regulations for nurse prescribing. The thinking has been that there will be three levels of prescribing where nurses will have access to specified drugs to manage minor injuries and diseases—likely according to protocols. These levels are

Staff nurse = level one

Professional nurse = level two

Specialist nurse = level three (only access for specialist area)

N. Geyer, personal communication, July 2, 2016.

---

supportive of the development of advanced nursing roles. This situation has interfered with legislative support for FNP practice and expanded nurse dispensing and prescribing (N. Geyer, personal communication, July 2, 2016).

Western Africa

The scope of practice for a NP in West Africa (WA) is very similar to that of a NP role described in other countries (Madubuko, 2016). However, even though more than 1,000 nurses have master's degrees, advanced education is not recognized in the nursing register. All registered nurses (RNs) possess a postbasic nursing education and clinical training in midwifery (registered midwife [RM]). Therefore, RNs have additional advanced education in at least one specialty area—for instance, in the psychiatric, perioperative, nurse education, orthopedic, gynecological, thoracic, or pediatric field. The WA College of Nursing has accredited the University of Benin Teaching Hospital's School of Ophthalmic Nursing for an 18-month master's degree for ophthalmic NPs that is consistent with the global NP movement. Hopefully, the nurses in WA—with time, explanation, and lobbying—will obtain official recognition for advanced education and clinical practice.

A RN or RM is certified by national certification examination and provides direct PHC. The scope of practice includes obtaining a history, performing a physical examination, diagnosing and treating common illnesses, performing illness prevention screenings, and promoting health. Education and counseling are provided in collaboration with other health professionals. Health-care reforms have supported an interest for more relevant health-care services in WA, thus providing an opportunity for RNs and RMs in NP-like roles and other health professionals (Madubuko, 2016).

The Americas: WHO-PAHO

The Pan American Health Organization (PAHO) is part of the United Nations system, serving as the Regional Office for the Americas of the WHO and as the health organization of the Inter-American System. The following descriptions provide examples of successful and emerging APN activity in this region.

Canada

The Canadian Nurses Association (CNA) continues to provide leadership for the development and implementation of ANP in Canada. In 1999, the CNA developed a framework for ANP that was subsequently revised in 2002 and 2008. The framework provides the following definition (CNA, 2008, p. 5):

> Advanced nursing practice is an umbrella term describing an advanced level of clinical nursing practice that maximizes the use of graduate educational preparation, in-depth nursing knowledge and expertise in meeting the health needs of individuals, families, groups, and populations. It involves analyzing and synthesizing knowledge; understanding, interpreting and applying nursing theory and research; and developing and advancing nursing knowledge and the profession as a whole.

According to this framework, it is the combination of graduate education and clinical experience that allows nurses to develop the competencies required in ANP (CNA, 2008, p. 6). Core competencies are described as essential to ANP with a list of competencies in four categories, outlined in the framework as clinical, research, leadership, and consultation or collaboration.

Nurses in Canada are regulated at the provincial or territorial level. The only advanced practice nursing role with additional regulation and title protection, beyond RN, is the NP. NPs can autonomously make a diagnosis, order and interpret diagnostic tests, prescribe pharmaceuticals, and perform specific procedures within their legislated scope of practice (CNA, 2009b, p. 1).

The implementation of the NP role regained momentum following an 18-month federally funded, CNA-led Canadian Nurse Practitioner Initiative (CNPI) conducted from 2004 to 2006. This initiative helped in the development of a framework for the integration and sustainability of the NP role in Canada's health-care system. Recommendations for practice, education, legislation, regulation, and health human resources planning were provided because of findings from the CNPI.

In 2009, the CNA consulted with stakeholders on the progress made in meeting the recommendations generated from the 2006 CNPI (CNA, 2006). The main purpose of the consultation was to compile information on the activities of governments, nongovernmental organizations, and other stakeholders at the federal and provincial levels in relation to the CNPI recommendations. The consultation process revealed that although more than half of the actions concerning the CNPI recommendations had been fully or partially completed, several key actions remained ongoing. The findings of the consultation process are outlined in *Recommendations of the Canadian Nurse Practitioner Initiative Progress Report.* Among the remaining challenges to NP integration, continued advocacy was needed on federal legislative or policy barriers (e.g., prescribing of controlled drugs and substances, distribution of drug samples, completion of medical forms for disability claims, and workers' compensation) (CNA, 2009b).

In 2016 CNA reported significant progress on several recommendations of CNPI and overall evolution of the NP role (CNA, 2016). NPs are now practicing in a wide variety of settings and in various models of care. There is expansion of their scope of practice as well as pan-Canadian title protection, a common role description, and professional liability coverage. In spite of this progress, there continues to be federal and legislative barriers for distribution of medical samples, medical forms for disability claims, and workman's compensation (CNA, 2016).

CNSs in Canada are "registered nurses who hold a master's or doctoral degree in nursing and have expertise in a clinical nursing specialty" (CNA, 2009a). The CNS role was introduced to respond to increased patient need, a demand for nursing specialization, and to support nursing practice at the point of care. The CNS role has been part of the Canadian health-care system for more than four decades (DiCenso, 2008); however, researchers in Canada report that CNSs are not fully utilized. Because the title is not protected, it is difficult to report accurately on the presence of the CNS (Kilpatrick et al, 2013). In 2014, 514 self-reported CNSs were prepared at the graduate level (Canadian Institute for Health Information [CIHI], 2015).

CNSs' practice varies in each health-care jurisdiction in Canada and the title *clinical nurse specialist* is used inconsistently. The CNA led the development of the first Core Competencies for the CNS in Canada (CNA, 2014). Roundtable discussion identified that the varied use of the CNS role stems from confusion about what it entails. Yet, there is significant evidence demonstrating the positive contributions that CNSs make to the health of Canadians (Canadian Centre for Advanced Practice Nursing Research [CCAPNR], 2012).

Several tools have been developed to assist with the implementation of Canadian ANP roles: the CNPI implementation and evaluation toolkit (CNA, 2006) and the Participatory, Evidence-Based, Patient-Centered Process for Advanced Practice Role Development, Implementation and Evaluation (PEPPA framework [Bryant-Lukosius &

DiCenso, 2004]). These tools serve as a structured and practical guide in assessing the need and readiness for ANP roles based on the population health needs of Canadians. In 2010, DiCenso and colleagues published research titled the *Clinical Nurse Specialists and Nurse Practitioners in Canada: A Decision Support Synthesis.* The report provides an understanding of the roles of APNs, the contexts in which APNs are being used, and the health system factors that influence the way in which advanced practice nursing is being integrated into the Canadian health-care system.

Although there continues to be a lack of understanding among health professionals and the public in relationship to ANP in Canada, the professional and policy environment in the country is generally receptive and progressively integrating ANP roles into the health-care system. Policy makers, decision makers, and nursing leaders continue to work together to face challenges as they refine and coordinate what ANP means in terms of health-care services (J. Roussel, personal communication, May 4, 2016).

Cayman Islands

The emergence of ANP services in the Cayman Islands provides an example of how NP-like roles evolve and develop in response to the needs of the people, as well as within geographical circumstances. The initiation of NP-like services started in 1930 with provision of care by a local midwife to meet community health needs. Physician services were scarce and conditions were primitive with populations residing in remote locations. NP services progressed with the official employment of a nurse experienced in midwifery and community health to provide PHC. Comprehensive health-care services were provided in homes, schools, and clinic settings (Slocombe, 2000).

Expansion of clinical expertise progressed rapidly during subsequent years, with the nurse as the main health-care provider on the islands. The nurse diagnosed, treated, prescribed, and dispensed what was viewed as necessary. Conditions receiving care were "whatever walked in through the door" (M. Slocombe, personal communication, 2002). Immunization, antenatal, well-baby, nutritional, diabetic, and hypertensive clinics were held, with backup consultation and collaboration provided by phone call to the nearest hospital or by appointment with periodic visiting physicians. The nurse took on the multifaceted role and duties of counselor, administrator, staff supervisor, health educator, accountant, and secretary. Absence of adequate

support by other professionals, lack of resources, and limited educational opportunities created frustration and obstacles to professional development.

The location of the three Cayman Islands, situated in the Caribbean Sea between Jamaica and Cuba, contributes to the diversity, as well as the uniqueness, of commonly seen conditions. Cuban refugees and rafters trickle in for health screenings and health care, periodic care for prison inmates is provided, and hurricane evacuation preparedness is essential for the health centers. The tourist industry, with visitors from more than 80 countries, requires the nurse to be knowledgeable about trauma and injuries related to deep sea diving (Slocombe, 2000). The Cayman Islands continue to register APNs and NPs to work at facilities on the islands (L. Joseph, personal communication, June 22, 2016).

Jamaica

In 1973 the Nurses Association of Jamaica (NAJ) held exploratory meetings with the minister of health (MOH) to discuss the training of NPs in the country. The interest in the NP concept came as a response to the shortage of physicians needed to provide cost-effective health care to the poor in rural and underserved areas. Following these discussions, NAJ then submitted a proposal for the establishment of a NP program that was accepted by the MOH. In 1977 the first NP program came into being under the joint auspices of the Ministry of Health and the Department of Social and Preventive Medicine within the Faculty of Medicine with the Advanced Nursing Education Unit (ANEU) providing a director.

The Ministry of Health with ANEU administered the program with the Department of Advanced Nursing (DANE) later having responsibility for the curriculum. The program was initially a certificate program. In keeping with the Ying Task Force on Education and also with current trends in nursing education worldwide, the program was transferred in 2002 to the Department of Advanced Nursing Education (now the University of the West Indies School of Nursing [UWISON]) where it is being offered at the master's degree level. Since the inception of the program in Jamaica many NPs from other Caribbean countries are educated at UWISON in Jamaica.

NPs in Jamaica have been providing nursing and medical care to all age groups within the health-care delivery systems and in communities since 1978. Most

NPs function in primary care health centers. As of July 2016 there are 80 NPs in clinical practice as family and mental health/psychiatric NPs. NAs are technically classified as NPs; however, even though the NA program started many years before the NP program, it has yet to evolve to the master's level.

Despite these achievements, NPs and NAs are not registered or licensed as APNs and have no prescriptive privileges. All NPs and NAs are registered as nurses or midwives. They have no official authority in the expanded role. Prescriptions must be countersigned by physicians. NPs, NAs, the Nursing Council of Jamaica, and other stakeholders on the island continue to work diligently to move forward an agenda to enact policies supportive of advanced nursing roles (D. Less, personal communication, July 20, 2016).

Latin America

Historically, in Latin America most nurses are trained to a baccalaureate level as licensed nurses or RNs. Nurses in rural areas often provide primary care services to underserved populations, essentially practicing in an advanced practice role. However, many lack formal skills training, a defined role, and graduate level education to support this degree of independent practice (Nigenda et al, 2010). In 2014 a PAHO strategy for universal access to health and universal health coverage was approved (PAHO, 2014) outlining key strategies for improving universal health, including an increasing interest in moving forward with an agenda for implementation of the APN roles.

In order to move this agenda forward, the Universal Access to Health and Universal Health Coverage: Advanced Practice Nursing Summit was hosted in 2015 by PAHO/WHO and the Collaborating Center in Primary Health Care & Health Human Resources at McMaster University in Hamilton, Canada. At this summit, participants from across the region representing health ministries, nursing associations, and nursing schools highlighted the contributions of nursing with specific focus on APN implementation and roles in different countries and outlined priorities for APN implementation (PAHO, 2015). The overall goal for this summit was to address the APN role in the promotion of PHC in the Americas. In addition to defining the scope of nursing roles and advanced practice nursing in Pan American countries, one specific objective

was to develop strategies for the implementation of the APN roles in Latin America in order to address gaps in health services and unmet population needs, changes in nurses' roles and responsibilities that can leverage APN expertise, and factors that might enable these changes in nurses' roles and responsibilities (PAHO, 2015, p. 4).

Five planning priorities were identified from the 2015 PAHO summit. They are:

- Establish master's level APN education programs
- Engage and influence decision makers, legislators, and other key stakeholders
- Focus on APN service delivery for underserved populations with high needs
- Establish a Pan American collaborative network to develop and implement the APN role
- Define and optimize complementary RN and APN roles in new models of primary health care (PAHO, 2015, p. 9)

A draft plan was created for each priority with 1-year (April 2016) and 3-year (April 2018) steps toward implementation identified. These planning priorities were designated to guide and unify advanced practice nursing implementation efforts in the region (PAHO, 2015). One result was the creation of a six-part webinar series in April 2016 titled "Advanced Practice Nursing: PAHO Activities and Strategy for Development in Latin America" (PAHO, 2016). The webinar was the collaborative endeavor of PAHO with McMaster University in Canada and was presented simultaneously in English and Spanish. The goal was to increase interest and awareness of the APN role for nurses and key shareholders in Latin America (PAHO, 2016). More than 300 individuals registered for the series representing nursing in more than 20 countries in the PAHO region.

An outcome of the 2015 PAHO summit was a meeting arranged by WHO-PAHO and the WHO Collaborating Center at the University of Michigan School of Nursing titled "Developing Advanced Practice Nursing Competencies in Latin America to Contribute to Universal Health." This meeting was built on the priorities set in 2015 to address APN competencies and curriculum development (Schober, 2016).

The 2015 PAHO summit promoted collaboration between nursing leaders and institutions in North America and those in Latin America. In February 2016, the Faculty of Nursing at Pontificia Universidad Javeriana in Colombia hosted a celebration of its 75-year anniversary titled "Posibilidades y Realidades de la Práctica Avanzada en Enfermería en Colombia Frente a la Cobertura Universal en Salud" (Possibilities and Realities of Advanced Practice Nursing in Colombia in the Face of Universal Health Coverage) in Bogota, Colombia. A PAHO representative participated and met with several nursing leaders and the Ministry of Health to discuss aspects that could facilitate advanced practice nursing in Colombia (Facultad de Enfermería, 2016; Schober, 2016).

In Chile, since the time of the PAHO 2015 summit, the University of the Andes has launched a master's degree Nurse Practitioner in Adult Acute Care program. Although the program is focused on the APN role in tertiary rather than primary care, it is a historical step as the first program in Latin America that will produce graduates in line with the ICN definition of an APN. The program is a collaboration with Johns Hopkins Hospital and School of Nursing in the United States. In addition to required clinical hours in Chile, students will have the possibility to participate in a 2-week internship at Johns Hopkins Hospital shadowing a NP or nurse specialist in order to understand the role and observe their practice (Magíster en Práctica Avanzada de Enfermería, 2016).

In an effort to initiate steps toward APN roles, representatives from the Federal Council of Nursing and the Brazilian Nursing Association came to PAHO headquarters in Washington, DC, in November 2015 to discuss and plan the future of APN in Brazil. A decision was made to join together and develop a document defining the scope of the APN role in Brazil in PHC to be subsequently presented to the MOH. An international seminar was organized in June 2016 with all nursing organizations in Brazil to increase visibility of the APN concept.

Along with recent success, challenges for APN implementation in the Latin American countries continue to need attention. These issues include lack of recognition of the significant role nursing has in strengthening health-care systems, the development of postgraduate nursing education in countries where there may not have been existing graduate nursing courses, and bringing changes to policy that would allow nurses in APN roles to practice to their full scope of practice (Schober, 2016).

Eastern Mediterranean Region: WHO-EMRO

The Eastern Mediterranean Regional Office (EMRO) of the WHO serves 22 countries and territories in the Middle East, North Africa, the Horn of Africa, and Central Asia. In June 2001, the regional director of nursing for EMRO convened the Fifth Meeting of the Regional Panel on Nursing to discuss ANP and nurse prescribing (WHO-EMRO, 2001). Countries represented at the 3-day workshop in Islamabad, Pakistan, included Bahrain, Cyprus, Islamic Republic of Iran, Iraq, Jordan, Lebanon, Oman, Pakistan, Saudi Arabia, Sudan, Syrian Arab Republic, United Arab Emirates, and the Republic of Yemen. Twenty-two representatives from nursing, medicine, pharmacy, and ministries of health gathered to begin to develop a regional policy framework for ANP and mechanisms for nurse prescribing. The regional panel highlighted factors leading to development of the roles, as well as identifying strategies for the region (WHO-EMRO, 2001). Obstacles and factors identified as supportive of development for ANP and nurse prescribing are provided in **Table 5.2.**

Strategies were formulated for ANP development and include the following:

- Assessment of need and cost-effectiveness for APN roles in the region
- Development of APN curriculum and standards of practice
- Definition of the role and identification of related revision of nurse practice acts to cover ANP

Significantly, there was consensus that authority for nurse prescribing within a range of essential drugs is an activity that could be allocated at some level to the competent general nurse and does not necessarily depend on the development of ANP. On the other hand, authority to prescribe was acknowledged as one of the many areas of expertise associated with APN roles. In addition, it was agreed that these nursing roles require advanced education, regulatory changes, and expansion of traditional nursing.

Recommendations were made for WHO-EMRO (2001) to provide guidelines to assist countries in the region that are in the process of developing and strengthening ANP at all levels of health care. Additional assistance was requested from WHO to initiate and coordinate pilot

TABLE 5.2	
WHO-EMRO Consensus on Factors Influencing Advanced Practice Nursing Development	
Obstacles	**Support**
Lack of a regional definition and role ambiguity	Increased population and community needs for health-care services
Absence of country-level educational or regulatory systems to support such roles	Improving levels of nursing education
No feasibility studies for ANP needs	Desire in the region to improve quality of care and access
No awareness of the role among the public and health professionals	Research studies from outside the region supportive of advanced nursing practice
Absence of nursing leadership at the policy level	Commitment of WHO toward development and use of nursing roles

Adapted from World Health Organization—Eastern Mediterranean Region. (2001). *Fifth meeting of the regional advisory panel on nursing and consultation on advanced practice nursing and nurse prescribing: Implications for regulation, nursing education and practice in the Eastern Mediterranean.* WHO-EM/NUR/348/E/L. Cairo: Author.

projects to evaluate the impact and cost-effectiveness of related change when introducing new nursing roles and nurse prescribing. As of July 2016 the progress in this region has been uneven and limited because of ongoing country conflicts; even so, there continues to be interest and progress toward the advancement of nursing. This initial meeting in Pakistan stimulated interest and discussion in the region that continues in Bahrain, Jordan, Oman, Pakistan, and the United Arab Emirates (F. Aldarazi, personal communication, June 21, 2016).

Bahrain

Because of the WHO-EMRO meeting in Pakistan in 2001, Bahrain received additional consultative support coordinated by WHO-EMRO to assess the country's readiness for ANP (Schober, 2007b). Consultation services found a stable organizational structure for health-care service provision within PHC. Two pediatric APNs educated in NP programs in the United States had started working in pediatric specialties in a hospital. Additional NPs, also educated in the United States, are faculty at the College of Health Sciences (CHS).

The CHS has had an RN-bachelor of science in nursing (BSN) degree for some years and established a 4-year BSN program in 2003. The BSN is now considered entry-level education for nursing practice in Bahrain. With proper planning, this places the CHS in an ideal position to develop an ANP master's degree program. Although the associate degree (AD) nursing programs have been discontinued, the majority of the current Bahraini nursing graduates come from these programs. Postbasic 1-year education, called *advanced practice programs,* is available in the country. Lacking a current option for a master's program within Bahrain, nurses interested in obtaining ANP education are sponsored by the Ministry of Health to study in the United States or elsewhere (A. Matooq, personal communication, March 14, 2008).

Bahrain faces certain challenges in developing an APN role suitable for its health services:

- Identifying services that could be provided by APNs or NPs
- Developing an educational plan that meets the needs of the current workforce while properly planning for potential APN roles
- Constructing strategies to ensure faculty are adequately qualified to deliver ANP education
- Establishing standards and regulations supportive of APN roles

In 2007 nurses were observed to be functioning in an advanced capacity in triage centers but were not using the terms *NP* or *APN.* Nurses were educated in the United States for NP roles. However, they were employed in hospital-based units and faced confusion by other health-care professionals as they worked to establish a new nursing role.

A survey of primary care physicians (PCP) conducted in Bahrain (Nasaif, 2012) to assess their knowledge of the NP role found the PCPs had a poor understanding of the NP role. The conclusion was that more education and orientation to the NP role was needed to fully implement this concept. As of July 2016 it is unclear the extent of progress toward inclusion of the NP role even though there has been interest in role development.

Iran

The first step toward advanced nursing in Iran occurred in 1976 with the initiation of a master's in nursing sciences (MNS) in the areas of nursing education and nursing administration with four subspecialties focused in psychiatric, pediatric, community health, and medical–surgical nursing. At the time, 14 schools of nursing offered a master's degree in nursing. In 1995, there were 10 doctoral degree (PhD) programs in Iran that graduated 40 individuals to be hired for clinical and academic positions in hospitals, community centers, and universities.

The Farsi term *Karshenasae-e-Arshad* translates to "advanced specialist" and is recognized by physicians in major cities for nurses practicing in advanced roles and direct patient care. In rural areas, Iranian nurses practice autonomously, similar to the way APNs in most states practice in the United States.

A practice permit is issued by the Iranian Ministry of Health that allows advanced specialty nurses to open their own private practice clinics as centers for nursing services. Medical supervision by physicians is not required at these centers because the state Ministry of Health monitors health-care practice; however, physicians supervise the scope of practice.

Society's needs for health-care services determine curriculum content in academic nursing programs. In 2008, advances were made through an addition of practice emphasis in geriatric, rehabilitation, women's health, neonatal health, military, and oncology nursing at the graduate level. Short-term continuing nursing education courses were made available by the Ministry of Health for positions in school nursing, home health, intensive care, wound care, ostomy care, HIV/AIDS, and geriatric care at various levels.

As of July 2016, there were 181 schools of nursing in Iran; 91 were government supported and 90 were privately owned. Seven thousand students graduate yearly with a baccalaureate of science in nursing (BSc). The number of postgraduate nursing majors has significantly increased with 10 nursing majors at the master's level in different specialty areas and one major at the doctoral (PhD) level similar to the doctorate of nursing practice (DNP) in the United States. In 2016 1,100 graduate students were admitted in 10 specialized fields for a master's degree at 49 universities and for a doctoral degree at 14 universities. The recent count shows that a total of 3,759 students graduated with a master's degree (MSc) in nursing and 259 earned a PhD (M. Fooladi, A. Heydari, & F. Sharif, personal communication, July 22, 2016).

Oman

Inspired in 2000 by a meeting of representative countries of the WHO Eastern Mediterranean Region (EMR) focused on advanced nursing capacity and nurse prescribing, nursing leadership in Oman developed an aim to introduce the APN/NP concept. The director of nursing services for WHO in Cairo simultaneously had an agenda to promote APN roles in the region including support for the interest in Oman. The driving forces for ANP in Oman included a shortfall in physicians, especially in the PHC settings, both in numbers and specific expertise. In addition, emerging health problems caused by lifestyle changes, increase in life expectancy, and the global trend of moving care closer and deeper into the community caught the attention of the Ministry of Health.

Active interest in the development of the APN role was initiated in 2004. Support for developing the role was articulated by a WHO short-term consultant following a review of the PHC delivery system in the country. A situation analysis was then conducted in 2005 followed by further consultations and workshops with health-care professionals and key stakeholders in 2006 and 2007. Reports provided to the WHO-EMRO and the Ministry of Health in Oman demonstrated high utilization and heavy patient load for physicians in larger health centers with resultant restricted access to PHC services resulting in potential poor outcomes and patient-provider dissatisfaction. In the many smaller and rural health centers nurses were found to function in a context that includes minor diagnosis and treatment. Thus, when there is no physician in the health centers, nurses are providing care beyond the scope of practice of their generalist nurse education. The WHO consultants noted these conditions and a proposal was made by the WHO-EMRO in 2008 to develop the APN role at the primary, secondary, and tertiary levels of care.

In 2010 and 2011 the Directorate General of Nursing Affairs for the Ministry of Health continued to gather information to support the development of advanced nursing capacity by utilizing techniques that engaged key stakeholders from service, education, and professional regulation. The discussions were supplemented by a review of relevant international literature. The results of these analyses and discussions continued to demonstrate support for the introduction of ANP. In 2012, another follow-up visit by two WHO consultants took place. The aim of this visit was to review and analyze previous documents and reports related to ANP and to meet with decision makers, educators, and practice nurses. Two recommendations resulted from the 2012 visit that emphasized actions to develop the APN role and to educate nurses already functioning in an extended capacity in PHC.

In 2016 a further WHO consultancy resulted in development of an "on the job training" (OJT) program for nurses practicing in an extended capacity and in development of the scope and standards of practice, service delivery structure, practice environment, and legal framework for the APN. In July 2016 the first advanced NP educated in a NP program in the United States began practice in Oman. Five more students in U.S. programs are scheduled to return to the country in December and further nurses are expected to enroll in U.S. NP programs. In addition, structure for the OJT training for nurses already working in health centers is planned to begin in 2017. There is long-term interest by the MOH to eventually establish an Omani NP program within the country (M. Al-Maqbali, personal communication, April 7, 2016; M. Schober, site visit, April 2016; S. Al Zadjali, personal communication, July 12, 2016).

Europe: WHO-EURO

The WHO Regional Office in Copenhagen, Denmark, serves the WHO European Region, which comprises 53 countries covering a vast geographical region from the Atlantic to the Pacific oceans. The European Union (EU) within this WHO region is composed of 27 different member states. The APN roles are connected with the historical and societal characteristics of each country.

In July 2016 BREXIT (British exit from the European Union) had just been announced. For the purposes of the chapter, development in the UK will be included with the other countries of Europe and as listed under the WHO designation. Note also that Israel is geographically located in the Middle East; however, when reviewing WHO-designated countries Israel is in the EURO region and as such is included in this section.

The European countries are at different stages in considering or implementing APN roles. The initial development in Europe was noted in 1991; the first NP educational program was introduced in the Royal College of Nurses in the UK (Sheer & Wong, 2008), thus catalyzing the development in the UK. In Ireland, the first "advanced NP" was accredited in 1996, and a career pathway toward ANP was established following a Commission on Nursing in the late 1990s (NCNM, 2005). The Netherlands has a nearly 20-year history with the Dutch version of NP. Other country initiatives are in the early stages, with dramatic growth shown within the past five to ten years. An example of a country in the early stages is Finland, which officially launched their initiative in April 2016, thus demonstrating the range of growth in Europe.

Increasingly, European universities are establishing advanced nursing degree programs at the master's level. For example, the University Medical Center, Groningen in the Netherlands has had a program since 1997 (Donato, 2009) with specialties on managing chronic illness, critical and intensive care, acute care, illness prevention, and psychiatric care. The University of Basel in Switzerland has established a program in the German-speaking part of Switzerland since 2000 with emphasis on managing chronic illness (Sheer & Wong, 2008). In French-speaking Switzerland the University of Lausanne and the University of Applied Sciences and Nursing Science offer a joint master degree. The program educates the nurse as a specialist nursing clinical practitioner that is similar to a CNS role (Schober, 2016).

The European Federation of Nurses (EFN) and Advanced Practice Nursing in Europe

The EFN is the independent voice of more than three million nurses in more than 34 national nurses associations (NNA), regulators, or unions at the European level. In 2011 EFN began to actively support advanced practice nursing following Directive 2005/36/EC that highlighted the need to update and modernize education requirements for nursing in Europe. The result was the strengthening of the nurse education requirements standards and the addition of a set of eight competencies. The EFN was very much involved in the clarification of those competencies, which were presented to the Parliament, council, commission, and stakeholders during a European Parliament roundtable on nurse education in October 2012. Now that Directive 2013/55/EU has been approved, EFN plans to ensure that appropriate changes occur in every member state for three categories of nursing: general care nurse (RN), specialist nurse (SN), and advanced NP (M. Sipilä, personal communication, April 28, 2016).

Finland

Significant social and health-care reform in Finland is providing momentum for the introduction of ANP in the country. The anticipated benefits of the APN roles are consistent with the main aims of the health-care reform: to decrease inequity of social and health services, to facilitate accessible health-care service provision for country populations, and to improve the management of health-care costs.

In Finland the concept of advanced practice nursing has historically not been officially recognized even though there are nurses in PHC and hospital settings who work in roles that have advanced clinical components. Advanced roles for RNs have been developed more systematically since the early 2000s. The first role associated with ANP at this time was that of the CNS. Limited authority to prescribe medicines was introduced in the country in 2010. Even so, the APN is in an early developmental phase in Finland.

A group of experts was selected by the Finnish Nurses Association in 2013 to assess the circumstances for APNs in Finland and to recommend actions for development. With great excitement and anticipation the report was presented in April 2016. In addition to suggesting the two roles of CNS and NP be considered, the report described a clinical career path for nurses in advanced roles. The report recommended:

- Establishing coherent titles for the roles with defined job descriptions
- Making legislative changes relevant to advanced nursing roles
- Establishing appropriate education for nurses to obtain relevant competencies

- Developing wages that are consistent with role responsibilities
- Defining a plan to evaluate the effectiveness of APN roles in the country
- Estimating the number of APNs needed in the country

The significance of these recommendations was highlighted by the presence at the launching event of the Ministry of Culture and Education, Ministry of Social Affairs and Health, the National Supervisory Authority for Welfare and Health, and the president of the Finnish Medical Association. This group of approximately 40 participants held a lively and productive discussion in support of establishing APN roles in the country. The next phase is a seminar when key stakeholders discussed education and implementation of strategies to promote the APN roles (A. Suutaria, personal communication, May 5, 2016).

France

France is facing an increase in health-care needs similar to many other Western countries. Current challenges to the health-care system include an aging population, a significant increase in chronic disease, scarcity of medical services, and emerging absence of medical services in some regions. National strategies are being developed to respond to these challenges, including the introduction of APNs.

As early as 2003 the report *Cooperation of the Health Professions: The Transfer of Tasks and Competencies* (Berland, 2003) listed strategies aimed at addressing the medical scarcity and envisioned the feasibility of the transfer of tasks in the French context. Pilot projects then followed. A series of reports ensued, allowing the *Haute Autorité de Santé* (HAS), the French authority for health, to formulate recommendations in 2008 (HAS, 2008). **Table 5.3** lists strategies for the adaptation of health-care services to compensate for challenges associated with implementing APN roles.

Two leading health organizations, HAS and *Observatoire National De La Demographie Des Professions De Santé* (ONDPS), appointed by the MOH in 2007, formed a working group to explore future education for NPs, or *infirmiere cliniciennes,* and to generate recommendations. They examined how roles of health-care professionals may be redefined through the transfer of tasks and competencies from MD to RN to allied health professional (AHP) with a

TABLE 5.3

Steps in Development of Advanced Practice Nursing in France

Year	Steps
1990s	Introduction of CNSs in the French context
2003	Berland Report: Consideration of task transfer between medical and nonmedical health professionals
2004	First trials aiming to transfer medical activities to nonmedical health professionals (five pilot projects)
2006	Second trials (10 new pilot projects and three renewed projects)
2007	Reports from a group of experts as to the modification of the fields of health professional competencies (focus: economic, legal, formation) of the *Haute Autorité de Santé* (HAS)
2007 (May/December)	Public consultation of the HAS, aiming to determine the functions between health professionals (334 testimonies)
2008	Recommendations of the HAS in the matter of the new cooperation between health professionals Mission: Reflection around the sharing of tasks and the competencies between health professionals (report not circulated)
2009	Adoption of the law for the patient health territories hospitals, introducing the new cooperation between health professionals (article 51 and application texts), launching of the first master's of science in clinical nursing intended for the education of APNs *(EHESP/Université de la Méditerranée)*
2011	Report related to midlevel professionals
2016	A new public health law officially introduces advanced practice for nurses and APNs Implementation of this law is still to come

Source: C. Debout, personal communication, June 17, 2016.

view of improving care and adapting interventions to actual health-care demands (HAS, 2007). Preceding the formation of this working group, five tentative projects to implement new task allocation between MDs, RNs, and AHPs in dissimilar areas of the country had been completed. Ten additional projects concerning role redefinition followed (C. Debout, personal communication, June 17, 2016).

Historically, although French nurses did acquire increased autonomy in 1978, they are still not considered a point of entry into the health-care system. Private practice nurses in contract with the French health insurance system *(infirmières liberales)* depend on a medical order to deliver professional nursing care. Recognizing that the current arrangement of the health-care workforce will be inadequate to respond to future health-care needs, the health authorities considered alternatives that included implementation of APN roles. Capitalizing on this situation, the French nurses association (ANFIIDE) conducted a

public information campaign on ANP, targeting nurses, authorities, and the public.

New cooperation: A model of substitution between MDs, RNs, and AHPS. The law *"Hôpitaux-Patients-Santé-Territoires,"* voted in 2009, authorizes in a local way and by name more flexibility in the competencies of the medical and nonmedical health professions while introducing the concept of "new cooperation" (Article 51, 2009). See **Figure 5.1.**

Although the question of transfer of activities of the medical profession toward the paramedical professions feeds the public debate, it is important to note that France is undecided about several structuring models. New cooperation, intermediary professions, and APNs are three concepts that coexist currently in discussions and reports without succeeding to be stable in France semantics and thus remain problematic. This lack of conceptual clarity generates a lot of confusion. Although the validation of a

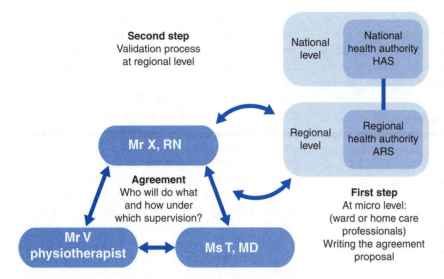

Second step
Validation process
at regional level

National level

National health authority HAS

Regional level

Regional health authority ARS

Agreement
Who will do what
and how under
which supervision?

Mr X, RN

Mr V physiotherapist

Ms T, MD

First step
At micro level:
(ward or home care
professionals)
Writing the agreement
proposal

FIGURE 5.1 Visualizing the concept of "new cooperation" in the French law, "Hôpitaux-Patients-Santé-Territoires."

protocol of cooperation imposes on the "delegated" nurse to combine required competencies to implement the designated activities, no qualifying education is required currently from a regulatory perspective.

The processes of revision of the diplomas of specialties certified by the Ministry of Health. The Ministry of Health engaged in a vast project aimed at revising the competencies and the education programs for three clinical specialty diplomas that it currently certifies: pediatric nurse, operating room nurse, and nurse anesthesiologist. This project is in line with the vast reformation of nursing education that seeks reconciliation with the university-based model coming from the Bologne agreements.

Initially, this project will develop a competence framework for every function from a descriptive and retrospective analysis of the activities of the professionals in these positions. The intent is to adopt a long-term approach that anticipates the evolution of the functions and activities of the professions wherein they address the health needs of the public. Leaders representing the professional specialty organizations requested that the specialties be viewed as advanced practice and that the recommendations developed by this network guide the revision of both education and practice (regulations, design of master's education, definition of autonomy). The negotiations related to the various points of view are in process, and decisions are still to come (C. Debout, personal communication, June 17, 2016).

Toward intermediary professions. A report relating to the new intermediary-level health professions, published in 2011, defines the characteristics of the APN in France (Henard et al, 2011).

A master of science in clinical nursing. The first master in science for clinical nursing was launched in 2009 jointly by the department of nursing science and AHP science section of *l'Ecole de Hautes Etudes en Santé Publique* (EHESP) and Aix-Marseille *Université* (faculty of medicine). In 2014, the department of nursing science of EHESP ended its activities because of budget restrictions; as of June 2016 this program was only implemented by Aix-Marseille *Université*. This program, a forerunner in France in the domain of the education of APNs, rests on a vision of advanced practice nursing in the international context but specific to France. When the Ministry of Higher Education approved this program, the Ministry of Health strongly supported this initiative. Currently three specialties are proposed: oncology, gerontology, and coordinator of complex health-care conditions. A second program was launched at the University of Versailles-Saint Quentin en Yvelines (school of medicine) offering three specialties: psychiatry and mental health, palliative care and pain control, and chronic diseases.

Many French universities had projects to develop similar programs in different parts of the country; however, as of 2017, the Ministry of Higher Education was opposed to giving approval to new programs in this field. The French government elected in 2012, especially the Ministry of Health, was not supportive of these projects. As a consequence, many graduates from the two earlier programs had difficulties using the competencies developed in the master's program because of a lack of implementation at the national and local level.

Unresolved issues. When examining the position of France, key words such as *protected title, qualifying education,* and *specific regulations* often associated with the APN roles are not yet observable. The methodology in the framework for the protocols of cooperation, while showing a response to local needs, makes development of national competencies difficult. No national directive existed in relation to this until January 2016. A national position to stabilize the APN concept and a defined regulatory process, including both education and practice, was urgently needed.

In January 2016, a new public health law was voted on by the French Parliament to modernize the healthcare system. In this law, one article introduces advanced practice for nurses and AHPs. The title of *advanced practitioner* will be protected. To practice as an APN an additional qualification will be required; however, the law does not specify whether this qualification will be at a master's level. APN practice will be regulated. Regarding their scope of practice, physicians in the hospital or in the community will strictly supervise them. The APN will have prescriptive authority but more as a supplementary prescriber rather than prescribing independently. As of June 2016 this article was still waiting implementation (C. Debout, personal communication, June 17, 2016).

Germany

As with other countries in Europe, Germany is emerging as a country in the early stages of ANP development. Evidence of this enthusiasm and progress was demonstrated in Munich in 2015 at the Third ANP/APN Congress for German-speaking countries. Delegates from Austria, Germany, and Switzerland represented German-speaking countries with an additional presence from Canada, Ireland, the Netherlands, and the United States.

The stimulus for ANP development in Germany is attributed to the expert group Sachverständigenrat zur Begutachtung der Entwicklung im Gesundheitssystem that recommended that nurses should widen their scope of practice (SVR Gesundheit, 2007). Additional support from key stakeholders representing nursing and higher education institutions paved the way for ANP developments across the country (Jeschke, 2010; Ullmann & Lehwaldt, 2013; Ullmann et al, 2011). According to Ullmann and Lehwaldt (2013) there are few master's level programs available across Germany that educate nurses for roles in advanced practice. Nurses with advanced clinical competencies in Germany commonly obtain these skills in other countries such as Ireland or those of the UK that have a longer history of ANP. Examples of programs based in Germany are at the University of Applied Sciences, Frankfurt am Main with an ANP master's program established in 2010 and the "Clinical Masters Programme at Hochschule für Angewandte Wissenschaften" in Hamburg established in 2013.

There is no legislation in place to award and protect the APN. The title *Pflegeexpertin APN,* which translated into English means "nursing expert APN," has been suggested for Germany (Ullmann et al, 2011). A legislative framework that formalizes a system for title protection, licensure, registration, and credentialing is needed. Without legislation to protect the title, as of July 2016, there is no consensus as to necessary roles and responsibilities that go with this title. Therefore, ANP in Germany seems to be developing from the bottom up as suggested by Teigeler (2015) who reported on 17 APNs who practice at a university hospital in south Germany. Hospital administrators are supportive of these APNs who work in direct patient care.

Deutsches Netzwerk APN & ANP g.e.V. was formed to offer nurses, institutions, and others with an interest in developing advanced nursing roles ongoing support. The activities facilitated by the Netzwerk include periodic international congresses, expert workshops, and an ANP/APN publication. With a goal to facilitate discussion and political debate, it is hoped that the necessary structures for ANP in Germany will continue to evolve and progress (D. Lehwaldt & P. Ullmann, personal communication, April 27, 2016).

Ireland

A Commission on Nursing in Ireland in 1998 acknowledged the need to provide a career pathway for nurses and midwives who wanted to remain in clinical practice and progress from entry level to clinical specialization linked to advanced practice. Subsequently, the National Council for the Professional Development of Nursing and

Midwifery (NCNM, 2001) provided a framework for the establishment of ANP and advanced midwife practitioner (AMP) roles and posts. This decision was a response to the national and international development of advanced practice in nursing and midwifery. Since these early efforts, research in Ireland has convincingly demonstrated that ANPs and AMPs provide quality care, improve health-care outcomes, and offer care that is acceptable to patients and cost neutral (Begley et al, 2010).

In 2011, once the NCNM was dissolved, the Nurses Act of 2011 provided for a distinct division for registered advanced nurse practitioners (RANPs). RANPs are now registered with the Nursing and Midwifery Board of Ireland (NMBI [Bord Altranais agus Cnaimhseachais na hEireann]). An applicant's portfolio must link the job description of the post or location site to the qualifications of the person seeking registration as an ANP. There must be clear evidence that the person who is applying for registration either as an ANP or AMP has the expertise, advanced knowledge and clinical skills, advanced clinical decision-making capabilities, leadership skills, research skills, and clinical wisdom to fulfill the advanced practice role. A master's degree (or higher) is required with evidence that reflects experience and preparation in a specialist area of practice (http://www.nmbi.ie/). As of May 31, 2016, NMBI reported there were 183 RANPs and 7 RAMWs in the country.

Updated Standards and Requirements for Advanced Practice (Nursing) and *Standards and Requirements Advanced Practice (Midwifery),* based on an interim report (WGAP, 2014), are due for publication later in 2017. In advance of these modifications, NMBI has made several changes: A new interim revalidation process has been established, all advanced practice forms have been reviewed and updated, updated guidelines for advanced practice portfolios have been developed, and updated information was developed in relation to advance practice posts. It is anticipated that the new guidelines will provide a more flexible structure for matching the RANP/RAMW candidate/applicant with the post or location site for practice (K. Brennan, personal communication, May 15, 2016).

The Irish Association of Advanced Nurse and Midwife Practitioners (IAANMP) was established in 2004 to provide a forum to support persons interested in promotion and development of ANP and AMP in Ireland. The association aims to support nurses practicing at advanced levels, provide a forum to debate issues and concerns, promote professional development, and link to other international organizations (http://www.iaanmp.ie).

Israel

As of July 2016 there was no nurse practice act (NPA) in Israel. All nurses practice under a clause of the Physician Practice Act passed during the establishment of the state in 1947 and revised in 1976. Therefore, the scope of nursing practice is not specifically defined by law but by executive order of the Ministry of Health and by institutional policies. The Division of Nursing within the Ministry of Health registers nurses who have successfully completed a course of study and have passed a qualifying examination. There are registries for licensed practical nurses, registered, postbasic nursing certification, and APNs (Ministry of Health, 2016b).

The introduction of APN occurred in 2009 by an executive order identifying the role of nurse specialist in palliative care (Ministry of Health, 2009). Requirements for the role are a baccalaureate and master's degree (where at least one degree is in nursing), postbasic certification in oncology or geriatrics, an advanced palliative care course, and successful completion of a theoretical and clinical examination. Thirty-five nurses with experience in palliative care and postbasic certification were grandfathered in as specialists (Ministry of Health, 2016a).

The role of geriatric nurse specialist was introduced in 2011. In 2013, the Ministry of Health published an executive order standardizing the specialist role within the health-care system (Ministry of Health, 2013) that not only defines the requirements for the role but also provides the scope of practice. Since 2013, additional specialist roles have been introduced and other specialties are in the planning phases (Ministry of Health, 2016a). As of July 2017, one geriatric specialist course is available that has graduated 19 nurses who are registered as geriatric nurse specialists.

The changes in Israel are positive and dynamic; however, qualified nurse specialists continue to work as staff nurses and not to the full extent of their scope of practice. In addition, education is usually not provided within an academic structure. In spite of this and a shortage of nurses in the country, development of the advanced practice role is progressing (F. DeKeyser Ganz, personal communication, May 4, 2016).

Netherlands

In the Netherlands the Dutch title that is used for the advanced nursing role is *nurse specialist* (NS). The concept of NP caught the attention of decision makers in the country nearly 20 years ago, but the words *nurse practitioner* could not be translated into the Dutch language. Since 1997, when the idea was introduced, there have been great strides in development in the country. Progress during the period 1997 to 2016 is because of multiple factors, but particularly support from the Dutch government.

In 2004 grants and supportive salaries were made available by the government for those nurses wanting to undertake advanced study. This plan was organized in collaboration with health-care institutions that took on the role of employer during the time the nurse was a NS student. In 2009 legislation was developed to guarantee the quality of education and work for the NS. The professional regulations provided title protection and stipulated standards for education, registration, and practice. In 2011 additional legislation expanded the authority for scope of practice for the NS with scope of practice and authority closely linked to the practice specialty chosen by the NS.

As of February 2016, approximately 2,750 NSs have been educated and registered in the country. Ten universities of applied sciences in the Netherlands offer a NS education program. In close collaboration, the universities have developed a competency-based program intended to be consistent across all universities in the Netherlands.

The shortage of physicians that prompted the introduction of NS roles in the Netherlands has been resolved, but the numbers of NSs continue to increase. At one point it was thought that the introduction of PAs would threaten NS development, but this has not been the case. The NS in the Netherlands has been accepted as a professional that provides high-quality care and friendly advice (J. Peters, personal communication, February 17, 2016).

Sweden

Sweden introduced the concept of advanced nursing roles as a strategy to improve access to PHC, especially care of the elderly in the community. Educational programs have been established with these clinical foci in mind. The title used in Sweden is *advanced clinical nurse specialist* (ACNS) (Lindblad et al, 2010).

In Skaraborg, the PHC authorities worked with the University of Skovde to develop a model and educational program that met the requirements of the National Board of Health and Welfare. The primary consideration was PHC for the community and care of the elderly with the ACNS as the vehicle to address these needs. The initial batch of students enrolled in 2003 faced challenges to introduce a new nursing role that fits the Swedish health-care system and is acceptable to all stakeholders. In the process, a definition for the ANP was negotiated (Schober & Affara, 2006, p. 6):

> An Advanced Nurse Practitioner in Primary Health Care is a registered nurse with special education as a district nurse with the right to prescribe certain drugs, and with a post graduate education that enables [the advanced nurse practitioner] an increased and deepened competence to be independently responsible for medical decisions, prescribing of drugs and treatment of health problems within a certain area of health care.

Prescriptive authority for nurses in Sweden has been in place since 1994, before the consideration and development of an ANP. Literature reveals that although there is interest in the idea of advanced nursing, demarcation of the role relative to physicians and appropriate integration of advanced practice nursing into the health-care workforce remains unclear (Jangland et al, 2014; Lindblad et al, 2010).

Switzerland

Advanced nursing practice was introduced in 2000 in Switzerland with the first master of science in nursing program at the Institute of Nursing Science (INS) at the University of Basel, Switzerland. A shift to master's level prepared nurses in clinical specialist roles and development of master's degrees at other academic institutions from 2004 further encouraged the introduction of APN roles in a variety of clinical settings.

A Swiss definition for ANP, based on the ICN definition, was announced in 2012. The definition was the result of a collaborative effort by the Swiss Nursing Association, the Swiss Association for Nursing Science, SwissANP, and the University Institute for Nursing Education and Research in Lausanne. Research on ANP in Switzerland has been conducted (Kambli et al, 2015; Müller-Staub et al, 2015;

Serena et al, 2015) and a framework for role evaluation has been developed (Bryant-Lukosios et al, 2016). In spite of this progress, APN roles are not yet legally protected or formally credentialed as of July 2017. Legislation to regulate health-care professions at the bachelor's and master's level for the entire country is in progress. There is interest to develop a legal framework for ANP (K. Fierz, personal communication, May 18, 2016).

The INS at the University of Basel has had a leading role in promoting the view of ANP education and role development in the German-speaking world, not only for Switzerland but also for other German-speaking countries. From French-speaking Switzerland there is early development in Lausanne for a specialist nursing clinical practitioner. As of July 2016, the University of Lausanne (http://www .unil.ch/index.html) and the University of Applied Sciences Western Switzerland (http://www.hes-so.ch/) offer a joint master of science in nursing sciences for this APN role.

United Kingdom (England, Northern Ireland, Scotland, and Wales)

The four countries of the UK (England, Northern Ireland, Scotland, and Wales) are developing ANP in different ways. The emergence of the NP movement in the UK has been described as a response to the changing demands within health-care systems and acknowledgment that the traditional medical model alone is not sufficient to provide comprehensive health care for community populations (White, 2001). A reduction in doctors' hours and an overall shortage of general practitioners in some areas accelerated the move toward NPs in acute and primary care settings. In addition, government-initiated pilot programs to address the needs of special groups, such as refugees, the homeless, the mentally ill, traveling families, and the elderly, increased the use of NPs and provision of services in a range of settings.

The NP degree program, originally developed by the Royal College of Nursing (RCN) in 1990, formed the basis for RCN accreditation of NP programs. In 2002 the first graduates from the RCN program celebrated their 10th anniversary. The initial 15 graduates paved the way for NPs now practicing throughout the UK (RCN, 2008). Different pathways of NP preparation still exist, ranging from a generic approach to a growing tendency to establish academic preparation at the master's degree level. As demand for NPs and APNs has increased, the number of universities providing such programs has escalated.

In November 2001, a decade after the first RCN NP course had begun, the inaugural meeting of the UK National Organization of Nurse Practitioner Faculties (NONPF) took place. Membership slowly increased and led to the establishment of a formal link with the national RCN Nurse Practitioner Association. In 2005, UK NONPF changed its name to the Association of Advanced Nursing Practice Educators (AANPE) and was formally re-launched as a new independent association. Since that time, AANPE participated in professional, regional, and country-specific advanced practice discussions, consultations, and policy development across the UK. In 2015, the association renamed itself as the Association of Advanced Practice Educators (AAPE UK) to reflect the growth and maturity of advanced practice in a broad multi-professional context in the UK.

Despite all the energy, dynamics, and growth in the UK, regulation of NP practice has not yet been established for NPs in the UK. The term *advanced NP* has been adopted by many NPs and is now the preferred term. A proposal to formalize and legally protect the NP role at the national level was scrutinized by the Department of Health and the Council for Healthcare Regulatory Excellence (CHRE, 2010). It was concluded that there was insufficient grounds for additional regulation for NPs who were already registered as nurses. Despite this, debate on the need for regulation of ANP continues (K. Maclaine, personal communication, February 15, 2016).

Southeast Asia: WHO-SEARO

The WHO South East Asia Region (SEAR) has 11 member states: Bangladesh, Bhutan, Democratic People's Republic of Korea, India, Indonesia, Maldives, Myanmar, Nepal, Sri Lanka, Thailand, and Timor-Leste. This section provides one example of APN development in the region.

Thailand

The Thailand Nursing and Midwifery Council (TNMC) adopted the ANP concept in 1998, and in 2003 the first group of 49 APNs was certified and awarded the title APN. The TNMC defines the APN as a RN with a master's degree who is qualified according to criteria set by the TNMC. The TNMC creates rules specifying which professional nursing organization certifications can be accepted for APNs and sets requirements for education, training, and experience. Terms accepted as advanced practice nursing include certified nurse-midwife (CNM), certified registered nurse anesthetist (CRNA), CNS, and NP. APNs work in one of ten specialist areas: medical/surgical, pediatrics, maternal/child, community care, elderly care, psychiatric, NP, midwifery, infection control, or anesthesia (P. Buaklee, personal communication, June 20, 2016).

In response to an urgent need for community health-care services, the country identified short- and long-term goals to offer 4-month education programs for general NPs to work in the community as primary care providers. Even though one of the first postbasic NP programs was established in the 1970s, it was health-care reform and the drive for a universal health-care coverage system, implemented in the country in 2002, that accelerated the development of NP educational programs. To identify the strategic approach of NP education Hanucharurnkul and colleagues (2007) conducted a study that explored characteristics and work settings of 1,928 NPs and provided a picture of those certified by the TNMC. Strategies derived from this study are as follows:

- Extend within 5 years the entry-level education to a master's level by acknowledging the 4-month programs that were originally initiated to respond to PHC needs of the country.
- Establish NP positions in the health-care system such that when APNs are master's graduates and certified, they are eligible for the title of APN/MN and have an associated increase in salary.

Results of a study on role development in Thailand conducted by Wongkpratoom and colleagues (2010) revealed that even though a certified APN role was functioning to some degree in the country, most APNs only occasionally served in an advanced practice capacity because of various organization, human, and resource issues. Major facilitators include supportive organizational policies, quality nurse administrators, well-functioning multidisciplinary teams, and financial resources. Conversely, study findings revealed that barriers included lack of a clearly delineated organizational structure and unclear organizational policies, poor administrative support for the APN (work assignments were not reflective of advanced nursing practice), and uncooperative team members. Study findings confirm

the complexities of role development and implementation when proceeding with the APN concept.

As of July 2016, there were two types of NP programs. The master's degree requires 42 credits to achieve APN accreditation and usually requires approximately 2 years of education. The curriculum is concentrated on an advanced graduate certificate designed for APNs. The second type of NP program involves specializing as a NP (primary medical care), which is a short course with 18 credits and a 4-month period of study (P. Buaklee, personal communication, June 20, 2016). To facilitate development, the Thai Bureau of Nursing recommended that the PEPPA framework developed by Canadian researchers Bryant-Lukosius and DiCenso (2004) be used as a guide for the introduction and evaluation of APN roles for further development in the country (Sathira-Angkura & Khwansatapornkoon, 2014).

Western Pacific: WHO-WPRO

The WHO Regional Office for the Western Pacific (WPR) is located in Manila, the Philippines, and represents 37 countries and areas in the Asia Pacific. The region stretches from the People's Republic of China in the north and west to New Zealand in the south to French Polynesia in the east. As one of the most diverse of the WHO regions, the WPR constitutes some of the world's least developed countries as well as the most rapidly emerging economies. It includes highly developed countries such as Australia, Japan, New Zealand, the Republic of Korea, and Singapore, as well as fast growing economies such as the People's Republic of China and Vietnam.

Australia

Australia first considered the development of NP roles in 1990 (Offredy, 1999). Pilot projects were conducted first in New South Wales (NSW) and then in most other states and territories of Australia. The results from the initial projects found that NPs are feasible, safe, and effective in their ability to provide high-quality health-care services in a range of settings (Gardner & Gardner, 2005; NSW Health Department, 1998).

In Australia, the NP title is protected and only nurses who have been authorized by the National Nursing and Midwifery Registration Board of the Australian Health Practitioner Regulation Agency may use the NP title.

A study by Gardner, Dunn et al (2006) recommended the master's degree as the required educational preparation for the role from two perspectives. Study findings suggested that a master's education is needed to meet the demands of the role and to also provide necessary credibility with the community and other health-care disciplines regarding the professional standing of these clinicians. The national registration board adopted this recommendation and mandates that a master's specifically for the NP is the minimal level of education required to practice.

The Nursing and Midwifery Board of Australia has two pathways for nurses to fulfill their educational requirements at the master's level for endorsement as an NP:

1. Successfully complete a board-approved NP program of study at the master's level
2. Complete a program of study at the master's level that is clinically relevant to the nurses' context of advanced practice nursing for which they are seeking endorsement as a NP and complete supplementary education that demonstrates equivalence and meets the national competency standards for a NP

Having the two educational pathways provides flexibility for nurses to choose an educational program that best meets their individual learning needs.

The Mutual Recognition Act of 1992 and the Trans Tasman Mutual Recognition Act of 1999 recognize nurses educated in all states of Australia and those educated in New Zealand regardless of differences within programs. In 2004, the Australian Nursing and Midwifery Council (ANMC) in conjunction with the Nursing Council of New Zealand commissioned a project to develop competency standards for the NP to further ensure delivery of safe and competent care (Gardner, Dunn et al, 2006). These competency standards were used to assess NPs educated overseas and by the Australian Nursing and Midwifery Accreditation Council (ANMAC, 2010) for accrediting universities and NP master's programs.

In 2014, the NP competency standards were reviewed and the following four standards were implemented:

- Assesses and uses diagnostic capabilities.
- Plans care and engages others.
- Prescribes and implements therapeutic interventions.
- Evaluates outcomes and improves practice.

As of September 2015, there were 1,287 endorsed NPs in Australia comprising a small but increasing component of the 261,582 nurses in the workforce (Schober, 2016). A study conducted in 2010 (Gardner et al, 2010) found that two-thirds of NPs in Australia reported their role was "extremely limited" because of a difference between state and federal governmental laws. These results were similar to those from an earlier survey undertaken in 2009 (Gardner et al, 2009). Until late 2010, NPs were able to write prescriptions and refer patients to other health-care professionals at a state level; however, at a federal level, NPs did not have access to the pharmaceutical benefits scheme (PBS) or the Medicare benefits schedule (MBS). Therefore, patients paid a premium when their prescriptions were filled at a pharmacy or when they had pathology tests undertaken. This situation placed patients at a disadvantage because they did not have equal access to government subsidies for health care. In November 2010, national legislation was enacted to enable NPs to obtain provider numbers, potentially reducing costs to patients. As of July 2017 this legislation is primarily limited to NPs in private practice.

In Australia, NPs are steadily being introduced throughout the country while continuing to face country-specific challenges. The Australian College of Nurse Practitioners (http://www.acnp.org.au/) has been established to provide a representative voice for NP role development in Australia (A. Green, personal communication, July 22, 2016).

Brunei Darussalam

The Nursing Services Department, Ministry of Health, Brunei Darussalam is proceeding forward in exploring ANP for the nurses in Brunei and for the health-care services in the country. To motivate the nurses and provide a strategic action plan to the MOH, a workshop and symposium were held in July 2011 to gain an understanding of ANP as an option for the future of the public. A resolution and recommendations were presented to the MOH for development of a nursing career pathway for clinical practice along with organization of a task force to promulgate criteria, standards, and regulations for ANP. Debate has been focused around alignment of NP roles with nurse-midwives under the ANP umbrella, as well as clarification of where the specialist nurse fits in the future scheme for Brunei Darussalam (M. Schober, site visit, July 2, 2011).

The MOH of Brunei, with the intent to strengthen the implementation of the registration of nurses into the Nursing Board for Brunei (NBB) and heighten the monitoring of nursing practices in the country, announced the Nurses Registration Act (Amendment) 2014. The amended Nurses Registration Regulations 2014 and Nurses Registration (Committee) Regulations 2014 were enforced in March 2014. The MOH highlighted that the new amendments in the act will protect the safety of nursing services and hoped that with the new nursing service scheme local nurses will reach the level of NP. As of July 2017 it remains unclear as to whether this role has become part of the health-care workforce in the country.

Hong Kong, China

Hong Kong has been pursuing the concept of the APN for many years while facing complicated governmental, clinical, and academic challenges. The Hospital Authority of Hong Kong, eager to motivate nurses to remain in clinical practice, introduced the NS position in 1994. As of 2014 a clear clinical pathway for nurses developing as a specialty with the APN title was available. Once a nurse has achieved APN status within the Hospital Authority System the next progression along the career path is as a nurse consultant.

Advanced practice nursing education is at the postgraduate level with APNs running more than 100 independent nurse clinics in Hong Kong. *The Hospital Authority Annual Report 2011–2013* indicated that there were 2,700 APNs and 70 nurse consultants. Nurses in Hong Kong endeavor to establish a statutory body to regulate ANP, with the Provisional Hong Kong Academy of Nursing set up in 2011 for this purpose (Wong, 2014).

Islands of the WPR (Fiji, Guam, Northern Mariana Islands, and Samoa)

NPs and other midlevel practitioners have provided health-care services for the populations of the Pacific Island countries for more than 20 years. The rural and remote nature of this region and a shortage of physicians encouraged governments to explore the most appropriate models to provide comprehensive health-care services. Demographics help determine the best approach for the Pacific Islands in initiating education and practice guidelines for NPs. Reasons for educating nurses for NP roles in

the Pacific Islands include the following (WHO-Western Pacific Region [WPRO], 2001):

- Nurses are already present in the workforce of most countries and usually comprise the largest category of health professionals.
- Nurses are currently living and working in underserved areas.
- Nurses are providing a wide range of preventive and curative services.
- Nurses are considered to be an adaptable, multitalented resource of the workforce.

Strategies recommended by WHO-WPR for developing and sustaining a midlevel practitioner workforce include the following (WHO-WPR, 2001):

- Legal protection
- Standard treatment guidelines
- Ongoing clinical supervision
- Continuing education
- Career structure or career ladder

Fiji

Fiji is made up of more than 300 islands, with more than 60% of the population living in rural or remote settings. Through an arrangement of health centers and nursing stations, authorities have attempted to address health-care challenges by providing preventive and PHC services supported by subdivisional and referral hospitals.

Staffing of facilities has been a major problem, especially in rural and remote areas. In response to this difficulty, an NP program was developed in 1988 and taught by staff within the then Fiji School of Nursing (FSN). In 2010 the school merged with the Fiji School of Medicine to form the College of Medicine, Nursing and Health Sciences within the Fiji National University. The NP program is now delivered as a two-semester, 13-month postgraduate diploma in nursing practice as a NP.

The program has a regional orientation and students are accepted from other islands in the WPR. In 2011, the Fiji government passed Nursing Decree 2011 that provided the legal framework for the establishment of the new Fiji Nursing Council to take over responsibilities from the Nurses, Midwives and Nurse Practitioner Board. Annual registration is now required by all NPs in Fiji (as well as student nurses, midwives, RNs, and specialist nurses) and evidence of annual engagement in relevant continuing professional development (CPD) activities is now expected.

NPs in Fiji have an established scope of practice and work under published protocols, allowing them prescriptive privileges. The Ministry of Health employs most NPs with postings for positions listed by the Public Service Commission. These nurses have been widely accepted by communities and other health-care providers. There is strong support from the directors of health services to continue the education program. Access to continuing education, an identified career pathway, and opportunities for locum relief are among the challenges facing NPs in Fiji (D. Lindsay, personal communication, June 30, 2016).

Guam

Guam is a 210-square-mile tropical island located 3,950 miles from Hawaii. Although Guam is a U.S. territory, it is in the WHO-WPR. It is designated as a rural area based on its population density.

Guam has one public hospital, the Guam Memorial Hospital (GMA); the Guam Naval Hospital (GNH); and the new private hospital, Guam Regional Medical Center (GRMC). There is a shortage of health-care professionals on the island, and Guam struggles to provide health care to the uninsured and those who receive public assistance for an estimated population of about 168,000.

The Guam Board of Nurse Examiners (GBNE) is a regulatory body of nurses appointed by the governor. A NP serves as the chair of the GBNE. The administrative rules of the Board of Nursing NPA were most recently revised and signed into law May 7, 2008 (Public Law 29-71). Article 5 includes the rules for an advanced practice registered nurse (APRN). An APRN is defined as a RN who is authorized by the board to perform ANP as a certified nurse practitioner (CNP), CNM, CRNA, or CNS.

Scope of practice for APRNs is in accordance with the functions and standards of the respective national certifying organization for each category. All APRNs in Guam are required to practice in accordance with protocols developed in collaboration with and signed by a physician licensed to practice in Guam. The board must approve a collaborative agreement between the APRN and physician. The collaborating physician provides consultation and agrees to periodic review of the services being provided by the APRN. The agreement must include a written protocol to be used by the APRN for the management of patients and for the referral of cases and the procedure for an alternative collaborating physician. Periodic review of the agreement must be done during the first year after signing the agreement and then every 6 months thereafter. If the collaborative agreement is terminated, either by the physician or the APRN, the APRN must inform the board in writing within 3 working days, and the license issued to the APRN will immediately terminate.

APRNs with a current license may apply for prescribing authority and must submit documentation of successful completion of advanced pharmacology coursework. In addition, the APRN must provide evidence of a minimum of 1,000 hours of practice as an APRN before application for prescriptive authority. The 1,000 hours must include clinical hours completed and verified by the collaborative physician within the past 24 months. When approved, a new APRN license card is issued indicating the qualification for prescriptive authority. Prescribing stipulations include legend drugs, diagnostic studies, and therapeutic devices as outlined in the protocols section. Controlled substances (Schedule II–V), defined by federal controlled substances lists, will be prescribed and administered or ordered as established in the protocols, provided that the APRN has an assigned DEA registration number.

The Guam NPA revisions are modeled after the National Council of the State Boards of Nursing (NCSBN) NPA in the United States. The NPA committee is working on revising the Guam NPA under the Guam Nurses Association (GNA) and the Guam Association of Advanced Practice Registered Nurses (GAAPRN). It is moving forward and hopes to be the next jurisdiction with full practice authority and APRN regulation with the major elements of the U.S. Consensus Model. There are several professional organizations that support APNs in Guam including the GAAPN, GNA, the Asian American/Pacific Islander Nurses Association, and the American Pacific Nursing Leaders Council.

Guam has been fortunate to have a strong relationship with three representatives of the American Association of Nurse Practitioners (AANP). All are dedicated to increasing access to high-quality health care for Guam's population. These three have made significant contributions as NPs in Guam and provide constructive energy to facilitate APRN practice in Guam and the Pacific Territory. Guam's nurses are very dedicated to their rural population's health care. They are cohesive, belong to the GNA, and meet in professional conferences twice yearly.

Men and women from Guam serve in the U.S. Army reserves. When not serving overseas in active duty or deployments, these veterans receive health care from the VA Clinic located in Guam. As of July 2016 there are two physicians, one psychiatrist, and one NP in addition to RNs, LPNs, and health technicians. Psychiatrists and APRNs from the United States have also served there for short periods because recruitment is a continual challenge.

The University of Hawaii School of Nursing (UHSON) and Veterans Administration (VA) in Hawaii collaborated on an interprofessional training opportunity at three rural VA sites: AMS, Guam, and Hilo, Hawaii. These sites were chosen because of the rural isolation and challenge of recruiting skilled and culturally competent health-care professionals. The goal is that they will ultimately choose to serve in these locations. The DNP program director from UHSON and the director of education at Hawaii VA collaborated to implement this grant program. The initial Rural Health Training Initiative (RHTI) grant was written as a 3-year pilot project that began in 2013. The UHSON sent students to Guam all 3 years (2013–2015) with a total of three students. The grant was renewed in 2016 with plans to send more students.

Interest in APN in Guam is increasing. In 2010 there were only a handful of APRNs including two to three NPs. As of July 2016 seven NP students were enrolled in a distance education program in Guam, but they faced a real challenge because of a limited number of preceptors. The GRMC has five NPs working in their emergency department. The GMH is now considering changing their hospital regulation to potentially hire NP hospitalists. There are six NPs at the GNH. Several NPs work at Guam Public Health and one in the Veterans Administration Clinic (L. Lorenzo, personal communication, July 29, 2016).

Northern Mariana Islands

The Northern Mariana Islands, officially the Commonwealth of the Northern Mariana Islands (CNMI), are located in the northwestern Pacific Ocean. CNMI is one of two U.S. territories with commonwealth status (the other being Puerto Rico). According to the 2010 census 53,883 people were living in the CNMI with the majority of the population living on Saipan, Tinian, and Rota.

The Commonwealth Health Center (CHC) on the island of Saipan is the only provider of comprehensive health-care services for the island and includes one hospital in addition to a wide range of public health services. The 86-bed hospital is staffed with three NPs, one CNM, and four midwives. Rota and Tinian also have health centers that are part of the CHC. A NP, one of 31 health center personnel on Tinian, has been the only medical provider for more than 10 years.

The CNMI Board of Nurse Examiners is the autonomous public agency known as the Board of Nursing. The governor appoints this regulatory body of nurses. The Administrative Rules of the Board of Nursing (Subchapter 140-60.1), also known as the NPA, were most recently revised and signed into law in May and June 2014. A NP serves on the Board of Nursing and has helped model the NPA for full practice autonomy.

An APN is defined as a RN who is authorized by the board to perform ANP as a CNP, CNM, CRNA, or CNS. Scope of practice is in accordance with the functions and standards of the respective national certifying organizations for each category. Before 2007, many APNs were certificate graduates and were grandfathered into the NPA. Since January 2007, a minimum of a master's degree in nursing is required. Documentation requires verification of graduation and certification in population foci of the education program and qualifications for prescribing. The scope of practice for a NP includes nursing functions as well as advanced assessment, diagnosing, primary care provider status, and admitting privileges for the hospital and other health-care services. NPs are independently responsible and accountable for the continuous and comprehensive management of a broad range of health care. The NPA scope of practice includes prescribing, ordering, dispensing, and administering therapeutic devices including legend drugs and controlled substances (PL 14-62 Section 2304) consistent with the definition of the practitioner's specialty category and scope of practice (L. Lorenzo, personal communication, July 30, 2016).

Samoa

American Samoa (AMS) is the southernmost territory of the United States with a total land area of 76.8 square miles, slightly larger than Washington, DC. The 2010 population of 66,000 qualifies AMS as rural. The health infrastructure consists of one hospital, five PHC centers, and a VA clinic. The U.S. federal match for Medicaid services is capped and the AMS government cannot bear the burden of paying for coverage beyond the match.

AMS Chapter 10 laws include the health services regulatory board, which includes any practice of medicine, dentistry, or nursing. The board is appointed by the governor and composed of the director of health, one physician, the public health officer, the director of nursing services, a medical officer, a dentist, a LPN, and a representative from the AMS community college nursing program. At least 50% of the board, excluding the chairperson, must be American Samoan. The board may carry out its functions through the use of committees that specialize in health services such as nursing, medicine, and pharmacy. The Nursing Committee establishes licensing and treatment, prescription, and other functions in collaboration with a physician or osteopath with established protocols, regulations, and process of licensure.

The practice of "advanced registered nursing" (ARN) means the performance of advanced level nursing actions by a nurse midwife, a NA, or a NP must have certification within the scope of practice and postbasic specialized education, training, and experience. The ARN may perform actions or nursing diagnosis and nursing treatment of alterations of health status. In addition, an ARN may perform actions of medical diagnosis, treatment, prescription, and other functions that are identified by their certification specialty in collaboration with physicians or osteopaths. The collaborating parties may establish by protocol higher levels of collaboration for specific acts or specific circumstances.

American Samoa participated in a 3-year RHTI offered to three sites in the WPR (refer to the section on Guam). A total of nine students from UHSON participated in this project (2013–2015) based in Samoa with plans to send more based on additional funding.

Setting precedence, a native from independent Samoa (Western Samoa) is the first Samoan NP to achieve a PhD in nursing and also earn her DNP. Therefore, she was bestowed the family title of a Fa'amatai (chief). Fa'amatai is the key sociopolitical system of governance and way of life (fa'a Samoa) in Samoan culture. As a faculty member she has served as a preceptor for NP students from the UHSON for the VA RHTI. In addition, she and her students live in AMS villages and serve at the VA clinic providing health-care services. One of the UHSON Samoan students plans to return, after graduation, to establish a NP practice in AMS (L. Lorenzo, personal communication, July 29, 2016).

Japan

An anticipated dramatic increase in the aging population in Japan and a shortage of physicians led faculty at Oita University of Nursing and Health Sciences (OUNHS) in Japan to stress practice-oriented nursing education at the graduate level. The aim of the promotion of academic education was to contribute to a health-care system that can provide patients in Japan with safe and timely opportunities for health care. With this in mind the Graduate School of Oita University established a course in 2008 to educate NPs in its master's program. This was the first such course in Japan, and the March 2011 graduates of the master's program became Japan's first NPs (Fukuda et al, 2014; OUNHS, 2016).

There are two NP majors in the fields of primary care with separate curricula in the Oita University Graduate School: the Geriatrics major, established in 2008, and the Pediatrics major, established in 2009. The objectives of the new majors are to train highly qualified NPs with higher levels of expertise and competence in practice who can contribute to clinical care in medical long-term care facilities in remote areas and work autonomously in collaboration with physicians (OUNHS, 2016). This program development provided momentum to move the government to amend the nurse practice laws. Policy and legal changes are needed to delineate the scope of practice for advanced practice nursing and to provide the foundation for NP education (Fukuda et al, 2014).

In order to support the establishment of a NP system in Japan, the Japanese Nurse Practitioner Association was established in 2008. The aims of the association are to standardize educational programs for NPs, to guarantee the quality of their performance, and to work for social understanding of the title of NP in Japan (OUNHS, 2016).

Following the initiation of the NP course by OUNHS, the university project team also submitted an application in collaboration with Oita Oka Hospital to arrange for a designated administration district system. In the system, NP students and graduates would be allowed to perform some of the designated activities for hospital patients under the supervision of and with physician orders. In addition, in 2013 the Ministry of Health, Labour and Welfare introduced plans for a new education system. The bill for the amendment of the nursing service law had not been changed for 66 years. Legislative discussions commenced in February 2014 with a hope for legal changes (Fukuda et al, 2014).

As of May 2016, there was no official professional designation of NP yet in Japan even though the Japanese Organization of Nurse Practitioner Faculties (JONPF) provided the certifying examination for the graduates from seven NP programs. Nursing and medical societies have opposed the policy and legal changes supportive of advanced practice nursing. Therefore, the activities of graduates from the NP programs depend on the physician in the institution where the graduates work (M. Suzuki, personal communication, May 9, 2016).

New Zealand

ANP was initially recognized in 1988 in New Zealand at two levels. The New Zealand Nurses' Organization's (NZNO) credentialing process certified nurses as nurse-clinicians or nurse consultants (clinical). Once the NP model was introduced in 2000, NZNO phased out and ceased its certification process in 2006 when regulation of NPs came under the jurisdiction of the Nursing Council of New Zealand (NCNZ) (S. Trim, personal communication, March 11, 2008).

A task force established in 1997 studied barriers to nursing practice and recommended the development of an advanced role. The NCNZ then set up a working group to develop a regulatory framework. Following significant consultation, a framework was agreed upon and published (NCNZ, 2001). The framework presented in 2002 and updated in 2014 included standards for the approval of specific master's programs and process for such approval, a title (NP), role competencies, and a description of the role and a process for endorsement (NCNZ, 2014).

The applicant formally applies to the council and must present a portfolio that includes a curriculum vitae, transcript of education preparation, research, publications, and evidence of clinical practice that includes descriptions, case studies, case notes from assessments, and endorsements of practice. The panel interview includes a presentation by the applicant describing relevant clinical practice and a response to panel questions that include clinical vitae and scenario testing (NCNZ, 2014).

The first NP in New Zealand was endorsed in late 2001. Initially title protection was achieved through trademarking; however, the trademarking concept is no longer in place. Before 2015 NPs in New Zealand were required to choose a specific area of practice that was then placed on the register as a condition. Following extensive consultation in 2015 regarding this stipulation, the Nursing Council has recommended changes that broaden the NP scope of practice and remove the requirement that restricts NPs to a specific area of practice. In 2016 a new scope of practice statement was introduced. The new scope of practice follows:

> Nurse practitioners have advanced education, clinical training and the demonstrated competence and legal authority to practice beyond the level of a registered nurse. Nurse practitioners work autonomously and in collaborative teams with other health professionals to promote health, prevent disease, and improve access and population health outcomes for a specific patient group or community. Nurse practitioners manage episodes of care as the lead healthcare provider in partnership with health consumers and their families/whanau. Nurse practitioners combine advanced nursing knowledge and skills with diagnostic reasoning and therapeutic knowledge to provide patient centred healthcare services including the diagnosis and management of health consumers with common and complex health conditions. They provide a wide range of assessment and treatment interventions, ordering and interpreting diagnostic and laboratory tests, prescribing medicines within their area of competence, admitting and discharging from hospital and other healthcare services/settings. As clinical leaders they work across healthcare settings, influence health service delivery and the wider profession. (http://www.nursingcouncil.org .nz/Publications/Consultation-documents/Decision-on-nurse -practitioner-scope-of-practice-and-further-consultation-2015)

NP candidates can focus on a specialty area of practice; however, this designation no longer appears on the register or on their practicing certificate. There will be a transition period to incorporate these changes and issues associated with the role of the Nursing Council of New Zealand's approval of educational programs.

Requirements to become a NP in New Zealand are the following:

- Registration with the Nursing Council of New Zealand (the Council) in the RN scope of practice
- A minimum of 4 years of experience in a specific area of practice
- The completion of an approved clinical master's degree program that includes demonstration of the competencies for advanced practice and prescribing applied within a defined area of practice of the NP. The program must include relevant theory and concurrent practice

- The completion of an equivalent program overseas, a clinically focused master's degree qualification that meets the previously specified requirement
- Passing an assessment against the NP competencies by an approved panel

—(NCNZ, 2014)

Prescriptive authority in New Zealand. The Medicines Amendment Act of 2013 designated NPs as authorized prescribers. The Misuse of Drugs Amendment Regulations of 2014 allow NPs to prescribe controlled drugs within their scope of practice for:

- Up to 1 month's supply for Class A and B controlled drugs
- Up to 3 months' supply for Class C controlled drugs (http://www.nursingcouncil.org.nz/Nurses/Scopes-of-practice/Nurse-practitioner)

Before July 1, 2014, NPs may have been registered without prescribing authority. From July 1, 2014, this group of nonprescribing NPs has a stipulation in the NP scope of practice identifying they are unable to prescribe. The stipulation reads "must not prescribe as an authorized prescriber (NP)." Nonprescribing NPs can achieve prescribing competency by either of the following pathways:

- Those with qualification that includes pharmacology and a prescribing practicum are required to complete 100 hours of supervised prescribing practice and a competence assessment by a medical mentor and a NP
- Those NPs who do not have the appropriate qualification must complete a Nursing Council approved pharmacology paper and a prescribing practicum that includes 100 hours of supervised prescribing practice and a competence assessment by a medical practitioner and a NP or supply a portfolio that demonstrates the equivalent knowledge and skills and complete a panel review

Nurse Practitioners New Zealand (NPNZ) is an organization that aims to offer a collective voice and act as a resource for the advancement of NP practice in the country (http://www.nurse.org.nz/npnz-nurse-practitioners-nz.html).

Philippines

Advanced practice nursing in the Philippines is partly recognized through the Nursing Specialty Certification Program (NSCP), which was formally launched through a Board of Nursing resolution in 1999 (Board of Nursing Resolution, 2002). Nursing leaders introduced the Nursing Specialty Certification Council, which credentials nurses and accredits organizations and educational programs highlighting the practice of specialized nursing. This is further enforced through the Comprehensive Nursing Specialty Program stipulated under the Philippine Nursing Law of 2002. Qualified nurses may be given certification in three levels—Nurse Clinician I, Nurse Clinician II, and Clinical Nurse Specialist—and may work under four major groups of nursing specialties: Medical-Surgical, Community Health, Maternal and Child Health, and Mental Health/Psychiatry (Philippine Board of Nursing, 2008). These policies provide for an informal category of nurses working in specialty areas across secondary, tertiary, and specialty hospitals. These nurses may or may not be credentialed under the NSCP. Most of these nurses are prepared through formal or informal education within their home institutions.

There are a large number of baccalaureate entry-level programs for nursing in the Philippines with an emphasis on education for export of its graduates, not only to the United States but also to the Middle East. In the midst of this situation, there are many master's degree programs in nursing with most emphasizing degrees in administration and at least three well-established nursing doctoral programs in the country (V. M. Manila, personal communication, June 18, 2016).

Currently, there is no policy that formalizes the position of an APN in the Philippines; neither are there explicit standards of practice for those who may be working as APNs. In most health institutions, the generalist and specialty area nurses have the same job descriptions with a similar sense of patient and professional accountability. These developments provide the motivation to formulate an APN framework in the Philippines that would define systems, scopes, and standards of practice, and ultimately contribute to better health for the public (V. Manila, personal communication, June 18, 2016).

Even though the system for a role similar to advanced practice nursing in the Philippines appears nonspecific, a form of APN is stipulated in four major policies in nursing: the Philippine Nursing Act of 2002 Article VI Sec. 28 and Article VII Sec. 31, and in Board of Nursing (BON) Resolution No. 99-13, 99-24, and 2002-118.

The Nursing Act Article VI Section 28 enlists the scope of the nurse to include "advanced nursing practice." A study conducted to evaluate coherence and outcomes to these policies and their relevance to ANP (Manila, 2013) revealed the following findings:

- Nurses in the Philippines function in specialized practice but with limited role expansion.
- Education for advanced practice is fragmented.
- There is an absence of a standard of advanced practice across institutions.
- There are notable similarities but foundational gaps compared with international APN frameworks.

These study findings contributed to the drafting of the new nursing bill which, as of June 2016, was being processed for new legislation that will incorporate a provision to include the term and position of *advanced practice nursing*. When signed into law the hope is that APN roles will be fully realized in the Philippines (V. M. Manila, personal communication, June 18, 2016).

People's Republic of China

Advanced practice nursing roles are informally being implemented across the People's Republic of China (PR China) in recognition of the need to expand the scope of nursing practice to meet changing population and health-care delivery needs. The Chinese government noted this situation and has given approval for clinical/professional degrees at the master's level aimed at training nurses to develop advanced practice competencies. By 2011 28 universities in PR China had recruited nursing students into clinical/professional degree programs in various clinical areas indicating a new developmental phase in graduate nursing education in PR China. In 2014, 58 new clinical/professional master's programs were approved. The total number of clinical/professional master's programs in nursing reached 84 by the end of March 2015 in China (Hill & Parker, 2015).

In 2015 the China Medical Board China Nursing Network (CCNN) sought expertise from Australian and American consultants for the development of the Chinese ANP program. Key recommendations included development of curricula for a clinical master of nursing program, suggestions for development of standards for APN roles, and a proposal to consider implementation of pilot projects with educated specialty nurses participating in the projects. The action plan included terms of reference for an oversight committee and key activities to initiate the project. CCNN planned an ANP program from May 2015 to May 2017, focusing on the education and a career development pathway for APNs (Hill & Parker, 2015).

Nursing in PR China is currently evolving toward increased professionalization. APNs with postgraduate education qualifications are an important component of this progress. In 2014 the Chinese Ministry of Education (MOE) approved 58 new clinical/professional master's of nursing programs. This means there will be more clinical nurses with a master's degree. The ANP program is being initiated to contribute to this advance in nursing. A Chinese ANP program Executive Committee composed of nursing deans from Fudan University, Peking Union Medical College, and Peking University and nursing directors from affiliated hospitals has been established to facilitate this process. This plan for nursing is consistent with the central government's 10-year plan to increase clinical training of physicians (M. Hill, personal communication, January 16, 2016).

Singapore

The National University of Singapore, under the auspices of the Yong Loo Lin School of Medicine, established an APN program in Singapore in 2003, offering academic preparation in acute care, adult health, and mental health, while viewing the course of studies as generic in emphasis. As of 2016 specialty offerings have expanded to critical care, oncology/palliative care, and pediatrics. Following graduation from the 2-year full-time master's program, students must complete the minimum of a 1-year internship in their specialty before applying for certification, licensure, and registration with the Singapore Nursing Board (SNB). Registration to practice as an APN is renewed on an annual basis with the SNB.

The APN Register established in 2005 by the Ministry for Health is expected to help with the systemic development of this category of clinical nurse, educated to a master's level in nursing, in becoming a key player in Singapore's drive to keep health care affordable while maintaining high-quality services. Consistent with this view and to support developing professionalism for nursing, the Ministry of Health established a clinical nursing career path that includes the APN roles. The clinical career track is similar to those that exist for management and education.

To renew the APN practicing certificate (PC), APNs must fulfill the requirements stipulated by the SNB to demonstrate that they have maintained their competency. Requirements include achievement of a minimum number of clinical hours related to their level of practice and years postcertification plus acquiring 30 Continuing Education (CE) points in every qualifying period (QP) in categories as stipulated by the SNB.

Key decision makers in education, policy, and administration are working to adapt models and frameworks from the United States while at the same time attempting to introduce APN roles to the public that are suitable for hospital and community settings in the country. Visibility and support for this advancement in nursing are evidenced up to the Ministry of Health level, where a request was made to have 200 APNs in place in various specialties in Singapore by 2014 (Ayre & Bee, 2014). In 2015 there were 172 registered APNs, mostly in the public sector in Singapore (MOH, 2016).

Republic of South Korea

It could be said that NP-like nursing roles have been in place in Korea since the time of the "medicine lady" in the 15th century. Care provided by the medicine ladies included deliveries, physical examinations, acupuncture, and prescribing of herbal medicines (J. Kang, personal communication, November 15, 2007).

CHNPs have been providing comprehensive primary health-care services in rural communities of South Korea since the health-care law for provision of health care for rural residents was legislated in 1980. CHNPs provide PHC to approximately 28% of the rural population in South Korea; however, this number is decreasing because it is more difficult to attract nurses to work in the rural areas (J. Tang, personal communication, November 15, 2007).

Haho Clinic, located 2 hours from Seoul between Yoju and Ichon, has provided clinic services for the community and the surrounding area since 1985. The scope of practice for the CHNPs includes diagnosis, prescriptive authority, and referral to other practitioners. In addition, home visits, health education, disease management, immunizations, school health services, and care for the elderly are part of the health-care service provision with additional support from nurses and community helpers. The nurse specialist system was formalized in Korea to fulfill changes in the medical environment. Anesthesia, public health, mental health, and home health-care nurses are approved for

practice under the Medical Service Law. A special law for agriculture approves the CHNP for practice as a nurse specialist.

Discussions attempting to clarify issues related to APNs began in the 1990s. In 2003, the medical law revision identified qualifications for the APN and designated 13 areas of specialization. Qualifications include master's-level education, passage of the certification examination, and experience in a chosen specialty. The first certification examination was given in 2005 (J. Kang, personal communication, 2007). As in many countries, the Korean Nurses Association faces difficulty obtaining consensus from the nursing community on scope of practice, educational requirements, and titling (Schober & Affara, 2006; Sheer & Wong, 2008).

While the APNs have also existed in the country for more than 20 years, a strong value of the physician role has inhibited the professional respect to allow APNs their own autonomy and peer collaboration. Lack of local support in Korea is represented by the fact that there is only one hospital in the country that employs APNs in the NP-like role, and even then the position reflects more of a senior nursing position (Maryland Nurses' Association, 2012).

Taiwan

Taiwan has a long history of nursing education and practice evolving from apprenticeship hospital-based programs to academic professional education in institutions of higher learning. Following the country's release from Japanese rule in 1945, nursing rapidly evolved in its development of university programs. The first master's of science (MS) program was started in 1979, with the first doctoral program in nursing offered in 1997.

In 1990 NPs were listed along with "professional nurse" as a legal position in nursing. In 1991 the Nurses Act was passed in an attempt to alleviate the nursing shortage and allow nurses to practice independently. NP programs were started in 2000 after an amendment to the Nurses Act made the NP title official (Chao, 2008). With passage of Paragraphs 3 and 4 of Article 23 of the Nurses Act, NPs became legally able to provide care (Chin et al, 2015). In general, practice guidelines allow NPs to practice more independently under hospital approval. NPs also can extend their practice to other institutions or community-based facilities; however, as of July 2016 the description for that possibility was unclear.

NPs have been educated in hospital training programs since the 1990s in an attempt to alleviate the shortage of physicians and lessen their workload. However, the NPs were functioning at first without guidelines and standards. The Department of Health (DOH), in conjunction with the National Health Research Institute (NHRI) and the Taiwan Association of Nurse Practitioners (TANP), has established standards for approving programs, curriculum guidelines, and preceptor guidelines. NP preparation remains predominantly based in hospitals with the faculty made up of physicians and health providers from other disciplines and the education focused on the medical and surgical domains. Even though the NP education model is still mainly hospital-based there are developing programs such as an academic model at Taiwan University and possibilities for education abroad. If participants achieve completion of those approved education programs, they can apply for the national examination to obtain an NP practice certificate.

The main work settings for NPs are in acute care hospitals with some positions in emergency room and ambulatory care settings with the possibility to extend their practice to long-term care. Continuing education is required for a NP to apply for a 6-year extension of the certification period. As of 2008 there were 857 certified NPs in Taiwan. Similar to other countries, certified NPs in Taiwan are seeking additional academic preparation to achieve professional status and credibility in their work settings and among professional colleagues. Several schools of nursing within universities are responding by offering master's-level NP programs. Additional universities are offering post-NP certificate transition programs toward a master's in nursing. There is a Taiwan Association of Nurse Practitioners. As of July 2016 there were association photos available with text only in Thai.

In a country with a NHI system that enrolls 99% of its citizens, it is estimated that there will be a health problem associated with an increase in the aging population that is expected to reach 4.76 million by 2026 (Tsay & Kuo, 2008). In response to the lack of medical labor the Ministry of Health and Welfare is deliberating a supportive measure to increase the number of NPs on a yearly basis (MOHW, 2014). Health promotion, disease prevention, integrated health care, and chronic disease management are all areas of upcoming need that will be addressed by nurses with advanced knowledge and skills. Advanced practice nursing

has a beginning with guidelines that have been established to ensure that nursing graduates will have sound preparation to provide quality care in Taiwan (R.T. Goodyear & S. F. Tsay, personal communication, June 23, 2016).

West Java, Indonesia

The Indonesian government and nursing associations have made efforts to enhance the professionalism of nursing through improvements of a higher degree of nursing education. Since 1985, nursing in Indonesia has moved from vocational to professional status through the opening of the first baccalaureate degree in the University of Indonesia (UI). In 1994, another baccalaureate program in nursing was opened at *Universitas Padjadjaran* (UNPAD) in West Java Province. Following the opening of baccalaureate programs, the UI opened the master of nursing programs that were integrated with specialization programs in 2003. These specialization programs consist of community nursing, maternity nursing, medical surgical nursing, psychiatric nursing, and paediatric nursing (Simamora, 2009). In Indonesia, master's of nursing and nursing specialization programs are dissimilar. The master's degree focuses on academics and research, whereas specialization programs focus on practice. The *Universitas Padjadjaran* has established a master's of nursing in critical care nursing and community health nursing in 2009, followed by a master's program in medical surgical nursing, nursing management, psychiatric nursing, and paediatric nursing. The University of Indonesia has been the only university in the country offering both master's and specialization programs. However, the specialization programs at UNPAD are planned to be established in 2017 and will include critical care nursing and community health nursing.

Indonesian nurses have the opportunity to open a private nursing practice that has been supported by regulation of the Ministry of Health since 2010. Moreover, in 2014, Indonesia has a Nursing Act that strongly supports private nursing practice. With advanced nursing education programs, the Indonesian government expects that the improvement of level of education can contribute to the improvement of nursing practice; however, the development of advanced practice nursing in Indonesia is relatively slow. No publications were found in July 2016 regarding the numbers of APNs in Indonesia nor the factors that contribute to the slow development of this practice. One possible explanation is that most of the students of the specialization programs are lecturers who use their special-ization skills to teach students, not to practice. Lecturers have difficulty practicing because of their high load of academic work. Therefore, a nursing centre (NC) model was established in West Java, Indonesia.

The NC model in West Java, Indonesia, is defined as a nurse-led clinic that integrates health-care services, education, and research through the optimal usage of all potential resources in the community health-care system (Samba, 2007). This NC is unique because it is co-located in the government-owned community health centers and places an emphasis on improving the quality of community health nursing services, education, and health outcomes for people in the community. A doctoral study (Juniarti et al, 2015) of the NC model in West Java, Indonesia, demonstrated that the NC model has made a positive change for nursing practice as well as people in the community (N. Juniarti, personal communication, July 25, 2016).

CONCLUSION

Descriptions of APN development in various countries and research reported in the international literature confirm the benefits of ANP and support the view that advanced nursing roles are feasible, sustainable, and provide high-quality, competent health care. Legislation and regulations often lag behind actual practice. Disagreement exists between practice acts of various health-care professionals and prog-ress supportive of ANP seems, at times, more similar to an intricate maze or puzzle than a picture of coordinated forward motion.

International momentum supportive of APN services is increasing; however, initiatives often face obstacles and challenges as leaders attempt to activate schemes that will ultimately change the profile of the health-care workforce and delivery systems. Role ambiguity and confusion regarding titling, scope of practice, educational preparation, and credentialing present questions that must be addressed.

For ANP to thrive in health-care systems globally, the authors believe that several areas need to be confronted and managed successfully. A well-developed scope of practice that engages APNs in a wide range of activities including health-care planning and policy development, in addition to health promotion, disease prevention, and diagnosis and treatment of illness, is essential. This involves the ability to embrace the diversity of health-care systems worldwide without losing ANP core characteristics. An international consensus on who an APN is and how the ANP concept fits in the health-care workforce would assist in speaking to the recurrent topic of role ambiguity. In addition, it is vital that any progress toward consensus take into consideration country-specific nursing, health care, and policy cultures.

Challenges lie in the capacity of ANP advocates and decision makers to achieve consistency across clinical and educational models. Continually evaluating and reviewing practice by adding competencies that reflect dynamic changes in health care and role development is fundamental. Increasingly, APNs will be asked to provide evidence that they are a cost-effective, valued, and sustainable addition to health-care teams and provision of health-care services. Research that provides evidence demonstrating the ability of APNs to provide care in partnership with patients and their families, within communities, and in collaboration with other health-care professionals will provide a strong foundation for the addition of this role to comprehensive health-care services.

2

The Practice Environment

Advanced Practice Nurses and Prescriptive Authority

Jan Towers

- Discuss advanced nursing practice and prescriptive authority.
- Summarize the evolution of prescriptive authority for advanced practice registered nurses (APRNs).
- Discuss the patterns of statutory and regulatory policy currently governing prescriptive authority for APRNs.
- Describe obstacles to achieving plenary prescriptive authority for APRNs.
- Explain the statutory and regulatory changes necessary to achieve plenary prescriptive authority.
- Distinguish prescriptive authority among nurse practitioners (NPs), clinical nurse specialists (CNSs), certified registered nurse anesthesiologists (CRNAs), and certified nurse-midwives (CNMs).
- Predict the future of prescriptive authority for APRNs.

DEVELOPMENT OF AUTHORITY TO PRACTICE

As professional nurses expanded their role to cross into traditional medical domains, the ability to prescribe medications became increasingly important. Although certified registered nurse anesthetists (CRNAs), certified nurse-midwives (CNMs), and clinical nurse specialists (CNSs) had practiced in advanced roles for some time before the birth of nurse practitioners (NPs), the advent of

NP practice in primary care influenced the authorization of all advanced practice registered nurses (APRNs) to prescribe medications. Before that time, CRNAs selected and administered anesthesia, but not other medications. Likewise, CNMs traditionally focused on childbirth and did not require extensive prescriptive authority. CNSs functioned in advanced practice nursing roles with diagnosed patients who were under the care of a physician. Although professionals in each of these roles made judgments regarding medications used by patients under their care, they relied mainly on physicians to provide prescriptions for medications when they were needed.

Nurse Practitioners and Prescriptive Authority

As NPs began to provide primary care services, they used these same traditional processes to provide medications for the patients that they served. Although primary care practice places an emphasis on health promotion and disease prevention, most patients coming for primary care services do so with a health problem for which they are seeking assistance. As time went on, it became evident that depending on physicians to prescribe medications created problems in the areas of patient access to care, continuity of care, and patient flow. When providing primary care, NPs assessed and diagnosed patients who needed prescription medications and treatments for their care.

The inability to sign one's own prescription, even if a physician was on site, was inconvenient for the NP, physician, and patient alike. It caused interruptions in the physician's interactions with patients, unnecessary delays each time NPs had to wait to get signed prescriptions from physicians, and often interfered with the credibility of NPs by rendering them dependent on physician signatures for medications that were being ordered based on their own diagnostic decision making. These problems were exacerbated when a physician was not on site. Patients then had to wait for prescriptions to be signed before they could be filled. If a physician was not available for a day or more, the implications for patient safety and health care were serious.

Methods were found to get around this stumbling block, such as calling prescriptions in to pharmacies or using other more questionable methods for obtaining a physician signature on the prescription so that the patient could pursue treatment in a timely manner. The need for the authority of NPs to prescribe under their own names became evident and pressing.

In the early days, NPs did not have title recognition other than that of registered nurse (RN) in their state regulatory systems. They were not alone; with the exception of CNMs and CRNAs in several states, no APRNs had title recognition in statutory or regulatory language in the state nurse practice acts or administrative rules. Likewise, there was no authority to prescribe medications. In fact, many nurse practice acts clearly prohibited the prescribing of medication by nurses regardless of specialty or status. Thus began the long journey of convincing legislators and regulators to change state statutes and regulations to give title recognition and prescriptive authority to APRNs.

Because licensure for all professions occurs at the state rather than the federal level, the movement to achieve these goals moved unevenly, as states with the most need moved forward to make changes. The movement was enhanced in the early days by an acute shortage of primary care physicians, and some states with higher primary care needs moved forward more rapidly than others. At that time, rural states were more likely to initiate statutory and regulatory adjustments than were states with large urban populations.

Convincing decision makers in the states was not without its problems. Then, as now, NPs had to demonstrate that they had the knowledge base to safely diagnose illnesses and prescribe medications. This meant that educational programs had to demonstrate that their curriculums prepared NPs for an independent prescribing role. Advanced pathophysiology and pharmacology and the development of differential diagnosis and clinical decision-making skills needed to be visible in the programs. With the advent of federal grants to prepare NPs, the content and quality of the preparatory programs was increasingly standardized.

In addition, to be credible in health-care systems, it was necessary for members of the medical community to advocate for the recognition of these professionals and their ability to prescribe medications independently. Many did, and through this window of opportunity NPs began to gain prescriptive authority state by state over subsequent years.

Initially, the authority to practice and prescribe was limited. In many of the early states where some form of prescriptive authority was conferred, boards of medicine and boards of nursing were authorized to jointly promulgate rules and regulations governing NP actions, including prescriptive authority.

States such as North Carolina and Idaho were among the first states with jointly promulgated rules. Even today a few states still fall under the regulation of both boards of nursing and boards of medicine. Some of those states (where the highest degree of controversy over scope of practice has traditionally existed) are limited to joint regulation of prescriptive authority. Recent attempts to change that regulatory pattern have been harder to achieve. Pennsylvania is the most recent state to move away from joint promulgation of rules to regulation solely by the board of nursing.

Initially, NPs were authorized to prescribe a limited number of medications under physician supervision. North Carolina was one of the first states to develop a limited drug formulary. Subsequently, states developed combinations of formularies and physician oversight under jointly promulgated rules or under rules developed by boards of nursing. The form of those rules depended largely on the persuasiveness of NPs and the attitudes of the legislators and governors of those states.

Currently, NPs prescribe legend drugs under their own signature in all 50 states and the District of Columbia. In addition, they prescribe controlled drugs in 48 states and the District of Columbia. Variation exists among states in the area of the authorization to prescribe controlled drugs and the relationship, if any, that must be maintained with a physician. Currently, there exists plenary prescriptive authority (no requirement for any physician involvement) in 22 jurisdictions (states) including the District of Columbia (National Council of State Boards of Nursing [NCSBN], 2016).

Nurse-Midwives and Prescriptive Authority

CNMs have had to undergo the same process as other APRNs to attain prescriptive authority. Because their educational preparation and role developed to include not only obstetrical and newborn care but also the general health management of their patients, the need to prescribe a broader range of medications also increased, making the previously described arrangement for prescribing under the physician's signature unreasonable.

Federal funding of CNM educational programs helped to implement the standards established by this discipline and facilitate the passage of statutes and rules that allow them to prescribe in 50 states and the District of Columbia with variable limitations in the area of controlled drugs.

In 23 of these jurisdictions the prescriptive authority is plenary (NCSBN, 2016).

Other factors that have assisted in this endeavor include an enthusiastic consumer population, especially pregnant women, who spread the word about the skills of CNMs. They have often packed hearing rooms and legislative chambers, bringing their babies and children, providing testimony regarding the worth and skill of the services provided to them by CNMs. CNMs have the same state-to-state variability regarding authorization to prescribe controlled drugs and required relationships, if any, with physicians.

Clinical Nurse Specialists and Prescriptive Authority

CNSs have more recently felt the need to prescribe medications for the patients they serve. Those particularly desirous of the authorization are the psychiatric and mental health CNSs who often have their own practices or function autonomously in mental health clinics and other specialty practices. The prescriptive authority need for practitioners in this field is particularly acute in agencies serving vulnerable populations.

The remainder of the CNS community has mixed responses to the need for authorization to prescribe medications. At the core of this ambivalence is the role played by the CNS in the employment setting, the scope of prescriptive authority needed when working in a particular specialty with patients who have already been diagnosed, the educational preparation required to allow for this authorization, and the risk of being unnecessarily placed under the supervision of physicians in states where such supervision is required. Some states do not provide title recognition for CNSs. There has been controversy regarding whether an additional title recognition is actually needed for CNSs. Therefore, the issue of prescriptive authority for CNSs has been more cloudy than that of NPs or CNMs (National Association of Clinical Nurse Specialists [NACNS], 2002).

Nevertheless, CNSs have begun to obtain title recognition (often driven by the need for recognition to receive reimbursement for services) and the authority to prescribe within their scope of practice. Currently, two-thirds of the states authorize CNSs to prescribe medications in one fashion or another, and 29 offer plenary authority (NCSBN, 2016). Variability in recognizing who may qualify, scope of prescriptive authority, ability to prescribe controlled substances, and required relationships with physicians occur from state to state. In some states the statutes and regulations are similar to those of NPs and in others they are not. A few states have extended prescriptive authority to psychiatric and mental health CNSs only. A few have grouped all APRNs under one set of regulations, whereas most have kept the four clinical groups separated under an APRN umbrella that allows for regulatory variability among APRNs in their states.

Nurse Anesthetists and Prescriptive Authority

The authority of CRNAs to select and administer anesthesia has long been recognized. Until recently, CRNAs have been less involved in the struggle to obtain prescriptive authority than the other three disciplines. Some representatives from the CRNA community have maintained that ordering and administering anesthesia does not fall under the rubric of prescriptive authority in its traditional sense (American Association of Nurse Anesthetists [AANA], 2016). Increasingly, however, CRNAs are becoming involved in pain management of patients in the practices they serve and thus have the need to prescribe. Currently, nurse anesthetists have prescriptive authority in 30 states; 23 of those states still require collaboration with or supervision by a physician, and 28 award plenary authority (NCSBN, 2016). As with the other APRN groups, CRNAs have found that they have to work to convince legislators and governors of their knowledge and skills. Their availability in rural areas has enhanced their ability to obtain these privileges even in the presence of opposition from the medical community. As with NPs, CNMs, and CNSs, they have had to demonstrate the strength of their educational programs and the safety of their practice to obtain privileges in this area.

THE ROAD TO STATUTORY AND REGULATORY CHANGE TO AUTHORIZE PRESCRIPTIVE AUTHORITY

To alter state statutes and regulations, APRNs had to educate state legislatures, executive officers, and regulators regarding the role of the APRNs they represented. In addition, they had to demonstrate a need for APRNs

to prescribe and prove that prescribing by APRNs was safe and contributed to the well-being of the population.

There are a variety of ways to authorize prescriptive authority within a state. Changes (amendments) may be made to nurse practice acts (statutes), new statutes may be developed separate from nurse practice acts, or changes may be made in states' administrative codes through the development of regulations promulgated by the appropriate regulating board (in most cases the board of nursing).

In the case of new statutes or statutory changes, legislation must be introduced that amends or adds to current law to give title recognition and prescriptive authority to APRNs (NPs, CNMs, CNSs, or CRNAs). Once legislation is introduced, it is referred to a committee of jurisdiction (usually a professional licensure committee) for consideration. Once the legislation is in committee, the chair of that committee generally calls for a hearing to allow proponents and opponents of the legislation to give testimony regarding the introduced legislation. After hearings are conducted, at the chair's discretion, the committee votes on the legislation and passes it out of committee. In some states, proposed legislation must also go through the appropriations committee of at least one of the voting chambers to determine cost and evaluate the fiscal impact on the state. After passing through all appropriate committees, the legislation, at the discretion of the majority party leadership, is taken to the floor of the voting chamber for a vote. Sometimes this is done simultaneously in both chambers of the state legislature; in others, the legislation passes through one chamber at a time. Once the legislation has been agreed on (passed) by both chambers of the legislature it is sent to the governor to be signed or, in the case of some states, to be vetoed.

During this process language changes in proposed legislation are often made or negotiated to satisfy other interested parties. For this reason, the language of authorizing statutes varies to a certain extent from state to state. This is particularly true in the sections (a) defining procedures to be followed and requirements that must be met to be recognized as an APRN; (b) defining the relationship, if any, that must be held with a physician to prescribe; and (c) determining the scope of prescriptive authority of the APRN, particularly the authorization to prescribe controlled drugs (schedules I through V). As statutes are passed, much time and energy goes into attempting to negotiate language that is acceptable to the advanced practice community, involved legislators, governors, regulatory bodies, and other interested parties. Once statutes have been passed and signed by the governor of a state, rules and regulations are developed and approved by the authorized regulatory body or bodies.

When regulations are developed, they are first written as proposed rules and are placed in a public register for comment. The comment period covers a limited time, after which the promulgating boards consider the comments and make appropriate changes in the proposed rule at their discretion before publishing a final rule. In most states, such regulations must then be approved by some arm of the legislature, often committees of jurisdiction, sometimes by one or the other legislative chamber, before approval by the governor. For this reason, APRNs and regulatory bodies are often embroiled in negotiations similar to those encountered in the legislative process that result in alterations that make for variance in regulations from state to state. These variations are in the same general areas where there is variability in statute.

Because the purpose of state regulatory bodies, such as boards of nursing, is to protect the public (in this case, the public health), boards of nursing vary in their advocacy of advanced practice roles in the regulatory process. In most states governors appoint the members of the professional licensure boards. Having APRNs who understand the roles of NPs, CNMs, CNSs, and CRNAs appointed to these positions can help the regulatory process when issues such as prescriptive authority are considered.

Several states, rather than introducing or altering statutes to authorize APRN prescriptive authority, have instead developed and instituted regulatory changes in the administrative code by which the advanced practice disciplines must abide. Although regulation cannot override statute, statutes are often worded broadly enough for regulations regarding title recognition and authorization to prescribe drugs to be developed by the regulatory body or bodies without disturbing statutes.

Patterns of Statutory and Regulatory Authority

Four basic patterns of regulation regarding prescriptive authority have evolved over time:

- The use of an established formulary or lists of drugs that the APRN can prescribe

- A negative or exclusionary formulary that allows the APRN to prescribe all drugs with the exception of a short list of forbidden drugs
- An individualized collaborative formulary established by the APRN with a collaborating physician
- Unlimited authority with no formulary or collaborative requirements

Regulator Established Formulary

An established formulary was used in the early days of APRN prescribing activity to determine an agreed-on list of drugs that APRNs could prescribe. As new drugs came onto the market, updating of these formularies was needed to allow prescribing according to current practice standards. Although this quickly became a cumbersome process, it is still in use today in a few states.

Negative or Exclusionary Formulary

Exclusionary formularies were found to be a more practical approach to regulation of prescriptive authority. By creating a short list of forbidden drugs (e.g., chemotherapy, gold treatments), the APRN had more flexibility in choosing appropriate treatments for patients. This has been particularly important in the primary care setting.

Collaborative Formulary

More flexible than the established formulary and, to a certain extent, more flexible than a negative formulary, a collaborative formulary allows the APRN to create a formulary most useful to his or her practice in collaboration with an identified physician who serves as a collaborator. Although this has worked well in some states, in others, where the formulary must be shared with the regulatory board, it has sometimes become a nightmare. Requirements regarding information to be included in formularies and updating formularies can be, to say the least, cumbersome and obstructive.

Open Formulary

The most flexible framework for prescriptive authority is the open formulary, in which APRNs have no limitations regarding what they can prescribe. In these cases, APRNs prescribe according to their own specialty scope of practice, just as physicians prescribe within their own scope of specialty practice. The majority of states that have implemented this framework in their regulations have done so without difficulty or negative repercussion. Overall, the trend toward the removal of barriers to prescribing has resulted in the removal of limitations of drugs to be prescribed and the requirement for physician collaboration to do so. Although barriers in a few states still exist in the authorization to prescribe controlled substances, the limitations of authorization to prescribe legend drugs have disappeared.

Advanced Practice Nurse–Physician Relationships in Statute and Regulation

The requirement of some sort of collaborative arrangement with physicians to prescribe is often coupled with the prescriptive authority patterns discussed previously. Whereas many states do not require formal collaborative arrangements with physicians, the remainder have some requirement for collaborative or supervisory agreements with physicians to practice or prescribe medication. For NPs, approximately one-third of the state statutes and regulations have no requirements, less than one-fourth require supervision or have delegated authority, and the remainder require some kind of collaborative or consulting arrangement with a physician. These arrangements range from identifying a consulting physician to submission of a written agreement to the regulatory board(s) for filing or approval (AANP, 2016). CNMs have a similar pattern: Approximately one-fourth have no requirements, approximately one-fourth require a supervising physician, and the remainder require some kind of collaborative or consulting relationship in statute or administrative rule (ACNM, 2016). CRNAs have supervising or cooperating physicians in most states (AANA, 2016), whereas CNSs, in the states in which they have prescriptive authority, tend to have the same requirements as NPs (NCSBN, 2016).

Some of these requirements stem from a desire on the part of legislators or interested and influential parties for physician oversight to prescribe; others have been driven by reimbursement laws and policy that calls for physician oversight of APRNs. Sometimes rules are made for APRNs that reflect the supervisory relationship required of physician assistants (PAs) without considering the fact that APRNs are accountable under their own license, carry their own liability insurance, and in the majority of states are not required to be supervised by physicians, as are PAs.

BARRIERS TO PRESCRIPTIVE PRACTICE

The roads traveled by APRNs to obtain prescriptive authority have not been without struggle. There is no denying that the majority of barriers to practice have roots in organized lobbying by certain parts of the medical community to limit the autonomy of APRNs. This move has often been couched in the language of "protecting public safety." Therefore, some legislators and governors have seen fit to set limitations in statutes and administrative rules governing APRNs. The literature is replete with studies that report on the clinical safety of APRNs. In the studies that have been conducted, patient safety has been found to be as high with APRNs as with physicians and often have been found to be higher with APRNs than with physicians (Brown & Grimes, 1995; Laurent et al, 2006; Office of Technology Assessment [OTA], 1986). The ratings on quality of care have also been consistently high. APRNs, particularly NPs, have been studied and scrutinized in multiple studies with consistently positive reports (AANP, 2016).

The biggest barriers to practice for all groups have been the limitations set in state statutes and regulations. Of those, the requirements for formalized agreements with physicians to prescribe or practice have created the most frustrating barrier. This has been particularly true for NPs and CNMs who, to practice and receive reimbursement, must find physicians who will agree to serve as collaborators. CRNAs, particularly in rural areas, suffer from similar problems.

Once a physician has agreed to serve as a consultant, both the APRN and physician often find the reporting rules to be frustratingly cumbersome. Although it now occurs infrequently, requirements to list types of patients that may be seen, consultation patterns to be maintained, types of drugs to be prescribed, and identification of physicians to serve as backup in the absence of the identified collaborating physician still sometimes plague APRNs. Although, generally speaking, pharmacists have been cooperative and NPs report a good working relationship with pharmacists, issues such as continued use of the collaborating physician name as the prescriber on a medicine bottle label and requests for the name of the "supervising physician" before dispensing a prescription have frustrated APRNs, physicians, and patients through the years. The requirement of a Drug Enforcement Administration (DEA) number by insurance companies to pay for prescriptions is still problematic, particularly in the two states where APRNs are not yet authorized to prescribe controlled drugs. This problem lands on the pharmacists' doorstep when they cannot obtain reimbursement for dispensed drugs from insurance companies without an accompanying DEA number. Although this practice is a misuse of the DEA number, which is to be used for the prescription of controlled drugs only, it has become common practice for insurance companies and pharmacies to use this number as an identifier because of its uniformity for physician identification throughout the country.

Mail-order pharmacies sometimes create barriers for APRNs. Occasionally, patients cannot obtain prescriptions from these entities without the name or signature of a physician. Although this is no longer a problem with most mail-order pharmacies, those with warehouses located in states where laws for this form of dispensing require the order of a physician still occasionally pose difficulties for patients with prescriptions written by APRNs.

Confusion about the role and scope of practice of an APRN through the grouping of NPs, CNMs, and PAs as "midlevel practitioners" has created problems for APRNs. It is often assumed that the required supervisory arrangements for PAs is the same for NPs and CNMs, so that policies related to practice, including prescriptive authority and ordering of medications for patients, are often based on the statutes and rules governing PAs rather than the APRNs. Because most regulation of PAs stems from a state's medical practice act, insurance companies, institutions, accreditation entities, and pharmaceutical companies sometimes assume that the PA administrative rules apply to APRNs and do not seek information regarding APRNs from a state's nursing practice act and supporting regulations. Because APRNs are authorized to practice more autonomously in most instances, this assumption, and the actions taken based on it, create barriers for the APRN, particularly in relation to prescribing controlled drugs.

PRESCRIBING PATTERNS

The AANP has conducted several national surveys that examined the prescribing patterns of NPs throughout the United States (Goolsby, 2005, 2009; Towers, 1989, 1999a, 1999b). Those studies found that an NP's prescription patterns reflected the specialty and the practice setting of the NP. In these studies the mean number of prescriptions per day for all NPs was approximately 19, with family, adult, and emergency NPs among the highest daily prescribers.

Drugs most frequently prescribed by all specialties in these studies were antimicrobials, anti-inflammatories, and analgesics. Antihypertensives, bronchodilators, and cardiovascular drugs were prescribed most frequently by adult, family, and gerontological NPs. Contraceptives were most often prescribed by women's health NPs. The vast majority of NPs practicing in emergency department settings prescribe analgesics, anti-inflammatories, and antimicrobials most often, and in the Department of Veterans Affairs (VA) hospital setting, the vast majority of NPs prescribe antihypertensives and cardiovascular drugs most frequently, followed by diabetic medications, gastrointestinal medications, and analgesics. Among NPs authorized to prescribe controlled drugs, the majority of adult, family, gerontological, and psychiatric and mental health NPs prescribe them at least once a week with the highest percentages being in the hospital and VA hospital setting.

CNM prescriptive activities center on medications needed for prenatal care, such as vitamins, and intrapartum and postpartum care, such as analgesics. In addition, their prescribing practices are similar to those of women's health NPs. They include contraceptives and other hormone therapies, vaginal preparations, and antimicrobials, as well as anti-inflammatories, analgesics, and vitamin therapies (Towers, 1999a). The CNSs who most often prescribe medications at this time are the psychiatric and mental health specialists. In a study conducted by Talley and Richens (2001), psychiatric and mental health CNSs authorized to prescribe controlled drugs were reported to most frequently prescribe antidepressants (selective serotonin uptake inhibitors and tricyclic antidepressants). The next most frequently prescribed medications were antiparkinsonian drugs and antihistamines for neuroleptic side effects and sleep, followed by mood stabilizers such as lithium and carbamazepine.

Among CNSs of other specialties, prescribing activities appear to function around already diagnosed conditions and altering, adjusting, or refilling physician-prescribed medications in stable patients. The lack of authorization and the desire to maintain autonomy in nursing practice led many CNSs to choose not to obtain authorization in settings in which such authorization is attainable.

The position of the NACNS is that CNS prescriptive authority should be optional and that when prescribing is to be undertaken, the CNS should meet the requirements of any other APRN (Lyon & Minarik, 2001; NACNS, 2005).

THE FUTURE FOR APRN PRESCRIBING

Authorizing APRNs to prescribe medications is no longer a controversial issue; however, obsolete statutes and regulations still need to be changed in some states to guarantee the unencumbered ability for APRNs to prescribe needed medications for all patients. Toward this end, two important documents have been developed that reinforce the authorization of APRNs to function at their full educational scope, which includes unrestricted prescriptive authority for APRNs. The APRN Consensus Model (2016), endorsed by 46 states and 48 national nursing organizations, provides recommendations for the education and certification of APRNs (NCSBN, 2016). Likewise, the Institute of Medicine (IOM) report, *The Future of Nursing: Leading Change, Advancing Health* (2011), reinforces the need for APRNs to be authorized to practice to the full extent of their education and training. Both documents reflect the culmination of the APRN's evolution to full prescriptive authority that generally exists today.

CONCLUSION

Prescriptive authority is now generally recognized as an integral part of advanced practice nursing. Although totally unfettered authority by all APRNs has not yet been achieved, the experience of prescribing medications for patients under the care of these providers has been found to be safe and beneficial. The arguments put forth to limit their prescribing activities grow weaker with each advance that APRNs make. The practicality, the enhancement of quality of care, and the cost-effectiveness of the practice of these groups has enhanced the logic and desirability of giving prescriptive authority to APRNs nationwide.

7

Credentialing and Clinical Privileges for the Advanced Practice Registered Nurse

Ann H. Cary and Mary C. Smolenski

Learning Outcomes

Learning outcomes expected as a result of this chapter:

- Describe the purpose of credentialing for providers, institutions, regulators, and the public.
- Evaluate the *Consensus Model for APRN Regulation: Licensure, Accreditation, Certification and Education (LACE)*.
- Explain the federal and state regulatory impact on the processes of credentialing and privileging required by institutional providers and payers.
- Justify the direct relationship between the processes and documents required for the APRN credentialing process and the decisions for scope of practice or clinical privileges made by the employing institution.
- Discuss the unique aspects of credentialing and privileging in telehealth and telemedicine as well as during disasters.
- Justify the creation and maintenance of the APRN portfolio as a documentary tool for use in credentialing.
- Discuss challenges that the APRN may experience related to the changing nature of institutional and regulatory requirements.

INTRODUCTION

Credentialing and privileging of health-care providers, and advanced practice registered nurses (APRNs) in particular, is the initial and ongoing mechanism employed by regulatory and voluntary oversight and delivery systems to ensure protection of the public and quality patient care during the delivery of health-care services. According to the U.S. Department of Health and Human Services (DHHS) credentialing is "the process of assessing and confirming the qualifications of a licensed or certified health care practitioner" (HRSA, 2001, 2006). The independence and autonomy of APRN services necessitates the same degree of attention to the processes of credentialing and privileging as accorded to physicians and other providers. The process is a critical dimension of any risk management plan and is reflected in the level of responsibility assumed by the governing board, medical staff organization, or top administrator of the institution. APRNs are increasingly being granted privileges in acute care and hospice settings and participate in provider networks as primary care practitioners. In some states APRNs are eligible to bill as primary care providers (Center for Advancing Provider Practices, 2016).

Credentialing certification of providers, verifying provider credentials, establishing privileges, and accrediting institutions serve five purposes (adapted from Cary, 2015):

1. Public protection
2. Quality assurance and risk management
3. Consumer information and choice
4. Competitive advantage
5. Economic advantage

The Institute of Medicine's (2011) *Future of Nursing: Leading Change, Advancing Health* has challenged nursing and society "to allow nurses to practice to the full extent of their education and training" (p. 4). Recommendation #1 asserts that in order to master this challenge, barriers to the scope of practice as detected by actions in Congress, state legislatures, the Centers for Medicare and Medicaid Services (CMS), the Federal Trade Commission (FTC), and the Department of Justice (DOJ) must be removed. In addition, organizational barriers of the APRN employer may be equally oppressive to those at the macro level. APRNs who experience these barriers often encounter them during the process of credentialing and as an outcome of the privileging process. Credentialing and privileging

outcomes have a dramatic and common impact on the APRN's ability to execute the full scope of practice and thus has resulted in the AARP (formerly the American Association of Retired Persons) issuing a warning: "barriers (to APRNs) . . . are short-changing consumers" (IOM, 2011, p. 106).

For almost a decade there has been a plan and model to remove barriers to APRN practice with the issuance of the *Campaign for APRN consensus: Model for uniform national advanced practice registered nurse regulation* (2008) and the credentialing and privileging processes for providers issued by CMS and The Joint Commission (TJC) (2012). The Consensus Model for APRN Regulation: Licensure, Accreditation, Certification and Education (NCSBN, 2008) or LACE promotes uniformity of national standards and regulation by the states to promote mobility of APRNs and access to APRN care. The APRN Regulatory Model includes (O'Sullivan, 2011):

- Licensure: The granting of authority to practice
- Accreditation: Formal review and approval by a recognized agency of educational degree or certification programs in nursing or nursing related programs
- Certification: The formal recognition of knowledge, skills, and experience demonstrated by the achievement of standards identified by the profession
- Education: The formal preparation of APRNs in graduate or postgraduate programs

Because credentialing verification includes the education, certification, and licensure of the APRN and accreditation of the educational institution from which the APRN graduated, the LACE model under consideration by the states for uniform APRN preparation and credentialing, once executed, can reduce APRN barriers to practice. Each state board with jurisdiction over APRN education and practice will need to adopt the LACE approach in order to foster a standard approach to APRN education, certification, and practice regulation. The impact of full implementation of the LACE model will simplify the credentialing process required by the APRN and the employer. Most of the states have adopted some aspects of LACE but it is far from fully implemented to date. The reader can access the model and explanation at www.ncsbn.org.

To assure consistency of standards and processes for providers, both the CMS and TJC have undergone regulatory changes related to the issuance of uniform processes and allowances for the credentialing and privileging of medical and allied health professionals (including APRNs and physician assistants [PAs]). Although an institution can be more restrictive in privileging it cannot be less restrictive than the CMS Conditions of Participation (CoP). Because CMS no longer recognizes an equivalent process for credentialing and privileging of certain providers who provide "medical level of care," APRNs providing this level of care must now be processed through the medical staff standards process at the institution or system (Cheung, 2011). This process includes recommendations of the medical staff, approval of the governing body, and implementation of review performance processes such as the initial focused professional practice evaluation (FPPE) and ongoing professional practice evaluation (OPPE). If the APRN does not provide "medical level of care," the APRN can be processed through an "equivalent" process (Cheung, 2011).

This chapter discusses credentialing and privileging as separate mechanisms with the understanding that analysis of the data about the APRN's application process of credentialing is a precursor to the decision about the nature of activities (specific procedures or treatment of specific conditions) for which privileging will be awarded (Pelletier, 2015). Issues related to credentialing and privileging for APRNs within the health-care arena are also presented. The reader is advised to maintain access to new developments in these areas because barriers to executing full scope of practice for APRNs appear to be rapidly changing in federal and state regulations, as well as voluntary, employer, and provider groups.

CREDENTIALING

The prelude to any discussion on credentialing is grounded in the fact that the graduating APRN today must have an earned graduate degree or postgraduate coursework in the additional area of focus once a graduate degree is conferred. The institution conferring the degree must be accredited by a regional accreditor of higher education and, in most cases, a nursing accrediting organization recognized by the U.S. Department of Education. Once a student graduates and meets all educational requirements— master's, post-master's, or doctoral program—for preparing the APRN graduate, the student must achieve a passing score on the certification examination.

Certification confers the initial, specific voluntary credential for the APRN. There is yet to be uniformity among the states as to whether an additional regulatory (nonvoluntary) credential process is required to practice in a particular state based on the certification credential, such as obtaining a second state license as an APRN. The value of the LACE model described earlier is to regulate uniformly among the states how nurses and educational institutions are credentialed based on a national standard and how these are recognized as equivalent among the states. However, the LACE model in total has not yet been adopted by the majority of the states. Renewal of APRN certification, for all except the certified registered nurse anesthetist (CRNA), is conferred by a combination of practice hours, continuing education, and academic coursework in accordance with the requirements of the respective (re)certifying organization.

The new model, structure, and process of recertification for CRNAs was initiated August 1, 2016, by the National Board of Certification and Recertification for Nurse Anesthetists (NBCRNA): the Continued Professional Certification program (CPC). This shift in recertification was driven by the expectation of consumers for the measurement of continuing competency in the recertification of health-care providers and may well portend a shift in the recertification process of all APRNs in the future. One difference in the recertification of the CRNA relates to the addition of an examination to the process of the recertification cycle. To obtain the most current information about the recertification process and the phased timeline for the CRNA certification and recertification access http://nbcrna.com/certification (Box 7.1).

Credentialing involves the collection, verification, and assessment of information determining the eligibility and qualifications of the APRN provider to provide health-care services and includes three categories: current licensure and certification; education and training; and experience, ability, and current competence to perform the work (TJC, 2008). Whereas privileging decisions are based on the initial and ongoing evaluation of the applicant's credentials and performance competencies, the credentialing process itself guarantees the integrity of the data issued for the APRN and serves as the basis of decisions regarding privileging authorization for scope of practice and appointment of the APRN in a facility or system.

Box 7.1

Organizations Offering Certification and Recertification for APRNs

American Academy of Nurse Practitioners Certification Programs (AANPCP)

American Association of Critical-Care Nurses Certification Corporation (AACNCERTcorp)

American Midwifery Certification Board (AMCB)

American Nurses Credentialing Center (ANCC)

National Board of Certification & Recertification for Nurse Anesthetists (NBCRNA)

National Certification Corporation (NCC)

Pediatric Nursing Certification Board (PNCB)

The American Board of Comprehensive Care (ABCC)*

*This organization is not recognized or used for regulation.

Box 7.2

Categories of Data Required to Be Satisfied for Credentialing Application

Personal and practice demographic information

Education and training

Clinical performance

Work history

State(s) licensure history (including state-controlled substance licenses)

Certifications

Drug Enforcement Agency (DEA) certificates

Provider number or ID

Criminal background report

Liability insurance and claims history

History of sanctions and penalties imposed on practice and voluntary relinquishment of licenses and certifications

Disclosures of physical, mental, substance, or criminal problems

Attestation of information completeness and accuracy

Authorizing statement to collect any information necessary to verify application

---

The types of data gathered during the credentialing process are directed by federal and state regulations; professional standards; facility requirements, policies, and procedures; and voluntary oversight bodies. Medicare CoP guide federal and many state-regulated processes; standards of practice guide the professional standards; institutional bylaws, policies, and procedures mandate the specific application of the credentialing and privileging processes for the employed, independent contractor or a licensed independent practitioner (LIP)—an APRN can be a LIP; and voluntary or semiregulatory accreditation standards mandate the institutional processes. At a minimum, TJC standards require credentialing and privileging of all LIPs and APRNs who deliver a "medical level of care" permitted by law and the organizational bylaws to provide patient care without supervision or direction (Pelletier, 2015). Regardless of the particulars of data required to support the APRN application, there are common data elements that the APRN can expect to see on the application.

Credentialing Application and Procurement of Data: Preapplication and Application

Data that are required to support the application for APRN appointment or reappointment to a clinical position fall into several general categories. **Box 7.2** lists the common categories included in the credentialing

application process. Organizations may use a two-step process for credentialing: preapplication and application. A preapplication typically will address any disciplinary actions or sanctions by regulatory or professional organizations; current unrestricted license; criminal history; board certification; clinical specialty requirements; and health status information compliant with the American Disabilities Act (MedPro, 2014).

A written application must be submitted to the authorized department or person in an institution. The application may be lengthy, and completeness and accuracy of information are critical to ensure timeliness of processing. Review of the application examines both the submission of information by the APRN and source verification as well as consistency of information among all sources. Any gaps in information or inconsistency are further investigated by the institution before a decision is made for appointment. The APRN is responsible for adding information as needed and answering queries for incomplete or inconsistent data. In circumstances where changes in status occur (e.g., licensure renewal, registration, additional education and certifications, recertification, voluntary or involuntary termination of staff membership, reduction or loss of privileges), the provider is obligated to submit the respective information to the credentialing body immediately for review of appointment status. Falsification of information or intentional omission of information on the application may be grounds for termination of the process, disciplinary action, or dismissal. If credentialing is denied, this is typically reported to the National Practitioner Data Bank (NPDB) (Pelletier, 2015). For APRNs working in managed care organizations (MCOs) credentialing for most health plans is largely conducted by a vendor such as the Council for Affordable Quality Healthcare, Inc. (CAQH) (Buppert, 2015).

Verification of Advanced Practice Nurse Application Data

Two types of verification of data sources, primary and secondary, are conducted on an application in accordance with the rules and regulations of the accountable body for credentialing within the institution and as directed by the institutional accreditation process. Primary source verification attests to the accuracy and authenticity of the APRN's credentials based on evidence obtained from any source issuing the credential or the attestation of clinical performance. Examples include verification of licensure by state agency and certifications by certifying bodies, letters by authorized personnel at the professional school, letters from individuals personally acquainted with the APRN's skills, and database queries. Secondary source verification relies on verification actions of the APRN credentials based on data obtained by means other than direct contact with the issuing source of the credential (Utilization Review Accreditation Commission [URAC] 2011, 2016). Examples include unofficial copies of documents or reports on patient satisfaction statistics by the applicant. It can also include peer references or quality data information from past employer organizations.

Some credentialing processes allow for documentation secured by Internet or telephone verification. State nursing licensure boards are continuing to evolve technologically and many have online license verification processes such as *Nursys*. In addition, some health-care institutions contract

with credentialing verification organizations (CVOs) to collect the primary and secondary data on which the decision for appointment will be made. For example, CAQH has more than 1.3 million physicians and other health-care professionals engaged in CAQH ProView™, an online Universal Provider Datasource (UPD) that allows providers to self-report updates in credentials to a database that can be accessed by employers (CAQH, 2016). The institution contracting with any CVO is responsible for monitoring the quality of service provided by the CVO and may require the CVO to be accredited by one of the national accrediting bodies such as URAC. The institution is not relieved of liability resulting from decisions based on contracted CVO data and processes for credentialing of APRNs. In addition, the institution remains accountable for the accreditation standards issued by its accreditation bodies such as TJC.

Analysis of Credentialing Application

Upon completion of the APRN application review and verification processes, the final step is institutional decision on appointment. This is guided by institutional policies and procedures related to structure of the decision-making body; roles of the members; risk management and legal reviews; due process mechanisms; documentation requirements for decisions; and reporting mechanisms to the institutional board of directors, clinical directors, and the applicant. In some institutions, the human resource department processes the data for credentialing, whereas in other institutions certain providers are credentialed by the medical staff. An organizational model at the University of Rochester, The Margaret D. Sovie Center for Advanced Practice, serves as a centralized coordination center for the core APRN functions related to regulation, institutional requirements, and credentialing with a direct line to the medical staff office. The center also functions as a repository for credentialing information, state licensure, prescriptive authority, and DEA numbers. See more information on the Sovie Center at www.urmc.rochester.edu/strong-nursing/sovie-center.

In most institutions, the credentialing committee is composed of physicians. As more APRNs become credentialed, their representation on medical staff committees will need to be embraced and the bylaws adjusted to expand governance for APRNs as part of provider panels and teams. The credentialing process is time consuming because of the importance of adhering to principles of good data integrity and decision making. It can often take 90 to 120 days (Monarch, 2002). It behooves the APRN to obtain a copy of the policy and procedures for the credentialing process, committee member list, schedule of meetings, anticipated action on the application, and due process mechanisms. Rapid responses to queries facilitate the completion of data collection and decision making. Also, alerting primary sources of the impending request by the verification body can facilitate the response for information.

When a credentialing process results in an appointment to the staff, the length of appointment and reappointment procedures are guided by institutional policy. It is wise to obtain copies of the reappointment process and criteria and continuously compile the necessary evidence to meet the criteria for reappointment. As new technologies and procedures become common, the APRN needs to understand the minimum criteria for credentialing in new procedures and document accordingly (TJC, 2008).

Decisions for emergency credentialing of volunteer LIPs have been revisited since 2002 because of national and local emergencies. For example in 2002, TJC created a standard that allows the institutional chief executive officer, medical staff president, or his or her designee to grant emergency privileges when an emergency management plan has been activated. Implications for credentialing focus on data integrity: acceptable sources of identification, including a current license to practice, current hospital identification with the license number, or verification of identity by a current hospital or medical staff member (TJC, 2012). Joint Commission Emergency Management (EM) standards for providers include:

EM.02.02.13 During disasters, the hospital may grant disaster privileges to volunteer licensed independent practitioners.

EM.02.02.15 During disasters, the hospital may assign disaster responsibilities to volunteer practitioners who are not licensed independent practitioners but who are required by law and regulation to have a license, certification or registration.

Time limitations are always imposed for credentialing providers in this status.

Organizational Standards for Credentialing Advance Practice Nurses in Institutions

APRN practices can be found in almost all venues of health-care delivery. Appointment and privileging oversight mandates from credentialing organizations have broadened the standards to include LIPs in hospitals, ambulatory care organizations, subacute long-term care, hospice, mental health, and MCOs, regardless of practice structures. Credentialing for other delivery systems is on the horizon. Because the standards of sponsoring organizations can change annually, the reader is advised to consult the many Web sites related to these topics to obtain the most current information possible on standards for accreditation as they relate to credentialing and privileging of the APRN's practice.

Once the application for credentialing is approved, a subsequent decision is made by the institution to authorize the specific practice activities (privileges) of the APRN. In some instances a separate privileging application is required. Consult institutional policies for their procedures.

PRIVILEGING

Once a process that hospitals used to "award" physicians the right to admit and perform clinical activities within their facility, privileging is now a process faced by many APRNs as they apply for positions within health-care facilities, MCOs, mental health and substance abuse treatment facilities, and even doctors' offices (if the APRN will be following private patients in the acute-care setting). Privileging is used by a facility or employing organization to authorize a provider's specific scope of patient care services that are consistent with an evaluation of the provider's clinical qualifications and performance for specific diagnostic or therapeutic services within well-defined limits. The granting of privileges is based on the following factors: state practice acts, agency regulations, licensure, education, training, experience, competence, health status, and judgment. It should be noted that just because the state practice act authorizes a particular activity (e.g., prescribing narcotics), a particular institution may be more restrictive and may not allow this privilege or may require a secondary signature by a physician. Monarch (2002) identifies seven categories of staff privileges within health-care facilities and systems. These are shown in **Box 7.3.**

Staff Privileges Categories

Active—allows the health-care provider to admit patients and participate in other hospital programs.

Courtesy—awarded when a limited number of patients will be admitted and when the health-care provider is an active member of another medical staff.

Affiliate—awarded when the health-care provider is no longer active, but has a longstanding relationship with the hospital.

Outpatient—awarded when the health-care provider is regularly engaged in the care of patients in outpatient settings or in programs sponsored by or on behalf of the health-care organization.

Honorary—awarded when the health-care provider is no longer active, but has outstanding accomplishments or reputation. Honorary staff privileges are distinguished from affiliate staff privileges in that honorary staff privileges permit the health-care professional to continue to admit patients to the organization.

House—allows a health-care professional to admit patients within a specialty area with the approval of an active staff member.

Allied Health Professional—permits nonphysician health-care providers to provide specified patient care services.

Rationale and Background

Privileging is a component of the credentialing process of health-care facilities. As mentioned previously, national accrediting bodies such as URAC, the National Committee for Quality Assurance, TJC, and the Accreditation Association for Ambulatory Care establish both the credentialing and privileging standards and processes by which organizations are accredited. In the early 1980s TJC (then the Joint Commission on the Accreditation of Healthcare Organizations [JCAHO]) revised its definition of medical staff and broadened the scope of practice rules to include permissive language that allowed hospitals to include other licensed individuals (permitted by law and by the hospital) to provide patient care services independently in the hospital. These privileges usually include clinical and admitting practices. TJC also established a mechanism to monitor these privileges and charged the hospital to establish criteria for clinical privileging and a process to ensure that competent individuals are providing patient care. Some facilities may have a list of "core privileges" that are appropriate for a particular type of provider or specialty practice. For example, HCPro provides sample core privilege forms that facilities can use for APRNs in dermatology and emergency rooms, acute care nurse practitioners (NPs), clinical nurse specialists (CNSs) in psychiatric mental health, and for CNMs (HCPro, 2016b). TJC is not prescriptive as to what process should be used for privileging nor do they endorse or devalue the use of "laundry lists" or core privileges. However, TJC requires evidence that the facility does indeed evaluate whether the individuals are qualified and competent to perform the privileges they are granted by the process (TJC, 2012).

The standards of TJC speak to the issue of hospital privileging in the sections on Leadership (LD) and Medical Staff (MS). The standards speak to the process itself and to the mechanisms that must be in place, executed, and outlined in the hospital bylaws. These processes must include the time frames, the appeals processes, criteria for appointment and determining specific privileges, those responsible for the credentialing and privileging process, the reappointment process, temporary privileging, telemedicine privileges, disaster privileges, and the quality improvement process. "Those who provide 'medical level of care' must use the medical staff process for credentialing and privileging, making all [medical staff] standards applicable (including recommendation by the organized medical staff and approval by the governing body, OPPE, and FPPE). APRNs and PAs who provide 'medical level of care' must be credentialed and privileged through the medical staff standards process. APRNs and PAs who do not provide 'medical level of care' utilize the human resources 'equivalent' process detailed in HR.01.02.05, EPs 10-15 (TJC, 2012)."

One area of credentialing and privileging approved by the CMS concerns the approval of TJC's requirements for telemedicine practitioners in hospitals and critical access hospitals as published in the 2012 Update 1 to the

Comprehensive Accreditation Manual for Hospitals and the *Comprehensive Accreditation Manual for Critical Access Hospitals.* These new standards appear as Standard LD.04.03.09 and MS.13.01.01 (The Joint Commission Perspectives, 2012). Several areas bear attention (The Joint Commission Perspectives, 2012): The originating site (where the patient is located) must have a written agreement with the distant site (where the provider is located) assuring compliance with Medicare CoP related to credentialing and privileging of providers. The governing body of the originating site grants privileges to a distant site independent practitioner based on the originating site's medical staff recommendations, which rely on documentation provided from the distant site if that site is a Joint Commission-accredited organization. The distant site practitioner must hold an active license that is issued and recognized by the state in which the patient is receiving the telemedicine services. The originating site collects evidence of internal review of a practitioner's performance of the privileges and sends this information to the distant site to assess quality of care, treatment, and services. Such information includes documented adverse outcomes related to sentinel events as well as complaints by patients, providers, and staff at the originating site.

In the case of a disaster, an APRN may be granted disaster privileges through a modified process. This process is typically granted for two conditions: when a disaster management plan has been activated and when the organization is unable to meet immediate patient care needs. At a minimum, verification of license and oversight of care treatment and services must be provided (TJC, 2016).

Continuing education is also mandated in TJC standards, as are four core criteria: current licensure, relevant training or experience, current competence, and ability to perform privileges requested.

Six areas of competence inform the evaluation of a practitioner in TJC standards for the credentialing and privileging process. These are:

1. Patient care
2. Medical and clinical knowledge
3. Practice-based learning and improvement
4. Interpersonal and communication skills
5. Professionalism
6. System-based practice

In addition to incorporating the aforementioned concepts into the overall evaluation of an individual's credentialing

and privileging file, two other processes also allow for closer evaluation. The first is a FPPE. As specified in TJC Standard MS.08 the FPPE is implemented for all initially requested privileges using performance criteria to judge competency. It can be subsequently used via a performance monitoring process when patient safety issues concerning competency, behavior, and ability to perform are documented. The second process is the OPPE; it supports an evidence-based approach to maintain credentialing and any decision to maintain, revise, or revoke existing privileges. Hospitals use a variety of approaches to assess APRN competency including physician review, peer review, focused case review, direct observation, coworker review, charts and documentation, and simulation testing (Center for Advancing Provider Practices, 2016). APRNs are subject to the credentialing, privileging, and monitoring processes, as are physicians, in accordance with applicable bylaws, rules, and regulations using the providers' scope of license and related standards.

When the process is done correctly, credentialing and privileging provide protection for the facility, the patient, and the practitioner. The process attempts to decrease risk for the facility and the practitioner by ensuring that the practitioners providing care to patients are currently licensed, have been educated for the role in which they are working, and are safe and competent in the scope of care they are authorized to provide. The intent is that patients ultimately benefit from well-educated, safe, competent practitioners. The process in an accredited organization also provides some security for the practitioner because federal law regarding participation in Medicare requires that staff membership and professional privileges in a hospital are not dependent solely on certification, fellowship, or membership in a specialty body or society (42 C.F.R. 482.12 (a)7) (Buppert, 2015). TJC also spells out that an appeals process must be in place if privileges are denied. The process provides for time frames and feedback to the practitioner and provides mechanisms for temporary or emergency privileging. Finally, privileging provides data for determining the economic effect of provider practice on the health-care system.

As stated in the definition, there are several factors that affect the outcome of privileging: state practice acts, agency regulations, license, education, training, experience, competence, health status, judgment, the culture of the medical staff, and the medical staff's bylaws. The factor that affects

APRNs most is the scope of practice outlined in the state practice act for the state of licensure and authorization. Each state continues to regulate the practice of APRNs differently at this time (although it may dramatically change with full implementation of the Consensus Model), and the scope of practice outlined in state regulations or statutes can be broad or narrow. Some practice acts define what APRNs can do and what specific drugs they may or may not prescribe, if they have prescriptive authority. The health-care agency regulations for credentialing and privileging are usually defined by the medical staff and hospital board and may restrict APRNs from performing certain procedures. The license and authority to practice as an APRN is tied to scope of practice issues outlined in each state practice act. Education provides the theoretical and experiential components to develop specific outcome competencies (as determined by the professional organization and the profession in scope and standards of practice). For example, the outcome competencies for a pediatric NP would not be the same as those for a geriatric NP, although there may be some overlapping competencies.

It is important to document education, training, and experience as practitioners progress in their careers because not everything essential for practice can be learned in the formal education process. A portfolio approach is essential to establish and maintain. However, just because a practitioner learned a particular procedure does not mean he or she is legally allowed to perform it because the procedure may be outside the scope of practice and license. Health requirements (both physical and mental) are evaluated and certain restrictions may apply. Untreated substance abuse problems and physical impairments may interfere with the performance of a particular role. Competence and judgment become a little more subjective when evaluating and reviewing a privileging file. Many of the components of the provider file are taken into consideration when making an overall determination of competence and judgment, and the credentialing panel may want to establish a period of observation and performance evaluation.

Process

Therapeutic and diagnostic patient care services that fall under the privileging framework are usually defined by the particular medical or surgical specialty area within the health-care facility, and criteria are established that outline safe practice. Delineation of the specific types of privileges may be presented in a variety of ways, and each facility may have its own guide of core privileges. Among the basic types of approaches are the following: category, "laundry list," severity or complexity of care, and hybrid form. The first, category, usually defines privileges along specialty lines and can vary significantly across types of specialty programs because of curriculum. The listing of privileges and skills, or the laundry list approach, is used mainly for procedures and is less appropriate when specific diseases are referenced because of the variability of presentation. For example, some of the specific tasks or procedures identified by Kleinpell and colleagues (2008) in a sample privilege request form for which an acute care NP might want to obtain hospital privileges include ventilator adjustments, managing resuscitation, digital block, chest tube insertion, and insertion of arterial or central venous catheters. The severity or complexity of care is the third form, and the fourth is a variation or hybrid of those previously mentioned.

The credentialing panel or peer review panel who reviews the credentialing files may also determine the applicant's privileges, or there may be a separate panel composed of members, including peers, from the particular service or area. The ideal panel includes an interdisciplinary group with APRNs represented. This group determines if a candidate applying for particular privileges meets the criteria based on the information submitted in his or her credentialing package and application. They may allow the practitioner independent privileges or supervised privileges depending on the evaluation. Other strategies that provide support for the credentialing and privileging of APRNs besides representation on the credentialing panel include representation in the development of any policies and procedures relevant to the process and communication networks for periodic updates on changes or alterations in APRN credentialing and privileging practices (Kleinpell et al, 2008).

Accreditation requires that the privileges and credentials files be reviewed every 2 years at a minimum to ensure currency and competence. However, clinical privileges are reviewed, revised, or updated for a variety of reasons other than at the time of reappointment. Evaluations of performance may warrant privileges being expanded or reduced. Nonuse of privileges may indicate that specific privileges are not needed and competency cannot be maintained. Finally, as technology and innovation emerge across hospital procedures and in the treatment of various diseases, the scope of privileges also change. Privileging is an ongoing process; new privileges may be added and some may be removed based on performance.

Temporary privileging may need to occur from time to time when a particular provider becomes ill or disabled, necessitating that another provider be recognized to take over certain duties of care. Recently recruited providers whose skills are specialized and needed in the facility may be awarded temporary privileges while the formal process of credentialing continues. These privileges are time limited and primary source verification of licensure and competence are allowed through phone calls until the full credentialing process occurs.

The NPDB serves an important role in the credentialing process. "The NPDB Public Use Data File contains selected variables from medical malpractice payment and adverse licensure, clinical privileges, professional society membership, and Drug Enforcement Administration (DEA) reports (adverse actions) concerning physicians, dentists, and other licensed health care practitioners and updated four times annually. It also includes reports of Medicare and Medicaid exclusion actions taken by the Department of HHS Office of Inspector General" (HRSA, NPDB, 2014).

In a survey of NPDB users, Waters, Warnecke, Parsons, Almagor, and Budetti (2006) found that many institutions use this inquiry process to make decisions about credentialing and subsequently privileging in a timely manner. Fewer than 10% of institutions indicated they had reached a credentialing decision before receiving the NPDB report, whereas up to 30% of respondents receiving a NPDB report did not grant privileging applications as requested. However, the issue of incidents not being reported to the NPDB still remains a barrier to the NPDB process as a leverage to comprehensive access to provider performance. Clearly multiple methods of data access and analysis are needed to achieve the goals of any credentialing and privileging system and the use of the NPDB is an essential component of data on credentialing of APRNs.

THE PROFESSIONAL CAREER PORTFOLIO

Portfolios continue to play a role in the world of competence assessment. Portfolios are used in a variety of ways by facilities, regulators, nursing organizations,

certifying bodies, and educational institutions. Hospitals use them for evaluation and career ladder programs. Regulatory agencies use them for assuring the public that practitioners are competent, such as in Ontario, Canada. Dietitians use them for their recertification processes. Certifying bodies use them for recertification or reactivation of credentials. Educational institutions use them for advanced placement of RNs into bachelor's of science and graduate programs and for compiling clinical practice evidence for doctoral projects. Professional career portfolios serve as the foundation of the credentialing and privileging application process used in today's health-care system.

Evidence-based practice provides a scientific, justifiable rationale for patient care therapeutics, whereas "practice-based evidence" provides a rationale for authorizing a practitioner to perform specific patient care therapeutics. Documentation of this practice-based evidence provides the information needed for making decisions regarding the privileging component of the credentialing process as currently outlined.

Tracking the events in our own lives becomes more and more complex, even though one would think it should be easier with all the technology available. As we add new experiences and roles to enrich our professional careers, work with new practitioners in a variety of settings, learn new skills, and pursue a path of life-long learning, it becomes more and more imperative to document where and when we did what, and where and when we learned what from whom. Establishing a professional credentialing portfolio as the APRN begins his or her advanced practice education and career can make the credentialing and privileging process easier and save time and money. It may even assist the APRN to be more adequately compensated by allowing him or her to achieve a higher status within a health-care facility because of practice-based evidence. The credentialing and privileging portfolio described here can build on this process. For students or early professionals building a portfolio, Beauchesne (2007) suggests including some of the following items (pp. 34–35):

- Résumé
- Personal statements on practice and scholarship
- Case studies and research activities
- Health-care project descriptions

- Brief papers and assignments
- Publications and presentations
- Evidence-based examples
- Clinical practice logs or reflections
- Video clips
- Certificates of participation
- Letters of support and recommendation
- Continuing education activities
- Evaluations and competency reviews
- Course syllabi and transcripts

An online portfolio is an excellent way to build a professional career history that can serve multiple purposes, including the credentialing and privileging process. The CAQH UPD (www.caqh.org) provides one example of a provider database, CAQH ProView, that can help health-care organizations and providers maintain accurate provider information. Registering with a database such as UPD is free for providers. Licenses, certificates, transcripts, and documents can be scanned or uploaded to the online portfolio, eliminating the need for paper copies. Although some of the materials collected during the student educational process (course syllabi, clinical logs, reflections) may not seem pertinent for the professional career portfolio, it is easy to archive these data through an online portfolio, making them available at a later time only if necessary. It is better to collect more information and not use it than to need it and not have it. Individuals can access their files anytime, anywhere with Internet access. Fear of misplacing documents or having them destroyed by unforeseen natural disasters (i.e., floods, hurricanes, or fires) can be eliminated. Stronger security of online materials has resulted from files that can be password protected. In addition, a compilation of particular documents can be sent to credentialing committees via e-mail or they may be provided Internet access to them. Updates can be added to the portfolio as new knowledge and skills are acquired, making the portfolio a living document. For those who are "Internet-phobic," the same documents can be stored on a flash drive, carried place to place, and updated when needed. Just be sure to purchase a flash drive with enough memory to store all current data and have room to spare for updates.

The purpose for which a portfolio is used determines the elements it should contain. Although many of the components are similar across portfolio types, some things are unique to the credentialing and privileging portfolio. Keeping the idea of credentialing and privileging in mind, the following format is suggested for developing this professional career portfolio. The professional career portfolio is composed of four major components: (1) the practitioner contact information page, (2) the practice-based evidence component used to assist in determining specific privileges, (3) the credentials component section, and (4) the attestation page.

Practitioner Contact Information

An introductory page with the practitioner's name, address, contact information, identity, and photo (if desired) is included.

Practice-Based Evidence Component

This area provides evidence to support the six areas of general competencies being evaluated during the hospital credentialing process and includes aspects of patient care, medical and clinical knowledge, practice-based learning and improvement, interpersonal and communication skills, professionalism, and system-based practice. The practice-based evidence component should include the following:

1. Copy of the state practice act governing scope of practice in the state of licensure
2. Core competencies for the APRN specialty
3. A sampling of references on the cost effectiveness and quality of care provided by APRNs
4. Copies of all job descriptions, especially where clinical privileges were awarded
5. Specialty procedures or processes learned and verified:
   a. in the educational process
   b. on the job
   c. through continuing education
   (See the sample of verification form, **Figure 7.1,** which could be used to validate these procedures.)
6. Letters of support and verification of practice competence in the areas outlined; include both peers and supervisors or employers
7. Employment history, identifying significant responsibilities

Provider Name:

Specialty:

License Number and Certification:
_____

Date(s) of performance _____
Procedure(s) or activity:

Description/elaboration:

Verification:

I, the undersigned, have observed ————————*(name)*———————— and can verify that he/she can safely perform the above outlined procedure(s) independently/with supervision *(circle one)*.

Provider/verifier: _____

Title: _____

License: _____

Facility: _____

Address: _____

_____

_____

Phone: _____   **Date:** _____

FIGURE 7.1 Sample verification of practice form.

8. Any performance outcome data that may have been collected at places of employment (e.g., number of patients seen per day, revenue generated, patient satisfaction)
9. Copy of the Consensus Document

Credentials Component

The credentials component should include the following:
1. Education (transcripts and diplomas)
2. Military history (if any)
3. Licenses (numbers and expiration dates or copies)
4. Certification(s) (national role specialty and subspecialty, if applicable)
5. Additional certification(s) (e.g., advanced cardiac life support, basic cardiac life support, pediatric advanced life support, trauma nurse coordinator)
6. DEA and Medicaid numbers
7. National Provider Identifier (NPI) number
8. Insurance coverage and any liability history
9. Immunizations and dates
10. Languages spoken, written, and understood (identify beginning, average, or advanced levels)
11. Research in progress or completed
12. Publications
13. Continuing education (no more than 5 years' worth or length of certification)
14. Professional organization membership and offices held in those organizations
15. References (professional and personal)
16. Certified Background Report results
17. Any previous denials of hospital credentialing or privileging

Attestation Page

The final page, or the fourth component, should include a statement that is signed and dated by the provider attesting to the information contained in the portfolio. This should be updated every 2 years or more often as any changes occur, as should the entire portfolio.

Sample

I,_____, attest to the authenticity of the information contained in this portfolio and verify that I am in good health

and able to perform the clinical privileges I am requesting. I permit the employer or gaining party of this portfolio to verify any of the information provided if necessary.

Signed_____

Date_____

CHALLENGES TO FULL SCOPE OF PRACTICE

Although APRNs are joining the staff of various facilities in greater numbers, there remain several areas that continue to challenge the APRN full scope of practice and the process to achieve it in clinical settings. The issues presented here are not exclusive, but provide a springboard for fuller discussion and solution generation in a manner in which APN scope of practice can benefit consumers.

Maintaining Data on Clinical and Administrative Performance

APRNs are held to standards of performance that include clinical practice and administrative standards. Both have economic implications for decisions to appoint or reappoint APRNs to an institutional staff. The institution may find that clinical performance falls outside established benchmarks if patients under the APRN's care have excessive lengths of stay, repeated and lengthy delays in appointments, quality of care issues, and additional exposure to liability resulting from variation in performance. Patient satisfaction may be easily tied to performance. Institutions will need to more closely track coding practices of APRNs in order to capture the actual practice of APRNs and subsequent outcomes. Without this data and analysis, performance cannot be understood or managed in ways comparable with other providers.

APRNs are wise to monitor their performance against the targets of the organization and colleagues and use the feedback to initiate personal or systems-wide performance improvement strategies. Maintaining documentation of outputs and accomplishments, patient acknowledgments, and cost savings are important assets for the APRN's portfolio. It is also important that APRNs be aware of the information and reference data about activities that are required to be verified as part of the credentialing process. Losing track of certification and licensure renewals has immediate repercussions for the credentialing process. Determining the accuracy of any inputs into the NPDB or other databases is important to verify before an institutional query on the APRN occurs. Opportunities to correct information are less stressful when the APRN is not abutting an institutional deadline.

Decreasing Barriers to Continuity of Care

Although the numbers of APRNs holding hospital privileges has accelerated, two reasons stand out as rationales to seek out and obtain privileges that will help to decrease barriers to continuity and seamless patient care. One is that some insurance companies and MCOs require their primary care provider (PCPs, or in this case APRN) to hold hospital privileges as a prerequisite to credentialing and billing or receiving payment. The other is that a PCP who does not have privileges within a hospital cannot review the chart or care provided for a patient once that patient is admitted to the hospital. Although the provider may make a friendly visit and ask questions of the patient, he or she cannot validate or follow the treatment, tests, and outcomes in the patient record because of the Health Insurance Portability and Accountability Act (HIPAA). Being the provider of record and in many cases the one who will eventually continue to follow that patient upon discharge would make that transition back to the community a much more seamless process. This is especially important for independent NPs who carry their own panel of patients and is also complicated by the fact that hospitals may not notify APRNs when one of their patients is admitted. They may not identify the APRN as the provider of record either, partly because of lower reimbursement levels for the hospital. It is important to emphasize to both the patient and his or her family that they must inform hospital staff if admitted and to notify the APRN of the admission. If the whole process is more transparent and collaborative and the provider can "hit the ground running" when the patient is once again placed in his or her care, the patient will be the one who benefits.

Managed Care Panels

Health-care providers work in a competitive environment where more than one type of provider may be able to provide the same scope of practice or provide partial activities within another scope of practice. The ability to be credentialed and apply for legal scope of practice privileges rests in the hands of the credentialing structure. Professional medical societies are flush with complaints from physicians who perceive they have been excluded from MCO provider panels, and these exclusions present a glass ceiling for APRNs as well.

Sometimes the exclusion of APRNs is because of lack of knowledge concerning the full scope of APRN practice parameters; at other times there is a perception of anticompetitiveness or restraint of trade action (IOM, 2011). APRNs are well advised to provide documentation about APRN performance outcomes compared with other providers through the use of evidence-based reports and articles and quality reports, especially ones published in the provider's representative journals. Seeking advocates and allies at the institution to which the APRN is applying can assist in the politics of selection for worthy candidates. Where warranted, legal consultation may prove helpful to understand the issues and the APRN's rights.

Another issue intertwined with managed care panels is reimbursement. Medicaid managed care in particular becomes tricky when (a) state laws affect recognition of NPs as PCPs, (b) federal Medicaid law permits pediatric and family NPs to be used in primary care management but does not require it, and (c) the law is silent regarding the inclusion of these providers in Medicaid managed care provider panels. Whether NPs, who serve more than half of all Medicaid beneficiaries, can be designated PCPs in MCOs is dependent on states' policy choices and individual MCO credentialing policies (Van Vleet & Paradise, 2015).

Credentialing of the APRN Across Multiple Organizations

When working in a health-care system or between two or more entities, the APRN may be confronted with replication of the credentialing application process for each entity. This can be extremely time consuming and result in lost opportunities. It is important to gather perceptions from other providers and administrators about expectations and ramifications for productivity given duplication in processing of multiple credentialing applications. Create a solution team to construct alternative approaches to reduce redundancy and be prepared to gather support from colleagues on alternative proposals to present to the governing board. As discussed previously, maintaining an online professional portfolio will also help. Providers are reminded quarterly to update their information and attest to its accuracy. Other regulations and organizations are on the horizon to limit redundancy in credentialing and privileging and streamline the business of health care. Consulting the CMS rules and regulations intermittently can facilitate your ability to meet the changes in processes in a timely manner.

Uniform Adoption of the Consensus Model for APRN Regulation

Although 2015 has passed, the number of states adopting all the components of the APRN Consensus Model document is still low. However, it is difficult to evaluate because there are multiple components that must be addressed to fully comply and many require legislative change. The NCSBN has been tracking states by each component and scoring each state as it reaches compliance. In general, NCSBN is tracking recognition of all four roles, graduate education, national certification, and uniform titling (APRN). As of 2017, less than one-third (1/3) of states have reached full compliance with all the components of the Consensus Model (see the maps on the NCSBN Web site at https://www.ncsbn.org for the latest details). Currently, credentialing requirements for APRNs vary among states as to the mechanism for title protection and scope of practice differences. The NCSBN proposed that it is appropriate for APRNs to be legally regulated through a second license for their role and population focus because their activities are complex and involve role and population competencies, independence, and autonomy (NCSBN, 2008). Most state models now require an application, RN licensure, completion of a graduate degree with a major in nursing or a graduate degree with a concentration in the advanced nursing practice category, and professional certification

from a board-approved national certifying body. Graduate education includes the doctorate of nursing practice (DNP) degree. The Comprehensive Care Certification (CCC) for DNP graduates administered by the American Board of Comprehensive Care (ABCC) and promoted by Columbia University grants the Diplomate of Comprehensive Care (DCC) credential. It is currently not an NCSBN-approved certification nor is it recognized by the Consensus Document or joint dialogue group as an appropriate certification for uniform regulation of APRNs. The CCC examination is based on Step 3 of the National Board of Medical Education Examination. Adoption of the (NCSBN, 2008) allows the APRN role and population focus to be regulated at the state level and the specialization focus to be credentialed by specialty organizations rather than by state licensure. The CCC currently falls into the "specialty" certification realm. The examination was first given in 2008 at which time 22 of 45 individuals taking the examination received the credential. From the initial 2008 examination through 2012, 135 individuals took the examination for the first time, with an average pass rate of 50.8% (range of 33% in 2012 to 70% in 2011). Although no results have been posted since 2012, the Web site indicates that the next testing date is anticipated to be in 2017. See further information at http://abcc.dnpcert.org/exam-pass-rates.

APRN Representation on the Medical Staff and Adjusting Bylaws

As APRN privileging becomes more common, the APRN should seek governance representation on the medical staff and ensure the medical staff bylaws embrace full representation of APRNs. There are exemplars for this movement: The Center for Advancing Provider Practices (2016) reported that 54% of Medical Staff Credentialing Committees have at least one APRN or PA as a member, representing a growth of 186% from 2013 to 2015 in APRN and PA representation among 37 organizations. Early on in Ellenville Regional Hospital in New York, an APRN, Bob Donaldson, was invited to review and revise the medical staff bylaws; he was ultimately elected president of the medical staff in 2009, with another NP serving as secretary of the medical board (Hendren,

2011; http://www.ellenvilleregional.org). As privileging of APRNs continues to grow across the country, more will assume positions and contribute to the leadership of institutional privileging.

All 50 states currently address advanced practice in public policy in some manner. For the most part, state boards of nursing hold authority over advanced practice. Where the prescription of medications is a sanctioned activity, additional education in advanced pharmacology is required. By this arrangement many state boards of nursing have deferred to the profession's right to recognize its specialists through certification and to develop and promulgate the standards of practice on which certification is based.

CONCLUSION

It is clear that credentialing and privileging are important processes that can be time consuming, complex, frequently changing, and influenced by multiple factors. But these processes can have a significant impact on both the scope of practice and economic status of the practitioner. As you think about eventual changes in credentialing and privileging, be aware that no change is insignificant. Each change holds both personal ramifications and implications for the profession as a whole. It is always wise to follow the dialogue and plan around national regulatory initiatives that will direct your scope of practice.

8

The Kaleidoscope of Collaborative Practice

Alice F. Kuehn

Learning Outcomes

Learning outcomes expected as a result of this chapter:

- Summarize the history of physician–nurse and nurse–nurse changing relationships and collaborative efforts.
- Describe the myriad aspects of collaborative practice.
- Distinguish between multidisciplinary, interdisciplinary, intradisciplinary, and transdisciplinary practices.
- Identify the status of collaboration in each of the four advanced practice nurse (APN) roles.
- Describe a framework for collaboration (concept and components).
- Explain the historic and current barriers to health professional collaboration.
- Propose strategies for developing a successful collaborative team.
- Compare the traditional and emerging collaborative practice models.

The future of nursing and health care depends on partnership. One of the four key messages of the Institute of Medicine (IOM) report on the future of nursing states that "nurses should be full partners with physicians and other health professionals in redesigning health care in the United States" (2011, p. 7). The adoption of the APRN Consensus Model (APRN Joint Dialogue Group, 2008) is identified as a key factor in regulatory change, noting that the resulting consistency in regulation of advanced practice nursing across states is facilitating steady progress in legislative reform (Pearson, 2011; Phillips, 2011). In Phillips's 2016 report, although

22 states plus the District of Columbia (DC) now allow for full NP scope of practice (SOP), meaning no collaborative agreements with a physician are required, 28 states still require some sort of agreement for prescribing and advanced clinical practice. Phillips noted that there were "significant state legislative accomplishments in the areas of APRN practice authority, reimbursement, and prescriptive authority. During the past year, exceptional progress continued through strong and successful partnerships made possible by APRN professional associations, Boards of Nursing (BON), and the Future of Nursing: Campaign for Action" (p. 21). Current trends in health care reflect an ever-increasing call for collaboration, consensus building, coordinated care, and shared decision making (SDM) as new models of care delivery such as medical homes, nurse-managed clinics, SDM, and accountable care organizations (ACOs) continue to emerge (American Nurses Association [ANA], 2010b; Haney, 2010; Hughes, 2011; McCarter et al, 2016; Rice et al, 2010). In the ANA's Social Policy statement, collaboration is described as a partnership in which all partners are valued for their expertise, power, and distinct areas of practice. The statement also acknowledges their shared areas of practice and mutual goals and emphasizes that the "nursing profession is particularly focused on establishing effective working relationships and collaborative efforts essential to accomplishing its health-oriented mission" (ANA, 2010b, p. 7).

The role of the APRN has evolved along a continuum of collaborative interactive models of increasing complexity (Kuehn, 1998). Just as a kaleidoscope creates a constantly changing set of colors and patterns, collaboration is a constantly changing aspect of health-care practice, moving from little interest to a great demand, from frustration to success, and sometimes back again. The interactions among members of a health-care team present a new picture each time the group, situation, time, or environment changes. This chapter reviews the history and examines myriad aspects of collaborative practice. It compares and contrasts multidisciplinary, interdisciplinary, intradisciplinary, and transdisciplinary practices, using examples to clarify the distinctions and similarities. The values, barriers to, and strategies by which collaborative practice is being developed are presented and the continuing and expanding evolutions of collaborative practice models are examined.

A HISTORY OF CHANGING RELATIONSHIPS

Our world continues to change so rapidly that change itself has become the constant. This sense of change in every aspect of life was described by Alvin Toffler in his classic 1970 publication *Future Shock,* a term he created to describe the "shattering stress and disorientation" resulting from too much change too quickly. Our response to change has historically been slower than the change itself. However, with today's rapidly increasing pace of change, the lag between the change and our response is growing, and this is what Senge (1994) calls *future shock.* Much of our human behavior flows from our ability to embrace or to fight the pace of life. Ours is a world of transience: a series of short-term relationships with people, things, places, workplaces, and information itself. In a situation in which the duration of relationships has been shortened, our sense of reality and of commitment and our ability to cope are seriously challenged. The flow of change is not linear, and we are being forced to adjust to novel situations for which we have not been prepared. Because we are living in a health-care world demanding collaboration, cost effectiveness, and high-quality care, the relationships among professionals are rapidly changing, demanding flexibility and collegiality. A key recommendation of the IOM report *Keeping Patients Safe: Transforming the Work Environment of Nurses* (2004) was for health-care institutions to move away from a hierarchal approach to shared decision making and increased support of interdisciplinary collaboration. It should be noted here that the Patient Protection and Affordable Care Act (PPACA) introduced in 2010 has had a major impact on the manner of health-care delivery today and continues to influence the development of new more collaborative models of care. However, although it supports efforts to increase the number of APNs, there remain challenges to the delivery of care by APNs because of continuing inconsistencies between federal and state policies resulting in practice restrictions (Carthon & Sarik, 2015).

Physician–Nurse Relationships Over Time

In 1859, Florence Nightingale described the role of nursing as a specific set of relationships to medicine and hospital administration set within the social structure of the times. Placing the nurse as a care provider subservient to the physician established and formalized a role structure that, after nearly 150 years, continues to define society's general sense of the nurse role as within the role of the physician (Partin, 2009; Workman, 1986). A statement issued at the 2009 American Medical Association (AMA) House of Delegates meeting supporting this hierarchical role structure called for physician supervision of nurses, noting that the nurse role, even though it is important, must be supervised. The nursing response drafted by the ANA and some APRN organizations stressed that the concept of physician supervision of APRNs is out of date, is inappropriate, and creates a major barrier to the access of care (Partin, 2009; Sorrel, 2009). The challenges physicians face in understanding, supporting, and embracing the reality of the advanced practice role is a result of "cognitive dissonance," a rejection or denial of information that challenges their preconceptions of the nurse role.

In examining the historical roots of collaborative experiences between physician and nurse, the years between 1873 and the 20th century saw the relationship of nurse to physician become more a scenario within a hospital setting. The triad of physician–nurse–hospital superintendent never truly evolved in equilibrium as the Nightingale model envisioned because the scenario of a nursing superintendent reporting separately to the hospital trustees challenged the deference given to physicians and administrators in practice and would have undermined both their authority and the use of student nurses as workers. The ongoing development of hierarchical relationships within the hospital between physicians, nurses, and administrators resulted also from changes occurring in nursing itself. Nursing sought to gain more professional status through a rigid hierarchical management style of its own within a continuing hospital attitude of paternalism (Markowitz & Rosner, 1979; Reverby, 1979, 1987). Collaborative relationships with physicians, hospitals, and foundations serving the health-care system began to develop during and following the Great Depression as evidenced by the following: medical society participation in the Committee on Nursing of the Association of American Medical Colleges as they endorsed the Committee on the Grading of Nursing Schools; a manual on hospital nursing service administration, sponsored by the American Hospital Association (AHA) and the National League for Nursing Education (NLNE), published in 1935; and a

survey of nursing schools in psychiatric hospitals under the auspices of a joint committee approach by the American Psychiatric Association (APA) and the NLNE. It should be noted, however, that these examples are not of individual collaborative relationships but of organizations, and were tenuous at best; the medical society withdrew from the Committee on Nursing shortly after their endorsement (Roberts, 1959).

The ANA code of 1950 spelled out a relationship of nurse to physician as a complex mix of dependent and independent responsibilities. Roberts (1959) stated, "The nurse is obligated to carry out the physician's orders intelligently, to avoid misunderstandings or inaccuracies by verifying orders, and to refuse to participate in unethical procedures" (p. 563). However, if every nursing decision made must come from within the orders flowing from another profession, the relationship cannot be collaboration but instead becomes supervised delegation. Kinlein (1977) identified the dilemma in nursing as a blockage of the ability of nurses to initiate nursing diagnoses, design nursing care, or establish a distinctive practice when the power of the medical judgment is the prime source of all decision making regarding patient care. Nursing judgments thus become delegated medical judgments because they are aimed at a medical goal and have to agree with that goal. Kinlein describes an example of a physician snatching a chart from her hands while she was teaching a student regarding a treatment regimen. The doctor stated, "What are you doing, talking about that? That's none of your concern. Just teach those students to give bedpans and then to remove them" (1977, p. 30), leaving both nurse faculty and student to conclude that either the nurse has to learn more and become a doctor or learn less so that he or she is prepared merely to carry out orders. In this situation, Kinlein notes, the nurse was expecting the physician to be knowledgeable, the patient expected both physician and nurse to be knowledgeable, and the physician expected the nurse to have no knowledge. This is an unacceptable situation, as well as a clear example of noncollaborative, unidisciplinary practice, with no communication between the two sets of providers except through a hierarchical, supervisory relationship.

The current system of care delivery has been described as supporting professional individualism and separatism of roles, often resulting in defensiveness, lack of continuity, competition, redundancy, excessive costs, fragmentation, little cooperation or teamwork, grossly inadequate and outdated systems of communication, and underutilization of APRNs (Fischman, 2002; Goodman, 2007; IOM, 2011; Norsen, Opladen, & Quinn, 1995; O'Neil & Pew Health Professions Commission, 1998; Spitrey, 2016). However, calls for collaborative practice have continued to grow and intensify, requiring physicians, nurses, and all health professionals to begin working through the relationship-building process required to establish a collaborative team approach. Pearson (2011) noted that "the irony of our continuing struggle with organized medicine is that, even while we fight against medicine's inappropriate domination over our practice, we must maintain and enhance our working relationship with individual physicians, for patients are best served when providers work together" (p. 22). This requires a team effort within an environment of mutual respect and valuing of each professional's role. As Cooper reminded us, "Ultimately, the success of each discipline will be judged by how effectively it participates in a continuum of care that meets the needs of patients and of the health care system overall" (2001, p. 58).

"The credible evidence showing that collaboration improves health care outcomes for patients entreats the two professions to put cooperation before professional roles" (Phillips, Green, Fryer, & Dovey, 2001, p. 1325). An increasing number of health-care studies continue to affirm the need for and value of collaboration, emphasizing that efficient delivery and high quality of care may depend on the level of collaboration among professional care providers (Donald et al, 2009; Hojat et al, 2003; Hughes, 2011; Rice et al, 2010; Zwarenstein & Bryant, 2000). Maier and Aiken (2016), in examining the expanding clinical roles for the nurse globally, noted that the "focus of research and policy debate in the U.S. is shifting away from *whether* NP-provided care is safe, to *how to* reduce barriers to practice and maximize access for those most in need" (p. 2, italics added).

Status of Collaborative Practice in Advanced Practice Roles

The growth and acceptance of the APRN role has hinged on the willingness of the profession to acknowledge and support the role; provide advanced education and experience; and promote a clarity of role that facilitates development of a sense of identity and clear understanding by other disciplines, policy makers and legislators, and the public. As each of the four APRN practices—certified registered nurse anesthetists (CRNAs), certified nurse-midwives (CNMs), clinical nurse specialists (CNSs), and nurse practitioners (NPs)—has moved toward autonomy in practice, establishing positive relationships with the medical community has been key. Stanley (2005, p. 34) notes that "consumer satisfaction and physician advocacy have proved to be powerful stimuli" for operationalizing the APRN role. Applying Benner's (1984) competencies and domains of nursing practice from novice to expert levels to advanced practice, Fenton and Brykczynski (1993) identified additional domains and competencies and verified the high level of expertise of APRNs. However, the SOP flowing from this model of expertise needs to be clearly identified. It is critical for the practice of all APRNs, while maintaining clinical practice distinctions, to be conceptually united, stressing commonalities while acknowledging differences in practice patterns but promoting an interdisciplinary focus in their practice (Stanley, 2005). Once the role is clarified, SOPs delineated, common practice elements of APRNs made known, and support from professional colleagues and consumers ongoing, the challenges faced in establishing collaborative practice will be greatly minimized. This is the hope of the APRN Consensus Model (APRN Joint Dialogue Group, 2008). Without these foundational components, the challenges of creating truly functional teams will continue to be significant. The following section provides a brief overview of role development challenges, achievements, and approaches to collaboration for each of the four APRN practices as well as three additional provider roles affecting primary care delivery: the PA, pharmacist, and the "patient navigator."

The Certified Registered Nurse Anesthetist

Clarity of role and a reach for autonomous practice were forged early in the development of nurse anesthetists. In a study of surgeon–nurse anesthetist collaboration in surgery between 1889 and 1950, Koch (2015) noted that the success of nurses in anesthesia duty during the Civil War led to the formal collaboration between nurses and surgeons at the Mayo Clinic and the beginning of a long and continuing surgeon–nurse collaboration that helped advance surgery in the United States. Alice Magaw, a pioneer in the field who worked at the Mayo Clinic in the early 1900s, supported the separation of nurse anesthesia from nursing service administration, emphasizing its need for recognition and requirements for specialized education. During World War II, the role was identified as a clinical nursing specialty within the military field, and in 1945 a formal national certification process was established. The SOP of the CRNA has been described by the American Association of Nurse Anesthetists (AANA) as a practice in collaboration with legally required professional health-care providers. This description noting a "legally required collaborator" has led some to regard the legal status of nurse anesthesia as a "dependent function" under physician control and continues to result in considerable challenges in development of a high-level collaborative practice model (AANA, 2006; Bigbee, 1996; Faut-Callahan & Kremer, 1996; Taylor, 2009). Some states use the term *collaboration* to define a relationship in which each party is responsible for his or her field of expertise while maintaining open communication on anesthetic techniques. Other states require the consent or order of a physician or other qualified licensed provider to administer the anesthetic. The Centers for Medicare and Medicaid Services (CMS) required physician supervision for nurse anesthetist services to Medicare patients. However, in late 2001, a rule published in the Federal Register allowed a state to be exempt from this physician supervision requirement for nurse anesthetists after appropriate approval by the governor. By 2007, 14 states had opted out of this federal requirement (Blumenreich, 2007, p. 93). Recent literature focuses on the term *anesthesia care team* (ACT) to indicate a practice by a CRNA with an anesthesiologist in a medically directed environment. Jones and Fitzpatrick (2009) identified four possible types of current inpatient anesthesia team arrangements in the United States: an all-anesthesiologist staff, an all-nurse anesthetist staff, a mixed staff of the previous two, and a team of anesthesiologist and anesthesiologist assistants (p. 431). In their study of collaboration among members of these teams, they found satisfaction with collaboration expressed by both nurse-anesthetists and physicians. However, they noted that there are still issues with role conflict; unclear expectations and limits on SOP with mixed teams; and a component of exclusion from hospital, departmental, and anesthesia group responsibilities when only physicians can participate in hospital committees or represent the group. The challenge for CRNAs is to work with physician colleagues to achieve fullness of practice for each member of the anesthesia team while working together to continue the advancement of surgery (Koch, 2015).

The Certified Nurse-Midwife

In the colonial and pioneer history of the United States, midwives were respected members of both settler and Native American communities. However, since the early 1900s the role has had a stormy history caused in no small part by the low status of women, sparse education, religious intolerance, and increased domination of physician obstetricians with the movement toward birthing in hospitals. In 1921, the Maternity Center Association of New York and the Henry Street Visiting Nurse Association proposed establishing a school of nurse-midwifery. However, strong opposition from medicine, nursing, and the public arose, mainly because of a generally held negative view of the role of midwife as an exemplar of inadequacy, little education, and social incompetence. In 1925, the role moved to a new level of recognition and respect with the inauguration of the Appalachian clinics of Kentucky (Frontier Nursing Service) by Mary Breckenridge (Dorroh & Norton, 1996).

The number of CNMs has increased from just 275 in 1963 to more than 4,000 by 1995 and 7,000 in 2011 (American College of Nurse-Midwives [ACNM], 2011). CNMs consider interdisciplinary practice as a *sine qua non* of their practice, and this position has been affirmed in their standards of care and formal definitions of practice (ACNM/ACOG, 2002). In 1971, the ACNM, the American College of Obstetricians and Gynecologists (ACOG), and the Nurses Association of the ACOG issued a joint statement supporting the concept of obstetrical team practice. However, the teams were to be "directed by a physician," formalizing a hierarchical practice pattern that continues to pose challenges to development of a collaborative approach to practice (Bigbee, 1996). The ACNM statement on collaborative management defines *collaboration* as "the process whereby a CNM or certified midwife (CM) and physician jointly manage the care of a woman or newborn that has become medically, gynecologically or obstetrically complicated" (ACNM, 1997). The need for collaboration is indicated by the health status of the client rather than by statute or edict. However, the number of viable practices currently differs considerably state by state because of legal and legislative requirements for collaboration and the parameters of required collaborative practice protocols, which vary from state to state.

Because of lack of support from physicians and hospitals, CNMs are often unable to practice or their practice is severely limited because of economic competition and differing views on the meaning and value of collaboration. A study from New Zealand offers a model of midwifery care in which midwifery-led maternity care is the dominant model and 75% of the New Zealand women choose a midwife as their "lead maternity caregiver" (LMC). When midwives did refer to an obstetrician, 74% indicated they continued providing care in collaboration with the obstetrician and the relationships between professionals were satisfying (Skinner & Foureur, 2010). This model starkly contrasts with the description by Goodman (2007) of the "marginalization of certified nurse-midwives in the United States" where in 2007 midwives attended only 7% of births.

The issue of economic competition is another hindrance to CNM practice. In a conversation between a nurse-midwife and an obstetrician with whom she had a good working relationship, the physician commented, "I don't have any problems with you personally, but the fact is that my practice is not full, and until it is there is not going to be a nurse-midwife that will get privileges at this hospital" (Goodman, 2007, p. 616). Another economic factor threatening the future of the collaborative relationship is malpractice insurance cost. For example, in a discussion with one CNM/physician practice group, the CNMs noted that the cost of malpractice insurance increased from $18,000 to $40,000 during 1 year, and their practice group could not afford to cover the additional costs. Individual CNMs did not get paid for all the calls they took, nor were they able to attend enough births to cover the cost of their own insurance. This inequity of practice compensation coupled with the lack of 100% support of a practice by their physician group resulted in the midwives no longer practicing midwifery but being limited to providing other women's health services.

In October 2002, the joint statement between the ACNM and the ACOG was revised for the fifth time in 30 years. An ongoing concern of many CNMs and physicians had been the language and the inferences of previous documents readily open to multiple interpretations. The leadership of ACNM and ACOG decided to develop a statement more reflective of the current status of each profession, as well as contemporary realities within the women's health-care system. The 2002 ACNM/ACOG joint statement was endorsed by both parties as a document "that promotes respect and collaboration between CNMs/CMs and [medical doctors] and encourages individual practices to work collegially together to meet the needs of individual patients" (Shah, 2002, p. 2). The simplicity of the statement was perhaps its greatest asset. By not dictating specific protocols or responsibilities, professional accountability is placed where it rightfully belongs: "on each respective profession and the individual women's health care professional" (p. 3). The most recent joint statement of the ACNM and ACOG alliance in 2011 reaffirms their shared goals regarding women's health and continues its simplicity of language and approach, emphasizing the need for a health-care system that facilitates communication among providers and across settings (ACNM/ACOG, 2002). The positive take on this statement, the review of APRN outcomes by Newhouse and colleagues (2011) confirming the high-quality care delivered by CNMs in the United States, and the evidence provided by the 2012 American Midwifery Certification Board noting that nearly 50% of recent CNM/CM grads were providing some primary care services either independently or collaboratively stress the continuing need for developing collaborative approaches in the practice setting as well as for greater clarity of SOP (Phillippi & Barger, 2015).

The Clinical Nurse Specialist

The CNS role, which originated in the late 1930s, was formalized as a nurse-clinician to be prepared in graduate nursing programs. Its emergence represented a major shift of focus in graduate education from the choice of a functional role of primarily teacher or administrator to the selection of a clinical specialization in practice. Of the multiple specialties represented by the CNS role, psychiatry was the first to move to graduate education and is among the most highly respected. Some have attested that collaborative activities with physicians seemed to come more naturally for this group because of their graduate-level education, which allowed CNSs and physicians to more readily relate to each other as peers (Bigbee, 1996). A review of literature published between 1990 and 2008 on care provided by CNSs gave supporting evidence of their value in acute care settings in reducing length of stay, cost, and rates of complications (Newhouse et al, 2011).

Key elements of CNS practice identified by the American Association of Critical-Care Nurses (AACN, 2007) include "collaborating with other disciplines to provide interdisciplinary best practices" (p. 7). Collaboration is one of the eight CNS competencies considered essential for nurses providing care in the acute-care setting. These competencies are part of the AACN synergy model for patient care, recommended as a guide for clinical practice in acute care. The model is predicated on the fact that patient outcomes are optimal when patient characteristics and nurse competencies are in sync (Kaplow, 2007). One CNS described her collaborative practice level as a real partnership with a great deal of mutual caring and respect between providers. Each partner grounded interactions in self-confidence and personal mastery, and they planned together "always." Yet another CNS noted that her collaborating physicians needed some education on what the CNS could and could not do, but they learned as they jointly practiced, and a real comfort level occurred after about 6 months. A hematology-oncology APRN group, which formed a successful collaborative practice over a period of 7 years, identified effective leadership and shared development of goals and communication as critical for establishment of a viable structure (Schaal et al, 2008). Another collaborative partnership of the CNS and the nurse manager of an oncology unit described the key element of success as development of mutually acceptable goals (Gaguski & Begyn, 2009). In 2016 Spitrey reported on the reaction to the Department of Veterans Affairs proposal to allow full practice authority for all APRNs working within the VA system as a means of increasing veteran access to care. She noted the resistance is still strong in some sectors despite nursing's track record of safe and effective advanced nursing care delivery. The key to the future of a positive and productive collaborative practice for all APRNs with physicians and other health professionals is a relationship that becomes more mutually valued and partner driven.

The Nurse Practitioner

The role of the NP has been described as an innovative role in primary care, grown from the role of the public health nurse and possessing a high degree of autonomy in practice (Bigbee, 1996). Since its inception in the 1960s, a considerable expansion of the concept of the NP role has occurred, as NPs have moved into a multitude of settings that are not necessarily primary care such as long-term and acute care. Because of the unique and varied ways in which the role has developed—coming from certificate programs, many within medical schools, and gradually moving into graduate nurse programs—the history of collaboration is a patchwork quilt. Support of and opposition to the role has come from both medicine and nursing. Martha Rogers (1972) opposed the role as demeaning to nursing in deference to medical practice, and this view, supported by many nurse educators at the time, created serious divisions within the nursing profession as NP educators worked to enhance the role and move it into graduate-level education. Medical opposition, which existed from the beginning, is often couched in terms of *patient safety,* despite the fact that it often is more related to issues of control and competition in practice. Because of these powerful sources of opposition, the focus on collaboration has been both a boon and a boondoggle to NP practice. The importance of the interdisciplinary team and the responsibility of the NP to assist in collaborative team development have been consistently emphasized (Buerhaus, 2010; Hanna, 1996). However, as the term *collaboration* found in some state nursing practice acts often conveys a concept of "supervision," there are many who would strike the word from any statutory documents. The evolving acute-care NP (ACNP) role requires a very explicit differentiation of medical and nursing domains within a collaborative practice. Strong support from nursing service—and better yet, having the ACNP housed within the nursing department—allows for easier differentiation of role by each partner. This promotes a team in which each partner comes from a solid professional sense of self and can then join with others to fuse into an autonomous, interdependent team of providers. In contrast, when the ACNP is "supervised" by a resident or is employed by a medical specialty department, it becomes more difficult for the practitioner to participate equally in decision making and to be considered a full partner in the practice (Lott, Polak, Kenyon, & Kenner, 1996).

The role of the NP within managed care systems has evolved into a process of collaboration, coordination, and negotiation, requiring the creation of new relationships among a wide range of personnel. Role negotiation is a key component of this type of practice, in which the required interaction between professionals for the specific purpose of changing the other's expectation of one's role can result in increased job satisfaction, reduced role conflict, and a more positive team relationship (Miller & Apker, 2002). A professional partnership promoting collaboration replaces competition with shared responsibilities in which each partner brings a unique and necessary set of knowledge and skills to the practice. The fear of loss of professional uniqueness is met head on by a practice in which the expertise and unique abilities of each team member, when combined into a synchronous whole, deliver a high level of care not possible through the efforts of a single provider (Norsen, Opladen, & Quinn, 1995).

A review of two rural Ontario primary care practices consisting of NPs and family physicians (FPs) found comparable involvement of both in health-promotion activities and considerably greater focus of NPs on disease prevention and supportive care. However, the review also found NPs were underutilized in relation to curative and rehabilitative services, with referral patterns being largely unidirectional from NP to FP. The authors noted that such a one-sided referral process does not reflect collaboration, which demands shared, reciprocal practice patterns (Way, Jones, Baskerville, & Busing, 2001). In addition, the regulated drug list required for Ontario NPs does not permit NPs to renew medications for stable chronic illnesses, limiting their SOP and hampering the ability of the NP to assist patients in the management of their chronic illnesses (Way et al, 2001). Rationale offered for drawbacks to a full collaborative practice included unclear medico-legal issues affecting the ability to "share responsibility," an absence of interdisciplinary education at both undergraduate and graduate levels, and lack of knowledge and practice experience regarding the scope of NP practice. The Missouri Nurses Association (2011) reported that the health-care access and needs of rural Missourians were currently strained and any discussion of solutions must include considering the role of NPs and physician assistants (PAs). They stressed that the "future economic stability and health status of rural Missourians depends on . . . [considering] options that allow for increased use of the expertise of advanced practice registered nurses" (Becker & Porth, 2011, p. 9). Panelist Charlene Hanson summarized the state of NP practice when she noted that "physicians and NPs at the grassroots have worked out a comfortable, collaborative, professional relationship that benefits both. But the relationship at the policy and organizational state and national levels is much more divisive" (Buerhaus, 2010). Expanding this thought, Marshall (2016) noted that obtaining full

practice rights for APRNs does not come from any federal action so much as from state legislative changes. Despite challenges to NP practice, their value is continuing to be acknowledged and the health system delivery process is changing and requiring a greater focus on teamwork (Maier & Aiken, 2016).

A FRAMEWORK FOR COLLABORATION

The Concept

Collaboration is a "dynamic, transforming process of creating a power-sharing partnership" (Sullivan, 1998, p. 6). As a dynamic process, it includes the flexible distribution of both status and authority, and requires both relationship building and shared decision making. A distinctive interpersonal process, it requires that the partners recognize and acknowledge their shared values and commit to interact constructively to solve problems and accomplish identified goals, purposes, or outcomes. Using the consensus process, where participants are not coerced as in compromise or "majority vote" but helped to reach an agreement they can approve, even if they do not agree with all points, facilitates high levels of agreement and team satisfaction. Shared power, a key component within a collaborative practice, requires the active contribution of each participant, respect for and openness to each other's contributions, and use of consensus in forming new approaches to practice that use the strengths of each participant (ANA, 2010a; APRN Joint Dialogue Group, 2008; IOM, 2011; O'Brien, Martin, Heyworth, & Meyer, 2009; Rice et al, 2010).

The Components

A viable and high-level collaborative practice may be readily identified by the existence of four essential components: separate and unique practice spheres, common goals, shared power control, and mutual concerns. **Table 8.1** presents the components essential for a positive practice, the key attributes of a highly collaborative practice, and practitioner competencies contributing to success. A phenomenological study of how APRNs and physicians perceive and describe their sense of collaboration identified four key behaviors as essential for collaboration: approachability, interpersonal

TABLE 8.1		
Components of Collaborative Practice		
Essential Components	**Key Attributes**	**Competencies**
Separate and unique practice spheres or scope of practice Common goals Shared power control	Autonomous, trusting relationship Confidence in a partner's skill Bidirectional referrals and consultation	Assertiveness Communication skills Conflict management Cooperation
Mutual concerns	Consensus-driven decision making	Coordination
	Equitable reporting lines and evaluators	Clinical skills Mutual respect
	Mutually defined goals of the practice	Decision-making skills Positive attitude
	Open, informal communication Parity between providers (physical space, caseload, and support staff) Positive support by colleagues, support staff, and consumers	Trust Willingness to dialogue

skills, listening, and verbal message skills, each of which reflects either the attributes or competencies identified by O'Brien, Martin, Heyworth, and Meyer (2009).

1. *Separate and unique practice spheres.* Both physician and nurse must identify components of their practice that are separate and unique (SOP) and components that they share. A high-level collaborative practice requires an autonomous, trusting relationship within which bilateral consultation and referrals are the norm. Autonomy exists within each practitioner's skill and competence and allows for confident decision making. It is the trust of the team that empowers that person to practice independently within his or her defined scope of practice. As one APRN noted, "You must be willing to expand your boundaries but know your limitations and where you feel comfortable in your practice" (Bailey & Armer, 1998, p. 243). The existence of bidirectional referral and consultation reflects a high level of trust between practice partners. In one instance, the physician response to a consultation request was, "Now this is not what you have to do; this is what I'd recommend. But the final decision is yours because it's your patient" (Bailey & Armer, 1998, p. 243).

2. *Common goals.* When both partners agree to responsibilities for practice goals, the partners are well on their way to a synchronous relationship. As one provider in a highly collaborative practice noted, "Care by all providers is based on mutually defined goals of the practice" (Bailey & Armer, 1998, p. 245). All the participants cited by Bailey and Armer (1998) stressed that responsibility for patient outcomes was the key driving force in their collaborative actions. One APRN noted, "If there's a patient [I treated] who calls in and . . . says 'I'm just not better,' she'll [the physician] say things like 'If I had treated you, I would have given you the same thing.' It just sets the patient at ease because they realize that we're working together" (p. 245).

3. *Shared power control.* Each physician and nurse partner assumes individual accountability along with a shared responsibility for actively participating in the decision-making process as well as supporting the consensus-driven decisions and sharing in their implementation. In one situation, a nurse, commenting on a physician perceived as very collaborative, stated, "We started when the MD and PA called me to discuss his patient's care and asked for suggestions. . . . We examined the patient together, the MD described

what we were seeing in the wound . . . and I identified potential strategies for wound healing. . . . The MD/PA team acknowledged my expertise and came to me for assistance to assist the patient" (McGrail, Morse, Glessner, & Gardner, 2008, p. 201). Ongoing and consistent communication is key to building a shared-power practice. Providers must be comfortable sharing information about patient care, issues of collaboration, and team functioning. Collaboration is a powerful tool to build a team, but without shared decision making collaboration cannot exist (Gaguski & Begyn, 2009; Maylone et al, 2011; O'Grady & Ford, 2009; Sullivan et al, 1998).

4. *Mutual concerns.* To ensure mutual concerns are met, providers need to have skills of assertiveness, cooperation, and coordination. Assertiveness can be described as the ability to express a viewpoint with confidence and with attention to being factually accurate and focused on the patient need. The key aspect of team success is the knowledge and utilization of each member's expertise by the others. For example, in a surgical care situation, the physician is in charge of the operation; the physician and NP or CNS jointly care for the patient postoperatively; the NP or CNS is in charge of discharge planning; and in some settings the CRNA might also be on the surgical team, assuming full responsibility for anesthesia delivery, each one confident in his or her skills and able to speak up regarding patient needs and care direction as he or she sees it. Acknowledgment and respect of other opinions and viewpoints while maintaining the willingness to examine and change personal beliefs and perspectives stresses the interdependence of the practitioners on the team and underlies true cooperation. Collegial relationships replace hierarchical authority with equality and shared decision making. Decisions made by consensus are based on the expertise of each member; there are different levels of input, but it is always in the best interest of the patient. One APN noted, "There are many times the physician will say to me 'This is a nurse practitioner patient,' and it's somebody that has all kinds of sociological problems. Problems that I could coordinate, and that's good; that's a compliment to nursing. He actually has learned what we do" (Bailey & Armer, 1998, p. 243). Trust is the bond that unites all the components of collaboration. "Without the element of trust, cooperation cannot

exist, assertiveness becomes threatening, responsibility is avoided, communication is hampered, autonomy is suppressed, and coordination is haphazard" (Norsen et al, 1995, p. 45).

The Intensity Continuum

The level of collaboration within a practice can be found by identifying the intensity of professional relationships (high to low) and the type of collaborative structure found along a complexity continuum of unidisciplinary, multidisciplinary, interdisciplinary, or transdisciplinary practice. See **Figure 8.1.** The interactive complexity of the practice will increase as the structure becomes more complex, offering greater challenges to the team but resulting in even more positive and productive outcomes of practice.

Professional staff in any health setting (e.g., licensed practical nurse [LPN], RN, social worker, APRN, physician, radiology technician, and so on) are coming from a *unidisciplinary* base. As students, they were prepared for the interactive world of practice within the security of working with students, faculty, and practitioners of their discipline and program. They begin to develop personal mastery of professional knowledge and skill, an essential requirement for functioning effectively at the more complex levels of interactive relationships found in collaborative practice. Educational experiences with students of other professions are generally very limited, usually to clinical encounters. As the professionals begin to share responsibilities for the same patient or patient populations, they begin to interact with each other and a *multidisciplinary* practice model emerges. This is a level of information exchange with no presumption of shared planning. Each fulfills a discipline-specific role but communicates with others on an as-needed basis. This level exemplifies the "chimneys of excellence" approach in which work is accomplished not by team effort but by a collection of professionals working for the most part in "isolated splendor" (Kuehn, 1998, p. 27). However, within this multidisciplinary framework, an *interdisciplinary* relationship can begin to develop as two or more members begin to coalesce their roles toward a common vision or goal. There begins to be a sense of shared investment and a desire to plan together for a better outcome. As each professional shares discipline-specific expertise, cross-fertilization of ideas starts to occur and group ownership of

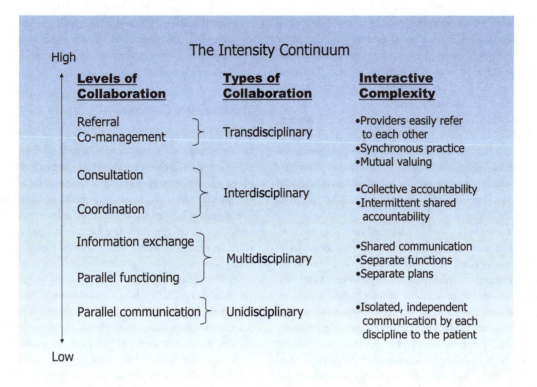

FIGURE 8.1 Intensity continuum.
(Data from Blais et al, 2002; Kuehn, 1998).

the practice begins to emerge. The dynamics that revolve around the emerging practitioner-to-practitioner relationships concern issues of leadership, power control, norms, values, group behavior, and conflicts and demand skills in communication, collaboration, and conflict resolution. Major growth in the complexity of interactive practices can be seen by the increased use of the terms *interdisciplinary* and *interprofessional* to describe this third level of team dynamics as a key requisite for high-quality care (American Medical Directors Association [AMDA], 2011; Donald et al, 2009; Parse, 2015; Rice et al, 2010). Parse (2015) describes distinctive differences between *interdisciplinary* and *interprofessional,* contrasting *discipline* as the body of scientific knowledge that is the basis of that discipline's practice and research with *profession* as those educated professionals committed to the vision and purpose of that vision. *Interdisciplinary* then refers to the joining of two or more disciplines in educational courses or projects, with each discipline preserving its uniqueness while being

complementary to the other(s). In contrast, *interprofessional* describes unique disciplinary knowledge applied in the service each discipline offers in a specific health situation. "Each professional comes to the situation with disciplinary knowledge and one profession does not preside over the others" (p. 5). The second basic tenet of nursing practice (ANA, 2010a) notes that "nurses coordinate care by establishing partnerships . . . collaborative interprofessional team planning is based on recognition of each discipline's value and contributions, mutual trust, respect, open discussion and shared decision-making" (p. 4).

The intensity of relationships is at a peak when a practice moves into a *transdisciplinary* level. It becomes a practice without professional boundaries, a synthesis of knowledge and practice. Here the practitioners are able to rise above fears of being subsumed and the individual visions of each become a shared vision with "laser-beam" intensity. All, including the patient, own the plan of care and the goal of high-quality patient care transcends any "turf" issues. As the number of participants increases, the resulting diversity, complexity, and intensity of relationship building requires that each participant feel that he or she "owns" the vision. The critical indicators of collaboration are now a part of each and a visible part of the whole. At this level communication through dialogue is the key to success. *Discussion,* coming from the same root word as *percussion,* implies a hard exchange of ideas bouncing back and forth, presented and defended with the need to come to a decision. In contrast, the art of *dialogue* allows for free exploration of ideas, issues, and innovations, with no sense of defensiveness and the ability to suspend personal viewpoints. When a team arrives at this point, they become in such close alignment that when working together they enter the "transdisciplinary" stage of collaboration in which they act as one and do not have to think about it. Senge (1994) offers an example using the Boston Celtics, a basketball team that won 11 world championships in just 13 years. The famed Celtics center Bill Russell described their team play not as friendship, but as a synchronous relationship among the players. He stated (p. 234) that sometimes during a game, it would

> heat up so that it became more than a physical or even mental game . . . and would be magical. . . . When it happened I could feel my play rise to a new level. . . . It would surround not only me and the other Celtics but also the players on the other team, and even the referees. . . . At that special level, all sorts of odd things happened. The game would be in the white heat of competition and yet I wouldn't feel competitive, which is a miracle in itself. . . . The game would move so fast that every fake, cut and pass would be surprising, and yet nothing could surprise me . . . during those spells I could almost sense how the next play would develop and where the next shot would be taken.

To develop positive relationships with other health-care practitioners, comprehensive care requires the collective contributions of many varied professionals with highly developed skills, including self-knowledge and traditions of knowledge in the health professions; team and community building; and work dynamics of groups, teams, and organizations. Practitioners must be familiar with the healing approaches of other professions and cultures, be aware of historic power inequities across professions, identify similarities and differences among traditions of community members, know the value of the work of others, and learn from having had experiences of working with

people from other disciplines and healing traditions. The key to team building is the affirmation by all of a shared mission, tasks, goals, and values (ANA, 2010a; IOM, 2004, 2011; Jehn, Northcraft, & Neale, 1999; Senge, 1994).

The "Iceberg" Effect

Where the team of APRN and physician falls on the collaboration continuum, as well as the intensity of the relationships, is determined by several critical factors. These factors can be visualized as an iceberg, with many factors visible and openly known and others that remain invisible or unacknowledged although still extremely significant in their effect on the success or failure of the collaborative effort (Pearson & Jones, 1994; Plant, 1987). See **Figure 8.2.**

The formal "visible" systems include many common components of practice such as organizational policies, clinic objectives, systems of communications, and role or job descriptions. These are accessible and changeable, and are readily addressed in open, rational discussion. In contrast, the "invisible," informal systems, including power networks, values, and norms, are not as accessible but subtly present, difficult to change, and often give a sense of being untouchable. Many of the barriers to collaboration are hidden here. Only through working together can a team become aware of the impact of this invisible system and work to eliminate the barriers. The barriers must first be identified and acknowledged, and then strategies applied to remove or neutralize them as the partners in practice work to become a viable team (Donald et al, 2009; IOM, 2011; Maier & Aiken, 2016; McCarter et al, 2016; Paradise, Dark & Bitler, 2011).

BARRIERS TO COLLABORATION

Barriers to collaboration hinder positive change and growth in our health-care system, frustrate the professionals trying to work as a team, and can negatively affect the future of health care (IOM, 2011; Kubota, 2011; Rice et al, 2010). Key barriers that continue to challenge collaborative efforts include educational isolation, professional elitism, organizational hierarchy, unrecognized diversity, expanding scopes of practice, role and language confusion, inadequate and inappropriate communication patterns, and professional dissonance.

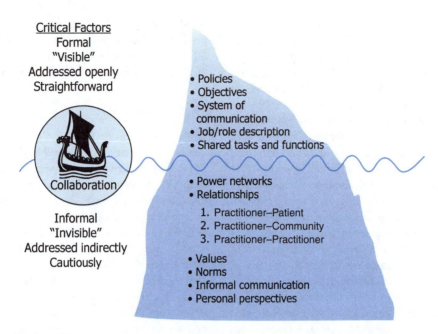

FIGURE 8.2   Iceberg factor. (Data from Kuehn, 1998; Pearson & Jones, 1994; Plant, 1987).

Educational Isolation

Despite an increasing call for an interdisciplinary approach to education in the health professions, many educators continue to use a traditional linear approach with built-in assumptions of bureaucratic organizational structures, standardized sets of relationships and roles, and systematized methods of record keeping, billing, and payment for services. Past studies exploring the status of interdisciplinary education have noted many inherent problems associated with developing interdisciplinary educational programs, citing workload stress, intense workload demands, lack of academic and institutional support, and often seemingly insurmountable complications with clinical arrangements (Kuehn, 1998). In the past, some nurse educators have expressed concerns that the traditional concept of a nursing workforce is challenged by calls for health care to be delivered by *interdisciplinary* teams, fearing that this focus has the potential of obscuring the unique contribution of nursing to health-care delivery (National League for Nursing [NLN], 1997). However, shared educational experiences can actually help clarify roles because as faculty and students work together, they begin to better understand the contribution each profession makes to the practice (Glasgow, Dunphy, & Mainous, 2010; Hojat et al, 2003). *Interprofessional* continuing education might focus on team building or on a specific patient care problem, helping health professionals acknowledge the value each brings to the situation and focusing on the patient rather than the discipline (Sauter et al, 2016; Trossman, 2014).

Professional Elitism

Educational isolationism easily leads to professional elitism as each profession educates "its own" with a sense of importance and unique worth. Professionalism consists of three components: professional ideals of knowledge and service, the professional occupation and the life career it provides, and the character of the work itself. The life career is the vehicle through which the ideals are put into practice, and the profession itself defines the character of professional work. The commitment to healing and to service is thereby limited by the definition of healing and public service crafted by the profession. Although "importance" and "worth" are valued aspects of self-identity, a pervasive sense of professional elitism running through this approach can result in the work of each professional taking priority over helping each other or putting the patient's needs first (O'Neil & Pew Health Professions Commission, 1998). In his classic discourse on medical dominance, Friedson (1970) claimed that the dominant position of the medical profession in the health division of labor "allows it to reinforce and protect itself from outside influence and to claim and maintain jurisdiction and control over many more areas than logic or evidence justifies. . . . It is 'professionalism' itself that seems to transform the ideal responsibility to serve the good of the general public into a limited concrete responsibility to serve the good of one's personal public" (p. 152). As Friedson (1970) cautioned, "A professional who is so qualified as to perform this extraordinary work of medicine . . . must himself be a rather extraordinary, gifted, person . . . as are his colleagues and his profession. . . . This professional pride leads the worker to consider himself to be quite different from, indeed superior to, those of other occupations. . . . The thrust of professional activity becomes a mission to build barriers that keep the profession and its clientele safe from those beyond the pale while seeking jurisdiction over all that cannot be excluded" (pp. 154–155). In a recent intervention study to improve interprofessional collaboration, physicians reported that they expected orders would be carried out without discussion. Nurses and other health professionals in the study agreed that this was the medical expectation and it limited the possibility of much collaboration (Rice et al, 2010).

Nursing should acknowledge that it, too, has been guilty of elitism and of exhibiting professional dominance and defensiveness, both in relating to other nurses with different levels of education and expertise and in working with other health-care professionals. Lack of understanding, failure to acknowledge roles and responsibilities of other professionals, and the very isolated nature of health professional education is the basis for much of the elitism still prevalent today (Glasgow, Dunphy, & Mainous, 2010; Rice et al, 2010).

Organizational Hierarchy

The key to the inadequacy of health services is described as "professional dominance," a situation in which health services revolve around professional authority, with a foundational structure of dominance by a single profession over a variety of other "subordinate professions" (Friedson, 1970). The two lines of authority in medicine and health care have historically been the administrative authority of the "office" and the medical authority of professional skills and expertise. The medical profession as an occupation with institutionalized privileges and authority granted by others on a basis of faith and trust holds a special form of legal "power" based on "expert status" because their knowledge and work are considered very complex and nonroutine, and subsequently has a position of dominance among other occupations providing health care. This results in professional control of information and suspicion of the value of what lies "outside" their domain. Friedson (1970, pp. 231, 234) suggests that this autonomy and dominance need to be and can be controlled by an administrative structure that stresses accountability for effective and humane services and is responsive to the patient:

> For a profession to be true to the ideal of a profession, members must let go of the total authority and control over the terms and content of their work and cease total dominance in favor of a division of labor. The physicians must temper autonomy and dominance with administrative accountability, accountability to the patient, self-regulated peer review and encouragement of other providers to assume responsibilities of health care . . . [However] no service using other providers is possible . . . without the active cooperation of the dominant profession. If the profession does not trust them, or if it resents and fears them, it will not refer patients to them, nor will it graciously receive patients referred from them. . . . Mere administrative fiat is not enough.

Supervision is defined as critically watching and directing activities or a course of action and is a mainstay of any hierarchical structure. Rationales given for supervision of health care include documented inadequacy; lack of knowledge, experience, or skills in relation to the person supervised; legal requirements; a lack of trust or confidence despite no legal limits requiring supervision; perceived safety needs of patient or provider; and history, tradition, or local institutional policy. In exploring the difference between "under the supervision of" and "ownership of practice decisions," it may be most helpful to view them not as polar opposites but as different levels of collaboration along a continuum of autonomous practice. Kinlein (1977) stressed that if a physician, a member of one profession, determines by his or her orders what actions a nurse, a member of a separate profession, will take, the practice is no longer the "essence of nursing" but becomes "medically directed care" delivered by nurses (p. 30). Supervised or medically directed care seems to fall within the framework of multidisciplinary interactions representing a very limited level of intensity of relationships and collaboration. Supervision may not preclude some level of collaboration, but it seems to severely limit its scope. The extent of collaboration possible within such a "delegated" mindset is questionable.

Unrecognized Diversity

Diversity in a health-care team can have a powerful impact on its success or failure as a cohesive workgroup. It can bring a wealth of helpful differences but can also be the cause of great conflict within the group. Cultural diversity may be easily recognized and acknowledged, but there are many complex aspects of diversity that may not be recognized and that can undermine team efforts. Three major categories of diversity are informational, social category, and value (Jehn et al, 1999). Informational diversity reflects the differences in knowledge and perspectives of team members flowing from their education, experiences, and levels of expertise. Social category diversity relates to age, race, gender, and ethnicity and is the aspect with which we are most familiar as cultural diversity. Value diversity reflects the differences in members' perspectives of the mission, goals, and values relating to the work at hand. A study of the impact of diversity on work-group performance found that different forms of diversity could result in different levels of performance within the team. Having high information diversity (differences in education and experience) can make a team quite effective because of the many professional perspectives that can be available to the team. However, if it is accompanied by high value diversity, the team may malfunction as a unit. Over time, age, gender, and race differences in a group become less important, but value diversity—differences in understanding of the mission, goals, and values— becomes the more important component as a predictor of conflict or success. The complexity of relationships within a team is heightened by the level and type of diversity. Often unrecognized or unacknowledged, value diversity may be the most critical factor in the success or failure of teamwork and collaboration (Jehn et al, 1999). The implementation of the PPACA seems to have brought

more intensity to the conflicts among health professionals regarding SOP and Gardner emphasizes that the most visible interdisciplinary fight is over SOP expansion, noting that "until there is an expansion of SOP, APNs in many states will not be able to provide services to the fullest extent of their training and knowledge, skills and experiences" (Gardner, 2010, p. 264). Gardner then notes that disputes are not only interest-based, but values-based and professional identity-based as well. *Identity conflicts* seem to relate to a professional's need to be treated with deference or one's difficulty in compromise; *value-based conflicts* arise when values relating to one professional culture differ from the other, such as in lines of communication being unidirectional; *conflicts of interest* seem to infer that one professional should get more (money, prestige, patient say) at the expense of the other. The challenge is to somehow address these issues using strategies such as mediation, clarifying SOP and interprofessional education.

Expanding Scopes of Practice

Nursing SOP is the extent of clinical actions, decision making, and patient management responsibilities authorized by state and federal law (i.e., the legal base of practice). However, SOP evolves and changes over time as variables change: nursing education, state and federal laws, professional standards and guidelines, policies of the workplace, experience of the nurse, changing needs of the community, expanding SOPs of other health professionals (such as pharmacists), and emerging models of health-care delivery that expand the role of non–health-care professionals. Schuiling and Slager (2000) described this as "freedom with limits" noting that determining one's SOP requires the health professional to first review the "inflexible boundaries" set down by professional standards of practice and core competencies and then examine the clinical reality and extent of his or her practice, considering the practice setting, education, years of experience, nature of collaborative relationships, and needs of the community. This latter is the flexible "grey area" that helps to better define and potentially change the "inflexible" current legal parameters of practice. Although the IOM's report (2011) on the future of nursing supported expansion of nursing's SOP and the ACA of 2010 opened the way for new models of care using nurses in expanding roles, the ability for APRNs to practice to the full extent of their education and expertise continues to rest in the hands of state legislators (Marshall, 2016). Nurses must continue to provide education to other health professionals and the public regarding the realities of their education and expertise. Clarity of SOP is key to team building and collaboration among practitioners and for full implementation of the nurse's practice potential.

Role and Language Confusion

The increasingly expanding scope of nursing practice being experienced across the United States continues to be hampered by inconsistencies of legal language and titling variations among states. Additional challenges to the clarity of health provider roles and SOP are also being experienced as pharmacists seek to provide patient education as well as independent prescriptive privileges and provision of immunizations in local pharmacies and CNMs seek legislative approval to provide primary care (Keely, 2002; Phillippi & Barger, 2015). In examining the role of "primary care provider," Starfield (1992b) identified three types of functions performed by nonphysician personnel: (a) supplementary, extending the efficiency of the physician by assuming the technical tasks, usually under the direction of the physician; (b) substitutive, providing services usually provided by physicians; and (c) complementary, extending the effectiveness of physicians by doing things physicians do not do at all, do poorly, or do reluctantly. Noting that the nonphysician role has not been clarified to the extent that the three functions can be differentiated, Starfield concluded that primary care is largely a physician-dominated effort. Although primary care cannot function without some teamwork involving other practitioner providers, she believed that there was little evidence supporting the concept of team practice and little research indicating when and under what conditions a team approach may be more effective than a singular practice approach. In conclusion, Starfield asserted that primary care should be provided by physicians and the concept of *teamwork* in primary care needed to be researched regarding (a) standards for different roles and relationships; (b) identification of which type of delegated function—substitutive, supplementary, or complementary—is most appropriately assumed by

what level or type provider; and (c) how well the attributes of primary care are achieved by nonphysicians in comparison with care by physicians. Concerns raised by Starfield's discussion of the primary care center were related to the language used, as well as her consistent adherence to the traditional medical viewpoint of the physician as the "captain of the ship." The use of the term *team* is quite perfunctory and seems to imply only a multidisciplinary collection of individuals gathered by the physician to facilitate his or her practice. The three functional types—supplementary, substitutive, and complementary—are each defined in relation to its ability to enhance physician effectiveness rather than as shared components of a joint practice. In addition, Starfield (1992a) frames the role of the nonphysician provider by tasks and functions, severely limiting the scope of advanced practice and the role of collaboration.

Collaboration, often used in statute, is frequently interpreted in rules and regulations as "supervision," implying a hierarchical relationship and a contradiction to the critical indicators of collaboration. For collaboration to consistently mean an egalitarian, collegial relationship, the legislative language must be more clearly defined. The question becomes whether power sharing can coexist with a supervision requirement in a practice. When collaboration is mandated, or termed *supervision,* the process of shared practice becomes one of forced negotiation in which the dominant profession, medicine, has the choice of collaboration, with no legal need for a collaborative partner, whereas the subjected profession, nursing, must obtain a collaborative partner to legally function within the full scope of its practice (Sullivan, Morgan, Heimerichs, & Scott, 1998). Physician involvement can be termed *collaboration, supervision, direction, delegation,* or *authorization,* and the meaning of each term can be ambiguous, particularly in statute.

Statutory requirements for collaboration for advanced practice nursing couched as "delegated" or "supervised" practice are not acceptable for several time-tested reasons. If patterns of practice are legislated, legislative judgment becomes limited by the parameters of the legal definitions, rules, and regulations of the state in which the practice is located. The flexibility needed for individual clinical situations may be seriously compromised by these legally defined parameters. The result is that, because of restrictive legislation, rules, regulations, and reimbursement policies, advanced nursing practice too often depends on the willingness of a physician collaborator, whereas the same limitations are not placed on the physician. "One can only imagine what the reaction of organized medicine would be if a state legislature attempted to delineate when and how internist physicians should refer patients to a specialist" (ANA, 1998, p. 4). Legislatively mandated collaboration often results in a conflict (Sullivan, 1998). In states where APRN practice is controlled by joint board decisions, the negotiation process of joint rule making can become very hostile because of an unequal balance of power among the parties. Further, when membership of the board of nursing includes representatives of each level of nursing, those members not in advanced practice may lack the knowledge base required for debating advanced practice issues such as prescriptive authority. The subsequent rules passed may be far more restrictive than had been imagined from the broader language of the statute. Reasons offered by Sullivan and colleagues (1998) for the failure of these disparate groups to accomplish an externally imposed power-sharing partnership are not difficult to understand. They state (p. 350),

> Because the participants did not share a common purpose or vision, and were forced to meet, it is not surprising that they did not work well together or achieve a satisfactory result—by any standards. Because the representatives were forced to come together and their Boards had their budgets held hostage to the process, it was not unexpected that despite the need to reach some level of agreement there was little commitment to a win-win situation. . . . Instead, representatives of each discipline worked to protect their distinctly different professional agendas. It became not a collaborative process but a legalistic and formalized process of enforced negotiation.

Collaboration has also been described as an interdependent, interdisciplinary practice in which the APRN role is "substitutive" in a primary care setting in contrast to the "complementary" role more applicable to acute-care settings (King, Parrinello, & Baggs, 1996). However, there are difficulties with the use of the term *substitutive* because it implies a temporary stopgap until the "regular" practitioner can be provided. More contemporary views of collaboration and interdisciplinary practice steer clear of the substitutive and complementary language and stress partnership and the unique areas of expertise of each member of the team (Donald et al, 2009; IOM, 2011). In a 2015 report, the Kaiser Family Foundation notes that 33 states no longer impose any statutory or regulatory

requirements on nurse practitioners for physician collaboration, direction, or supervision, reflecting a movement toward the autonomous nursing role and facilitating a teamwork approach to practice.

Another language issue relates to the use of protocols and clinical guidelines. *Protocols* are defined as the "detailed plan of a scientific or medical experiment, treatment, or procedure" (*Merriam-Webster's,* 1994). In research, they need to be followed "to the letter" to have accurate, consistent, and comparable sets of data. The concern with protocols comes with their use in statutes, rules, and regulations as a definitive set of boundaries restricting practice to sets of predetermined criteria. When the perception of nursing is a dependent practice under physician supervision, the mechanisms created for allowing advanced practice often include a system of protocols designed with the approval of the "collaborating" physician. However, this "solution" compromises the concept of nursing autonomy, suggests that the nurse is incapable of making accurate choices among treatment options, and becomes implicit "standing orders" reinforcing nursing dependency (Baer, 1993). In some states, neither protocols nor a collaborative practice agreement with a physician is required for full practice privileges. In others, if prescriptive authority is possible, a collaborative practice agreement with a physician may be required, but perhaps no protocols. Historically, clinical guidelines represented collective wisdom gathered over time and were considered no threat to autonomy. In contrast, guidelines today may not be as willingly accepted because of the fear that they might influence or "manage" provider behavior. If guidelines or protocols allow room for the exercise of provider judgment, they will support provider autonomy as well. The Agency for Healthcare Research and Quality (AHRQ) uses the term *clinical practice guidelines* to describe systematically developed statements to assist practitioner and patient decisions about appropriate health care for specific clinical conditions. They may be broad or very detailed based on literature review as well as expert opinion. These are written by independent multidisciplinary panels of private-sector clinicians and other experts supported by AHRQ. Practitioners must have clinical guidelines in place for reimbursement from Medicare (Newman, 1996), and they are viewed sometimes as an excellent tool for communicating the role to funding agencies (Way & Jones, 1994).

One additional aspect of language confusion is that of "titling" of APRNs. Many titles found in the different state statutes include advanced nurse practitioner (ANP), advanced practice nurse (APN), advanced practice professional nurse (APPN), advanced practice registered nurse (APRN), advanced registered nurse practitioner (ARNP), certified nurse practitioner (CNP), and registered nurse practitioner (RNP). The APRN Consensus Model for APRN Regulation—Licensure, Accreditation, Certification, and Education (LACE)—defines advanced practice and each specialty, describes the regulatory model, and identifies titles to be used. This document was created by regulators, nurse educators, APRN certifiers, and representatives of a large number of APRN professional organizations with the goal of creating national consistency regarding laws and rules regulating APRN practice. With some physician groups still insisting on supervision, the challenge remains to get past the language barriers and clarify roles to foster a collaborative approach to care. *The Pearson Report* (2011) encourages NPs to share the updated legislative information with their legislators to help them understand that NPs are competent and high-quality clinicians and to remove barriers to advanced practice nursing.

The launching of doctorate of nurse practice (DNP) programs has also created some language difficulties. The fairly recent nursing doctorate (ND) has been phased out and the DNP is now identified as the future expectation for all APRNs. One expected benefit of the DNP is the greater opportunity to fully participate on the interdisciplinary team. However, there are challenges to the concept suggesting that the educational and clinical residency requirements of the DNP do not prepare one for becoming faculty, assuming leadership roles, or conducting clinical research (Brar, Boschma, & McCuaig, 2010; Webber, 2008). In addition, the term *Dr. Nurse* is causing many physician groups to challenge not only the terminology but also the concept itself (Landro, 2008). In some states, legislation has directly challenged the nurses' ability to be called "Doctor" despite having doctoral credentials, simply because they are not "physicians." A report of a developing collaborative practice in the emergency department (ED) stated, "By performing the dual role of physician and nurse, the NP eliminates the fragmentation of care often seen in the ED" where patients see many different physicians, nurses, and staff members and there is no consistent provider (Covington, Erwin, & Sellers, 1992, p. 124). Instances in which the APRN is described as assuming the "dual role of physician and nurse" can

lead to a misconception of the nurse role. No nurse can assume the role of a physician, nor can a physician assume the role of a nurse. What is possible is that certain responsibilities, functions, and skills are learned and assumed by both providers. When the nurse assumes some of the responsibilities, functions, and skills traditionally assumed by the physician, if they fall within the scope of nursing practice, they are nursing. If they fall outside, they are considered medically directed acts, and the nurse in that instance is serving as assistant to the physician. It follows, then, that if a physician assumes some of the responsibilities, functions, and skills traditionally assumed by the nurse, they would be considered nurse-directed acts and the physician is serving as assistant to the nurse.

Inadequate and Inappropriate Communication Patterns

When physicians and nurses do not share information or concerns, when communication is a one-way street, or when there is an inadequate system of written and verbal communication, quality of patient care suffers. Poor communication patterns also affect working relationships and seriously hinder any attempts at collaboration, often resulting in separate professional decision making that can create confusion and safety issues (Clarin, 2007; Zwarenstein & Bryant, 2000). Inappropriate communication patterns may reflect a pattern of "physician abuse." In a survey of nurse–physician relationships (Rosenstein, 2002), the level of respect for nurse input and collaboration was rated significantly higher by physicians than by nurses. However, physicians rated the findings on how important the physician's disruptive behavior was in contributing to nurse dissatisfaction and low morale much lower than nurses did. These findings reflect a dissonance in perception that is often a result of poor communication and lack of trust, creating a defensive, noncollaborative practice environment in which the number of errors rises and patient safety and positive patient outcomes are threatened. Magnet hospitals, emphasizing collaboration between physicians and nurses, have been documented as having better patient outcomes and fewer problems relating to shortages, turnover, or abuse (Drenkard, 2010; Fischman, 2002).

Another aspect to consider is the line of reporting accountability. An NP-staffed "fast track" in the ED of Vanderbilt University Medical Center was designed using written protocols created collaboratively by the NPs and the medical director of the ED. Although the NPs reported to the ED nursing director and the physicians to the ED medical director, the collaborating practice was well established within a few months with a growing sense of confidence and trust between these distinct professional providers. However, the report made no mention of the effect of a parallel reporting system (Covington, Erwin, & Sellers, 1992). If reporting is different for each practitioner, does that negatively affect the practice?

Professional Dissonance

When diversity is not recognized and acknowledged, the result is professional dissonance with a serious negative impact on the capacity for teamwork. Confusion of language, differing communication patterns and ways of interacting, and difficulty respecting each other's skills and roles are inevitable. In a study of attitudes regarding teamwork by critical care nurses and physicians, a seven-item "teamwork climate scale" was developed. It found that nurses and physicians had distinctly different attitudes toward teamwork. The source of the differences was found to be status or authority, responsibilities, gender, training, and professional culture (Thomas, Sexton, & Helmreich, 2003). In a study of nurses and physicians in a medical intensive care unit (ICU), Baggs and Schmitt (1997) found that collaboration would occur only if the time and place were appropriate, the physician believed the nurse had the knowledge needed, and trust, respect, and sincere interest in teamwork were present. For example, the physicians believed the general medical unit nurses did not have the same level of knowledge about medical illness as the medical ICU nurses. This perceived knowledge level was a precondition to the physician's willingness to collaborate more effectively with the nurses in the ICU.

A study by Jones (1994) explored the nature of nurse–physician collaboration, examining the differences and similarities in their perceptions related to the four indicators of nurse–physician collaboration identified in the ANA social policy statement of 1980: mutual power control, mutual safeguarding of provider concerns, responsibility for practice, and practice goals. The findings offer an interesting portrait of the collaborative perspective of the partners. Although nurses and physicians were in agreement on power control, most affirmed that the physician initiated more communications

than the nurse, indicating a lack of mutual power control. In another study examining provider concerns, nurses and physicians were rated on the degree to which they achieved both assertiveness and cooperativeness, with high levels of both dimensions indicating collaboration. Nearly half of the responses reflected competition, compromise, or accommodation as the preferred method of safeguarding concerns. They did not agree on where responsibility for practice should rest—nurse, physician, or both—and they agreed on only 4 of 24 practice goals (e.g., maintain elimination patterns, promote cardiovascular healing). The conclusion reached was that nurses and physicians who cannot agree on provider responsibility regarding areas of practice and patient goals reflect a lower level of collaboration and will not be able to deliver the same high level of coordinated patient care as those nurse–physician teams who agree on the areas of responsibility (Norsen et al, 1995).

The Bottom Line

Barriers to collaboration hinder positive change and growth in our health-care system but do not need to be perpetuated. Organizational climate and culture are living, growing aspects of institutional work life that bind the organization together. Professions and professionals are not static. They can and must work to eliminate barriers to collaboration and create a new culture of team practice in health care.

STRATEGIES FOR SUCCESS

Collaboration is a developmental process that emerges slowly through a series of sensitive and delicate interactions. Members of a newly forged partnership join forces in the belief that the common need they recognize can best be met through their combined efforts. Levels of collaboration achieved depend on context, ability, and the desire of the prospective partners to skillfully develop the practice. Based on the conceptual framework of collaboration described in this chapter, the following are some key strategies for developing a successful collaborative team.

Create a Collegial Team

Teamwork is a critical need for today and the reality of tomorrow's practice. Peters and Waterman (1982), focusing on people as the means to achieve productivity, suggested that coworkers should be treated as partners. The reality of this shift of power from an authoritarian command structure to one of collegial teamwork can result in innovation, rapid response, and greater access by the customer. However, it requires a considerable mind shift by participants. The redesign of a health-care delivery model that supports a collegial, interdisciplinary team approach requires a radical way of thinking to acknowledge that this new model is not something "out there," but belongs to each of the participants as they confront their learned beliefs and perspectives. In addition, the participants must realize that they must undergo a significant cultural shift in accepting that they must become a community of learners, a "learning organization" that never "arrives" but continues to translate a shared vision into an ever-evolving practice (O'Brien, Martin, Heyworth, & Meyer, 2009; Rice et al, 2010; Senge, 1994). The key feature of this type of learning organization is a realization that the role of the "grand strategist" at the top is no longer possible because of the complexity and dynamic status of work. Instead, each individual participant's commitment and capacity to learn is tapped. Unlike a linear approach, the learning organization forges ahead based on shared understandings of interrelationships and patterns of change, thereby creating a common bond of commitment to the practice.

One approach to initiating dialogue to address professional conflicts of values, professional identity, and interests is through mediation. Gardner (2010) suggests that the mediator challenge key medical and nursing professionals to "acknowledge their core values, to facilitate discussions in which each side accepts those aspects of the other's values that it can agree with, and then build on those shared beliefs" (p. 266). In summary, five qualities are suggested as essential for participants in the "learning organization" that never "arrives" but continues to translate a shared vision into an ever-evolving practice (O'Brien, Martin, Heyworth, & Meyer, 2009; Rice et al, 2010; Senge, 1994):

1. *Personal mastery.* The practitioner is true to a personal vision while staying committed to the truth of the current reality.
2. *Use of mental models.* Learning is accelerated as we mentally consider alternative scenarios for care delivery. Participants do not become so attached to one scenario

because it could freeze them into rigid adherence to outdated approaches to care.
3. *Shared vision.* Shared vision is described by Senge (1994) as the "first step in allowing people who mistrusted each other to begin to work together as it creates a common identity and sense of purpose" (p. 208).
4. *Team learning.* Nurses, physicians, and others on the team learn to think together about complex issues, acknowledging that the whole is truly greater than any of the individuals. They develop what is termed *operational trust* and master the practice of both dialogue and discussion. The apex of "team" is at the transdisciplinary level.
5. *Systems thinking.* Foundational in teamwork, systems thinking forces a focus on the whole pattern of the collaborative practice rather than any isolated role. The structure or key interrelationships of the practice pattern influence behavior and decision making and are examined collectively.

Accept Growth and Development as a Joint Responsibility

For the concept of collaborative practice to grow and flourish, interdisciplinary education must be supported, affirming the values and roles of both physician and nurse. Educational institutions must reaffirm the value of education for interdisciplinary practice and implement the results of studies of the effect of collaboration on clinical outcomes. In practice, bidirectional referrals must be promoted and must include the expanded APRN SOP and "skill set" found in the APRN role description. Professionals and the public must be educated regarding the roles by both physician and nurse partners. Strategies recommended for physicians to address physician abuse and improve collaboration include physician education, zero tolerance policies, role playing, and changing the culture of the environment from defensive and hierarchical to supportive and collegial. Nurse responsibility for the problem—in tolerating the behavior, perpetuating the inequalities in the nurse–physician relationship, and sometimes countering with abusiveness—should be addressed with education, role playing, assumption of accountability, and an assertive capability to share the nursing perspective (Buerhaus, 2010; Fischman, 2002; Glasgow, Dunphy, & Mainous, 2010).

Use Protocols and Guidelines Wisely

In clinical practice, *protocol* is often used synonymously with *clinical guidelines* and is representative of a statement of agreement between an APRN and his or her collaborating physician. When the providers agree on a standard of care acceptable to both, the guidelines or protocols stand as their codification of acceptable criteria for diagnosing and managing an illness or condition. Classic texts such as *Patient Care Guidelines for Nurse Practitioners* (Hoole, Pickard, Ouimette, Lohr, & Powell, 1999) and *Gerontological Protocols for Nurse Practitioners* (Brown, Bedford, & White, 1999) offer excellent resources for practitioners, as well as sometimes serving as the basis for legal documentation to allow for treatment and prescriptive privileges through incorporation into the collaborative agreement as the agreed-to standard of care. More current articles on development of clinical protocols are increasingly available such as one by Martinen and Freundl (2004) describing the development of an interdisciplinary protocol for managing congestive heart failure in long-term care and another by Colon-Emeric et al (2007) identifying "Barriers to and Facilitators of Clinical Practice Guideline Use in Nursing Homes."

Clinical practice guideline development needs three aspects to accomplish its goal. First, identification of key decisions and their consequences must be outlined. In the case of the APRN, there are decisions to be made about when to call the physician with questions and when referral to an outside specialist is in order. The process of reviewing charts and prescriptions is the second aspect. Finally, reimbursement from insurance providers must be defined because of strict insurance policies and legislative mandates. Although state and federal statutes may allow for certain billing practices, the viability of the practice may be hampered when nurse professionals are limited to lesser reimbursement amounts or are refused reimbursement. Legislative language in many states must continue to be reworked to clarify the meaning of the terminology, role and scope allowed, and the effect on practice viability of protocols and clinical guidelines. Progress is ongoing regarding legislative and statutory language changes needed for clarification and full SOP. *The Pearson Report of 2011* noted there were 31 states reporting an expanded SOP for APRNs through legislative or regulatory changes in 2009, compared with 22 in 2008 and 19 in 2007. In 2015, three states completely eliminated collaborative and supervisory models of practice This brought the total to 22 states plus the District of Columbia (DC) that now allow for full NP SOP, meaning no collaborative agreements with a physician are required. However, 28 states still require some sort of agreement for prescribing and advanced clinical practice, underlining a need to continue to work to remove barriers to full SOP for APRNs (Phillips, 2016). The annual legislative reports of Phillips (2016) provide a benchmark and an incentive for regulatory reform and language clarity; however, practitioners must be careful to not eliminate a sense of collaboration as they move to eliminate restrictive collaborative agreement requirements.

Watch Your Language

Language is one of the most significant facets of relationships. In an editorial from *American Family Physician* (Phillips et al, 2001), a physician professor took aim at the use of the term *health-care provider,* noting that "calling me a 'provider' lumps my physician colleagues and me with individuals who are frankly less qualified and yet aspire to do the same work we do . . . the use of terms . . . although 'politically correct' diminish us as professionals" (p. 1342). That same year an article in the *Annual Review of Medicine* (Cooper, 2001) was titled "Health Care Workforce for the Twenty-First Century: The Impact of Nonphysician Clinicians." No APRN I have ever known has positively embraced the concept of his or her practice as being that of a "nonphysician clinician." In a forecast study of Missouri nursing (Kuehn & Porter, 1993), the first round of the Delphi brought together both nurse and nonnurse participants. One physician commented that it was the first time he had ever been called a *nonnurse* and found it rather demeaning. When he was reminded of the nurse correlative being termed a *nonphysician,* a shared understanding of the awkwardness of either term in supporting a sense of collegiality emerged. In stark contrast to Starfield's (1992b) language of dependency flowing from "delegated medical functions," nursing language stresses the need to avoid definition by function or tasks when describing role. Orem (1995) stresses that a task orientation for nursing disallows the focus on the person. To define oneself as a nurse, the following questions must be answered:

What do I do (scope of practice)?
How do I do it (methods of practice, tasks)?
Whom do I care for?
Why do they need or want my care?

The ANA social policy statement of 2015 reaffirmed collaboration as a standard of practice. Although advanced practice nursing texts have consistently addressed the concept of collaborative practice, undergraduate nursing texts on professional practice have not historically addressed collaboration. Often the word is not even found in the index, and if it is, it has nearly always referred to collaboration between nursing practice and education or between types of nurses within the same setting. However, this too is changing. A chapter in the 2002 text *Professional Nursing Practice,* "The Nurse as Colleague and Collaborator," noted, "changing models of health care have created a need for modification of traditional roles. Nurses and physicians have been especially affected by these changes and work more collaboratively" (Blais et al, 2002, p. 199).

In a spring 2001 report, *The Health Care Workforce in Ten States: Education, Practice and Policy* (American Federation of Teachers [AFT] Healthcare, 2001), 10 pilot states were studied regarding the status of their health-care workforce. Aspects compared were data collection status and process, practice issues, influences, and policies. In describing licensure and regulation of practice, the extent of physician supervision varied considerably among states and among types of providers. In one state, APRN practice called for both "independent judgment" and "collaborative interaction with other health-care professionals." However, neither collaborative interaction nor other health-care professionals was defined in their practice act (AFT Healthcare, 2001, p. 50). Although the effect of the enforced collaboration and supervision on APRN practice (noted in 9 of 10 states studied) was not addressed, researchers (AFT Healthcare, 2001, p. 2) affirmed that

> the greatest opportunities for influencing the various environments affecting the health workforce lie within state governments. States are the key actors in shaping these environments as they finance and govern health profession education; license and regulate health profession practice and health insurance; purchase service; pay designated providers under Medicaid programs; and often assume responsibility for

design and/or subsidy of programs providing incentives for health professionals to choose specialties and practice location.

Socialize Students to Communication Skills Needed for Collaborative Interactions

When education includes the process of establishing an interdisciplinary team, it helps to create a system for promoting collaborative practice and facilitates the use of essential communication skills. One point highly stressed is the insistence that interdisciplinary teams should be already delivering care and have a solidly positive practice in place before integrating students into the teams (Hanson & Spross, 1996; Hughes, 2011; Norsen et al, 1995). Alberto and Herth (2009) explored in depth the history, benefits, and challenges of interprofessional collaboration in education and practice, offering an excellent review of their experiences with collaboration in health-care education. Examples of interdisciplinary professional education initiatives may be seen in **Table 8.2.** Group dynamics, role theory, organization theory, change theory, negotiation strategies, team interactions, networking, and focus on the need for organizational leadership for supporting interdisciplinary programs are key factors in these interdisciplinary educational initiatives preparing students and enabling practitioners to function in a collaborative world.

COLLABORATIVE MODELS: EARLY PIONEERS AND EMERGING MODELS

For clarity, many of these models are described as they were implemented with specific populations and in specific settings. However, they are transferable to a variety of places where health care is practiced once the philosophy and concepts are extracted and understood.

Early Pioneers

Primary Nursing Model

A national project conducted by the National Joint Practice Commission (NJPC, 1981) required hospitals utilizing a primary nursing model of practice to demonstrate 100% registered nurse staffing, individual clinical decision making by the registered primary nurse, a joint practice

TABLE 8.2			
Interdisciplinary Professional Education Initiatives			
Project or Model	**Location or Clinical Area**	**Focus**	**Citation**
Interdisciplinary Educational Initiative	Vanderbilt University	Medical, APRN, pharmacy, and social work students learning together	Buerhaus, 2010
Simulation training	Freestanding children's hospital in the southeastern United States with teams consisting of pediatric residents and fellows and nurse volunteers	A study to determine the level of physician–nurse collaboration in pediatrics using simulation exercises	Messmer, 2008
Proposed transdisciplinary medical, nursing, and health professional simulation center	Multiple examples of models being tested in various clinical areas, nationally and abroad	Students from the health disciplines, nursing, health professions, and medicine who are exposed to the complexities of teamwork within a clinical setting	Glasgow, Dunphy, & Mainous, 2010
Continuing education in classroom and clinical settings	Baystate Health of Massachusetts	Strengthening collegial relationships	Trossman, 2014
Simulation labs	University of Alabama, Birmingham	Strengthening collegial relationships	Trossman, 2014
Annual emergency department "skills blitz" simulation exercises	Cone Health of Greensboro, North Carolina	Strengthening collegial relationships	Trossman, 2014

committee with equal representation of providers, an integrated patient record, and joint evaluation of patient care. The structural elements of integrated records, joint practice committees, and joint care review reflect the common goals, mutual concerns, and shared control identified as critical indicators of a high-level collaborative practice (see Table 8.1). Primary nursing, "the performance of clinical nursing functions by registered nurses with minimal or no delegation of nursing tasks to others" (NJPC, 1981, p. 11), is considered essential for enabling the nurse to better enter into a collegial relationship with the physician. The emphasis on the primary nurse role, coupled with the element of increased nurse responsibility for decision making, relates accountability directly with collegiality and individual clinical decision making by nurses and is considered to be a prerequisite for shared decision making—you cannot share what you do not

have (Devereux, 1981; Sullivan, 1998). The results from the four participating hospitals were positive in relation to improved doctor–nurse communications, increased mutual respect and trust between physicians and nurses, increased job satisfaction for physicians and nurses, and highly satisfied patients.

Differentiated Practice Model

In recent years, the cost effectiveness of the primary nurse model has been challenged based on the limited reality of achieving it amidst a nursing shortage. However, newly developing models of differentiated practice have converted the "primary nurse" concept into that of a patient care coordinator (PCC) who assumes 24-hour accountability for specific patients. The PCC, however, does not deliver all the care personally. Instead, a team of other nurses and ancillary help assume major responsibility for care delivery, each with specific roles and levels of accountability. Each nurse is paired with certain physicians and his or her patients, and trust and collaboration are more readily developed as nurse and physician work together. This collaborative system model of patient care delivery has reported higher levels of coordination, cost effectiveness, and patient and provider satisfaction than previously seen in less collaborative models (Devaney, Kuehn, & Jones, 2002; Koerner & Karpiuk, 1994).

Collaborative Practice Model in a Clinic Setting

A collaborative practice model established in the early part of 2000 in an inner-city clinic in Beirut, Lebanon, reported a positive impact on quality of care of patients with type 2 diabetes mellitus that was nothing less than amazing (Arevian, 2005). The researchers first identified four key elements essential for the model—"collaborative defining of the problems; joint goal setting and planning; providing a continuum of self-management and support services; and maintaining active and sustained follow-up" (p. 446). In developing the model, they determined that thorough preparation of the professional team members would be an essential factor for success. In addition, they developed provider support systems, including standardized guidelines for care management; provided for patient education in illness management skills; and provided consistent access to a single team member. The development process was proven to be very effective because teams reported a high level of enthusiasm, cooperation, willingness to share expertise, and acknowledgment of skills of other colleagues. As one physician said, "We were treating each other like colleagues, with mutually respectful relationships," and another noted that he gained insights into "how much and how well the other team members contributed to patient care" (p. 449). Outcomes reported included improved documentation, increased patient recruitment, and improved glycemic control, as well as decreased cost of care. The most amazing aspect of the clinic was the positive response of team members to each other's skills and expertise in a Middle Eastern culture in which nurses are still considered as "handmaidens" to physicians. In addition, the positive patient response to active participation in their care was surprising in a Lebanese culture that encourages "passive submission" to the physician authority figure (Arevian, 2005, p. 450). The development

process of this collaborative practice model can serve as an excellent template for clinics and provides additional proof of the value of interprofessional collaboration. Building on this concept, the Nurse-Managed Health Clinics (NMHCs) were established by the PPACA to serve underserved populations. This grant program requires the clinics to be led by APNs who are associated with a school, college, university or department of nursing, a federally qualified health center, social services agency, or independent nonprofit health agency (Haney, 2010).

Collaboration in Long-Term Care

For more than 30 years, collaborative practice models have been developing in long-term care (LTC). Collaborative models in LTC as described by the AMDA (formerly the American Medical Directors Association) Ad Hoc Work Group (2011) include different employment scenarios, such as the APRN employed by the physician, self-employed, or employed by the nursing home; a specialty APRN collaborating with a specialty physician; and the care manager.

The positive impact of NP–physician partnerships in LTC has been reported in studies of the Nursing Home Demonstration Project and the Teaching Nursing Home Project, among others. In the 1980s, two NPs developed the LTC model of care teams that focused on coordinated care of frail and elderly nursing home residents (Kappas-Larson, 2008). They founded the Evercare Company, whose facilities are now nationwide and whose model is used both in nursing homes and in the community where nurse–physician teams care for seniors who are still living independently at home. Seven specific practice roles of Evercare NPs are collaborator, clinician, care manager or coordinator, coach or educator, counselor, communicator, and cheerleader.

The NPs serve as the center of the interprofessional care team in which both physician and nurse are valued partners. It is required by Evercare that each NP establish a positive relationship with his or her collaborating physician. As physicians become more aware of and comfortable with the NP's skill and expertise, they grow more supportive of the role. Active participation by physicians in LTC patient care is reported higher in Evercare programs, perhaps because their increasing comfort in LTC care participation is caused by their confidence in their NP partner. Physicians have said that "one of the most important components of their experience with Evercare is the personalized and coordinated care patients receive, thanks in part to the quality of Evercare's NPs and care managers" (Kappas-Larson, 2008, p. 135).

Collaboration in LTC facilities should include other employees who are involved in patient care. For example, a recent educational program about heart failure for certified nursing assistants (CNAs) in a LTC facility designed and led by a NP focused on CNA clinical education and CNA–nurse communication, especially in regard to not only recognizing but reporting vital resident information in a timely manner. It was stressed that the CNA be included in all quality improvement projects to "promote CNA input and maximize buy-in" (Kim, Ea, Parish, & Levin, 2016, p. 34).

Emerging Models of Shared Professional Practice

Shared Governance

Shared governance is a collaborative *organizational model* in which management and staff acknowledge that their interdependence and power is balanced equally on issues relating to nursing practice (Porter-O'Grady, 1992). A recent model of shared governance on an oncology unit is focused on collaboration and mutually agreed on goals between the CNS and the nurse manager. It is described as an approach focusing on professional development, shared decision making, autonomy, use of evidence-based practice, and creating a "culture of excellence for nursing staff through role modeling, smart allocation of resources and the development of standards of excellence" (Gaguski & Begyn, 2009, p. 385).

Innovative Care Models (www.innovativecaremodels.com) is a program initiated in 2008 that identified 24 successful collaborative care models for *acute care* and *comprehensive aftercare* developed as part of a research project funded by the Robert Wood Johnson Foundation. One example is "Collaborative Patient Care Management," a multidisciplinary case management model in which certified RN PCCs and physicians co-chair practice groups targeting high-risk, high-cost patient populations.

Accountable Care Organizations (ACOs)

The ACO is a collaboration among primary care and specialist clinicians, a hospital, and other health professionals accepting joint responsibility for both quality and cost of care provided to their patients. Under the PPACA, ACOs are a facet of Medicare's cost-saving plan and members share in any bonuses received from meeting cost saving targets. The ACOs allow for greater nursing leadership and participation; however, CNMs and CRNAs are not included as "practitioner" participants at this writing. In addition, pilot projects are working on testing the model with both Medicaid and private payers. Key benefits for nursing include leadership and increased collaborative opportunities (Haney, 2010).

Medical/Health Homes

The Patient-Centered Medical Home (PCMH) model is a move away from the traditional primary care model as it seeks to provide coordinated care through an interprofessional team of health-care providers. The concept of a medical home is not new; it was introduced in 1967 by the American Academy of Pediatrics to better serve children with special health-care needs. The PPACA has served as an impetus for newly emerging community-based interdisciplinary and interprofessional teams. These teams must include physicians; have a patient-centered, whole person orientation; and provide a broad scope of coordinated-care services, expanded access, and provide quality, cost-effective, and culturally appropriate care across the age spectrum. These aspects aim to increase patient positive outcomes; reduce repeat hospitalizations; and promote effective, personalized, and timely access to care. Emerging models and pilot projects stress "care coordination" as the key to success to the medical home concept and offers nursing an excellent leadership opportunity for preparing teams to deliver "patient-centered care," a core aspect of nursing practice (Schram, 2010; Swartwout et al, 2014).

Emerging Model of Shared Decision Making

SDM is a collaborative model of health-care delivery in which patients actively participate in treatment decisions. The model places the nurse in a key role as patient educator, advocate, and facilitator of the exchange of information between patient and the health-care team as they work together to find a mutually acceptable treatment plan among patient, physician, nurses, and other providers. McCarter et al (2016) describes this model as the dominant delivery model in cancer nursing practice.

Box 8.1

TEN New Rules to Redesign and Improve Care

Recommendation 4: Private and public purchasers, health-care organizations, clinicians, and patients should work together to redesign health-care processes in accordance with the following rules:

1. *Care based on continuous healing relationships.* Patients should receive care whenever they need it and in many forms, not just face-to-face visits. This rule implies that the health-care system should be responsive at all times (24 hours a day, every day) and that access to care should be provided over the Internet, by telephone, and by other means in addition to face-to-face visits.

2. *Customization based on patient needs and values.* The system of care should be designed to meet the most common types of needs, but have the capability to respond to individual patient choices and preferences.

3. *The patient as the source of control.* Patients should be given the necessary information and the opportunity to exercise the degree of control they choose over health-care decisions that affect them. The health system should be able to accommodate differences in patient preferences and encourage shared decision making.

4. *Shared knowledge and the free flow of information.* Patients should have unfettered access to their own medical information and to clinical knowledge.

Clinicians and patients should communicate effectively and share information.

5. *Evidence-based decision making.* Patients should receive care based on the best available scientific knowledge. Care should not vary illogically from clinician to clinician or from place to place.

6. *Safety as a system property.* Patients should be safe from injury caused by the care system. Reducing risk and ensuring safety require greater attention to systems that help prevent and mitigate errors.

7. *The need for transparency.* The health-care system should make information available to patients and their families that allows them to make informed decisions when selecting a health plan, hospital, or clinical practice, or when choosing among alternative treatments. This should include information describing the system's performance on safety, evidence-based practice, and patient satisfaction.

8. *Anticipation of needs.* The health system should anticipate patient needs rather than simply reacting to events.

9. *Continuous decrease in waste.* The health system should not waste resources or patient time.

10. *Cooperation among clinicians.* Clinicians and institutions should actively collaborate and communicate to ensure an appropriate exchange of information and coordination of care.

(IOM, 2001, Executive Summary, pp. 8–9)

An example of this model is the Patient Navigator program pioneered by Dr. Harold Freeman at Harlem Hospital to help eliminate barriers the minority communities encountered when seeking cancer screening, diagnosis, treatment, and ongoing care. It can be either hospital or clinic based. At present, patient advocacy or navigation is not regulated in its own right, there is no national or state licensure or credentialing, and the navigator is not necessarily a nurse. Hospital-based navigators are often nurses working for the hospital. Private navigator services may or may not be paid for by insurance or advocate

funding and often are not provided by nurses. One blog describes the navigator as one who "works with patients and families to help them at many points along the health-care continuum: disease research, insurance problems, finding doctors, understanding treatment and care options, accompanying them to visits, serving as coach and quarterback of their health-care team, working with family members and caregivers, mobilizing resources, managing medical paperwork and almost anything else you can think of" (Russell, 2013). The role sounds similar to nursing and more nurses and even physicians are becoming private navigators or advocates. However, many models described in the literature stress that they prefer a nonmedical or lay person with interpersonal skills and some experience in service-oriented fields (de la Riva et al, 2016; Loskutova et al, 2016). Nurses need to understand the role and work with the navigators as lay members of the team. In addition, they might consider reshaping their clinical role to have the advocate or navigator approach.

CREATE THE FUTURE

The call for collaboration continues to accelerate, driven by consumer and insurer demands for high-quality care at low cost; the existence of fragmented, disorganized, impersonal, and inaccessible care; numerous reports and commissions recommending collaboration; and the demands of some accrediting agencies for collaboration (Bodenheimer, 2008; IOM, 2011; Maier & Aiken, 2016; Marshall, 2016; Zwarenstein et al, 1998). The IOM Committee, in its call for the design of a new health-care system for the 21st century that better meets patient needs, recommended that health-care processes be redesigned in accordance with 10 new "rules" listed in **Box 8.1** (IOM, 2001). The rules speak to a system of care delivery focused on continuous healing relationships, shared knowledge and decision making with patients, and cooperation among professional providers as reflected by active collaboration and communication, emphasizing cooperation in patient care as more important than professional prerogatives and roles. This emphasis on

teamwork is repeatedly stressed in the IOM report, *The Future of Nursing* (2011). Collaboration is considered intrinsic to nursing, the norm for professional practice, and "a health care imperative" (Sullivan, 1998, p. 62). With health care increasingly provided in complex systems, the interactions of various providers are not only inevitable but also essential for high-quality holistic care. However, agreement on basic definitions of medical and nursing practice is the *sine qua non* of collaboration between the sets of providers.

During the tumultuous years of the mid 1990s, amid national debates regarding comprehensive federal health-care reform, the leaders of the AMA and the ANA drafted the following joint definition of collaboration (ANA, 1998, p. 2):

> Collaboration is the process whereby physicians and nurses plan and practice together as colleagues, working interdependently within the boundaries of their scopes of practice with shared values and mutual acknowledgment and respect for each other's contribution to care for individuals, their families and their communities.

Although the ANA board of directors adopted this definition in 1994, it has yet to be adopted by the AMA. In considering strategies for successful collaboration, perhaps revisiting this mutually developed definition with medical and nursing organizations and practice boards on a state-by-state basis will provide the groundswell for a truly meaningful sense of shared practice relationships. The ongoing work of adopting the APRN Consensus Model state by state is a positive step in that direction (O'Grady & Ford, 2009).

9

Participation of the Advanced Practice Nurse in Health Plans and Quality Initiatives

Rita Munley Gallagher

Learning Outcomes

Learning outcomes expected as a result of this chapter:

- Support the potential for advanced practice nurses (APNs) to improve both patient experience and health plan (HP) profitability.
- Recommend skills needed for APNs to be successful in the managed care environment.
- Illustrate the relevance of value-based pricing strategies to APNs.
- Demonstrate the benefits of participation in quality reporting programs.
- Explain the barriers to autonomous practice by APNs inherent in the health-care delivery system.
- Illustrate the relevance of value-based purchasing (VBP) strategies to APNs.
- Support national organizations engaged in quality efforts and participate in quality initiatives.
- Present the benefits of integrating measurement into professional nursing practice at all levels.
- Propose the utilization of data to mobilize consumer support for their services.
- Defend the need for marketing skills.

INTRODUCTION

Advanced practice nurses (APNs) continue to be conspicuous by their absence from health plan (HP) provider panels. In addition, their efforts have not been fully recognized in activities within the national quality enterprise. Is this because of their predominantly employee status? Are they reluctant to take on the full responsibility of a primary care provider, fearful of accepting accountability, hesitant to mobilize consumer support on their own behalf? Or, is it a more fundamental issue—an issue of respect?

Today's evolving health-care environment has transformed the way many health-care services are provided and compensated. The approach to health-care service delivery has undergone a significant alteration in both its contracting and reimbursement mechanisms. Fee-for-service is no longer the primary source of pricing but has been overtaken by prospective payment, global pricing, capitation, and value-based purchasing (VBP). Along with these changes has come a significant increase in financial risk to the provider. By taking on liability not only for service delivery costs but also for level of use, providers have assumed roles historically reserved for insurance carriers. In addition, demonstration of practitioner accountability for quality has moved into the forefront of health-care delivery. More than 260,000 APNs (National Council of State Boards of Nursing [NCSBN], 2012)—and their numbers are growing—are carving out a larger role in delivering safe, effective, patient-centered, timely, efficient, equitable health care. This chapter focuses on the involvement of APNs within HPs and within the national quality enterprise and offers suggestions for increasing their visibility within both.

APNs possess the education and expert clinical knowledge to practice in multiple settings. The expertise of APNs serves to complement other practitioners within the health-care arena. "Nurse practitioners (NPs) are proven to be excellent health-care providers. More than 40 years of research has established that NPs provide high-quality, cost-effective and personalized care. The body of evidence regarding the quality of NP practice supports the notion that NP care is at least equivalent to that of physician care. When NP care is compared with that of other providers such as physicians, NP patients are more satisfied with their care and say that, in addition to providing excellent health care, their NP excels in giving health advice. They are expert at assessing and diagnosing problems. The treatments they prescribe result in positive outcomes" (American Academy of Nurse Practitioners, 2010). Still, they are often underutilized by health insurance plans.

HEALTH PLANS

HPs have become the overseers and administrators of health-care services for most Americans. HPs are nearly ubiquitous, having assumed the management and control of the overwhelming majority of health-care services provided throughout the entire United States. In 2014, nearly 90% of the U.S. population was covered under HPs; the majority (55.4%) were covered in commercial plans with approximately 35% covered by Medicare or Medicaid (Smith & Medalia, 2015).

HP leaders are in a position to improve both patient experience and the HP's bottom line by including more NPs in a greater number of HPs. APNs are highly cost effective. Their care results in decreased hospital admissions, increased adherence to treatment protocols, and improved patient outcomes (Swan et al, 2015). The number of APNs is increasing as is the physician shortage, especially in medically underserved areas. Furthermore, APNs are already caring for these vulnerable patient populations in large numbers (Buerhaus, DesRoches, Dittus, & Donelan, 2015).

Given these findings, understanding the rationale for not including significant numbers of APNs in HP provider panels is difficult (Miller, 2014). Almost all HPs have some sort of managed care program to help control health-care costs. Managed care includes programs "intended to reduce unnecessary health care costs through a variety of mechanisms, including: economic incentives for physicians and patients to select less costly forms of care; programs for reviewing the medical necessity of specific services; increased beneficiary cost sharing; controls on inpatient admissions and lengths of stay; the establishment of cost-sharing incentives for outpatient surgery; selective contracting with health care providers; and the intensive management of high-cost health care cases" (National Library of Medicine, 2011). At least in theory, managed care is designed to foster the effective, appropriate, and efficient monitoring of a specific population's health. Managed care calls for providers to assume responsibility and accountability for the health-care needs of a specifically defined population while at the same time agreeing to accept the financial risk inherent in taking on that responsibility. In a managed care system, the insurer determines, under written standards, the medical necessity of medical services and directs care to the most appropriate setting so as to provide high-quality care in the most cost-efficient manner. To control benefits, HPs require preauthorization of certain services, careful review of payment of claims, and maintenance of a provider network. Each of these administrative functions contributes to lowering the cost of care by managing benefits closely (Richards, 2010). "In America, we strictly ration health care. We've done it for years," says Dr. Arthur Kellermann, professor of emergency medicine and associate dean for health policy at Emory University School of Medicine. "But in contrast to other wealthy countries, we don't ration medical care on the basis of need or anticipated benefit. In this country, we mainly ration on the ability to pay. And that is especially evident when you examine the plight of the uninsured in the United States" (Horsley, 2009).

In managed care, the burden of risk is shared. Unlike traditional indemnity plans in which the insurance company bears the financial risk and burden of enrollees requiring more complex and costly care, various incentive plans and capitation place the risk (and burden) on the managed care provider—whether that be a plan, APN, physician, mental health provider, or other practitioner (Managed Care, 2008). In addition to point-of-service (POS) plans, the most common types of HPs include health maintenance organizations (HMOs) and preferred provider organizations (PPOs), a component of which are exclusive provider organizations. All of them are grounded in provision of care to a specified cohort of enrollees at an established per member/per month rate. See **Box 9.1.**

The initial goal of managed care was to improve quality of care and population health by increasing use of preventive services while controlling costs (Chernof, 2013). This mission has not always been readily apparent in practice or necessarily shared by all HPs. However, as systems of managed care have continued to develop, the goals have expanded to include, among others, a focus on outcomes analysis, development of practice guidelines, the creation of provider panels with a host of practitioners, and the coordination of service provision among providers

(Medicaid and CHIP Payment and Access Commission [MACPAC], 2011).

State governments have been moving to increase their regulation of HPs. Many states have passed laws expanding patient rights; guaranteeing access to care; requiring POS options, including whistleblower clauses; and establishing provider due process protections. However, several self-insured HPs have successfully challenged state health insurance regulations under the Employee Retirement Income Security Act (ERISA) based on their contention that they are self-insured employee health benefit plans. Therefore, these types of plans are exempt from many state regulations, such as any willing provider and nondiscrimination provisions (Berkery & Vann, 2013).

With a background in patient education and certification in a specialty at the master's level, the APN is well equipped to provide high-quality care in a cost-effective environment (American Academy of Nurse Practitioners, 2010). Yet APNs continue to be underrepresented on HP panels, thereby limiting enrollee access to their services. This gives rise to suspicions of lack of respect for APNs and for nursing overall. Managed care has become a way of life for all health-care practitioners and must include APNs.

Competencies Necessary in the Managed Care Environment

Clearly managed care is here to stay. However, although the fit between its stated health promotion and disease prevention goals is in line with those of the APN, HPs place emphasis on the "bottom line" in an often very competitive market. To prosper in such an arena, several skills are needed. These include marketing, advertising, and finance, which are generally considered as being beyond the components of (and, therefore, not included in) the basic nursing curriculum.

To form an optimal system of "managed" care, a new paradigm of professional practice may be needed. In this "new" system, the practitioner needs to be capable of integrating the traditional curing focus with an ability to manage the health of individual enrollees and the covered cohort overall. In addition to appropriate credentials, APNs must possess the following skills to be successful in managed care:

- Clinical accountability
- Communication skills
- Leadership skills
- Team-building abilities
- Negotiation and conflict resolution skills
- Ability to engage in quality management activities
- Financial acumen

APNs who see themselves as possessing these competencies can improve their chances of successfully negotiating a contract with a HP by doing the following:

- Highlighting communication; enhancing documentation; becoming familiar with the "ins and outs" of the contract
- Being ready to follow through with commitments
- Educating HPs on the value—both quality value and efficiency value—of their services
- Improving fiscal and management system capacities
- Being creative, flexible, and willing to work with the HP to meet mutual goals

To operate successfully in the HP environment, it is crucial that APNs work collaboratively with case managers, identify gaps in service that they are capable of filling, and hone the skills necessary (see the previous list) to succeed in contracting with the HP as well as in securing needed benefits on behalf of their enrollees (Centers for Medicare and Medicaid Services [CMS] Medicare-Medicaid Coordination Office, 2013).

HPs are interested in a provider's ability to furnish financial and cost data cross-referenced by client characteristics. These characteristics include clinical complexity, resource utilization, therapy and pharmaceutical use, length of stay, and outcome criteria. In addition, the APN must be able to

detail the processes established to ensure quality improvement and outcomes of activities. Administrative expertise is needed and quality and financial reporting mechanisms must be in place. Operating standards focused on efficacy and outcome measurement criteria along with practitioner performance evaluations are also closely scrutinized by the HP (Anthem Blue Cross, 2015). At a minimum, it is assumed that all parties preparing to enter into a contract do so voluntarily and knowingly having read and fully understanding the document. Failing to read the contract critically, as well as failure to have it reviewed by an attorney, can result in significant problems for the APN at a later date.

Contracting With Health Plans

Several challenges are inherent in providing health-care services, which makes the decision to enter into a contractual agreement with a HP particularly attractive and also potentially difficult. Such challenges may also result in a significant number of APNs continuing in the traditional role of employee, albeit with an HP as employer instead of the traditional hospital or nursing home. The majority (74.7%) of respondents to the American Association of Nurse Practitioners (AANP, 2015) compensation survey were salaried, whereas 22.5% were paid an hourly rate and 2.8% were self-employed.

When an APN *does* consider entering into a contract with a HP, numerous questions arise (Jones & Mills, 2006): Does the HP need additional APNs in your geographic area? Is the HP planning to bid on an employer group whose employees heavily utilize your specialty? Do you offer any unique services that will benefit the HP and its members? These and other relevant issues must be clarified by the APN before contractual integration into any HP system. Clearly prospective planning is critical in the decision-making process preparatory to contracting with an HP. See **Box 9.2.**

APNs must know whether the HP with which they are negotiating does the following:

- Confronts the realities of providing adequate care to clients
- Supports strong research and development programs
- Promotes health education and disease prevention
- Strongly integrates the perspectives of relevant enrollee groups
- Promotes collaborative care

Following are six tips for successful contracting with a health plan (HP):

1. Do your homework! Know as much as possible about the plan before you start to negotiate a contract. If you can, talk with other practitioners already on the provider panel.

2. Be a tough but fair negotiator up front and then a team player once you have signed on. If you want to make changes in the contract, do it before signing, not after.

3. Evaluate the "attitude" of the plan and cultivate a relationship with its officials. Do not expect plans to improve after you have signed on.

4. Clarify ambiguous language. Refine issues prospectively rather than trying to negotiate substantive changes after signing. Start with the less important issues when negotiating. It is important to know what you want and to know your limits.

5. Pay particular attention to any specific processes required by the HP in relationship to the transfer of a patient (Buppert, 2008).

6. Finally, seek competent legal advice to avoid contracting pitfalls. The health plan does.

- Supports patient engagement
- Collects and disseminates accurate data
- Advocates for financing reforms that better fund primary care
- Does a thorough job of attending to psychosocial factors
- Promotes palliative care, when appropriate
- Educates the public on the benefits of a healthy lifestyle
- Incentivizes APNs commensurate with the risks they accept

Reimbursement

When Medicare and Medicaid were first enacted in 1965 by amendment of the Social Security Act, few nurses were practicing independently; thus, no provisions were made for direct payment to them. Enactment of the Omnibus Budget Reconciliation Act (OBRA) of 1989 allowed for Medicaid coverage of services by family NPs and pediatric NPs and extended Medicare Part B coverage to NPs in skilled nursing facilities only (with no provision for coverage of services provided by clinical nurse specialists [CNSs]) and with the payment going to the facility, not directly to the NP. Medicare Part B coverage was extended to services provided by both NPs and CNSs in nonmetropolitan statistical areas (i.e., rural areas) by OBRA '90, establishing NPs and CNSs as Medicare providers. The 1990s saw several attempts by the American Nurses Association (ANA) and others to expand coverage for APN services, culminating with the signing of the Balanced Budget Act (BBA) of 1997 by President William Jefferson Clinton. The BBA extended reimbursement opportunities for APNs by removing geographical and practice site restrictions (ANA, 2016). However, significant barriers to full and autonomous practice for APNs remain firmly entrenched in the health-care delivery system. Federal (and many state) laws do not provide adequate support for the removal of barriers to practice for APNs that are created by policy makers, health-care institutions, insurance payers, or HPs. These barriers include denial of claims from third-party payers; failure to include APNs on preferred provider panels; institutional and provider policies that inhibit the objective and accurate assessment of the quality of care and benefits provided by use of APNs; and institutional and provider limitations on APN scope of practice (SOP), including contracting with HPs. Although the BBA did allow for direct Medicare reimbursement for services provided by NPs and CNSs regardless of geographical location or practice setting, it was at only 85% (80% for CNSs) of the amount that Medicare reimbursed physicians. This inequity resulted in continued billing for APN services as "incident to" the physician (i.e., allowing a service provided by an APN to be billed at 100% of the fee schedule when the physician is on site and available for consultation, if necessary) adding to the "invisibility" of APNs.

Also of relevance is Medicare's payment system, which has historically rewarded quantity rather than quality of care, providing neither incentive nor support to improve health-care quality. Conversely, the current system of VBP links payment more directly to the quality of care provided. This strategy transformed the payment system by rewarding providers for delivering high-quality, efficient clinical care. The Centers for Medicare and Medicaid Services (CMS) launched its VBP initiative through several public reporting programs, demonstration projects, pilot programs, and voluntary efforts in hospitals, physicians' offices, nursing homes, home health services, and dialysis facilities. There is administrative as well as evidentiary support for VBP. Higher spending does not equate with higher quality, and VBP is working to improve quality and avoid unnecessary costs.

In 2006, Congress passed Public Law 109-171, the Deficit Reduction Act of 2005 (DRA), which under Section 5001(b) authorized CMS to develop a plan for VBP for Medicare hospital services commencing with fiscal year 2009 when CMS added additional conditions to the hospital-acquired conditions provision (DRA Section 5001[c]). Scoring in the hospital inpatient VBP program is based on whether a provider meets or exceeds the performance standards established with respect to selected measures. In adopting this program, CMS rewards hospitals based on actual quality performance, rather than simply reporting data for those measures (Department of Health and Human Services, 2011, May 6). Therefore, CMS (and several other third-party payers) no longer make higher payments for selected conditions such as complications of surgery or hospital-acquired infections that were not present at the time of hospital admission (CMS, 2012).

Although early VBP strategies were focused solely on hospitals, there are also aspects directed to home health care and to practitioners, including those related to resource use that should be particularly relevant to APNs. On December 20, 2006, Public Law (PL) 109-432, the Tax Relief and Health Care Act of 2006 (TRHCA), was signed. Division B, Title I, Section 101 of the law authorized the establishment of a physician quality reporting program by CMS. The Physician Quality Reporting System (PQRS) (initially the Physician Quality Reporting Initiative [PQRI]) is a quality reporting program that encourages individual eligible professionals (EPs), including APNs and group practices, to report information on the quality of care to Medicare. PQRS gives them the opportunity to assess the quality of care they provide to their patients. By reporting on PQRS quality measures, APNs can also quantify how often they are meeting a particular quality metric. In 2015, the program began applying a negative payment adjustment to those who did not satisfactorily report data on quality measures for Medicare Part B Physician Fee

Schedule (MPFS)-covered professional services provided in 2013. APNs who report satisfactorily for the 2016 program year will avoid the 2018 PQRS negative payment adjustment (CMS, 2016).

The Patient Protection and Affordable Care Act (PL 111-148) (ACA) links payment to the quality of patient outcomes and calls for transforming the health-care delivery system, in part through VBP, to foster improvement in the quality and efficiency of health care. "Demonstrations to test payment incentive and service delivery models that utilize physician- and nurse practitioner-directed home-based primary care teams designed to reduce expenditures and improve health outcomes are but one example of programs being instituted. P.L. 111-148 also allows nurse practitioners and clinical nurse specialists to order post-hospital extended care services. Access to care provided by certified nurse midwives is improved through increased reimbursement for their services. Nurse practitioners will have the ability to write orders so that patients can continue to receive hospice services" (Gallagher, 2010).

In addition to the potential impact on reimbursement, participation in quality activities is important because it can improve health care. Health-care professionals, including APNs, can participate in several quality activities, including those sponsored by CMS. The CMS programs are voluntary activities that indicate health-care professionals and group practices have a commitment to quality care. In addition to Hospital Compare, the CMS quality programs include:

- Physician Quality Reporting System (PQRS)
- PQRS Maintenance of Certification Program Incentive
- Consumer Assessment of Healthcare Providers & Systems (CAHPS) for PQRS
- Electronic Health Record (EHR) Incentive Program
- Million Hearts®

Showing a commitment to quality is the first step in achieving quality care.

Advanced Practice Nurse Participation in Health Plans

Great strides have been made in recent years to establish APNs as independent practitioners providing health-care services. Health-care consumers are accepting APNs' practices more widely than previously. Research has continued to demonstrate over time that APNs have established and built on a record of delivering high-quality health care. Despite this fact, there are continuing indications that APNs face significant barriers in the health-care marketplace, including the absence of full access to HP provider panels. Despite the 2012 creation of the Council for Affordable Quality Health Care Universal Provider Datasource, designed to simplify the provider credentialing process, APNs continue to experience significant barriers in the credentialing process with HPs, to inclusion on HP provider panels, and to being listed in HP provider directories. The result of these barriers is that consumers' choice of providers is limited. Furthermore, the APN's role is relegated to employee in many cases, as opposed to that of independent contractor, as is the case of most other classes of practitioners. In addition to barriers to inclusion on HP panels, insurers and employers have also added arbitrary restrictions to APNs' practices such as adding physician supervision or needless patient record cosignatory requirements. These requirements are not necessarily in adherence with state practice laws and increase the cost of APNs' services, thereby creating disincentives to employers and consumers to use APNs.

A secondary issue is that there is little data collection regarding the role of APNs in HPs. Most HMOs do not have formal methods for estimating and reporting nonphysician provider care, thus making it difficult to track APN use, efficiency, quality, and credentialing. With disparities in prescription labeling, it is equally hard to track APN prescribing patterns. These impediments make APNs the "invisible providers," caring for many patients and generating revenue without recognition of their efforts (O'Grady, 2008).

The practice environment in the states in which they are chartered influences the policies of HPs. The legal definition of APN SOP, the type of physician collaboration required (or not required), prescription-writing authority, and state insurance laws may all affect the reimbursement and use of APNs. As health-care delivery systems evolve into increasing numbers of multistate HPs, the procedures and policies affecting APNs are not always clear. In some cases, the multistate corporations may elect to establish their own sets of rules instead of following state law. Multistate policies tend to diminish use of the separate states' APN scopes of practice, sometimes substituting stricter physician collaboration policies or limiting nurses' prescriptive writing authority to HP formularies. Yet, inconsistent

application and interpretation of state insurance law can adversely affect reimbursement and HP plan inclusion of APNs. To lend conformity and simplify regulatory compliance, HPs have generally resorted to application of the most rigorous (and hence most restrictive) rules promulgated among the states in which they provide services. The "Nondiscrimination of Health Care" section of the ACA (Section 2706) states that an insurer "shall not discriminate with respect to participation under the plan or coverage against any health care provider who is acting within the scope of that provider's license or certification under applicable state law." The intent of this provision is to provide patients with access and choice of health-care provider, including such providers as NPs, without discrimination. By complying, HPs are acting in their own best interests as well as the best interests of patients (Miller, 2014). APNs must continue to direct their efforts toward ensuring that additional states enact such legislation and that HPs allow them the recognition they so richly deserve. Whether the APN intends to work as an employee of an HP or to seek inclusion on an HP's provider panel by contracting with one, there is a need to develop a base of consumer support.

The issue is not one of APNs' competence or of the quality of the care they provide. Decades of reports have documented the high quality of NP practice (AANP, 2013). Nurses have topped Gallup's honesty and ethics ranking every year but one since they were added to the list in 1999. (The exception is 2001, when firefighters were included on the list on a one-time basis, shortly after the September 11 terrorist attacks. Firefighters earned a record-high 90% honesty and ethics rating in that survey.) With an 85% honesty and ethics rating—tying their high point—nurses have no serious competition atop the Gallup ranking (Gallup Organization, 2015). Yet, it has been said that nurses—not just APNs, but all nurses—are invisible in health care (Davis, 2012). However, that perspective is changing. A 2002 poll commissioned by Johnson and Johnson found only 25% of those polled had ever heard of a NP (Johnson & Johnson Poll, 2002, p. 14). Conversely, most respondents (90%) to a later survey knew about NPs and the majority had seen a NP for their care. Eighty-two percent of NP users were satisfied or very satisfied with the care they had received compared with a 70% satisfaction rate for other providers (Brown, 2007). Nevertheless, the skills of many APNs remain underutilized.

As ANA and the state nurses associations continue to advocate for the right of APNs to fully practice within their scope without arbitrary barriers, physicians have stepped up efforts to confine the practice of APNs. For decades, organized medicine has fostered comprehensive grassroots and media campaigns to promote supervised, collaborative practice between physicians and APNs and has increased its public opposition to the expanded scope and independent practice of APNs (Mukherjee, 2013).

One of the latest assaults of organized medicine was directed at APNs practicing in the Department of Veterans Affairs (VA), which proposed a rule to grant full practice authority to APRNs when they are acting within the scope of their VA employment. Full practice authority would help optimize access to VA health care by permitting APRNs to assess, diagnose, prescribe medications, and interpret diagnostic tests. This action proposed to expand the pool of qualified health-care professionals authorized to provide primary health care and other related health-care services to the full extent of their education, training, and certification to veterans without the clinical supervision of a physician. All VA APRNs are required to obtain and maintain current national certification. According to VA Under Secretary for Health Dr. David J. Shulkin, "Implementation of the final rule would be made through VHA policy, which would clarify whether and which of the four APRN roles (certified registered nurse anesthetist (CRNA), certified nurse-midwife (CNM), CNS, certified nurse practitioner (CNP)) would be granted full practice authority. At this time, VA is not seeking any change to VHA policy on the role of CRNAs, but would consider a policy change in the future to utilize full practice authority when and if such conditions require such a change" (VA, 2016). Organized medicine decried the proposal because, according to the American Medical Association (AMA), "it runs counter to physician-led, team-based care, which it called the best approach to improving quality" (Lowes, 2016). In late 2016, the Department of Veterans Affairs issued a final rule allowing certain APRNs—CNPs, CNSs and CNMs—to practice to the full extent of their education and training within the agency. Among other provisions, the rule defined the scope of full practice authority for the three APRN roles, which are consistent with the nursing profession's standards of practice. The rule excludes CRNAs but requested comment on whether access issues or other unconsidered circumstances might warrant the inclusion of CRNAs in future rulemaking (American Hospital Association [AHA], 2016).

Yet another strategy that has been put forth by organized medicine is advocating for the relaxation of antitrust laws as they apply to health-care professionals. Legislation has also been introduced on both the federal and state levels to provide collective bargaining rights for health-care professionals. Only those employees deemed nonsupervisory under the National Labor Relations Act are accorded the rights to collectively bargain; however, these legislative proposals would provide physicians the right to enter into joint negotiations with insurance companies to work out payment arrangements, clinical practice conditions, and more. Such activity is currently forbidden under state and federal antitrust laws and is considered anticompetitive collaboration among competitors. In some instances the courts have held that such collaboration on prices and market access are illegal boycotts. Changes in law being advocated by physician organizations would not only allow negotiation, but also would weaken the ability of the APN to prove antitrust violations by physician competitors, thereby ignoring their ability to take part equally in the competitive managed care arena regardless of the quality of the care they provide.

Examples of other barriers include limitations on prescriptive authority, such as the ability to prescribe only a 30-day supply of Schedule II drugs, and opposition to removal of the APN-to-physician ratio. "This high degree of variation across the states for APN regulation has spotlighted the need to ensure that regulation serves the public, promotes public safety, and does not present unnecessary barriers to patients' access to care" (O'Grady, 2008, p. 8).

NATIONAL QUALITY EFFORTS

The public concern for error and patient safety together with the continuing "quest for quality" has created renewed responsibility and accountability for the outcomes of patient care. The National Quality Forum (NQF), a private, nonprofit, voluntary, consensus standard setting organization composed of more than 400 organizations (including several nursing organizations, the first of which was the ANA) and individuals from federal and state governments and private sector entities is prominent in the national quality arena. NQF is governed by a board of directors representing health-care consumers, purchasers, providers, HPs, and experts in health services research. The NQF board also includes representatives from four federal agencies: the Agency for Healthcare Research and Quality (AHRQ), the Centers for Disease Control and Prevention (CDC), CMS, and the Health Resources and Services Administration (HRSA) (NQF, 2016b).

The mission of NQF is to lead national collaboration to improve health and health-care quality through measurement by:

- Convening key public- and private-sector leaders to establish national priorities and goals to achieve health care that is safe, effective, patient-centered, timely, efficient, and equitable
- Working to ensure that NQF-endorsed standards will be the primary standards used to measure and report on the quality and efficiency of health care in the United States
- Serving as a major driving force for and facilitator of continuous quality improvement of American health-care quality (NQF, 2016c).

Nursing is active in all aspects of NQF efforts on steering committees and their technical advisory panels: the National Priorities Partnership, the Consensus Standards Advisory Committee (CSAC), and the NQF board of directors. The central activity of NQF is the endorsement of performance measures as "voluntary" consensus standards and the identification of gaps in health-care quality research.

Voluntary consensus standards, although relatively new in the health-care arena, are not new to other industries. Moreover, since passage of the National Technology Transfer and Advancement Act of 1995 (Public Law 104-113) voluntary consensus standards have legal standing. The voluntary consensus process, even in the face of strict requirements as to periods and transparency, is timelier than is the federal rule-making process. One key component of the act is the obligation of the federal government to use voluntary existing consensus standards, thus encouraging the federal government to take part in the NQF process. Federal agency involvement in NQF serves to encourage both public and private purchasers, accrediting bodies, practitioners and providers, and the public to also take part.

NQF recognizes the value of nursing to health-care quality. The NQF nursing care performance measures project established consensus on a set of evidence-based measures for evaluating the performance of nursing in acute-care hospitals (NQF, 2007). It also addressed the implementation of those measures within health-care organizations to improve nursing care and patient outcomes and designated a subset of measures that are appropriate for public reporting (such as on the Web site Hospital Compare, which was developed by the Hospital Quality Alliance [HQA] in which the ANA was a principal).

HQA developed and launched Hospital Compare to provide information to the public on hospital quality. HQA worked to increase hospitals' voluntary participation in public reporting and expand the set of quality measures being reported. The information on Hospital Compare helps patients determine how often individual hospitals provide the specific care that most patients should receive for certain conditions, such as giving heart attack patients an aspirin on arrival at a hospital. Although only a limited number of nursing measures are included in Hospital Compare, the sheer number of nurses and their primacy in caregiving are compelling reasons for measuring their contribution to patients' experiences and the outcomes that are attained (NQF, 2007). See **Box 9.3.**

The Joint Commission engaged in a "comprehensive test of the NQF nursing-focused performance measures to determine whether they could be used nationally to identify opportunities to improve the quality of patient care provided by nurses. The project was funded by a grant from the Robert Wood Johnson Foundation. Testing of the integrated set of measures led to refined technical specifications. The resultant measures then underwent NQF investigation and most were re-endorsed. They are now available for use by hospitals nationwide and included in quality initiatives used by the CMS and/or The Joint Commission" (Hill, 2007). The information available to assist consumer decision making (such as is provided on Hospital Compare) would be greatly enhanced by the inclusion of the full portfolio of NQF-endorsed nursing-sensitive measures. See **Box 9.4.**

Advanced Practice Nurse Participation in Quality Initiatives

In addition to the NQF-endorsed nursing-sensitive measures, other clinician-level quality measures are of relevance to APNs, including those developed by the Physician Consortium for Performance Improvement (PCPI) convened

Box 9.3

The Value of Measuring Nursing Care

To increase the value of information provided to consumers regarding the quality of nursing care by nursing-sensitive measures, interested parties should focus on the following points:

1. Nurses represent the largest single group of health-care professionals.

   - Registered nurses held about 2.8 million jobs in 2014 (Bureau of Labor Statistics [BLS], 2016).
   - In initially endorsing voluntary consensus standards for nursing-sensitive care, the National Quality Forum (NQF) noted nurses, as the principal frontline caregivers in the U.S. health-care system, have tremendous influence over a patient's health-care experience (NQF, 2004).

2. Decades of evidence demonstrate nursing's impact on the provision of care that is safe, effective, patient centered, timely, efficient, and equitable:

   - RNs play key roles in hospitals' systems for early detection of threats to patient safety and for prompt remedial intervention (Dubois et al, 2013).
   - A high level of evidence indicated better serum lipid levels in patients cared for by NPs in primary care settings (Stanik-Hutt et al, 2013).
   - Patient outcomes on satisfaction with care, health status, functional status, number of emergency department visits and hospitalizations, blood glucose, blood pressure, and mortality are similar for NPs and MDs (Stanik-Hutt et al, 2013).
   - Increasing RN staffing could reduce costs and improve patient care by reducing unnecessary deaths and reducing days in the hospital (Stone et al, 2007).
   - A 10% increase in the number of patients assigned to a nurse leads to a 28% increase in adverse events such as infections, medication errors, and other injuries (Weisman, 2007).
   - Understaffing of RNs in hospital intensive care units increases the risk for serious infections for patients, specifically pneumonia (Hugonnet, Uçkay, & Pittet, 2007).

   - According to The Joint Commission (2005), "quantifying the effect that nurses and nursing interventions have on the quality of care processes, and on patient outcomes, has become increasingly important to support evidence-based staffing plans, understand the impact of nursing shortages and optimize care outcomes."

3. Measures of quality have been fully developed, are in use, and have been previously vetted. The endorsement of the nursing-sensitive measures by NQF was an initial (albeit significant) step toward standardized measurement of nursing care, detailing its relationship to the quality (and efficiency) of health care.

   - Nursing-sensitive indicators are widely used as a barometer of quality care by CMS, the Patient Care Link, and the Magnet Recognition Program (Erickson, 2011). Collectively, the measures "provide consumers a way to assess the quality of nurses' contribution to inpatient hospital care, and they enable providers to identify critical outcomes and processes of care for continuous improvement that are directly influenced by nursing personnel" (NQF, 2004).

4. There has been a public call for information about nursing care quality.

   - Enhancing the initial nursing-sensitive measure set through the inclusion of additional measures will increase the overall value of the set.
   - Consumers will benefit from information regarding the impact of nursing care as they make decisions regarding care.

5. Evidence exists that public reporting stimulates quality improvement and choice.

   - Making performance data public results in improvements in the clinical area reported on (Hibbard, Stockard, & Tusler, 2005).

6. Measuring and publicly reporting health-care quality information results in higher-quality care for patients (MN Community Measurement, 2015). There is agreement among diverse health-care stakeholders

that the NQF-endorsed nursing-sensitive measures should be incorporated into national and state hospital performance measurement and reporting activities.

- Interviews were conducted with nearly three dozen national health-care, hospital, and nursing leaders, principals of nursing performance measurement efforts, and hospital representatives to determine their interest in and use of the NQF's nursing-sensitive measures. Recommendations derived from the data gathered from these interviews and published by NQF (2007) point to several

complementary and incremental actions that can be collectively undertaken by health-care stakeholders to advance hospital performance measurement and accelerate our collective understanding of nursing's key role in quality. Among these recommendations is a "call" to health-care leaders to fully integrate the nursing-sensitive measures into national and state hospital performance measurement and reporting initiatives, including, but not limited to, Hospital Compare (NQF, 2007; USDHHS, 2012).

Box 9.4

National Quality Forum–Endorsed® National Voluntary Consensus Standards for Nursing-Sensitive Care[1]

Patient-centered outcome measures:

1. *Death among surgical inpatients with serious, treatable complications (PSI 4):* In-hospital deaths per 1,000 surgical discharges, among patients ages 18 through 89 years or obstetric patients, with serious treatable complications (deep vein thrombosis/pulmonary embolism, pneumonia, sepsis, shock/cardiac arrest or gastrointestinal hemorrhage/acute ulcer). Includes metrics for the number of discharges for each type of complication. Excludes cases transferred to an acute care facility.

2. *Pressure ulcer prevalence (hospital acquired):* The total number of patients who have hospital-acquired (nosocomial) category/stage II or greater pressure ulcers on the day of the prevalence measurement episode.

3. *Patient fall rate:* All documented falls, with or without injury, experienced by patients on eligible unit types in a calendar quarter.

4. *Falls with injury:* All documented patient falls with an injury level of minor or greater on eligible unit types in a calendar quarter. (Reported as injury falls per 1,000 patient days.)

5. *Restraint prevalence (vests and limb):* Total number of patients who have vest and/or limb restraint (upper or lower body or both) on the day of the prevalence measurement episode.

6. *National Healthcare Safety Network (NHSN) catheter-associated urinary tract infection (CAUTI) outcome measure:* Standardized infection ratio (SIR) of health-care-associated, CAUTI will be calculated among patients in bedded inpatient care locations, except level II or level III neonatal intensive care units (NICU). This includes acute care general hospitals, long-term acute care hospitals, rehabilitation hospitals, oncology hospitals, and behavior health hospitals.

7. *Percent of residents with a urinary tract infection (long-stay):* This measure reports percentage of long-stay residents who have a UTI in the 30 days before the target assessment. This measure is based on data from the minimum data set (MDS 3.0) OBRA, PPS, or discharge assessments during the selected quarter. Long-stay nursing facility residents are identified as those who have had 101 or more cumulative days of nursing facility care.

8. *Risk-adjusted urinary tract infection outcome measure after surgery:* Risk-adjusted, case mix adjusted UTI outcome measure of adults 18+ years after surgical procedure.

9. *Urinary tract infection admission rate (PQI 12):* Admissions with a principal diagnosis of UTI per 100,000 population, ages 18 years and older. Excludes kidney or urinary tract disorder admissions,

Continued

Box 9.4

National Quality Forum–Endorsed® National Voluntary Consensus Standards for Nursing-Sensitive Care[1] *(Continued)*

other indications of immunocompromised state admissions, obstetric admissions, and transfers from other institutions.

10. *National Healthcare Safety Network (NHSN) central line-associated bloodstream infection (CLABSI) outcome measure:* SIR of health-care-associated, CLABSI will be calculated among patients in bedded inpatient care locations. This includes acute care general hospitals, long-term acute care hospitals, rehabilitation hospitals, oncology hospitals, and behavioral health hospitals. Nursing-centered intervention measures—system-centered measures:

11. *Skill mix (registered nurse [RN], licensed vocational/practical nurse [LVN/LPN], unlicensed assistive personnel [UAP], and contract):*

   • NSC-12.1—Percentage of total productive nursing hours worked by RN (employee and contract) with direct patient care responsibilities by hospital unit.
   • NSC-12.2—Percentage of total productive nursing hours worked by LPN/LVN (employee and contract) with direct patient care responsibilities by hospital unit.
   • NSC-12.3—Percentage of total productive nursing hours worked by UAP (employee and

contract) with direct patient care responsibilities by hospital unit.
   • NSC-12.4—Percentage of total productive nursing hours worked by contract or agency staff (RN, LPN/LVN, and UAP) with direct patient care responsibilities by hospital unit.

12. *Nursing hours per patient day:*

   • NSC-13.1 (RN hours per patient day)—The number of productive hours worked by RNs with direct patient care responsibilities per patient day for each in-patient unit in a calendar month.
   • NSC-13.2 (Total nursing care hours per patient day)—The number of productive hours worked by nursing staff (RN, LPN/LVN, and UAP) with direct patient care responsibilities per patient day for each in-patient unit in a calendar month.

13. *Practice Environment Scale–Nursing Work Index (PES-NWI) (composite and five subscales):* PES-NWI is a survey measure of the nursing practice environment completed by staff RNs, which includes mean scores on index subscales and a composite mean of all subscale scores.

[1]Endorsed as of July 8, 2016 (NQF, 2016a).

---

more than a decade ago by AMA. Its goal is to improve patient health and safety by:

• Identifying and developing evidence-based clinical performance measures and measurement resources that enhance the quality of patient care and foster accountability
• Promoting the implementation of effective and relevant clinical performance improvement activities
• Advancing the science of clinical performance measurement and improvement

Consortium activities are carried out through cross-specialty work groups established to develop performance measures

from evidence-based clinical guidelines for select conditions. Membership is open to any organization or individual who is committed to health-care quality improvement or patient safety and who participates in the development, review, dissemination, or implementation of performance measures and measurement resources. The PCPI balances its work efforts among new measure development, maintenance and enhancement, specifications, measure testing, and implementation. New measure topics are reviewed and selected against criteria including addressing gaps and unexplained variations in care, quality improvement, patient safety, appropriateness of care, and key priorities of the current health-care environment. The multiple step process for measure development begins with a review of evidence and selection of a work group and continues through public comment and member voting. Specifications and eMeasures (standardized performance measures specified in the accepted standard health quality measure format) are developed for implementation into an EHR. Practitioners of all relevant disciplines of medicine—as well as other health-care professionals for whom the care topic is within their SOP, including APNs—are involved in each measure work group (Kmetik, 2007). The PCPI eSpecification, which provides the requirements for writing and calculating the measure in an

electronic environment, includes *human readable* format, and the PCPI eMeasures translate the eSpecifications into a *computer readable* format. The PCPI tests many of its performance measures for feasibility, reliability, validity, and unintended consequences via PCPI-convened testing networks (AMA, 2016). PCPI is the sole developer or a collaborating party for a portfolio that includes measurement sets in 47 clinical areas and preventive care and more than 350 individual measures (AMA, 2016a, 2016b). See **Box 9.5.**

Nurses are the primary caregivers in all health-care settings. As such, they are critical to the provision of high-quality

---

Box 9.5

Physician Consortium for Performance Improvement: Quality Measures Relevant to APNs

Physician Consortium for Performance Improvement (PCPI) measurement descriptions and specifications are available for the following 48 clinical topics and conditions:

1. Acute otitis externa (AOE)/otitis media with effusion (OME)
2. Adult sinusitis
3. Anesthesiology and critical care
4. Asthma
5. Atopic dermatitis
6. Atrial fibrillation and atrial flutter
7. Care transitions
8. Chronic obstructive pulmonary disease
9. Chronic stable coronary artery disease (Updated as of April 2016)
10. Chronic wound care
11. Community-acquired bacterial pneumonia
12. Dementia (Updated as of December 2015)
13. Diabetes—adult
14. Emergency medicine
15. Endoscopy and polyp surveillance
16. Eye care I and II (Updated as of August 2015)
17. Gastroesophageal reflux disease
18. Geriatrics
19. Heart failure (Updated as of April 2016)
20. Hematology
21. Hepatitis C (Updated as of June 2016)
22. HIV/AIDS

23. Hypertension
24. Kidney disease—adult
25. Kidney disease—pediatric
26. Major depressive disorder—adult (Updated as of September 2015)
27. Major depressive disorder—child and adolescent (Updated as of December 2015)
28. Maternity care
29. Melanoma
30. Nuclear medicine
31. Obstructive sleep apnea
32. Oncology (Updated as of September 2015)
33. Optimizing patient exposure to ionizing radiation
34. Osteoarthritis
35. Osteoporosis
36. Outpatient parenteral antimicrobial therapy
37. Palliative care
38. Pathology
39. Pediatric acute gastroenteritis
40. Percutaneous coronary intervention
41. Perioperative care
42. Prenatal testing
43. Preventive care and screening (Updated as of April 2016)
44. Prostate cancer (Updated as of September 2015)
45. Radiology
46. Rheumatoid arthritis
47. Stroke and stroke rehabilitation
48. Substance use disorders

care. "Gaining a more in-depth understanding of the role that nurses play in quality improvement and the challenges nurses face can provide important insights about how hospitals can optimize resources to improve patient care quality" (Draper, Felland, Liebhaber, & Melichar, 2008). All nurses must have thorough evidence-based knowledge of the impact of the care they provide on the outcomes that patients experience. Measurement must be integrated into professional nursing practice at all levels, including the practice of APNs, and not simply considered to be a separate activity.

RECOGNITION AND CONSUMER SUPPORT

APNs are health-care professionals who do the following (The University of Tennessee Health Science Center College of Nursing, 2016):

- Provide high-quality health-care services
- Diagnose and treat a wide range of health problems
- Stress both care and cure, using a unique approach
- Focus on health promotion, disease prevention, health education, and counseling
- Assist patients to make wise health and lifestyle choices

Simply put, APNs engage in many of the care practices that patients are seeking. APNs focus primarily on health promotion and disease prevention—factors frequently overlooked by traditional primary care providers. They have significant experience in both the acute and ambulatory care arenas. These abilities coupled with APNs' possession of case management skills make them ideal for involvement in HPs not merely as employees but as fully credentialed members of the HP's provider panel. Why, then, are HPs not clamoring to engage their services? How can APNs increase HPs' demand for their services? In short, how can APNs market themselves (and their advanced practice roles) to both the HP and its enrollees?

Although continuing emphasis is placed on quality, managed care's focus on reduction of costs has often resulted in a type of "managed competition" in which enrollees' benefits are restricted through limitation of their access to a variety of providers. It is within this trap that APNs frequently find themselves. To flourish in the managed care environment, APNs must market themselves to the HP and to enrollees.

Marketing begins with a survey of the desires, needs, and expectations of the "customer," which in managed care is the enrollee. Armed with that information, APNs should then structure a plan to meet those needs. Because most APNs practice in a specialty area, the marketing plan should focus on the provision of related services, known as a *market segment*. An APN can choose to focus on a population with a single condition (e.g., individuals with insulin-dependent diabetes), a specific enrollee need (e.g., rehabilitation following amputation), or a particular population (e.g., older adults). A primary decision centers on whether to engage in provision of services to a single population, a variety of populations, or to all plan enrollees.

Marketing principles are sometimes referred to as the "four Ps": product, price, promotion, and place (NetMBA, 2008). The first "P," product, encompasses the specialty practice services APNs provide amplified by health promotion and disease prevention skills. The APN's product is self-evident. Thorough understanding of the second "P," price, is essential to the success of the APN, be it within an HP or in independent practice. Although the marketplace itself has a significant impact on demand for an APN's services as well as on how much it is willing to pay, the APN is the final arbiter regarding price. It is critical that the APN has full knowledge of the costs of *all* the components of the services delivered, not just personal compensation. The most difficult "P" for many nurses, not just APNs, to engage in is promotion. Nurses do not usually excel at "tooting their own horns." Self-promotion, or marketing, is unfamiliar to most nurses. Nurses generally operate from a mindset that views all health-care providers as doing their utmost to provide high-quality care. To increase recognition as well as consumer or enrollee support, APNs must be willing to call attention to the positive aspects of the safe, effective, patient-centered, timely, efficient, equitable care they provide. Finally, APNs must make an informed decision as to the last "P," place; that is, whether or not to engage in providing care as an employee, as an independent practitioner, or as a contractual partner in an HP.

CONCLUSION

Today's health-care delivery system, with increased merger activity between insurance companies and health-care systems and the biased policies of providers and HPs, has created an environment in which APNs experience significant barriers to their ability to practice. Strategies are needed to unite the collaborative efforts of ANA, constituent member associations, other national APN organizations, individual APNs, and consumers. There is an ongoing need to identify trends related to exclusionary behavior and to develop an effective multipronged approach to address anticompetitive policies and practices.

Nurses have looked to antitrust protections for relief from practices that block their full participation in the health-care market. CNMs and CRNAs used federal antitrust laws to limit boycotts and expand their market share. The Federal Trade Commission (FTC) has rendered opinions that provide the foundation for anticompetitive action by registered nurses. The Department of Justice and the FTC have issued joint guidelines for antitrust enforcement in the health-care industry that offer general direction about those practices that are (and that are not) likely to trigger action by these enforcement agencies.

Restrictive policies at the state level must be addressed by a comprehensive state-based strategy to better define and combat state-based anticompetitive behavior. Such strategies should include the state insurance commissions, state boards of nursing, and consumer and regulatory entities to enforce the law and to challenge anticompetitive activities.

It is crucial that nurses in general, and APNs in particular, work to gain recognition for the high-quality, cost-effective care they provide. ANA and other nursing groups remain committed to monitoring state and federal activities of organized medicine to counteract their effectiveness. To the extent that organized medical societies focus their efforts on opposing or supporting legislation, even through the use of exaggerated arguments and legislative strategies, the major option available to nursing is to oppose those efforts and to respond to them by ensuring that legislators and the public hear the facts about APN practice.

APNs continue to be notably absent from HP provider panels and from the national quality enterprise. This is likely due, in part, to their predominantly employee status. In moving to contracting independently with HPs, APNs can take on full responsibility as managed care providers. In addition, APNs can engage in the collection and reporting of data, using measures related to the quality of care they provide. Those data, in addition to informing nursing practice, can help purchasers and consumers decide where to look for high-quality, effective, efficient care. Using data, APNs can mobilize consumer support for their services, thereby increasing respect for themselves and on behalf of nursing overall. It is up to individual APNs, to professional nursing, to NQF, and to all who have interest in the provision (or receipt) of high-quality health care to advance quality in a collaborative, coordinated way. After all, health-care quality really is an art . . . "more like ballet, than hockey" (Crosby, 1979).

10

Public Policy and the Advanced Practice Registered Nurse

Marie-Eileen Onieal

- Understand agenda setting and policy design.
- Explain the interdependence of policy and practice.
- Describe the importance of the political process in shaping health-care policy.
- Integrate sociological, economic, and political perspectives into an understanding of health policy issues.
- Describe and discuss the impact of politics and economics on the health-care delivery system.
- Analyze the current health-care policy environment and its effect on advanced practice registered nurse (APRN) practice.
- Participate in influencing political decisions that affect APRN practice.
- Advocate for APRNs within the policy and health-care communities.

INTRODUCTION

To begin a chapter on policy, one must first understand there is much ambiguity regarding its definition. Derived from the Greek word *polis* meaning city-state, a society is characterized by a sense of community and obligation to participate in its government, religious cults, defense, and economic welfare and to obey its sacred and customary laws (Merriam-Webster online; Encyclopædia Britannica® Online). Policy is also defined as principles or actions derived toward specific ends. In simple terms, policy is the rational attempt to achieve common (often complex) objectives. It is important to know that all policies reflect the values of those making the policy.

Public policy is about communities trying to achieve something as a community despite any conflicts within the goals (Stone, 1997). It encompasses the choices that society as a whole, or a segment of society, makes regarding those goals and priorities, which can be a "public interest." In that construct, there can be two sides; one of self-interest and one of public spirit. Regardless, the underpinning of the policy is for the good, and in some instances the protection, of the community.

Public policy is the group of authoritative decisions made in the legislative, executive, or judicial branches of government at either the state or federal level within the jurisdiction of those entities. The decisions, intended to direct or influence the actions or behaviors of others, can be laws, rules, or operational criteria. Public policy is the government's solution to resolve the problems of society (Harrington & Estes, 2008). A component of the policy making process is the formulation of the problem and the identification of possible solutions. The selection of the solution, based on an analysis of alternatives, forms the policy.

THE ADVANCED PRACTICE REGISTERED NURSE

Advanced nursing practice is broadly defined by the American Association of Colleges of Nursing (AACN, 2004) as "any form of nursing intervention that influences health care outcomes for individuals or populations, including the direct care of individual patients, management of care for individuals and populations, administration of nursing and health care organizations, and the development and implementation of health policy" (p. 2). The advanced practice registered nurse (APRN) title consists of four roles: certified nurse practitioner (CNP), certified nurse-midwife (CNM), certified registered nurse anesthetist (CRNA), and clinical nurse specialist (CNS) (National Council of State Boards of Nursing [NCSBN], 2008).

The history of the APRN can be traced back to the mid 20th century, a time when barriers of access to health care were increasing. The combination of the decrease in the number of nurses and physicians being deployed to Viet Nam and the growth in population stressed the health-care provider community. At the same time, Americans were clamoring for health care to be a fundamental right rather than a privilege, and the need for primary care providers (PCPs) was increasing. APRNs quickly began to fill the need for PCPs, especially in rural areas where poor and low-income families, lacking access to health-care services, were woefully underserved.

APRNs are a testament to the nursing leaders who preceded them. Trailblazers such as Florence Nightingale, Lillian Wald, and Margaret Sanger championed the cause of improved health care, especially for the disenfranchised (Piren & Reinhard, 2009). Following in the footsteps of those pioneers, Loretta Ford blazed the trail for the nurse practitioner (NP) role to meet the health-care needs of society. In 1965 Loretta Ford, EdD, RN, PNP, and Henry Silver, MD, saw the need for better access to care for children and launched the first program to educate nurses in the advanced practice role. From that seed, the profession grew and brought with it a new paradigm in health care. The birth of the advanced nursing practice role was instrumental in solving the health-care access crises faced in the mid 1960s.

Throughout nursing history people considered nurses as a "group set apart to serve society" (Sellew & Neusse, 1951, p. 391). The public also looked to nurses for community service and leadership (Dock & Stewart, 1929, p. 361), leaving nurses with a moral obligation to society. That obligation constituted a type of social contract that, in addition to assurance of competence, concern for the well-being of patients, integrity, and accountability, is the responsibility to participate in formulating public policy that affects not only the scope of practice for APRNs but also the access to APRNs as PCPs and integral members of the health-care team.

Policy and the APRN

In 1985 Senator Edward Kennedy astutely noted that "Nurses are America's largest group of health professionals, but they have never played their proportionate role in helping to shape health policy, even though that policy profoundly affects them as both health providers and consumer" (Mason & Talbot, 1985, p. xxi). He was a tireless supporter of, and endless believer that, all Americans deserved the opportunity to have access to health care. More than that, Senator Kennedy understood and supported the roles played by nurses, specifically APRNs, in making that access a reality.

Responsibility for working toward meeting the health-care needs of society lies with every APRN. As a member of the profession, every APRN has an ethical and moral obligation (the social contract) to influence both public and health policy so that the health of the public is both protected and promoted. Far too often in the past, the idea of becoming "politically active" has been frightening to many APRNs. Perhaps they lacked the confidence to get involved or confidence regarding how to advocate at the policy level, or they preferred to stay on the sidelines. Today, with health policy and leadership essential components in all nursing education, not just APRN education, the barriers to becoming an active participant in policy development are decreasing. It is imperative for APRNs to recognize and undertake the responsibility of the potential to contribute to the development of health policy through political action, thus meeting the obligations of the social contract.

APRNs have long used the policy making process when reaching decisions—perhaps not as a formal method, but surely informally as the process of gathering the alternative options for solving the problems at hand, such as going through a sequence of mental operations to achieve the desired outcome, weighing one option against another, and choosing the one that most likely will achieve the goal. In this policy making process, it is imperative that the APRNs be participants in those processes that occur in the public arenas and impact the practice of APRNs. It is equally imperative that the APRN role is represented at every policy table—it is often said, "If you are not at the table you are on the menu." Being involved in the discussion of alternatives gives the APRN a voice and ensures that voice is heard on issues in state and national legislation that potentially affect APRNs, their patients, or access to health-care services. Those issues that affect the future development of the profession are of specific concern, specifically the requirement in some states that APRNs practice in collaboration with a licensed physician.

Professional nursing organizations worldwide have mandates and processes for nurses to engage at some level in policy development. Provision 7 of the 2015 Code of Ethics for Nurses with Interpretive Statements (American Nurses Association [ANA], 2015) requires nurses, in all roles and settings, to advance the profession through research and scholarly inquiry, professional standards development, and the generation of both nursing and health policy.

The latter underscores the nurse's responsibility to lead or serve on institution, local, state, regional, or global civic or organizational policy making committees (Lachman, Swanson, & Windland-Brown, 2015). As a component of that, APRNs must act on their responsibility to be leaders, serving and mentoring others on policy committees in their practice settings, and serve as health-care consultants to local, regional, and state representatives.

Entities that credential APRN programs, or provide guidelines for those programs, also have mandates that the curricula include content that provides for the APRN to become competent in the policy arena. Those bodies (National Organization of Nurse Practitioner Faculties [NONPF], AACN, and Commission on Collegiate Nursing Education [CCNE]) acknowledge that political activism and a commitment to policy development are central elements of professional nursing practice (Ehrenreich, 2002). Engagement in the process of policy development includes the ability to influence policy makers to improve health-care delivery and outcomes. An essential component of that engagement is that APRNs understand the relevant state legislative agenda and how it affects their scope of practice.

Political competence is requisite within nursing to (a) intervene in the broad socioeconomic and environmental determinants of health, (b) intervene effectively in a culturally diverse society, (c) partner in development of a humane health-care system, and (d) bring nursing's values to policy discussions (Warner, 2003). In 2007, the ICN described the APRN's policy making role and asserted that APRNs should contribute to public policy pertaining to the determinants of health (Carnegie & Kiger, 2009). One reason APRNs need to assume a political role is a shift in focus from the individual as patient to communities experiencing health inequalities. APRNs must get involved at the political level and where advocacy and citizenship are located within a community role.

APRNs must advocate for their autonomy, educate legislators on both the economic and societal value of care provided by APRNs, and strive to convince legislators to remove barriers to their practice. APRNs need to be more involved in policy making, which influences the delivery of care. Professional associations have traditionally fulfilled key roles by acting on behalf of the profession's individual members to "establish a contract with society" and influence health-care policy (Dollinger, 2000, p. 28); however, it is incumbent upon the individual APRN to take an active role in advocating for those policies that promote access, equity, quality, and cost, all of which require removal of barriers to practice.

APRN Regulation: The Consensus Model

In July 2008 the *Consensus Model for APRN Regulation* was published. The rationale for the APRN Consensus Model was to align the processes of license, accreditation, certification, and education to alleviate concerns about patient safety in light of the increasing numbers of APRNs performing in roles with constantly changing expectations.

The model is the product of many years of substantial work conducted by the Advanced Practice Nursing Consensus Work Group and the National Council of State Boards of Nursing (NCSBN) APRN Committee. The task of the committee was to develop and validate nationally recognized educational standards, nationally recognized role competencies, and nationally recognized specialty competencies. The members of the consensus group represented 41 nursing organizations. The document defines APRN practice, describes the APRN regulatory model, identifies the titles to be used, defines specialty, describes the emergence of new roles and population foci, and presents strategies for implementation.

The *Consensus Model for APRN Regulation* was endorsed by those nursing organizations that participated in the APRN Consensus Work Group and the APRN Joint Dialogue Group with unanimous agreement on most of the recommendations (2008). It includes the following essential elements: licensure, accreditation, certification, and education (LACE).

- *Licensure* is the granting of authority to practice.
- *Accreditation* is the formal review and approval by a recognized agency of educational degree or certification programs in nursing or nursing-related programs.
- *Certification* is the formal recognition of the knowledge, skills, and experience demonstrated by the achievement of standards identified by the profession.
- *Education* is the formal preparation of APRNs in graduate degree-granting or postgraduate certificate programs.

The recommendations within the Consensus Model reflect a necessity and intent of collaboration among regulatory bodies to achieve a sound model and continued communication with the goal of increasing the clarity and standardization of APRN regulation. In addition, the group recognized the need to continuously and regularly discuss issues related to nursing education, practice, and credentialing. The model must remain a living document that can be easily updated to respond to changing societal needs and the desire for consumers to have unfettered access to care provided by APRNs. In addition, the model provides a formal, ongoing communication mechanism that allows transparent and aligned communication among the key stakeholders having an interest in advanced practice nursing.

Implementation of the recommendations for an APRN Regulatory Model was intended to occur incrementally (NCSBN, 2008) and be fully implemented by 2015. The model, now 9 years postendorsement, has been enacted in more than 40% of states. Those 21 states have adopted full practice authority licensure and practice laws for APRNs. Under these laws, APRNs practice independently and are accountable "for recognizing limits of knowledge and experience, planning for the management of situations beyond [their] expertise; and for consulting with or referring patients to other health care providers as appropriate" (Fairman, Rowe, Hassmiller, & Shalala, 2011). The enactment of major Consensus Model elements by a sufficient number of states now should create the momentum to encourage the remaining states to align. Continued attention and persistence along the Consensus Model elements demonstrates that full practice authority removes barriers to APRN practice.

The societal benefit of implementing full practice authority for APRNs is in providing patients with full and direct access to all the services that APRNs are prepared to provide. Full practice authority for APRNs is supported in reports from several entities. Along with the Institute of Medicine (IOM), which specifically targets regulatory barriers, organizations such as the Macy Foundation support broader scope-of-practice boundaries. One of the largest consumer groups, the AARP (formerly the American Association of Retired Persons), also supports an expanded role for APRNs in primary care as well as care provided in secondary and tertiary settings. From an economic benefit standpoint, strengthening access to primary care by increasing use of APRNs expands the availability of primary care at a lower price. In addition, it has the potential to decrease the incidence of sequelae related to illness and disease that has gone untreated because of access barriers. In Massachusetts alone, research shows that allowing APRNs to practice at their full capacity demonstrated a savings of $4.2 billion to $8.4 billion over 10 years and that greater use of retail clinics staffed primarily by APRNs could save an additional $6 billion (Eibner et al, 2009).

Since the 1960s APRNs have enabled the expansion of community health centers. By 2011, there were 7,354 sites throughout the country that provided care for more than 16 million people (Aiken, 2011). In addition, millions of American families received care at more than 1,100 retail clinics staffed primarily by APRNs, easing the burden on emergency departments (EDs). Moreover, several health-care reform initiatives are contingent on APRNs' filling a range of new roles in primary care, prevention, and care coordination (Aiken, 2011).

The Affordable Care Act and the APRN

The ability to access health-care services, regardless of setting, is a longstanding concern for both consumers and government. The IOM Primary Care Reports consistently define accessibility as a cornerstone of care (IOM, 1978, 1993, 1996). The 2000 IOM report, *America's Health Care Safety Net: Intact but Endangered,* recognizes that the United States fails to provide timely and adequate access to health-care services for vulnerable populations.

In March 2010 President Obama signed comprehensive health reform, the Patient Protection and Affordable Care Act (ACA), into law. The law was designed to increase the number of Americans covered by health insurance and decrease the cost of health care. Its enactment was the end of decades of attempts to enact comprehensive health insurance. Many arguments have been made both before and since criticizing the passage of this law, calling it too costly and too quickly implemented without sufficient planning or thought. Many have also denigrated the law as being a step toward "socialized medicine," whereas others warn it encourages "big government," a historically distrusted approach to solving problems.

Improving access to affordable health insurance, and by extension to care, is one of the main goals of the ACA. With its enactment came wide-ranging changes to the U.S. health-care system not seen since the 1965 development of the Medicare and Medicaid programs. Because of these laws, the United States has the opportunity to transform its health-care system and provide higher quality, safer, more affordable, and more accessible care than ever before. That said, fulfilling the vision of the ACA requires a transformation of many aspects of our health-care system, particularly those pertaining to APRNs (Cella & King-Jensen, 2011).

Although the enactment of the ACA has improved access to the services provided by APRNs, barriers to full implementation still exist. Case in point: APRNs have been authorized Part B Medicare providers since 1998. Despite this recognition, APRNs with patients who need home health-care services still have to locate a physician to certify that the APRN has conducted the required face-to-face certification examination to document eligibility for care. APRNs can provide face-to-face assessments of the patient's needs, yet the requirement that a physician document the encounter still exists. Such requirements increase costs and delay necessary care, which is contrary to the intent of these authorizations.

Since the full implementation of the ACA, 18 million uninsured people have gained health coverage (Assistant Secretary for Planning and Evaluation [ASPE], 2015). The ACA has also improved access to health-care services provided by NPs evidenced by the nondiscrimination provision acknowledging APRNs as PCPs. Having access to a regular source of primary care is associated with more effective provision of preventive services and better management of chronic disease. The Department of Health and Human Services (HHS) estimates that another 10.5 million uninsured Americans are eligible for coverage through the public insurance exchanges, and a push will be made to enroll them (Pear, 2015). These factors and an aging and growing population contribute to the demand for primary care. A shortage of PCPs, acute in some areas of the country, is expected to significantly grow in the years ahead. These are solid reasons to support full-practice authority for APRNs with favorable and fair reimbursement policies.

According to the IOM's landmark 2011 report, *The Future of Nursing: Leading Change, Advancing Health,* the ability of APRNs to meet the nation's health-care needs and practice to the full extent of their education and clinical preparation continues to be limited by significant barriers in federal law and regulation. Further, the report recognizes unique attributes of the nursing profession, including our adaptability, close proximity to patients, and scientific understanding of care processes.

Healthy People 2020 outlines multiple determinants of health; they include "policymaking, social factors, health services, individual behaviors, and biology and genetics" (HHS, 2011). APRNs are educated to address individuals in light of the social, economic, and environmental factors that influence their health—in close keeping with the recommendations of *Healthy People 2020* (Pericak, 2011). Moreover, the evidence is compelling that APRNs already have a significantly growing role in U.S. primary care delivery (Pohl, Barksdale, & Werner, 2015).

State-to-State Comparisons

Different states have adopted different titles for the advanced practice nurse, including NP, advanced nurse practitioner (ANP), advanced registered nurse practitioner (ARNP), clinical nurse practitioner (CNP), and registered nurse practitioner (RNP). Title variation by state increases the confusion about the APRN role. This inconsistency in titling has proven to be very confusing to the public (Fotsch, 2016). Further, the differences in how certification bodies direct APRNs to specify their credential (i.e., FNP-C, CPNP) adds to the confusion. There is no uniform model of regulation of APRNs across states. Although the Consensus Model is a step toward eliminating that lack of uniformity, each state independently determines the APRN legal scope of practice, the roles that are recognized, the criteria for entry into advanced practice, and the certification examinations accepted for entry-level competence assessment. These have all created a significant barrier for APRNs to easily move from state to state and has decreased access to care for patients.

The ACA recognizes APRNs as PCPs eligible to receive grants and primary care bonus payments with no mention of collaboration or supervision requirements (**Figure 10.1**). Acknowledging APRNs as PCPs is paramount to the success of the ACA. Yet the barriers for APRNs to practice independently continue. Restrictions on scope of practice limits the supply of labor, restricts competition, and increases the cost of services. Utilizing APRNs to the full extent of their knowledge and competence extends the paradigm of health care. APRNs must be acknowledged as full partners with physicians and other health-care

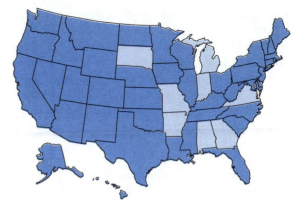

Legend

■ Yes: 42 states
(May include recognition in Medicaid or in other insurance laws)

□ No: not explicitly recognized:
8 states + DC

*Note: Not all states grant full-practice authority to ARNPs.

FIGURE 10.1 Recognition of ARNPs as primary care providers in state law.*

professionals in redesigning health care in the United States to achieve better health outcomes.

Within the constructs of practice authority are three categories: full, reduced, and restricted. When the APRN role was in its infancy, states with the most need for PCPs, particularly those with large rural areas, were more apt to mitigate statutory and regulatory barriers. A full practice license allows the APRN to evaluate patients, diagnose, order and interpret diagnostic tests, and initiate and manage treatments—including prescribing medications. This is significant because in those states the right to full practice is under the exclusive licensure authority of the state board of nursing, not a regulated collaborative agreement with another health discipline. This is the model recommended by the IOM and the NCSBN. Today, across the 50 U.S. states and territories, in only 21 states and Washington, DC, do ARNPs have the authority to practice the full extent of their preparation.

Reimbursement

The Centers for Medicare and Medicaid Services (CMS) regulate federally supported insurance programs. Medicare provides insurance for people age 65 or older, people under age 65 with certain disabilities, and people of all ages with end-stage renal disease (permanent kidney failure requiring dialysis or a kidney transplant).

Medicaid provides health insurance coverage for our nation's most vulnerable individuals and families. Medicaid, a shared state and federal program, is regulated differently than other insurance providers. Each state sets its own guidelines for eligibility, services, and reimbursement (CMS, 2016).

Effective January 1998, services provided by primary care ARNPs became reimbursable by Medicare. Although the reimbursement rate was 5% lower than that for physicians, this was a breakthrough in mitigating barriers of access to care based on payment. Despite this achievement, challenges to reimbursement for APRNs continue to exist. In addition to Medicare and Medicaid, many third-party payers, whether a managed care organization or other commercial insurer, recognize APRNs as qualified health-care providers. However, differences in the reimbursement and coverage policies can be extensive. This conundrum is compounded by the restrictions of Medicaid and other private insurers, as well as restrictions within states and policies related to direct reimbursement and supervisory requirements by another health-care provider. Each entity has its own set of billing criteria and within them exist challenges for the APRN.

It is imperative that reimbursement policies for all payers be updated to guarantee that APRNs are eligible to participate and are directly accessible to patients. Moreover, reimbursement should reflect true costs associated with providing quality care and promote the effective and efficient utilization of the health-care provider workforce (Nurse Practitioner Roundtable, 2010). The IOM (2011) echoes the sentiment of the APRN community in their recommendations that all third-party payers participate in direct reimbursement for APRNs who provide services within their scope of practice.

The requirement for collaborative agreements in many states limits the ability of APRNs to have a self-governing license. Lack of consistent reimbursement across states has kept APRNs largely invisible and minimizes the quantity and quality of care they currently provide. Moreover, reduced Medicare reimbursement for APRN services, which is already low, makes financial solvency difficult.

In July 2016 there were 683 bills in the legislatures of the 50 states and territories that directly affected APRN-delivered care. An additional 112 bills dealt directly with primary care. Within each bill was a recommendation to remove barriers that make it difficult for APRNs to serve as PCPs and leaders of patient-centered medical homes or other models of primary care delivery. Those barriers included reimbursement policies, scope of practice and controlled substance prescriptive authority, required supervision by another health-care provider, and discrimination by individual health plans. State and national regulatory and reimbursement policies must be amended to remove barriers that make it difficult for NPs to serve as PCPs in all models of care delivery.

CONCLUSION

Over the years, studies have consistently demonstrated that APRNs provide high-quality, cost-effective health care to patients of all ages in all walks of life in all settings. It is crucial that reimbursement policies and systems be re-engineered to reflect the true costs of care and promote sustainable practice.

APRNs must be prepared to participate in the political arena. They must stay focused on national and local contexts in order to encourage policy development that includes APRNs as key players in the delivery of quality care to the American public. It is a component of their social contract to maintain accountability to their communities to provide high-quality and affordable care.

It is easy to forget that the APRN role, established in 1965, is a relatively young one when compared with the nursing profession as a whole. Despite its relative youth, it has grown to become one of the most important roles in the health-care community. APRNs have a rich history of providing effective and essential care to patients and the public. As we look to the future, we must celebrate and draw upon our rich, if comparatively brief, history. And all APRNs must continue to be active participants in the political process.

11

Resource Management

Eileen Flaherty, Antigone Grasso, and Cindy Aiena*

Learning Outcomes

Learning outcomes expected as a result of this chapter:

- Interpret profit and loss (P&L) statements.
- Explain the drivers of operating revenue.
- Distinguish relationships between reimbursement and payer mix.
- Describe types of expenses: salary, nonsalary, and depreciation.
- Understand fundamental considerations in creating a budget.
- Recommend strategies to maximize revenue.
- Illustrate cost containment strategies.
- Demonstrate the impact APRN practice can have on revenue generation and expenditure of resources.

INTRODUCTION

In any setting, the advanced practice registered nurse (APRN) influences and is influenced by the environment of an organization. The organization provides the structure in which the APRN's clinical practice goals will be pursued.

The underlying assumption for any organization is that its reason to exist is to produce some product or service (output) that is of value. The corollary assumptions are that, because the output is of value, it will generate revenue and that the revenue generated will both cover the costs of the resources expended (input) and provide some level of profit. Profit is necessary to ensure the continued viability of the organization, for example, to upgrade existing facilities, to replace outdated equipment, to expand services or to add new programs, and, in for-profit organizations, to provide a return for investors or owners and encourage continued investment. If this does not occur, the organization will not survive. To succeed

*Earlier versions of this chapter were authored by Christina Graf.

in its mission, the organization must secure its financial viability through appropriate prioritization of outcomes and effective utilization of resources.

Organizational decisions can affect both the content and direction of the APRN's practice or in fact determine to what extent APRNs are able to practice within the organization. The absence of effective input from clinicians can result in inappropriate or ineffective expectations of the clinician. Similarly, clinicians' decisions can generate unintended consequences that undermine the health and strength of the organization. Therefore, the APRN needs to understand the business and financial structure and systems of the organization. For example, how does the APRN's practice affect revenue generation and expenditure of resources? To what extent do business and fiscal policies enhance or constrain clinical practice?

STRUCTURE

In accomplishing its mission, an organization engages in a series of transactions that it tracks and manages through its financial system(s). These transactions are categorized according to the chart of accounts, a matrix structure that organizes the transactions. One axis of the matrix, the account codes, aggregates transactions according to type (e.g., patient care revenue, salaries, office supplies, maintenance contracts). The other axis, the cost center, revenue center, or responsibility center, aggregates transactions according to function and may be identified by service line (cardiac center, cancer care center), physical location (patient care unit, outpatient clinic), or activity (blood bank, hemodialysis). The detailed designations in the chart of accounts are specific to each organization and, as such, not only aggregate transactions for better information and management but also provide a picture of the organization and its internal structure. The aggregated transactions are summarized in a statement of operations called the profit and loss (P&L) or income and expense (I&E) statement that also quantifies the operating margin or the gain or loss (income minus expense) from operations. See **Figure 11.1.**

Most health-care organizations use accrual accounting in preparing financial statements. Accrual accounting specifies that revenues are recognized when services are provided and expenses are reported as resources are used. The matching principle requires that, when revenues are reported, the associated or matching expenses are reported. Thus, revenues reported for activities within a particular cost center are matched to the expenses generated in producing those revenues and reflect the activity and resource utilization that occurred in that reporting period regardless of when actual monies for services are received or bills for resources are paid.

REVENUE

Revenue refers to the income that an organization receives and can be broken into two main categories: operating and nonoperating. Operating revenue includes the income from the primary activities of the organization. For a hospital, this might include patient revenue, retail activities (retail pharmacies, parking, and cafeteria), and research-related income. Nonoperating revenue is from other sources that benefit the organization through activities such as investments and philanthropy.

Operating Revenue

Revenue that is generated primarily from the day-to-day activities of the organization is termed *operating revenue.* In health-care organizations, the majority of the operating revenue is related to patient or client services rendered and may come from a variety of payers: the federal government (Medicare, military, and veterans benefit programs), state governments (Medicaid, health insurance exchanges, and other state programs), other third-party payers (Blue Cross/Blue Shield, health maintenance organizations, fee-for-service insurance plans), or the recipient of the service (self-pay).

Revenue or income refers to the monies received for services provided and reflects the volume of output of the organization. It is based on the price or charge allocated to each specific service, activity, or item (also referred to as gross patient service revenue). The organization's charge master is a list of the prices charged, which are intended to reflect the related costs plus some margin of profit. However, charges are usually discounted or bundled under a global fee for most payers, entirely waived

PROFIT AND LOSS STATEMENT
FISCAL YEAR 2017
(In Thousands of Dollars)

	Actual	Budget	Variance	Variance Percent
Gross Patient Services Revenue				
Inpatient	$515,994	$496,843	$19,151	3.9%
Outpatient	$341,769	$332,764	$9,005	2.7%
Total Gross Patient Services Revenue (GPSR)	$857,763	$829,607	$28,156	3.4%
Deductions From Revenue				
Contractual Allowances	$498,732	$479,560	−$19,172	−4.0%
Charity Care	$23,760	$22,230	−$1,531	−6.9%
Net Patient Services Revenue	$335,272	$327,818	$7,454	2.3%
Indirect Research Revenue	$31,555	$30,951	$605	2.0%
Other Operating Revenue	$16,089	$15,126	$964	6.4%
Total Operating Revenue	$382,916	$373,894	$9,022	2.4%
Expenses				
Salaries & Wages	$152,628	$151,908	−$720	−0.5%
Employee Benefits	$26,517	$26,726	$209	0.8%
Supplies	$58,682	$56,421	−$2,261	−4.0%
Utilities	$9,503	$10,187	$685	6.7%
Other	$81,249	$77,487	−$3,762	−4.9%
Depreciation	$27,300	$27,468	$168	0.6%
Provision for Bad Debt	$8,758	$10,126	$1,368	13.5%
Interest	$4,956	$5,485	$529	9.6%
Total Operating Expense	$369,592	$365,806	−$3,786	−1.0%
Income (Loss) from Operations	$13,324	$8,088	$5,237	n/a
Percentage of Total Revenue	3.5%	2.2%		

Note: Positive variances are favorable to budget; negative variances are unfavorable to budget.

FIGURE 11.1 Sample profit and loss (P&L) statement.

for charitable care, or not collected from those who are not expected to pay (bad debt). Therefore, charges are not necessarily an accurate reflection of actual income (net patient services revenue) from the service provided (Gapenski, 2012).

Medicare revenues are determined not by charges on individual services but by a prospective payment system that allocates a fixed payment based on an episode of care (Cleverly, Song, & Cleverly, 2011). The payment is determined for inpatient episodes of care by the discharge diagnosis (diagnosis-related group [DRG]) and is adjusted for variations in regional cost of living, urban versus rural setting, and organizational involvement in medical education. Except for some small amount of adjustment for cost or length-of-stay outliers, the payment to an organization for each DRG is constant regardless of costs incurred. This prospective payment system is not applicable to psychiatric and rehabilitation units or hospitals, children's and cancer hospitals, or long-term care facilities; these are reimbursed on a reasonable cost basis, with some limits, for Medicare-eligible patients. For outpatients, Medicare has developed a similar prospective payment system using ambulatory payment classification groups (APCs) that aggregate services that are similar clinically and with respect to resource requirements. Medicare reimburses providers for services based on prior fixed rates for the APCs (Rimler, Gale, & Reede, 2015).

Medicaid and other state-sponsored payment programs reflect not only the intent of the program but also the economic and political environment of the state and thus vary widely from state to state. The state determines what will be covered and the level of reimbursement, and may limit payments through global or flat-rate fees for episodes of care, exclusion of certain services from coverage, discounting of specific charges, or targeted spending caps.

Many nongovernmental third-party payers negotiate contracts directly with health-care organizations. These contracts may include DRG-like prospective payment systems, discounted or adjusted rates, risk-sharing agreements such as flat-rate payments per member per month for all defined care needs, prior authorization requirements, or other mechanisms that minimize the cost to the payer and distance the revenue from the charge. These payers, primarily managed care organizations, also include in their reimbursement systems copays, specified dollar amounts per episode of care, deductibles, and identified annual dollar amounts or deductibles that are paid directly by the consumer. Fee-for-service insurance payers typically reimburse based on a negotiated percent of charges, but there also may be copayments or deductibles, payment ceilings, or service exclusions that shift the burden to the insured. In any case, fee-for-service insurance provides only a small percentage of the income of health-care organizations. Even smaller is the proportion of self-pay patients who are able to afford health care. The number of uninsured, who have no access to federal, state, or private coverage, generates charitable care for many health-care organizations. However, it is important to note that with the implementation of the Affordable Care Act in 2010, the number of uninsured Americans has gradually decreased. Other reductions to expected revenue come in the form of denials and bad debt, where either the insurer determines that services provided did not meet the eligibility requirements or a patient who was expected to pay, in the form of copayments or deductibles, defaults on those payments. As health-care costs increase and all parties become more cost conscious, it becomes important for providers to understand the rules and meet all requirements to ensure they are getting paid for all services rendered.

In addition to the many reimbursement methods that currently exist, new payment mechanisms continue to emerge. For example, many payers link quality measures, outcomes, and utilization measures with reimbursement incentives, also referred to as pay-for-performance and shared savings programs. The intention of such programs is to encourage cost management while maintaining continuous improvement in the quality of care delivered in all health-care settings. In these arrangements, health-care organizations and their providers are held accountable not only for achieving defined quality standards to receive full payment for services but also to decrease unnecessary costs. Efforts around population health management and medical homes are designed to improve performance on these measures.

Another example of linking reimbursement to quality is the October 2008 Centers for Medicare and Medicaid Services (CMS) reimbursement policy that denies Medicare reimbursement for specific hospital-acquired conditions (HAC) that were not present on admission; this list of HACs was further revised in 2013. See **Box 11.1.** CMS named these medical errors "never events" because they should never occur for any patient. As health-care organizations are required to assume responsibility for the cost consequences of preventable complications, more emphasis is being placed on the leadership role nurses can play in reducing medical errors. More specifically, many of the "never events" such as pressure ulcers and patient falls are nursing sensitive, which further underscores the importance of high-quality nursing care in protecting patients and securing revenues. Intended to motivate hospitals to improve patient safety, CMS has encouraged state Medicaid programs to follow Medicare's lead. In addition, many commercial health plans are also seeking to implement payment plans that will hold hospitals financially accountable for preventable errors (Austin & Pronovost, 2015).

In addition to revenue from patient services, organizations may generate operating revenue from other

---

Box 11.1

Hospital-Acquired Conditions (HAC) List

- Foreign object retained after surgery
- Air embolism
- Blood incompatibility
- Stage III and IV pressure ulcers
- Falls and trauma
- Manifestations of poor glycemic control
- Catheter-associated urinary tract infection (UTI)
- Vascular catheter-associated infection
- Surgical site infection, mediastinitis, following coronary artery bypass graft (CABG)
- Surgical site infection following bariatric surgery for obesity
- Surgical site infection following certain orthopedic procedures
- Surgical site infection following cardiac implantable electronic device (CIED)
- Deep vein thrombosis (DVT)/pulmonary embolism (PE) following certain orthopedic procedures
- Iatrogenic pneumothorax with venous catheterization

"Hospital-Acquired Conditions." Centers for Medicare and Medicaid Services, 2016.

---

day-to-day activities in areas such as the parking garage or the cafeteria, or indirect research revenue, the overhead received from research sponsors for providing facilities and administrative support for research projects. Total operating revenue is net patient services revenue plus other operating and research revenue and reflects the total reimbursement in actual monies that the organization expects to receive from operations.

Nonoperating Revenue

The organization may also generate nonoperating revenue that is not tied directly to the services provided. Nonoperating revenue is managed and reported separately from operating revenue. This revenue is not included when reviewing the financial implications of day-to-day operations nor included in the operating margin. Interest income may be generated on cash or investments. Gifts or donations may be given to a not-for-profit organization for a specific purpose or for the general purposes of the organization. If the gift is in the form of an endowment, the principal (the original amount of the gift) is invested and only the interest income on the investment may be used.

EXPENSES

Expenses are costs incurred in providing services. Wage and salary expenses are the costs of personnel, the labor costs required to deliver care and other activities within the organization. Salaries are determined by the organization, subject to regulation regarding minimum wage and fair labor practices and, in some organizations, union contracts. They include base wages plus any differentials, premiums, bonuses, or other monetary rewards. Fringe benefits fall into two categories: those mandated by law, such as unemployment insurance and workers' compensation, and those specific to the organization, such as health insurance and pension benefits. Other benefits that incur costs are related to the organization's personnel policies regarding sick, vacation, holiday, and other paid time off. In addition to the obvious salary cost for the employee receiving paid time off, there is an additional expense if the work of that employee must be covered by another individual. If the work of the employee is not fully covered, there may be a productivity cost associated with volume or revenue that is not realized. In a practice, if practitioners are functioning at efficient levels, the absence of one practitioner on a paid leave will result either in loss of revenue for patients not seen or increased costs for a temporary replacement for the practitioner. Note that this relates to paid absence. Unpaid absence leaves unspent wages available to support a temporary replacement or provides a cost offset to unrealized volume and associated revenue.

Nonsalary expenses are those nonpersonnel costs for consumable supplies, minor equipment, and related activities used in the delivery of service. Some are directly related to patient care activities, such as medical supplies, drugs, and blood products. Others are related to supports for the care process (office supplies, telephone charges), the environment (maintenance contracts, utilities), personnel (seminar registration, consultation fees), or interest on loans.

Another type of expense is depreciation or the recognition of the cost of capital assets (Gapenski, 2012). Capital expense refers to major investments in durable assets, such as facilities, equipment, and machinery. Capital assets are expected to have a value and useful life significantly greater than that of minor equipment. The threshold for determining what is capitalized is set by the organization and usually describes both a monetary value and an expected life span. For example, the threshold for capital might be equipment that costs more than $5,000 and has a useful life greater than 3 years. Under these guidelines, neither a $100 intravenous (IV) pole (monetary threshold) nor $1,000 worth of instructional videotapes (life span threshold) would be considered capital.

Because capital assets are expected to be used over an extended period of time, their full purchase price does not appear as an operational expense at the time of purchase. Rather, in each reporting period for the duration of its useful life, the I&E report reflects the capital depreciation or use of the capital asset during the period. For example, if a capital purchase of $12,000 is expected to have a useful life of 10 years, one-tenth of its value is estimated to be used each year. Therefore, the financial statement would report depreciation of $1,200 per year or $100 per month.

COST CONCEPTS

A variety of cost concepts are relevant in understanding resource management and utilized when making decisions about long-term planning (Cleverly et al, 2011).

Variable Versus Fixed Costs

Variable costs are those related to the volume of activity and fluctuate based on changes in volume. Fixed costs are those that remain constant regardless of fluctuations in volume. In personnel, the staff nurses may be considered variable—more are needed when the unit is at 90% occupancy than when it is at 75% occupancy—whereas the clinical nurse specialist (CNS) and nurse leader are fixed—one allocated to the unit(s) regardless of the number of patients. Similarly, medical supply expense is variable based on patient volume and acuity whereas maintenance contract expenses may be fixed based on the terms of the contract and not driven by volume. Some expenses may be step-variable, that is, fixed over a short range and variable over a longer range. For example, one secretary may be sufficient for a practice with up to four clinicians, but a second secretary may be required if an additional clinician enters the practice. In that case, the number of secretaries is fixed at two unless the number of clinicians increases beyond eight. In general, all costs that are fixed in the short run are variable in the longer run. See **Figure 11.2.**

Direct Versus Indirect Costs

Direct costs are those related to the process of producing a product or service. Indirect costs are those incurred in supporting that process. In practice, the identification

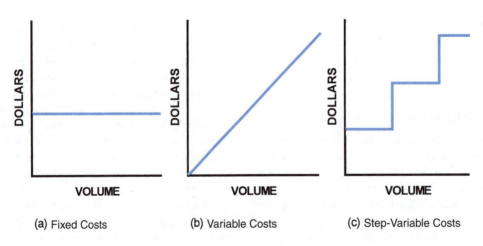

(a) Fixed Costs   (b) Variable Costs   (c) Step-Variable Costs

FIGURE 11.2 Fixed versus variable costs.

of expenses as direct or indirect depends on the context. In addressing an individual patient, caregivers—nurses, therapists, practitioners—would be considered direct whereas the leadership and support staff—secretaries, CNS, or nurse leader—would be considered indirect. In considering patient populations aggregated by clinical care unit or practice, the entire staff of that unit or practice could be considered direct whereas support departments—human resources, environmental services, finance—are identified as indirect.

Total Versus Unit Costs

Total cost is the aggregate cost incurred within a given time period for all volume of activity in that time period. Unit cost is the cost of one unit of volume, calculated as the total cost divided by the total units of volume. Marginal cost is the additional cost required to produce one more unit of volume. Because the total cost includes both variable and fixed costs, economies of scale can be achieved by increasing volume—and variable costs—on the unchanged fixed cost base. For example, if a clinical care unit can increase its occupancy, it will expend more in variable direct care staff, but the cost per patient day will decrease because the fixed costs are spread over more patient days. Marginal cost for each additional patient day is equal to the cost of the variable staff and supplies for that patient day.

Incremental Versus Opportunity Costs

Incremental cost is the added cost incurred for an activity that would not be expensed if that activity did not occur. These costs may be variable or fixed, but they are essentially new costs and do not include current costs that may be redirected to the new activity. For example, if a CNS proposes to teach a new series of classes on pediatric cardiac life support, incremental costs could include items such as demonstration mannequins, audiovisual aids, books, or other informational material and supplies for practical application. These would all be incremental costs because they would be incurred specifically for the purpose of the program. The participants' salaries are incremental if they are paid beyond their usual or regular hours to attend the program. If the program is to be given within the participants' regular working hours and it will be

necessary to provide additional staff hours to cover those in class, these replacement costs are also included in the incremental costs. The CNS's time in preparation and teaching, and the facilities or space in which the classes are taught, would not be considered incremental costs because—if the classes were not given—the CNS's salary and the cost of maintaining the facilities would still be incurred. The incremental costs would be calculated for the number of students and programs presented over a given period of time.

Opportunity cost measures the loss of the effect of the next best alternative use of the resources allocated to a particular use. If the previously described program is approved for implementation, what activity will the CNS forego to implement the program? If the participants are taking the course during their regular working hours and replacement is not required, what will they not be doing that might otherwise have been done? If the incremental resources were not allocated to this program, how would they be used instead? The answers to these questions describe the opportunity costs. Identification and quantification of opportunity costs can provide important information in setting priorities and analyzing alternatives (Finkler, Jones, & Kovner, 2013).

BUDGETING

Effective management presumes that an organization, in planning for its continuing existence, is able to describe and project the level of activity or production of services or products it will experience and anticipate the resources that will be required for that level of activity. The budget is the translation of that plan into quantities and dollars. The conceptual plan on which the budget is based may describe the projections for the entire organization or for some particular sector or activity and will determine the scope of the budget including the time frame and the level of detail.

Types of Budgets

Strategic planning is likely to be translated into a long-range budget that addresses the direction of the organization over the next 3 to 5 years or more. For this type of budget, the projections of volume and resources will be at a high level, with estimations of revenue and expense totals, but not at an extremely detailed level. The major drivers of volume and resources will be described and quantified and include items such as anticipated changes in the patient mix, Medicare reimbursement rates, treatment protocols, and inflationary cost increases as well as incorporating any new major strategies such as new programs and service lines or adding capacity. Other factors will be estimated in the aggregate based on current experience. The strategic plan and long-range budget are schematic representations of the direction of the organization rather than detailed blueprints. They need to be reviewed and refreshed at regular intervals to ensure that the organization continues to move in its preferred direction and to respond to significant changes in the health-care environment.

The operational budget, on the other hand, addresses the detailed, day-to-day activity of the organization. This type of budget looks in extensive detail at the projected volume and resources and the associated revenue and expense over a prescribed period of time. Usually the operating budget is constructed for the fiscal year, the organization's 12-month accounting cycle. The budget describes anticipated activity based on the specific operational goals and plans of the organization for that period of time and incorporates assumptions that will affect revenue and expense, for example, changes in reimbursement or inflationary increases in the cost of utilities or supplies. The budget is prepared at the detailed level of account within each cost or revenue center. Throughout the fiscal year, actual performance is reported against the budget for each month and cumulatively for the fiscal year to date, and is reported for each cost or revenue center and account code. However, each fiscal year's operating budget is independent of other years, that is, the positive or negative variance and the unspent budgeted monies from one fiscal year are not carried over into the next. The operating budget as a plan is valuable at the detailed level, the level at which the work occurs and at which the activity and resources must be managed. Aggregation of the budgeted and actual revenue and expense at the organizational level is also useful in providing overall direction and evaluation for the organization as a whole.

The capital budget reflects the projected expense for necessary facility improvement or acquisition of major durable equipment. Funding for the capital budget comes from the profit generated from operations, or from loans, which are also dependent on the organization's ability to generate a profit from operations. Although the capital budget may be prepared in yearly cycles, unlike the operating budget it is contained by the time frame of the project rather than of the budget year. Thus, capital funds may be allocated over several budget years for a particular remodeling project or equipment replacement proposal, and, unlike the operating budget, the funds will carry over from year to year until the project is completed. The capital budget is based on the plans and projections of the organization and will address the facilities and equipment needed to expand or upgrade services. These can include the need for new or added clinical equipment such as cardiac monitors and ultrasound equipment; major software (electronic medical record, provider order entry system); and facilities improvement (renovation and remodeling). The capital budget also needs to address the maintenance needs of the organization and therefore will also include such things as replacing existing equipment (such as ventilators that have reached the end of their useful life) or facilities maintenance (such as the heating, ventilation, and air conditioning [HVAC] system). Finally, in preparing the capital budget, it is important to consider any additional operating costs that will be incurred because of the use of the capital asset. For example, purchase of a monitoring system, clearly a capital expense, can also generate operating costs in the form of replacement leads or probes, batteries, or electrocardiogram (ECG) tracing paper, as well as potentially salary costs if additional personnel hours are required to review the monitors or file the tracings. These expenses must be identified and incorporated in the appropriate operating budget.

Frequently, organizations will consider initiating new activities or expanding or changing existing ones. The program budget is useful for this purpose. This type of budget isolates one activity or program from all other organizational activities to evaluate its effectiveness. The basis for the program budget is the conceptual plan of the program, or the program proposal, which also determines the time frame for the budget as well as the types of expenses to be included (e.g., total costs, incremental costs, opportunity costs). For example, a plan to expand the hours of service for a medical urgent care clinic, using existing facilities and equipment, may be adequately described in a program budget that looks only at incremental volume, resources, revenue, and expense for the current fiscal year. Evaluation of the fiscal viability of the plan would consider the extent to which incremental revenue exceeds incremental expense. A plan to add a neonatal intensive care unit in a service that previously provided only routine and intermediate care would require a more extensive program budget. The quantification of activity would need to address potential volume—both numbers of neonates and clinical conditions—and probable income based on payer mix and reimbursement rates. Resource requirements would include both capital expenditures for facilities and major equipment and operational expenses for personnel, supplies, minor equipment, utilities, and overhead. Because of the time required to set up the program and the anticipated ramp-up from opening to full occupancy and utilization, the program plan would cover an extended period of time. Fiscal estimates would then need to be adjusted for the effect of inflation and reimbursement changes. Evaluation of the program would include a calculation of breakeven, that is, the point at which the average total revenue for an admission is equal

to the average total cost. Before breakeven, the program generates a loss for each admission. After breakeven, the program generates net revenue for each admission. See **Figure 11.3.**

Determination of the value of a program considers more than the fiscal benefit, for example, opportunity costs, social benefits and costs, or public relations value. These factors are difficult to quantify and are therefore not part of the program budget although they would be contained in the program proposal. When a program budget is approved and implemented, it becomes part of the operating budget for the implementation period and for all subsequent years. However, it is also useful to evaluate actual performance against the original program budget.

The projection of the cash budget is critical in the life of the organization. In the other types of budget, one of the guiding principles is matching revenue to expenses, that is, identifying the income for the activity that occurred in a particular time period and the expenses related to that activity that were incurred in that time period. Typically, however, the actual receipt of the revenue and the payment

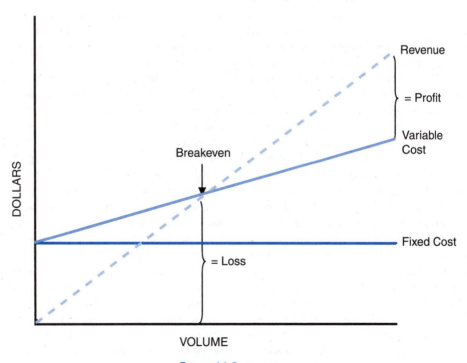

FIGURE 11.3 Breakeven.

of the expenses do not occur in the same time period. Services are billed to third-party payers but the actual revenue is received weeks or even months later. Supplies are ordered, delivered, and used but the organization may be billed days or weeks later and the bills may be paid on a 30-, 60-, or 90-day payment cycle. Thus the revenue and expense projections for a particular accounting cycle in the operational budget may not reflect that cycle's cash flow, the actual cash coming into and going out of the organization. The cash budget projects this flow over the course of the fiscal year to ensure that there will be sufficient money in the organization to meet its obligations to its employees for payment of salaries, to its suppliers for payment of bills, and to its lenders for repayment of loans.

The Budgeting Process

The budget process is based on the conceptual plan, goals, and objectives of the organization. The first step in this process is the identification of the activity that generates revenue and drives resource utilization. Within the health-care system, there are typical volume statistics that are used to quantify activity: admissions, discharges, patient days, patient visits, procedures, and tests. In the aggregate, however, these measures do not have the level of precision needed for accurate prediction of revenue and expenses. For purposes of predicting revenue, the volume needs to be further defined to reflect the basis of payment—by payer, by service, by product line, by DRG, or by test or procedure code.

In contrast to revenue, different categories may be needed for the purposes of predicting resource utilization. DRG payments, for example, reflect medical condition and interventions but do not as clearly reflect nursing care needs of patients. Therefore, patients in the same DRG—and generating the same revenue—may have different nursing care needs based on age, functional capabilities, communication issues, or learning needs and thus generate different levels of resource utilization. Payment systems may be based on global fees (e.g., for normal pregnancy and delivery) or on panels of patients (with the practice or organization receiving a per patient per month payment regardless of utilization of services) that are not reflective of the individual variability in care needs and resource requirements. It is necessary, therefore, to develop workload measures that identify both the resource drivers, that is,

the significant activities that generate resource utilization, and the elements that account for individual variation within those drivers. For example, in the cancer infusion unit, the primary measure may be the patient visit or the therapeutic protocol. However, resource utilization may vary based on whether this is a new or returning patient, the length of the treatment, the patient's response to the therapy, or other issues or concerns that the patient raises in the course of the visit. Although it may not be possible to implement a workload measure that addresses this variability in minute detail, it is possible to develop measures that differentiate among patients and aggregate those with similar resource requirements. For patients with the same medical condition or undergoing the same therapeutic protocol, it may be possible to identify variations in resource utilization based on age, stage of treatment, functional level of activity, or other indicators. Using these indicators as well as the primary volume indicator of the visit or protocol to describe patient populations, one can then generate a more accurate projection of required personnel and resources. The patients can be aggregated into groups with similar resource requirements and the groups can be weighted based on their average utilization relative to one another. For example, in a particular practice, patients receiving a specific intervention may require 15 minutes of the clinician's time. However, a follow-up patient may only require 10 minutes and a new patient may require 40 minutes. All patients, however, may require 5 minutes for documentation and 5 minutes for follow-up. The intervention patient, therefore, will consume 25 minutes of time and the others 20 minutes and 50 minutes, respectively. If the intervention patient is the benchmark and weighted at 1.0, the follow-up patient is weighted at 0.8 (20/25 (1.0)) and the new patient at 2.0 (50/25 (1.0)). Projecting visits by patient type and applying the appropriate weights will give a more accurate representation of the anticipated workload than projecting the visits alone.

Similarly, although there has been a current focus on considering mandated nurse–patient ratios as a way of ensuring adequate levels of care for patients, the ratios ignore the differences among patients in their need for nursing care. Identifying and measuring these nursing care requirements, often referred to as patient acuity, can be valuable information in managing and allocating nursing resources. To do so, many acute-care settings have implemented patient classification systems as a methodology for quantifying nursing workload. Such systems, which classify patients according to their needs for nursing care (examples may include activities of daily living, medication administration, physiological assessment or intervention, communication support, medication preparation), enable organizations to capture actual nursing workload and to measure productivity by looking at the relationship between nursing hours and workload over time. This approach can provide a new dimension for managing resources beyond the more simplistic but common measure of workload as patient days and nursing hours per patient day (Finkler et al, 2013).

Variable personnel and material resource requirements are based on the projected workload volume. Using historical and current data, it is possible to construct a ratio of resources to volume—personnel hours per unit of work or supplies per unit of work. The personnel hours will include more than the direct care hours because there is indirect time in the form of orientation for new staff, continuing education for current staff, practice or departmental meetings, teaching or precepting, or other organizational activities that are a necessary part of the working year. In addition, the personnel hours must reflect the impact of benefit time because the individual on sick, holiday, or vacation time is not available to attend to the workload. Therefore, the personnel budget should be constructed first on the ratio of direct care hours to workload, that is, projected workload multiplied by the required hours per unit of work. Indirect time is added to this based either on a specific identification of the hours in the year that will be allocated to these activities or on a current ratio of indirect to direct care hours. For example, if clinicians are currently spending an average of 36 hours per week in direct patient activities and 4 hours per week in other organizational activities, the 11% (4/36) needs to be added to the calculated direct care hours to project the total worked time. In the same way paid time off must be added, calculated as the number of paid absent days projected, or, if there is variability, current paid absent days as a percent of total worked days.

Variable supplies can also be projected using a ratio of current utilization to workload and projecting that same ratio into the future. This approach assumes that future utilization rates will mirror current ones. Changes in procedures, practices, or products could affect this, however, and to the extent that those changes can be quantified, it is possible to adjust the ratio. Current utilization relevant to the change can be replaced with the anticipated utilization and the ratio recalculated. Personnel and materials that are not volume-driven are projected based on function and analysis of current utilization. It is important to remember that all fixed resources become variable over the long range, so it is important to look at the overall growth of volume and workload to determine whether the level of fixed resources continues to be sufficient.

When the projections of activity and resources have been completed, they are translated into dollars. The simple definition of total revenue is volume times price. However, this must be adjusted for the payer and previously noted contractual variations. Personnel expenses are based on the salaries for the positions identified, including the cost of differentials, premiums, and fringe benefits. Nonsalary expenses will incorporate the existing cost for projected materials and supplies adjusted for anticipated price increases and general inflation. The revenues and expenses are totaled for the organization and the profit identified. If there is no profit—if the projected expense exceeds the projected revenue—or if the level of profit is not at the level needed to achieve its fiscal goals (i.e., repayment of debt, cash for capital expenditures), the organization moves into the negotiation phase of the budget process. This is the most difficult phase of the process because the organization reviews its objectives and identifies steps to be taken to resolve the issue. If the conceptual plan, goals, and objectives for the budget were well thought out and clearly stated at the outset, and the activity and resources projected and quantified in relation to the plan, the negotiation phase is more likely to produce the budget plan that is most beneficial for the organization and its mission. Individual participants need to speak to the priorities and requirements of specific departments or programs but also evaluate them in relation to the requirements of other areas and of the total organization.

The final stage of budgeting, and the most important one, is implementation with evaluation. The plans developed and refined through the rest of the process—initiatives, practice changes, productivity improvements, and new or expanded programs—now move into the operational life of the organization.

Ongoing analysis identifies the extent to which actual performance matches budget projections. The organization can thus adjust as needed to unanticipated events that may affect overall outcomes. The analysis of actual to projected performance can be either fixed or flexible. Fixed budget analysis compares actual revenue and expense to the calculated budget. Variances may be favorable to budget—better than anticipated, that is, more revenue or less expense—or unfavorable to budget—not as good as anticipated, that is, less revenue or more expense. It is also important to understand the relationship between variances and the overall impact to the hospital. For example, unfavorable expense (such as increased staffing needs) may be related to favorable revenue (higher patient census). Whether the net of those two is favorable or unfavorable is key rather than looking at one in isolation.

The limitation of this type of analysis is that it assumes that the budget is static, unaffected by events or activities that differ from budget assumptions. Flexible budget analysis assumes a more dynamic budget, one in which the new information is incorporated but maintains a similar profile as the fixed budget. For example, staffing is aligned with patient days in the fixed budget. If patient days increase, it is expected that staffing will need to change. A flexible budget maintains the relationship but changes the budget to reflect the updated assumptions. As an illustration, if six intensive care patients require four nurses to care for them, a 3:2 patient-to-nurse ratio, nine patients will require six nurses. On a fixed budget analysis, the output—patients served—is favorable to the budget because there are more patients served, and presumably more revenue, than projected. The input, however, is unfavorable to the budget because there are more staff, and presumably more expense, than projected. On a flexible budget analysis, however, the 3:2 ratio of output to input remains constant and the performance mirrors the budget. If the nine patients require only five staff, the ratio is 3:1.8 and the actual performance is favorable to the budget on a flexible budget analysis even though the output and expense are unfavorable to the budget on a fixed analysis.

Clearly there is a place for both types of analysis in evaluating actual performance against projected. As noted in the discussion on cost concepts, although in the long run all costs are variable, in the short run some costs are variable and some are fixed. It is appropriate, therefore, to use a fixed budget analysis to evaluate fixed costs and a flexible budget analysis to evaluate variable costs (Finkler et al, 2013).

MANAGING RESOURCES

The objective of financial management is to ensure that the organization generates a profit that is sufficient to maintain viability. The purpose of ongoing budget analysis is to determine the extent to which the organization is meeting its targets over a given period of time or for a particular program or activity and to correct or improve its performance. Prudent management demands that the organization maximize revenue and contain costs to generate profit or margin. Because both revenue and expenses are initially generated primarily by the clinicians who are providing services, it is important that all clinicians, including APRNs, understand and appreciate their contribution to the fiscal soundness of the organization. In this context, it is necessary to emphasize that fiscal considerations do not drive the activities of the organization; it is the mission, vision, and goals that determine direction and activities. However, the financial structure provides the framework for these activities and ensures the long-term viability of the organization.

Maximizing Revenue

Revenues are a composite of volume (the number of services provided) and price (income received for each service provided). Effective organizations ensure that they are generating as much income as possible. Fraudulent or deceptive practices such as billing for services not provided or providing unnecessary, expensive services clearly must be avoided. However, ethical strategies for maximizing revenues can be employed and can relate either to volume issues or price issues.

Once an organizational activity passes the breakeven point—that is, the point at which revenue equals expense—any additional volume will generate profit, all else being equal. It is not surprising, therefore, that there is so much emphasis, especially in practices, on how much volume and revenue the individual practitioner generates. In fact, in incentive practices within larger organizations, financial rewards to practitioners are based on volume and productivity. The measurement for identifying the individual practitioner's contribution to the organization most frequently is based on services billed. There is a desire, and in many situations even a demand, to demonstrate that the individual clinician is generating enough revenue to cover salary and to contribute to profit. This has driven the very appropriate efforts of nurse practitioners to secure billing privileges. (See Chapter 6 for a more extensive discussion of reimbursement issues.) However, this direct billing is not available in all settings or through all payers. Even where it is available, it may not be advantageous to the practice for the nurse practitioner to bill directly. Regardless, it is imperative to demonstrate the nurse practitioner's contribution to the practice and to develop other measures of volume and activity that can be used to evaluate the extent to which the nurse practitioner is generating revenue. These measures will be internal to the organization but need to be regularly reported and evaluated in relation to the overall success of the practice. Such measures will be required as well in other circumstances where capitated or managed care payment systems do not accurately reflect through the billing system the volume of activity generated for the practice by the nurse practitioner.

In other organizational settings, volume may be measured by charges generated for particular procedures, tests, or services. This often leads clinicians to look for new ways of charging for various activities, assuming that this will maximize revenue and at the same time demonstrate their impact on revenue enhancement. Increasing charges results in increased revenue potential from only a relatively small percentage of payers because of the decline of fee-for-service payment systems. Even this potential may not be realized because of exclusions or payment maximums set by the insurer.

Rather than focusing on charges, therefore, it is more effective for APRNs to address issues with systems or practices that affect the volume of activity that is the basis for payment. Under Medicare's prospective payment system, for example, payment is based on the number of patients discharged within specific DRGs. If the length of stay per discharge can be reduced, a greater volume of patients can be admitted. What are the systems or practice issues that increase the length of stay without adding therapeutic value for the patient? What processes could occur before admission or subsequent to discharge that would reduce the length of stay? What services need to be provided that will attract patients to the facility? Consideration of these questions has led to a variety of approaches that ultimately result in increased volume, for example, preadmission testing and evaluation with same-day admission for surgical patients; telephone triage and follow-up or home visit programs; clinical pathways, case management, and discharge planning programs; protocols to prevent or promote early identification and treatment of complications of hospitalization such as nosocomial infections or decubitus ulcers; or enhancing and expanding specific services such as cardiology or oncology. APRNs in the inpatient setting are uniquely positioned to influence the efforts that affect volume. The APRNs can identify approaches through study and analysis of existing systems and research on best practices. They can have significant input into the development of programs or protocols as part of the multidisciplinary team. They may support the implementation of changes through clinical evaluation, consultation, and education. Finally, the APRNs may be the most appropriate clinicians to manage the particular program or activity.

Another mechanism to both increase revenue and reflect the level of services provided to a patient is to assure that all services rendered are reflected on the bill with the appropriate charge. "Charge capture," or documenting and charging for all billable services, can be a time-consuming and administrative burden. However, accurately capturing services not only improves reimbursement in the short term but is also used by external agencies to impact reimbursement rates as well as calculate and publish quality and acuity scores. Therefore, these additional services become key to accurately reflecting the resource allocation for the level of care that is being provided.

In addition to adding volume, revenue can be increased by increasing reimbursement rates, the amount that the organization is actually paid for each product or service. However, this deceptively simple strategy is constrained by regulatory, contractual, and economic considerations. With the increasing trend in price transparency, public opinion can also be a constraint. Actual reimbursement is determined by government regulation, contract negotiation, or organizational definition. Government-regulated reimbursement, such as for Medicare or Medicaid, is not organization specific and, although concerted lobbying efforts may have some impact, the potential for change is limited. Organizations may present evidence that they qualify for certain levels of reimbursement, for example, for direct medical education benefits, but otherwise will have little opportunity to affect payment levels. Reimbursement rates set through contract negotiations have a greater potential for change but only during the period of open contract negotiations. Because the negotiation outcome needs to be satisfactory to both parties, and because both parties as business organizations are interested in maximizing their profit, rate increases preferred by one party may need to be tempered to be acceptable to the other party. Charges defined by the organization can be increased but the associated reimbursement rates may not change based on contract terms related to price increases (Finkler et al, 2013).

To maximize revenue, organizations must successfully implement strategies to ensure that the organization receives all the revenue to which it is entitled under the existing regulations, contractual obligations, and pricing structure. Payment for services is contingent on the organization's demonstrating that it has in fact provided the relevant service or product. Different payers have varying requirements in the way that claims are processed, the forms that are used, and the specific data that are included. It is important, therefore, to understand what is required, where it needs to be recorded, and how it is presented to the payer.

All payers will require some level of detail on the services provided. This may be in the form of an itemized statement of all billable charges for an episode of care or the specification of relevant codes. Current Procedural Terminology (CPT) and Resource-Based Relative Value Scales (RBRVS) are coding systems developed by the American Medical Association (AMA) and adapted by the government to identify cost procedures and services provided by clinicians. The *International Classification of Diseases,* tenth modification *(ICD-10),* is developed by the World Health Organization (WHO) and adapted for use in the United States by the federal government. It classifies diseases by system or category (e.g., blood disorders, neoplasms, infectious diseases) and may be used alone or in conjunction with other classification systems. DRGs and APCs as discussed earlier are used for Medicare claims for inpatient and outpatient hospital services and for selected nongovernmental payers.* Certain payers may also require evidence of preauthorization for specific procedures or treatments or referral authorization for specialty evaluation and management. Clinicians in many

practices or in ambulatory settings may be more directly involved in identifying the appropriate code for the services rendered and must have a thorough understanding of the coding system and the relationship of codes to services provided. In other settings, coding may not be done by the clinicians; rather, the codes are determined based on information that the clinicians provide. The source document for information for coding and billing is the patient's medical record. Documentation in the medical record validates to the payer that the billed services were provided and justifies the organization's claim for payment. Inaccurate or incomplete documentation can lead to lost revenue opportunities if the coders are unable to identify all the services that can appropriately be charged (Finkler et al, 2013).

Reimbursement is negatively affected by payer denials and delays. Payers may deny reimbursement for services not covered (excluded from reimbursement based on the patient's policy or the contractual agreement with the organization) or for services not authorized (lacking required prior approval from the payer or from a designated clinician). Payment may also be denied for services deemed by the payer to be incompatible with the diagnosis, medically unnecessary, or not adequately validated. Payers who reimburse for hospital care on a per diem basis may carve out days for payment denial if delays in scheduling tests or consultations or in initiating discharge planning and referrals result in additional, otherwise avoidable inpatient days. Billing challenges by payers may also result in payment denials if supporting documentation does not appear in the medical record that the billed services were in fact rendered. Payers will audit records to validate that billed services have been provided even after payments have been made. If there is not adequate supporting documentation, the organization is at risk not only for repayments but also for additional financial penalties.

Inadequate documentation can lead to delays in billing if additional information needs to be accumulated before coding determinations can be made. Lack of compliance with payers' filing requirements may also result in denial of payment. Claims that are questioned initially may be resubmitted with additional evidence of the validity of the claim; however, this involves rework and delays. In addition, most payers have a filing limit, a defined period of time in which a "clean" bill is presented in order for the organization to be reimbursed at all. Delays in processing

---

*Case mix classifications are used for reimbursement in other sectors of the health-care system by both governmental and private sector payers: Home Health Resource Groups (HHRGs) and the Outcome and Assessment Information Set (OASIS) in home care; the Minimum Data Set (MDS) and Resource Utilization Groups (RUGs) for long-term care (Cleverly et al, 2011).

and submitting bills and generating reimbursement, whether related to incomplete documentation or because of other systems issues, may also result in a lost income opportunity for the organization. Money that the organization has received can be invested to generate interest income. Money in accounts receivable—that is, income that is anticipated but not yet received—does not generate any additional revenue for the organization.

The APRN in a practice setting that bills directly or indirectly for the practitioner's clinical activity needs a clear understanding of the requirements and systems for billing—what can be billed, how it is processed, what documentation is required, and time frames for billing. By following through on these requirements, the APRN is able to contribute directly to the timely and accurate generation of income. In other settings, the APRN with an understanding of the systems for reimbursement to the organization contributes indirectly by providing and promoting accurate and complete clinical documentation, identifying systems issues that can generate delays in the billing cycle, and supporting practices that enhance the potential for maximizing revenue. For example, in the inpatient setting, an APRN caring for a complex patient with multiple comorbidities may be able to increase reimbursement by assessing and documenting each of the patient problems and interventions. Addressing the patient's DRG alone may limit reimbursement and not acknowledge expenses generated from additional care needs.

Containing Costs

The volume of products or services produced drives the total expenses of an organization. These costs are a function both of intensity, or the extent of resources required for each unit of volume, and of price, or the cost to the organization of individual resource units. Cost containment focuses on identifying the least costly alternatives for supplying the personnel and materials to produce these services or products. In addressing cost containment, the organization evaluates the alternatives not only in terms of total expenditures but also in relation to potential impact on other aspects of the organization. It is less costly to pay lower salaries, but if salaries are not competitive in the market, costly vacancies and turnover are likely to result. Inferior products that are less costly to purchase may initially save money but in the long

term may generate additional expense in replacement, rework, decreased customer satisfaction, and loss of business. The desired alternative therefore is the least costly alternative that is consistent with the mission and goals of the organization.

Wage and salary expenses constitute a significant proportion of the costs in health-care organizations. Market forces, regulatory requirements, and ethical personnel management practices provide a framework for personnel expenditures. Within this framework, however, the organization has flexibility in controlling expenses related both to intensity and price of personnel resources used. Intensity addresses the number of personnel or staff hours required to manage a given patient population. The volume and type of patients and their particular care needs—the workload generated by that patient population—drive the personnel resources required. Measuring and managing workload variability can provide opportunities for cost containment. For example, scheduling staff in consideration of daily, weekly, or seasonal volume variations can minimize expensive "down time," as well as staff frustration resulting from inadequate staffing at busy times. This requires an ongoing analysis of workload patterns and trends to identify recurring variations. Unexpected variations may be addressed with the use of overtime or outside agency personnel. Both of these alternatives are more expensive than the normal personnel costs for the workload involved but are justifiable for unpredictable workload variations. A consistent increase in activity, however, requires a consistent plan for managing the workload. If a practice is increasingly seeing patients later than the usual scheduled hours and incurring overtime and other increased costs because of it, it is worthwhile to analyze the cause of the variation. System inefficiencies may be delaying patient throughput and thus generating additional unnecessary expenses that can be eliminated by addressing the inefficiencies. Patterns of patient scheduling may be changing, resulting in fewer visits scheduled earlier in the day with more down time, suggesting that scheduled staff hours need to be adjusted to accommodate patient preferences. However, the variation may be the result of a net increase in numbers of patients and visits. If this is so, an analysis of the fiscal impact of the increased revenue and increased expense may demonstrate that adding regular staff to cover the increased activity will be more cost effective than continuing to use overtime.

Intensity of personnel resource utilization may also be related to inefficient clinical practices. Routines, procedures, and protocols that are based on tradition ("we've always done it this way") rather than on analysis or research-based evidence may include unnecessary and time-consuming activities that do not add value for desired outcomes. How are medication administration times determined? What are the indicators that determine the level of support for activities of daily living that each patient requires? How frequently is it necessary to monitor vital signs on postoperative patients? In what circumstances are isolation precautions instituted and under what circumstances can they be discontinued? How effective are the standard protocols for preparation for tests? Do the standard patient teaching tools and programs result in patient learning? Does the timing of drawing blood for laboratory tests make sense in relation to the timing of meals or medication administration or other treatments? It may be instructive to evaluate the care that patients with the same condition receive from different caregivers or in different settings to determine whether differences in practices result in differences in outcomes. In some circumstances it may become evident that practices in one setting are more resource intensive but do not add value and can be adapted or eliminated.

For personnel resources, price is generally equated with the cost of salaries and benefits. Containing costs by reducing salaries or benefits is not often possible given market conditions and the mobility of today's workforce. It is possible, however, to ensure that the least costly resources are used in any given situation. Overtime, for example, is a very expensive way to staff. It is effective for the occasional unanticipated increase in workload, but extensive, continuous use of overtime requires identification of causes and alternative approaches.

In addition to volume increases, variability in workload practices, or system inefficiencies, overtime may be related to the capabilities of the staff involved. For example, inexperienced staff may need assistance with complex patient issues or with development of organizational skills, or experienced staff may be struggling with unfamiliar procedures or patient conditions. For these staff, education and mentoring can promote developing competencies that also increase efficiency and ultimately reduce the overtime. The mix of staff may not be appropriate or the total numbers of staff may not be sufficient for the workload

experienced. In these circumstances, it can be less costly to provide more skilled staff or more total staff at regular salaries than to continue with overtime.

One approach addresses the mix of personnel and the perceived advantages of reducing the numbers of professional staff and substituting less expensive unlicensed assistive personnel (UAP). In some circumstances, this may be effective; however, given the increasing acuity of patients, such substitution may be counterproductive. In acute care settings, for example, patients are requiring more and more complex care, most of which cannot be delegated to unlicensed staff. In addition, unlicensed staff increase the workload of the professional staff because they assume the added responsibility of directing and supervising the UAP. For direct care, it may be less costly to have a higher percentage of licensed staff and fewer total numbers than to have a lower percentage of licensed staff and greater total numbers. However, if the professional staff are responsible for clerical or environmental tasks that can appropriately be delegated to less costly personnel, providing those supports can be an effective cost management approach.

Cost containment efforts can also address some of the hidden costs in personnel management. Turnover generates significant costs in recruiting, hiring, and orienting new personnel. Additional costs may be incurred before the new employee is available if vacancies need to be covered with overtime or more expensive outside agency personnel. Programs to promote staff retention can therefore be valuable in reducing turnover and its associated costs. Absenteeism can also be costly. Some level of unanticipated absenteeism caused by illness is anticipated. However, staff dissatisfaction, unmanageable workloads, frequent excessive overtime requirements, or on-the-job injuries can also contribute to high levels of absenteeism. The cost is increased by the need for replacements, again often with overtime or agency personnel. In addition, costs to the organization for workers' compensation are directly related to the number of claims filed out of the organization. Cost can be lowered—and, potentially, staff satisfaction and efficiency increased—by identifying and addressing the factors contributing to absenteeism and on-the-job injuries.

Similar to wages and salaries, the costs for supplies and equipment are affected by market issues and regulatory requirements, as well as by the volume and intensity of services provided. Intensity in this context refers to the number and kind of materials used for these services. Cost containment looks at the least costly alternative to providing the services. This can be addressed on two levels. What are the specific supplies and equipment required for a particular procedure, protocol, or service? In addition, given that a specific item is required, which is the best product to select among the alternatives available? In relation to the first question, it is important to look at the work and how it is accomplished. Materials assumed to be necessary for the service provided may incorporate items that are no longer necessary, do not add value, or are useful only to a subset of the patients receiving the service.

With the materials necessary for a service identified, the focus moves to selection of specific items among those available. Product evaluation requires the involvement of clinicians and others in the organization. Inherent in the identification of an item as necessary for a particular service is the description of its purpose and how it is to be used. The primary concern in product evaluation is how well the different products under review meet these criteria. Other criteria also need to be considered such as availability from the manufacturer and storage and maintenance requirements. A product that meets all clinical criteria but cannot be produced and delivered on a timely basis or has high maintenance (and associated down time) potential may not be preferable to a less exotic but more available and reliable product.

Prices for materials and supplies are negotiated with vendors. Organizations may identify cost containment opportunities in the course of these negotiations through volume discounts or as part of purchasing groups. This raises the issue of managing the tension between standardization and customization. Frequently, standardizing supplies and equipment across service areas has significant benefits in reducing the expense for purchasing, storing, distributing, and using specific products. Although this limits the range of products available to the clinician, it also limits the time needed to become familiar with the product, to develop ease in working with it, and to use it in a variety of settings. It may, however, generate some level of waste if, for example, a standardized pack of supplies for a particular procedure contains items that are used in most but not all situations. Customization, on the other hand, matches the products specifically to the individual patient, clinician, or situation. It can have advantages in being more effective in achieving the

desired outcome or in reducing the potential for waste. However, customization sometimes is more a matter of individual clinicians' preferences than of value added for the patient. It is important, then, to evaluate the pros and cons of standardization or customization in specific circumstances to identify the least costly alternative. In general, for products and processes that are used in a variety of settings, standardization is preferable not only because of the cost and productivity benefits but also because it promotes consistency in providing services. Alternatives to standardization should be undertaken only after careful evaluation to ensure that the marginal benefit of customization—that is, the greater value that accrues from the alternative—outweighs the fiscal and operational benefits of standardization.

As the previous discussions suggest, the appropriateness of measures to contain costs cannot be evaluated in isolation from outcomes. Cost efficiency identifies the minimum expenditure necessary to achieve an outcome. Cost effectiveness identifies the minimum expenditure necessary to achieve the outcome that is consistent with the organization's mission and goals. Cost effectiveness, therefore, incorporates an element of quality that is not inherent in cost efficiency. Vacuum-assisted dressing for postsurgical wound healing is significantly more expensive than traditional dressings and would not be considered cost efficient in a simple analysis that only addressed the expense incurred for dressings until wound healing is achieved. However, because it accelerates wound healing, this intervention reduces the necessary length of hospitalization and extent of postsurgical follow-up. As such, it is certainly cost effective, with benefits for both the patient and the provider organization. In some circumstances quality measures are not sufficiently developed to allow precise measurement of cost effectiveness but, to the extent that such measures are available or can be approximated, they should be incorporated into analysis.

Cost effectiveness and cost efficiency are typically analyzed using productivity measures or cost-benefit analysis. Productivity is the relationship of inputs and outputs, of resources used and products or services produced. Productivity relationships are expressed as ratios and can focus either on the output or on the input. Focus on the output addresses the question, "What does it take to produce the output?" and is the ratio of input to output, or resources divided by products or services.

Examples of productivity measures focusing on output include hours per patient day, cost per procedure, and visits per episode of care. Focus on input addresses the question, "How well are resources being used?" and is the ratio of output to input, or products or services divided by resources. Examples of productivity measures focusing on input include visits per full-time equivalent (FTE), tests per staff hour, and case hours per available room hour. Productivity improves when output remains constant and input decreases, or when output increases and input stays constant. Productivity declines when output remains constant and input increases, or when output decreases and input stays constant. Productivity ratios are of little value in isolation. Comparisons of productivity ratios to targets set during the budgeting process, to historical experience and trends, and to other internal or external benchmarks are valuable for analysis and identification of opportunities for increasing efficiency and effectiveness.

Cost-benefit analysis is frequently used to evaluate a particular program or project, or to compare programs, approaches, or activities competing for resource allocation. The analysis compares the revenues and expenses generated by the program to determine the net benefit (income minus expense) or the ratio of benefits to costs (income divided by expense). Determination of the value of the program to the organization, however, is not determined exclusively by analysis of the financial benefit. Benefits and costs that are difficult to quantify, such as social benefits and costs, opportunity costs, public relations value, and loss leader opportunities, may be of considerable importance to the organization and influence decisions to implement or continue specific projects and programs.

Productivity is often focused on personnel resource utilization, but the concept also applies to material resources and to the overall utilization of services. Length of stay or number of days per inpatient stay, for example, can be considered to be a productivity measurement that identifies the relationship between the episode of care (output) and the patient days, representing the aggregated resources required to provide for that episode (input). Comparisons are made among patients or groups of patients for a given time period or across multiple time periods, and against internal and external benchmarks. Productivity improves if the length of stay (and associated expense) decreases for the same level of activity.

Cost-benefit analysis can identify the impact of productivity improvements for the organization. Baseline analysis of the net benefit (revenue minus expense) identifies the profit margin. Productivity improvements are designed to increase the profit margin by reducing the cost (but maintaining consistent income) for each episode of care. Moreover, decreasing length of stay has the added opportunity of creating capacity for additional volume. That volume will generate additional income as well as additional expense. Assuming a consistent patient population, if the cost per episode of care remains the same, the total profit (income minus expense) will increase although the profit per case remains the same. However, the cost per episode of care may well decrease (as fixed costs are spread over more cases) and enhance both the total profit and the profit per case. Cost-benefit analysis can also identify potential negative aspects of productivity improvement efforts. Length-of-stay reductions must be consistent with good clinical practice. Early discharge of patients may be clinically premature and result in readmission of the patient for continuation of care. Obviously, for the patient this is an undesirable outcome and therefore could not be considered cost effective. It cannot even be considered cost efficient because many payers, particularly those who reimburse on a cost per case, identify a time period after discharge during which a readmission (for a condition related to the original hospital stay) will be bridged to the original admission. Additional expense will be incurred, but the merged admissions will be considered as one episode for the purposes of reimbursement and additional payment will be denied (Finkler et al, 2013).

IMPLICATIONS

Reimbursement levels and the associated incentives to contain costs are to a large extent payer driven. Reimbursement systems structured as fee-for-service include little incentive for the provider organization to contain costs. For a minority of payers reimbursement is generated by charges that are paid either in full or at some negotiated percentage so increased utilization results in increased revenue. The majority of payers, however, have built into their reimbursement systems some incentives for containing costs. Reimbursement at the per visit rate is an incentive to reduce resource utilization and increase efficiency for that visit. Reimbursement based on cases (DRG-based, for example) build in incentives to reduce the length of stay as well as the resource utilization during the stay. Capitated reimbursement systems create the additional incentive to reduce the number of episodes of care—admissions or visits. Individual payer variations add complexity for providers and consumers. Some, for example, may offer additional payments for achieving specific clinical quality outcomes with defined patient populations such as pediatric asthma patients or adult-onset diabetic patients. Others may have payment tiers for certain benefits with different consumer copayments for different levels of services (generic versus brand pharmaceuticals, for example) (Finkler et al, 2013).

Clinicians, however, generally are not attuned to incorporating reimbursement variables into clinical decision making for individual patients and prefer to provide care that is "payer-blind." They do have a responsibility, however, to promote efficiency in the allocation and utilization of health-care resources, and not only for the viability of the organization within which they practice. As health-care costs escalate, insured patients increasingly are at risk for higher out-of-pocket costs, including deductibles into the thousands instead of the hundreds of dollars before the insurer assumes liability, and they are entitled to value for their expenditure. In addition, social justice demands that constrained resources be used judiciously to ensure the maximum availability of health care to all members of society. In addition, with increased emphasis and transparency related to cost, patients are now making choices not only on clinical criteria but also on cost. The

most appropriate approach for clinicians, therefore, is to provide cost efficient and effective care for all patients regardless of payer.

Fortunately, in many circumstances, cost containment efforts developed to accommodate a given payment modality can be designed to benefit—or at least not disadvantage—patients of other payers as well. Programs to reduce length of stay, efforts to improve productivity, analyses to identify the most cost-effective products, and benchmarking to identify best practices may be initiated because of the structure of one payment methodology, but their beneficial effects need not be limited to patients of that insurer type. However, because resources are not unlimited, in different circumstances difficult choices need to be made. Organizations can rarely respond to all requests for resources and often are in the position of needing to select among competing priorities that may all be necessary and worthwhile. Should the organization expand the cardiac program or the pediatric program; replace the ventilators in the critical care units or the ultrasounds in the echocardiology laboratory; construct additional ambulatory facilities or additional inpatient facilities? The decisions will require compromise and consensus and a clear understanding of the benefits not only for the organization but also for the staff and, most important, for the patient. Advanced practice nurses have the knowledge and expertise to provide the clinical input and to advocate for the patient. To have a credible voice in this decision-making process, they must also have a clear understanding of the business and fiscal issues that affect resource allocation and management.

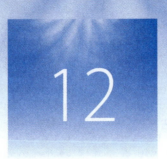

12

Mediated Roles
Working With and Through Other People

Thomas D. Smith, Maria L. Vezina, Mary E. Samost, and Kelly Reilly

Learning Outcomes

Learning outcomes expected as a result of this chapter:

- Explore the relational mechanisms of working with and through others as an advanced practice registered nurse (APRN).
- Apply the six APRN core competencies to practice.
- Compare and contrast models of APRN collaboration.
- Demonstrate APRN leadership roles in interprofessional teams.
- Develop a framework to align professional nursing connections.

ADVANCED PRACTICE AND PARTNERSHIPS

The four established advanced practice roles—certified nurse practitioner (CNP), clinical nurse specialist (CNS), certified nurse-midwife (CNM), and certified registered nurse anesthetist (CRNA)—reflect significant evolution of the nursing profession and nursing practice over the past five decades. Progress in role development and advanced practice registered nurse (APRN) integration into health-care teams has yielded positive outcomes; however,

barriers related to scope of practice (SOP) persist. The APRN Consensus Model addresses some of the issues of role definition and SOP for the four APRN roles (National Council of State Boards of Nursing [NCSBN], 2008). The implementation mechanism for the APRN Consensus Model is Licensure, Accreditation, Certification, and Education (LACE) (Stanley, 2009). The APRN Consensus Model/LACE serves the purpose of standardizing APRN SOP, increasing access, and promoting greater value and mobility for the APRN within the national health-care system (Rounds, Zych, & Mallary, 2013). It also serves to support one of the recommendations of the Institute of Medicine's (IOM's) report *The Future of Nursing: Leading Change, Advancing Health* (IOM, 2011) to remove SOP barriers (Stubenrauch, 2010). The Committee for Assessing Progress on Implementing the Recommendations of the IOM *The Future of Nursing* report found significant progress toward reducing SOP restrictions with increases in full practice status from 8 to 21 states (IOM, 2015). According to *Nursing's Social Policy Statement* (American Nurses Association [ANA], 2010), these roles involve specialization, expansion, advancement, and autonomy, suggesting the necessary skills of managing people, the organization, and the environment of care. According to the IOM (2011), "more than a quarter of a million nurses are APRNs who hold master's or doctoral degrees and pass national certification exams. APRNs deliver primary, acute and medical home care as well as other types of health-care services. For example, they teach and counsel patients to understand their health problems and what they can do to get better, they coordinate care and advocate for patients in the complex health-care system, and they refer patients to physicians and other health-care providers" (p. 52). Specifically, the CNS (APRN) role centers on the synthesis, integration, transformation, and translation of best practices as articulated in the literature (National Association of Clinical Nurse Specialists [NACNS], 2007). Davies and Hughes (1995) note that "the term advanced nursing practice extends beyond roles. It is a way of thinking and viewing the world based on clinical knowledge, rather than a composition of roles" (p. 157). This view of the world is an interactive process that emphasizes direct and indirect partnerships with both patients and a diverse group of health-care providers. In addition to clinical competency, the varied aspects of advanced practice also require socialization and interpersonal skills to form the foundation for collaboration, consultation, and clinical leadership. Although advanced practice roles require autonomy and authority to be fully enacted, the ability to achieve patient and system outcomes is dependent on partnerships with others to manage interdependent and interdisciplinary relationships. In fact, the NACNS (2007) concluded that "the synergy of working with, leading and coordinating teams of professionals in a highly communicative, focused care environment regardless of

setting, will continue to be the hallmark of practice into the future" (p. 8). According to Bleich (2011), APRNs, as either "master's or doctorally prepared clinical scholars, may not have the extent of formal education in advanced research methods and statistical techniques, but they are nonetheless critical to clinical inquiry at the point-of-care and evidence-driven decision making within the organizational context. Their clinical expertise and advanced knowledge of nursing practice can be used in partnership with nurses prepared with research based doctoral degrees. APRNs need to engage in a full range of scholarly activities that include research, evidence-based practice, performance improvement, teaching and learning, and dissemination to influence and improve the quality of care provided to patients, families, and populations (Pape, 2000). Inter- and intra-professional connectivity will optimize nursing's impact in advancing health via the synergy that bridges scientific knowledge generation with translational expertise at the point of care. This synergy may also serve to link nursing better with other health-care professions, giving nurses a stronger voice in decision-making forums and at policy tables" (Bleich, 2011, pp. 169–170).

CORE COMPETENCIES

APRNs function as clinicians using evidence-based knowledge to provide direct care, diagnose and manage health-care problems, coordinate services, educate patients and families, advocate for patients, and manage the health-care system in all its dimensions. This approach to care supports the continued focus on disease prevention, health maintenance, and resolution of functional problems (IOM, 2004). In *The Future of Nursing: Leading Change, Advancing Health,* the IOM (2011) stated that "nurses are developing new competencies for the future to help bridge the gap between coverage and access, to coordinate increasingly complex care for a wider range of patients, to fulfill their potential as primary care providers to the full extent of their education and training, to implement system-wide changes that take into account the growing body of evidence linking nursing practice to fundamental improvements in patient safety and quality of care, and to capture the full economic value of their contributions across practice settings" (pp. 53–54).

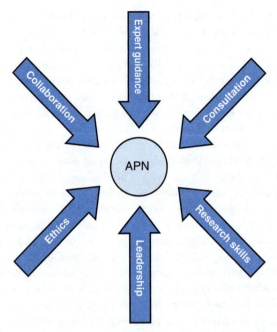

FIGURE 12.1 Core competencies of advanced nursing practice.

Accordingly, six core competencies, as shown in **Figure 12.1,** further define advanced nursing practice.

These competencies have consistently been identified as essential features of advanced practice (American Association of Colleges of Nursing, 1996; Davies & Hughes, 1995; NACNS, 2004, 2010; National Council of State Boards of Nursing, 2006):

1. *Coaching:* skillful guidance and teaching to advance the care of patients, families, groups of patients, other care providers, and the profession of nursing
2. *Consultation:* patient-, staff-, or system-focused interaction between professionals in which expertise is utilized for problem solving
3. *Research skills:* interpretation, translation, use of evidence, evaluation of clinical practice, and conducting and active participation in research
4. *Clinical and professional leadership:* the ability to manage change and empower others to influence clinical practice and political processes within and across the system
5. *Collaboration:* working with intra- and interdisciplinary teams toward achieving optimal patient and family goals

6. *Ethical decision-making skills:* identifying, articulating, and taking action on ethical concerns at the patient, family, provider, system, community, and public policy levels

Given this overview of core competencies, the theme of relationships within the health-care arena is evident. The ability to work with and through others is inherent within these competencies and consequently indicates a strong foundation for practice. Although not explicitly stated in definitions of advanced practice, there is an understanding within interprofessional teams that APRNs must be skillful and cognizant of the key elements of their partnerships with patients, families, and other health team members. Managing the interpersonal strategies of providing care is critical to success as an independent care provider in a competitive health-care environment. For example, care previously provided by APRNs in the complex, acute setting is transitioning into the community, thereby increasing the need for the APRN to assess his or her strengths to provide accountable practice while working successfully with other providers. According to the IOM (2004), the opportunities presented by the current practice environment can be met through a strong foundation of clinical practice, specialty expertise, and a rigorous graduate education.

With reference to the six core competencies, several interpersonal themes emerge:

1. Coaching, skilled guidance, and teaching of patients, families, other care providers, and the profession of nursing is both a formal and informal role for the APRN. As mentors, APRNs develop others to either take the lead or share the pathway of care. As formal teachers, APRNs assist in the application and evaluation of evidence-based practice in determining and improving the quality of health-care delivery.

2. Consultation is the direct involvement of another practitioner, which denotes the need to confirm findings, diagnosis, and plan of care. The responsibility for care, however, rests with the primary practitioner. It can require an overlap within the same specialty for an added opinion or a discussion with a specialist for another view or preference of treatment. In either situation, the partnership is necessary for optimal patient care and a deliberate approach in solving problems and managing care.

3. Research of a practice discipline includes conducting systematic and scholarly inquiry, interpretation, and use of evidence in clinical practice and quality improvement. APRN competencies in translating research into practice, designing innovations based on new knowledge, or integrating quality evidence are keys in achieving optimal outcomes (Riley & Omery, 1996). Innovative change is possible when health-care professionals come together to redesign clinical practices. APRNs also contribute in the care of research participants through supporting accurate, reliable, and ethical study implementation. Additionally APRNs need to participate and contribute in creating policies and procedures and care standards for implementing clinical research across the continuum of health-care settings (National Institutes of Health [NIH], 2010).

4. Clinical, professional, and system leadership can be powerful when approached in an interdisciplinary manner. Leadership competencies of APRNs are required for assessing and influencing nursing practice and patient outcomes in populations, health-care systems, regulatory requirements, and health-care finance. Although the unique roles of distinct professions are useful within the framework of individual competencies, in patient care the leadership of a team is a supportive experience for patients, especially for those with limited access to a health system and those with complex care needs. A focus on the specific patient and not on professional turf issues requires skill in leadership and change agency. In this realm, the blurring of roles is often helpful and not hurtful.

5. According to *Merriam-Webster's Collegiate Dictionary* (2003), collaboration means to work together, especially in a joint intellectual effort. The ANA (2015) *Guide to Nursing's Social Policy Statement* cites qualities of collaboration such as a common focus, recognition of another's expertise, and a collegial exchange of ideas and knowledge, and recognizes that nurses uniquely contribute to wider conversation to address the health needs of society. Hamric, Spross, and Hanson (2005) refer to collaboration as a "dynamic, interpersonal process in which two or more individuals make a commitment to each other to interact authentically and constructively to solve problems and to learn from each other in order to accomplish identified goals, purposes or outcomes" (p. 318). By definition, then, collaboration identifies relationships and involves an interpersonal process. The focus of the relationship needs to be positive and grounded in a problem-solving approach creating interdependence as a mutually fulfilling experience between the involved parties. Although collaboration is a cornerstone of many APRN roles, it eludes some clinicians. Consequently, models of collaboration have emerged to assist in structuring relationships and guiding the process of working partnerships.

6. Ethical decision-making skills are a central component of effective advanced practice. According to Thompson and Thompson (1985), "To be professional is to be ethical, and to practice ethically requires an understanding of ethics, values and oneself." The goal of ethical practice is to do the right thing for the right reason (Thompson, Kershbaumer, & Krisman-Scott, 2001). Although grounded in one's values and presentation of self, the inclusion of the team in ethical decision making is key to the holistic care of patients. Ethical clinical practice requires an atmosphere of trust, mutual respect, transparency, and commitment to critical

thinking and reasoning. To create this atmosphere, APNs, as the managers of care, need to work with others in an inclusive manner, so as to build a team whereby the ability to express values, feelings, beliefs, and knowledge can be encouraged and ensured as the ethical dimension of practice emerges.

MODELS OF COLLABORATION

The basis of collaboration is the belief that high-quality patient care is achieved by including the contributions of all care providers. In *The Future of Nursing: Leading Change, Advancing Health,* the IOM (2011) stated that "being a full partner transcends all levels of the nursing profession and requires leadership skills and competencies that must be applied within the profession and in collaboration with other health professionals" (p. 35). The Macy Foundation (2010) states that "mounting research shows that health care delivered by nurses, doctors, and other health-care professionals working in teams not only improves quality, but also leads to better patient outcomes, greater patient satisfaction, improved efficiency and increased job satisfaction on the part of health professionals" (p. 2). Collaboration is often cited as the "key to success" for any initiative that extends beyond an individual's scope of activity. Collaboration is therefore the foundation of effective patient care. According to Arcongelo, Fitzgerald, Carroll, and Plumb (1996), a variety of interpersonal attributes are necessary for successful collaboration. These include trust, knowledge, shared responsibility, mutual respect, positive communication, cooperation, coordination, and optimism (p. 107). See **Figure 12.2.** The authors define these attributes as follows:

- *Trust* among all parties establishes a high-quality working relationship; it develops over time as the parties become more acquainted and establish norms. According to Hamric, Hanson, Tracy, and O'Grady (2014) trust also depends on clinical competence (p. 306).
- *Knowledge* is a necessary component for the development of trust. Knowledge and trust remove the need for supervision.
- *Shared responsibility* suggests joint decision making for quality patient care and outcomes, as well as accountable practice, within the organization.

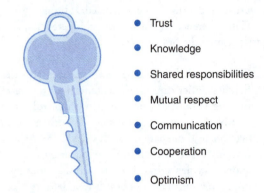

Collaboration Is the Key to Success

- Trust
- Knowledge
- Shared responsibilities
- Mutual respect
- Communication
- Cooperation
- Optimism

FIGURE 12.2 Collaboration attributes.

- *Mutual respect* for the expertise of all members of the team is a linchpin to successful collaboration. This respect is communicated to the patient.
- *Communication* that is not hierarchical but rather two way ensures the sharing of patient information and knowledge. Two-way communication between equals serves as a framework for difficult conversations. Questioning of the approach to care of either partner cannot be delivered in a manner that is construed as criticism, but as a method to enhance knowledge and improve patient care.
- *Cooperation* and *coordination* promote the use of the skills of all team members, prevent duplication of effort, enhance the productivity of practice, and improve the patient's experience of care.
- *Optimism* promotes successful teamwork when the involved parties believe that collaboration is the more effective means of promoting high-quality care.

Although these attributes are key in any collaborative relationship, it is primarily the unique contribution of each member of the team that determines a successful outcome.

Although there are several models of collaborative practice, they often are distinguished by the response to two questions:

1. How is the expertise of each team member used to the fullest?
2. Who is responsible for decision making and patient care?

Table 12.1 summarizes three practice models commonly used in primary care (Strumpf & Whitney, 1994) and one

TABLE 12.1

Models of Collaborative Practice

	Parallel Model	Sequential Model	Shared Model	Collaborative Model
APN role in patient care	Manage stable patients	Perform intake assessment	Manage patients identified by the physician to be less complex	Manage all levels of complexity
Physician role in patient care	Manage medically complex patients	Diagnosing and management of patients	Initial screening of patients Manage more complex patients	Comanage during unstable periods Collaboration between APN and physician in plan of care

collaborative model being adopted in various health-care settings (Arcongelo et al, 1996; Matthews & Brown, 2013):

1. The parallel model
2. The sequential model
3. The shared model
4. The collaborative model

In the parallel model, the APRN manages stable patients and the physician cares for those who are more medically complex. In the sequential model, the APRN performs the intake assessment and the physician assumes responsibility for differential diagnosis and management, or the pattern may be reversed with the physician screening all patients and delegating the care of patients identified as less complex to the APRN. In the shared model, the APRN and the physician care for an individual patient on an alternating schedule and based on patient needs. Arcongelo and colleagues (1996) identify a fourth model, the collaborative model, which involves the APRN as the primary care provider without regard for the complexity of the problem. The APRN and physician collaborate based on an "egalitarian partnership to deliver high quality disease management using APRN full abilities: a unique professional lens, expertise in team-based care and patient partnerships" (Matthews & Brown, 2013). The communication in this model is ongoing, may transition to a comanagement arrangement during an unstable or complex period, but always involves the input of the two professionals in establishing the plan of care. One outcome of this style is the ability for the APRN to expand his or her knowledge and skills within the complex realm of patient care and establish closer contacts with consulting team members while managing the complexity.

Regardless of the model of collaborative practice, the elements of trust and a positive working relationship are vital. Collaborative relationships are a "work in progress," not facilitated by inflexible expectations or boundaries. Over time, mutual expressions of expertise become grounded in an invisible pattern that is the glue of the successful relationship, reflective of growing skill, trust, and confidence among partners.

The advantages of collaboration often begin with negotiation by the involved professionals regarding which patients and conditions are best managed by the APRN or the physician. This process may seem to be a hurdle to competent and successful APRNs, but armed with data, performance indicators (both financial and clinical), and the maturation of one's practice, the process of collaborative decision making promotes effectiveness of care. For example, in the management of chronic illness, APRNs tend to prescribe fewer drugs, order fewer tests, choose less expensive treatments, and spend more time with patients (Fitzgerald, Jones, Lazar, McHugh, & Wang, 1995). According to hospital salary surveys, the cost of an APRN is often 50% of the physician's or less. Subsequently, an effective collaborative APRN/physician practice would enable physicians to spend more time with patients with more complex health needs while APRNs focus on the care of more stable patients, as well as helping patients traverse the health-care continuum in managing their complex diseases.

In all health-care settings, it is becoming an increasing challenge to provide the ongoing surveillance and case management that can support sick and frail patients to function at their highest level possible. In a study of elders, Naylor and colleagues (1994) found that acute-care nurse practitioners (ACNPs) were able to reduce posthospital complications and readmissions. The management of acute illness of established patients has also shown a decrease in complications and cost while maximizing the quality of life for patients. Physicians are then available to deal with those situations that require the clinical decision making and intervention of specialized medical care. It is becoming increasingly apparent that future trends in health-care reform and public reporting will require greater collaboration and role recognition among all health-care providers as a strategy to relate effectively and efficiently with all patients.

Although barriers to collaboration persist, progress has been noted in interprofessional practice. Advanced practice nurses (APNs) are leading interdisciplinary teams, improving primary care access, managing care of vulnerable populations, and improving patient and population outcomes (IOM, 2015). Barriers to collaboration have been rooted in the many traditions of the "Doctor-Nurse Game," which range from sex-role stereotypes to incongruent expectations of knowledge and skill acquisition. Intertwined within these concepts are those related to cultural, social, psychological, and financial complexities of the health-care system. Nonetheless, when patient-focused approaches to health care are endorsed and when interprofessional education and team-based collaborative practice models are adopted, the critical aspects of collaborative relationships, skills, and practices are uncovered. The opportunities in which patient-focused approaches fully engage among various health-care disciplines become self-evident over time. In other words, the dimensions of the physician-nurse relationship are fundamentally tied to the quality of patient care (Brandt, 2001). This observation alone provides the health-care system and clinicians with primary motivation to encourage effective relationships between professionals to identify opportunities for working through and with one other.

CLINICAL RELATIONSHIPS

The nature of advanced practice is such that most patient care can be managed because of the skill and knowledge of the practitioner within the role. However, each practitioner acknowledges the critical significance of consultation and referral when used in a timely and effective manner. Embedded in these partnerships are the issues of relationships within the health-care team, communication styles, trust, and the ability to interact within these clinical relationships without a hierarchical framework. Although many APRNs have formal consultative relationships within their SOP, others do not. In addition, these formal structures vary among states and health-care institutions with a range of directives from state boards, often from different disciplines. National efforts are underway to remove SOP barriers and allow for increased reimbursement for APRN services but they have not yet been implemented (IOM, 2015). Accordingly, these changes can result in significant savings and increased access, as well as performance improvement in patient safety and quality of care. With legislation and statute aside, the ability to work within a model of consultation and referral is necessary. Each member of the health-care team has knowledge and skills to offer the other and a partnership can often effect changes in practice and influence patient care outcomes that would not be possible if managed alone. Many consultative practices are also influenced by the environment whereby specialty and primary care is clearly differentiated. In these situations, consultative relationships are vital to improved care processes.

Often consultation and referral activities are confused with supervision, comanagement (the working together to manage a complex case), and direct oversight. In these situations, the accountability for practice may become lost and roles are blurred. The limits of one's practice expertise or the need to receive advice should be viewed as complementary, not as a deficiency or "take over" approach. The professional interactions inherent in consultation and referral expand the APRN's ability to work with and through others while maintaining autonomy over the situation until there is a mutually identified decision that a change in care is necessary. Although comanagement and referral (the relinquishing of care temporarily or permanently) may have different themes, the goal of care is still accomplished within a partnership mode. Hamric, Spross, and Hanson (2005) state that APRNs themselves are often confused about the differences. They refer to a more thoughtful definition of collaboration described as "a dynamic, interpersonal process in which two or more individuals make a commitment to each other to interact authentically and constructively to solve problems and to learn from each other in order to accomplish identified goals, purposes, or outcomes. The individuals recognize and articulate the shared values that make this commitment possible" (p. 318). Within this framework of collaboration, the varying processes of consultation, referral, or comanagement may assume the added dimension of a therapeutic, professional relationship acknowledging the role each member plays while supporting the complexities inherent in the delivery of high-quality patient care. Although knowledge, skill, and clinical expertise are all key factors in day-to-day practice, the elements of working with each other in this collaborative manner will determine and distinguish the best practices.

INTERPROFESSIONAL TEAMING

The need for integrated health-care teams is fueled by several factors, including patient safety; the increasing complexity of patient needs, especially among the growing population of elders; expansion in the continuum of care in various health-care delivery models; the sophistication of telecommunications and information networks; and changes in methods of health-care financing and reimbursement regulations. It is also evident that members of the interprofessional health-care team—physicians, APRNs, registered nurses (RNs), social workers, and other clinicians—often practice independently of one another, rendering care as if services for the same patient or groups of patients were unrelated. This can create an uncoordinated, conflict-laden environment resulting in a diminished voice for patients and families to participate in their own care. Ineffective teamwork and communication are primary root causes in medical errors becoming the third leading cause of death in the United States. Estimates of health-care costs for medical errors are more than $17.1 billion a year with an conservative total monetary loss of up to $73.5 billion a year based on the cost of quality-adjusted life year (QALY—an economic evaluation to assess the value of money for medical interventions) (Andel, Davidow, Hollander, & Moreno, 2012; National Patient Safety Foundation [NPSF], 2015). Interprofessional teaming differs from the multidisciplinary approach to care, which has been compared with the parallel play of children with limited interactive and intersecting activity (Clark, 1994). See **Figure 12.3.** According to Cronenwett and Dzau (2010), interprofessional training and teaming are critical

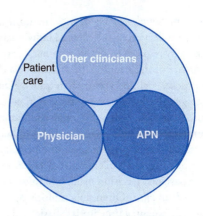

FIGURE 12.3 Multidisciplinary approach to patient care.

to meet the needs of patients, families, communities, and populations to provide the care they want and control costs in health care.

Interdisciplinary teaming, currently referenced as interprofessional collaboration, was proposed decades ago as an alternative model of care (Pfeiffer, 1998). Interdisciplinary teaming requires that the members of the health-care team integrate their disciplines' work and create plans of care together, centering this plan on the patients' needs. This form of teamwork, interdisciplinary care, has been defined as a "special form of interactional interdependence between health-care providers who merge different but complementary skills in the service of patients and in the solution of their health problems" (Tsukuda, 1990, p. 670). See **Figure 12.4.**

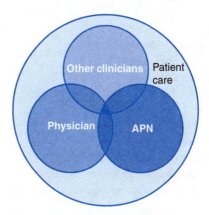

FIGURE 12.4 Interprofessional approach to patient care.

The term *complementary* defines the team approach. However, a collection of like-minded individuals does not automatically result in an interdisciplinary team. Because of the nature of this teaming, there must be a clearly defined purpose, goal, and approach to team activity, shared phraseology to ensure effective communication (e.g., SBAR communication), as well as the value and understanding that mutual accountability of each team member is crucial to the team's overall performance. The primary purpose of this type of team is collaborative decision making for and with patients. Decision making in this model occurs in a unified timeline. Often, in a multidisciplinary team approach, a sequential timeline is experienced as a dependent process in which the final decision is made by the "lead" member who pulls everything together. This type of decision making is limited, and potentially ineffective, when complementary activity is desired.

For the APRN, the influence of interdisciplinary teams is powerful when practitioners practice at the full SOP with clear roles and responsibilities and shared values. Creative teamwork can be achieved when the entire team caring for patients can actively participate in planning, decision making, problem solving, and include patients and families in their care. Changing the norms of practice, however, may be necessary. Interdisciplinary teams are the epitome of working with and through others while recognizing the importance of an individual's clinical expertise.

There are several dimensions to consider when implementing interdisciplinary team relationships. According to Howe, Cassel, and Vezina (1998), these dimensions include the following:

1. Skills
   - Conflict resolution
   - Team interaction
   - Communication
   - Leadership
   - Outcomes-focused care
   - Performance improvement
2. Attitudes
   - Respect for other disciplines
   - Respect for patient and family input
   - Respect for patient management and patient-focused care
   - Awareness of outcomes-based practice

3. Knowledge
   - Roles, responsibilities, and SOP for each discipline
   - Role of the extended team
   - Group dynamics
   - Application of clinical concepts and quality measures among disciplines
   - Up-to-date knowledge of the health-care environment, policy, and technology

Inherent within this interdisciplinary framework, collaboration underpins the field of day-to-day practice within a team concept. According to Tsukuda and Stahelski (1990), collaboration takes on the dimension of cooperation with others, adding trust as an essential component of this interactional style because patient outcomes are consistently dependent on the efforts of others. As a team member, one may ask the following questions:

- Are my own goals consistent with team goals?
- Do I advocate solutions for problems that will benefit team members?
- Do I work for consensus and focus on performance and measureable outcomes?
- Do I cooperate with other team members' activities?
- Do I do an equitable share of the group workload?
- Do I feel individual responsibility for the joint outcomes of the group members?
- Do I support the team in dealing with larger organizational and regulatory issues?
- Do I view my contributions as belonging to the group—to be used or not—as the group decides?
- Do I listen to team members in a positive and respectful manner?
- Do I actively participate in team meetings and assignments?

Advocates of interdisciplinary team approaches to care realize that there are many psychosocial influences on health and disease. This underscores the importance of relationship-centered care (Tresolini & The Pew-Fetzer Task Force, 1994) and patient-centered care (Coles, 1995), which are based on interpersonal communication techniques and a collaborative care model. A paradigm shift for all members of the health-care team may be necessary because new core competencies are required and need to be role modeled for the successful transition to occur. APRNs are often members of these teams and are positioned to initiate the transition to a more collaborative and patient-focused approach in their practice. APRNs often assume a mediator role to introduce these changes in the delivery of patient care and to assist the team in its growth and development in the core competencies of interdisciplinary team approaches.

APRNs may take a leadership role in influencing stages of team development. Their role is easily linked to the various members of the health-care team, allowing APRNs the advantage of connecting with each discipline, clearly expressing the similarities and the differences of each member's role and contribution. With this common ground set, the formation and development of a team can occur.

According to Tuckman (1965), four stages of team development are discussed:

- Forming
- Storming
- Norming
- Performing

As implied by the stages, the creation and maintenance of teams is personnel intensive with professional adjustments required by every member of the team. Successful outcomes also imply that at least four conditions are met: The task is suitable for teamwork, the team must include the right clinical skills to perform the task, team members must combine their resources effectively, and the organization must provide a supportive context for the team (Dow et al, 2013).

Roles and relationships will be challenged, but the team will also move to a new level whereby extraordinary achievements and improved patient care can occur. In this context, interprofessional teaming with its strong emphasis on relationship-centered care is a requisite skill for the 21st century.

PROFESSIONAL NURSING CONNECTIONS

Expanded roles for nurses span a century of growth and development, with the earliest days of clinical specialization in anesthesia, operating room, and obstetrical nursing. However, the knowledge and skills required in a basic nursing education lay the foundation for the advanced practice platform. Common ground skills and competencies include patient assessment, health promotion and maintenance, health education, advocacy, caring, accountability, continuity, and collaboration with other health team members. This overlap and sharing of skills create a bond of practice between RNs and APRNs—forming professional nursing connections. How do these two groups move together in partnership? Hopefully, they join together with respect for the value of each role, intending to effectively use the expertise of each professional while avoiding duplication of effort and promoting true collaborative relationships. Such connections can broaden the scope of health care and achieve professional satisfaction for both RNs and APRNs.

Regardless of the common ground, however, each advanced practice specialty has dealt with resistance from other nurses because advanced roles have often represented innovations in practice that shook the status quo of the nursing establishment and the overall health-care system (Bigbee & Amidi-Nouri, 2000). Rigid boundaries were often created and the struggle for recognition and acceptance followed. However, through organized and focused educational and political efforts, tensions were lessened and improved relationships flourished.

The roles of the RN and the APRN sometimes clash within the context of leadership for the delivery of patient care. Once an understanding of expertise and specialization is clearly reached and communicated, the contribution of each role can be qualified and recognized and a complementary approach to health care defined. Evaluative research can also assist in this recognition and educational process—providing data to illustrate the effect of advanced practice nursing care on quality patient outcomes. Together, professional connections between the RN and APRN can be fortified and not diluted by professional conflict.

The common ground between RNs and APRNs creates a powerful force in health-care delivery. The professional bonding that exists between both groups reinforces the image of the RN and the APRN as coleaders of care. By practicing together, the RN–APRN team can design approaches to care that recognize each other's respective strengths and expertise—resulting in a dynamic practice arena free of hierarchy.

EXEMPLARS: ENACTING ADVANCED PRACTICE ROLES

The enactment of the advanced practice roles of the APRN, the CNS, the CNM, and the CRNA are best detailed through the narratives set forth by the following exemplars. Using the standard set of interview questions listed in the text that follows, these enactments are related to existing practice settings. See **Boxes 12.1 through 12.6.**

Advanced Practice Nurse Interview Questions

To guide the interview process for chosen groups of APRNs, the following questions were used consistently for each group with the intent of assessing roles, expectations, and influences on practice.

1. How would you describe your role?
2. How would you describe your working relationship with physicians, other nurses, and other members of the health-care team?
3. What does *referral* mean to you?
4. What does *consultation* mean to you?
5. How open are members of other disciplines in taking direct referrals or consultation from you?
6. What degree of authority do you experience in these situations and in your role?
7. Do you observe that you bring about change and a higher order of knowledge to your practice area?
8. Can you discuss a situation that may exemplify your role, especially regarding your work through other people?

Box 12.1

The Acute-Care Nurse Practitioner

This group of acute-care nurse practitioners (ACNPs), situated within an oncology inpatient practice, describes their role as geared to management of their patient's experience of illness. The patient's diagnostic workup is often completed before admission in the ambulatory setting. Therefore, the patient's in-hospital experience focuses on the management of the acute phase of illness and treatment options as the goals of care. They describe their perspective as multidimensional. Using their RN background, they always view the patient in a holistic manner. Advanced practice clinical competencies engage their ability to case manage and guide patients and families through the complexity of health care. Within this framework, the ACNP's relationships with the health-care team are key because they spend significant amounts of time discussing medical management and locating resources, managing symptoms, integrating feedback from other disciplines, and identifying alternatives to the health-care system when challenged by the limitations of third-party payers. Given their range of activities, this group of ACNPs consistently relate to a variety of other disciplines, primarily medicine, nursing, and social work.

This group describes their autonomy as follows: "We feel that our common ground is the care of the patient. Working collaboratively with the interprofessional team in the lead position, "we decide the day-to-day care for our patients, and in acute or critical episodes, we often independently manage the process. Although critical incidents may be a time when the physician takes a more active role, this does not necessarily translate into the need to 'take over.' The goal is to work together—not to work around each other or without each other." The ACNP is usually the leader of care because of several factors, including the close relationship to the patient and family members, the advantages of consistency of care by the ACNP, and well-defined collaboration between physician and ACNP.

Regarding their relationships with RNs, the ACNPs state: "There is nothing better than working with a competent nurse. When this relationship occurs, there is such a strong bond that you firmly believe that there is absolutely nothing that can stand in the way of quality." On the other hand, ACNPs state that some nurses can become more passive about patient care when relating to an ACNP. Because the RN recognizes the "nurse" in the ACNP role, the RN may relinquish aspects of his or her responsibility for patient management or assessment to the ACNP. This transfer rarely occurs within the RN–physician relationship. NPs must therefore carefully assess the nature of the ACNP–RN relationship to avoid jeopardizing their ability to work through others while facilitating the advanced practice perspective.

Within the ACNP role, referrals are commonplace—ACNP to nutritionist, social worker, pharmacist, physical therapist, and home care services. Physicians often refer their patients to ACNPs, acknowledging their specialization, expertise, and consistency of care. Consultations are more informal within the inpatient setting. When acute patient situations occur, however, clinical consultation is common. ACNPs state: "Not a day goes by that I am not involved in a clinical consultation primarily focused on symptom management, such as pain control, the side effects of chemotherapy, nausea, vomiting, constipation, or palliative care." This type of consultation is almost always verbal for, it seems, "physicians want to maintain control of the written consultation process within the hospital experience." ACNPs consult other ACNPs as well, often involving clinical specialization expertise—usually within a verbal, face-to-face framework.

The degree of authority within the discipline of nursing is explained by acute care ACNPs in a variety of ways. ACNPs are integral in the decision making about their patients and have significant influence on the nursing care being delivered. Using a specialization approach, ACNPs take advantage of opportunities to teach about clinical sequelae and

implications. One ACNP states: "I often teach at the bedside about what is going on with the patient, and I am watchful for the types of questions the nurses have. This helps me observe the growth of the staff and assess their advancing competency. It is really a very rewarding experience for me." Through rounding with staff nurses, ACNPs also have the opportunity to clarify the patient story and often act as a facilitator of communication about patients among team members. ACNPs state their role as "performing the editing role"—distinguishing the critical elements of the patient story and routing the necessary data in a more concise and relevant way to obtain what is necessary for their patients. As one ACNP stated, "Our role within the interdisciplinary team is one of monitor of the communication patterns and the perspective at hand. We often translate what is going on into a relevant, concise language that evokes a rapid, clear understanding by those team members who need to hear the information."

According to this group, the design of the ACNP embraces many relationships within the health-care team and consists of these major components:

1. Gatekeeper
2. Decoder of the complexity of the situation
3. Director of care, delineating roles and responses
4. Problem solver, often suggesting alternatives when barriers arise
5. Provider of a secure environment for staff nurses to ask questions and learn
6. Guide for directing the patient care experience, providing the driving force behind what needs to be done, when, and why

Integral to these components is the ability to work with others, to recognize the many roles inherent within the health-care team, to value the team's input and contribution, and to recognize that influencing others should be always focused on the unified goal of high-quality patient care.

Box 12.2

The Clinical Nurse Specialist

The CNSs describe their role as multifunctional, defining their framework of practice as more focused within a nursing model rather than medicine. CNSs categorize their role into two primary domains: clinical and professional. Clinically, this CNS group describes their role as including a major teaching component and direct clinical practice to facilitate and influence care of complex patients. These functions are often intertwined because they routinely bring about change and a higher order of knowledge by role modeling, mentoring, and coaching staff to perform at "the next level." CNSs also intervene within the health-care team to make clinical recommendations to change the course of action or resolve conflicts for optimal patient care. Professionally, the CNS also assumes major responsibilities for the development of policies, procedures, protocols, and standards of care. Within this context, the education of patients in health promotion and maintenance is key. Standards of care are holistic in nature, spanning the physical, psychosocial, and spiritual needs of patients. The needs of nurses are also critical. The CNS encourages the professional growth of staff, often provides career counseling, and directs the building of expertise among nurses in a specific, individualized manner.

The CNSs describe their role with physicians as collegial with a defined focus on specialty patient care management, often receiving referrals for a specific patient population (e.g., diabetes) or an occurrence such as death or dying and bereavement. CNSs are consistent in their view of the "big picture," focusing not just on disease and pathophysiology but on the patient's response to the disease. With other nurses, CNSs describe their role as an enabler—one of camaraderie focused on patient care. CNSs also provide clinical, professional, and legal clarification regarding issues of care to ensure a safe patient environment.

When asked about autonomy, this CNS group cited self-direction and motivation as key elements in working with others. Several strategies are used to engage others in change and ultimately provide state-of-the-art, valid, and effective approaches to care:

1. Use benchmark data and national standards to energize staff to change or modify practices.

2. Develop and educate staff so they can question their patient care environment and relate to a higher level of performance through evidence-based practice and scholarly query.

3. Involve staff in various levels of patient care projects, moving forward together in change.

4. Ground all projects in the literature and best practices so as to base decisions on evidence and promote confidence in the process.

The CNS role engages an inclusive approach within these strategies that guarantees a successful and lasting outcome over time.

Referrals are routine in complex cases. The CNS is often the originator of referrals to other members of the health-care team but integral to bringing team members together to problem solve. Inclusiveness is again a key element of the CNSs' practice domain and a hallmark of their effectiveness in patient care through their ability to relate to others.

Consultation, on the other hand, is associated with the level of the CNS's clinical expertise and is often initiated by other members of the health-care team—physicians, nurses, and social workers. As an inductive thinker, the CNS has a clearly articulated interest in the patient experience of care. Using these tenets of practice and change—standards, safety, and ethics—the CNS is able to define a plan for care, engaging caregivers to undertake the plan and empowering others to assume an appropriate trajectory for the patient.

As the integrator of care, the CNS exemplifies how positive interdisciplinary relationships ensure positive outcomes for patients. CNSs are teachers, clinical experts, care providers, case finders, role models, mentors, patient advocates, coaches, team members, policy makers, project leaders, innovators, case managers, career counselors, and change agents. With a vision of best practices as their foundation for care, the CNSs hold the value of expertise and dynamic working relationships within the health-care team as critical elements to the success of their role.

Box 12.3

The Midwife

Midwives in a combined ambulatory and inpatient setting describe their advanced practice role as primary caregiver of women along the life cycle with a focus on low-risk obstetrical and gynecological care, health promotion, wellness, family-centered care, risk assessment, and management of common illnesses and acute conditions. Clinically, this group views their role as centered on direct care with a strong emphasis on patient education and health promotion. Their relationships with other members of the health-care team revolve around this focus. Midwives independently care for a patient caseload, often comanaging more acute conditions with physicians or employing the physician as consultant.

Regarding referral, midwives in this practice describe the process as formalized and often interchangeable with consultation. They define many of their referrals as transfers to the care of a physician because of a specialized need of the patient over time. Ongoing referrals to other disciplines are also common, usually engaging the services of social work and home care. In these instances, the midwife maintains the primary care responsibility for the patient. With consultation, the process is also formal. Using written communication, consultations are often provided through the required practice protocols that identify the consulting physician and the decision guidelines for the consultation. Within this collaborative relationship, the midwife is able to transition the care of the patient when a condition warrants. This can be accomplished in a comanaged arrangement or by a referral of the care responsibility to another caregiver. However, the midwife has an expectation to be involved in the communication of the plan of care and the ultimate follow-up of the patient being referred. The midwife explains that the "relationships with physicians in my practice are necessary and denote many shared responsibilities. I find this relationship to be within an interdependent framework because we both need to work together to manage the patient safely in given situations. I have

a consulting agreement with a primary physician for immediate feedback and intervention as well as with other physicians who are colleagues and can be employed for a less acute need. But I also have the need to maintain my primary care role for my patients."

Working with the nursing staff involves interdependence. The need for the RN to facilitate a plan of care and become integral in the assessment and the education of patients is key. One midwife states, "I find that once my role is accepted and understood, positive relationships follow and communication about patients is facilitated. I admit that I need nurses to ultimately deliver good patient care. I cannot do everything myself." Nurses and other health team members who seek out the midwife as primary caregiver ultimately improve the patient experience because the model of working together and understanding the role is achieved. One midwife states that over the past decade this recognition of the midwife role has improved tremendously, especially because of updated SOP legislation and changes in third-party reimbursement.

When asked about autonomy and authority over practice, midwives strongly identify that their influence over care processes is recognized by others. The primary reason for this influence is the public respect, acceptance, and demand for their roles and services. They add that this authority is stronger and more flexible in an ambulatory setting and can be less autonomous in a hospital-based birthing unit, especially when associated with a medical residency program. Interdisciplinary competition in these settings can affect the perceived authority and working relationships of the midwife with other clinicians, as well as patients.

When discussing their relationships with nurses, midwives were clear that within the specialty of women's health RNs do not abdicate components of their roles to midwives. RNs often question an approach to care, exchange ideas to complement care, and practice as team members. The specialty of women's health is

The Midwife (Continued)

often not characterized as illness-focused but within a health promotion or health maintenance framework, enabling the team approach to flourish. Respect for the team's contribution to the varied aspects of the needs of patients enables the nurse-midwives to work effectively with and through others. As one nurse-midwife

summarized her role: "Being on the same page in our plans for care is easily delineated within this advanced practice role. Thus collaboration is a natural outcome. Respect is key, and once earned, paves the way to collaborative practice."

The Primary Care Nurse Practitioner

This group of primary care NPs view their role as provider of a comprehensive holistic health-care experience for their patients. With independence and autonomy, the primary care NP has a threefold responsibility to assess, diagnose, and manage a variety of common and chronic illnesses within all the dimensions of the physical, psychosocial, and financial elements of care. "My caseload of patients" is a common reference point, delineating the accountability of this group of NPs for their patients over time—not limited to a hospital experience but to the continuum of care. In primary care, the NP possesses a leadership role in the practice generally by providing a surveillance function—a "third eye"—always watchful of the effectiveness of day-to-day patient care delivery. The need to evaluate systems and clinical outcomes is essential to the role.

The team approach in this type of practice is fundamental and involves a strong interdisciplinary, participative approach to care. Patients are independently managed, comanaged with physicians, or referred within their continuum of care. The need to relate effectively with all members of the health-care team is constant. Multidisciplinary options coexist within an interdisciplinary framework—creating many opportunities for therapeutic relationships among staff, patients, and family members.

Within the primary care practice, RNs are the "heart" of any clinical operation. The RN complements the APN role, especially in the areas of patient teaching,

patient monitoring, and data gathering. Although roles are often strongly delineated, sharing clinical activity among health-care team members is consistent and necessary.

Because of the primary care focus, referrals to specialists are commonplace. However, as one NP explained, "Losing the primary relationship with a patient to a specialist is a concern." The information and insight the specialist provides will enhance the care the patient receives from his or her primary care provider. There are also instances when a specialist and primary care provider work collaboratively on the health-care management of a patient over the longer term. Feedback on the means to best manage the patient is the expected outcome. One NP stated: "We expect to have our patients return to us for their care and to benefit from the expertise and evaluation by the specialist."

Consultations, on the other hand, are frequently engaged in by other caregivers. Within a mature primary care practice, a multidisciplinary team approach is often developed. Formal consultations usually occur within the practice. The opportunity to have "curbside" or "hallway" consultations with these same specialists or experts exists as well. This type of consultation is often informal. The NPs from this practice cited that the key criteria for successful and effective consultations of any type include the development of positive relationships, a clear direction of the plan of care, and a model of inclusivity among team members.

Primary care NPs describe their authority as an essential part of their potential for success in their role while maintaining autonomy and a knowledge base to provide sufficient holistic primary care to patients. Practicing side-by-side with physicians and other NPs creates opportunities for sharing advice or consultation. Leading patient care in this practice setting is very satisfying and empowering to this group of APNs. At the same time, however, this sense of control and satisfaction occurs only when interdisciplinary teamwork is achieved by doing the following:

1. Listening to others
2. Teaching others
3. Demonstrating the APN role in positive, creative ways
4. Communicating openly
5. Demonstrating expertise

Respect from other members of the team enables the primary care NP to facilitate and lead care effectively. When sharing the same mission within this framework of practice, advancement of learning and change occurs. By empowering and educating staff at all levels, the barrier of the "task" is removed and has been replaced with a "connection" to the patient's illness experience. Assisting staff to understand the rationale for care is a definitive way to initiate change and a higher level of performance. In addition, the primary care NP often exhibits his or her own clinical specialization and expertise, which may provide a different perspective of care, adding to the knowledge base of the staff. As educator, the NP is capable of working through other people, engaging the staff's interest in the mission and work at hand. Knowledge is power, and this power translates into effective practice.

Box 12.5

Rural Health Nurse Practitioner

This group of NPs works in isolated or underserved areas with patients who have limited access to health care. Some rural health NPs are the primary caregiver to an entire community. Rural patients have higher rates of chronic disease and have a higher utilization rate for Medicare and Medicaid compared with more populated areas. Access to specialty providers is more difficult as well, with the average patient driving between 20 and 60 miles to see a specialist; therefore, rural health NPs provide more extensive care compared with their primary care NP counterparts in large practices with easier access to specialists.

The role of rural health NPs is to diagnose and treat health disorders, promote health and prevent disease, and provide health education and counselling. They describe their practice as "highly autonomous, relationship-based, and extremely rewarding." Interprofessional collaboration poses challenges because of distance, outdated technology, and communication barriers. Quality of care is improved when the rural health NPs take on the leadership and management roles in patient care,

support communication and follow ups through the use of technology, and understand the rural cultures.

Rural health NPs cite the following requisite competencies for their specialty practice:

1. Home-based primary care to reduce the travel burden, increase the compliance of health regimens, and improve health outcomes for patients
2. Aligning patient care teams through relationships and technology
3. Telemedicine consults and digital communication to improve access to high-quality care that includes, but is not limited to:
   a. Acute care
   b. Radiology
   c. Pharmacy
   d. Psychiatric services
   e. Lifestyle coaching
4. Support for caregivers to increase coping and decrease stress

---

Box 12.5

Rural Health Nurse Practitioner *(Continued)*

5. Problem solving and innovations to generate solutions and overcome challenges with creativity and resourcefulness
6. Interprofessional learning and education

The ability of the rural health NP to manage complex cases in the home encourages patients to be partners in identifying health-care issues, discussing possible solutions, and developing and implementing plans of action together. "I get to the point where I look forward to Joan calling me on Wednesday afternoons. You know three o'clock comes and I know I have to be near the phone and be ready for her call, and then I give her all my numbers. She'll check with me to see if I have any pain, how the week went and so forth, which I find is good," explained rural veteran Oscar Bourbeau (retrieved from http://dph.illinois.gov/topics-services /life-stages-populations/rural-underserved-populations). Rural health NPs agree that discussing risk factors (i.e., smoking and nutrition, focusing on exercise, medication adherence, and stress management) encourages health promotion and involves community-based organizations in the care of patients. "When patients are hospitalized,

we need to make connections, understand the goals of care, make visits when they are discharged home, and implement an ongoing strategy for return to optimal health." The rural health NP must develop and practice at his or her full SOP to improve the health of rural populations. SOP barriers and outdated technology that were once a hindrance in providing high-quality care are now becoming opportunities and strengths within this growing profession. Rural health NPs have successfully lobbied in the years leading up to the Affordable Care Act and in the years after to increase access to quality rural health-care services and to remove barriers to NP SOP in many states to ensure there are a sufficient number of providers to take care of the rural and underserved populations of this country. "There is a great deal of satisfaction in the role, from building strong interprofessional and interpersonal relationships with all members of the health-care team, including the patient and their family, providing innovative and high quality care to individuals, families, communities, and populations, and having a lower cost of living with higher pay [compared with primary care NPs in large urban practices] that all make for a very rewarding profession."

Box 12.6

The Nurse Anesthetist

The role of the CRNA within a hospital practice is described as an advanced practice specialty with a strong and eventful history that has provided many benchmarks for nurses seeking expanded roles. As an anesthesia provider, the goal of the CRNA is to provide safe and comfortable anesthesia for all types of surgical procedures in multiple settings across the care continuum for patients of all ages spanning the American Society of Anesthesiologists (ASA) classifications of "healthy" to "gravely ill/impending death." In discussing this broad role definition, the concept of independence is also clearly expressed, especially because the CRNA often is able to administer anesthesia without the direct supervision of a physician, depending on state

regulations and the requirements of the employing health-care institution. For example, this CRNA stated that in her practice an anesthesiologist is required to practice in specified ratios with the CRNA and that an anesthesiologist must be present in the room at the start of general anesthesia induction.

The clinical relationship between the CRNA and the anesthesiologist is clearly described as one of a collegial and trusting nature with open communication. However, outside of the clinical arena, the political tension between the two disciplines is present with a long history of debate and interprofessional struggle and competition. With the demonstration of expertise, however, positive communication patterns and relationships have developed around the patient and quality care in institutional settings. The day-to-day operational framework has thereby demonstrated advancement over time in terms of professional acceptance and colleagueship.

Within the operating room, the surgical team assumes a vibrant interdependent structure. This CRNA stated: "Teamwork is the expectation in the operating room setting. The involvement with RNs, surgeons, and surgical technologists is intense and very focused on the individual patient and the procedure at hand and can sometimes be described as somewhat of an isolating relationship because of this directed focus." Regarding the relationship between the CRNA and RN, it is described as important but less influential in affecting the role of the CRNA when compared with the other team members such as the surgeon or technologist. The relationship with surgeons is described as one of respect for the specialization of anesthesia and sometimes is dependent during the course of surgery because the CRNA often leads patient stabilization efforts when a critical change in condition occurs.

In the specialty of anesthesia, the CRNA usually does not make referrals but is the recipient of referrals from other providers. With the exception of some specialized services such as pain management, CRNAs do not have their own patient caseload because the patients' primary relationship is with their surgeon. Consultations, on the other hand, comprise a major component of anesthesia practice. Consultations reflect clinical, legal, and medical aspects of the plan of care. Surgeons frequently request a consultation from a CRNA, respecting the expertise of this specialization to assess the risks of surgery. In this endeavor, the surgeon is dependent on the expertise of the anesthesia specialist. Within this activity, the CRNA attains primary patient and family contact, subsequently establishing the patient-family relationship.

Authority in practice is significant within the specialty of anesthesia. "Many other disciplines do not share a common ground in this specialty: thus my role is unique within patient care." The CRNA in this practice comments that she also identifies that through her unique expertise, the independence and influence of her role takes hold. "Other members of the health-care team recognize my competence, which directly affects my sense of autonomy and authority. I am called on to assist others in their clinical assessment of patients, as well as the advancement of professional knowledge and skills of residents and nurse anesthesia students. With this broad range of influence, my sense of authority is promoted."

The ability of the CRNA to influence change and a higher order of knowledge in the arenas of perioperative and perianesthesia practice is strongly affected through teaching by example, demonstrating competence, and role modeling professional behaviors to all members of the health-care team. Using this framework, the CRNA in this practice identifies that she is able to influence change and advance knowledge by relying on a clinical approach rather than an academic approach. In many practices, however, CRNAs also assume formal faculty roles within various levels of educational programs throughout the country.

Although working through other people is an expectation of any health-care professional role, interdisciplinary exposure is often more limited for CRNAs and can potentially contribute to isolation. Interdisciplinary relationships are strongest within the perioperative team of the surgeon, anesthesiologist, nurse, and technologist. Extending this relationship to other clinical staff and family members is challenging. In addition, CRNAs are often placed within a separate administrative structure within the health-care facility or practice, contributing to the isolation, especially from other professional nurse colleagues.

Within the context of advanced practice, the goal of the CRNA is to promote nursing, advance health care, and ensure a safe and high-quality patient care experience. As the earliest advanced practice role, CRNAs have successfully built a strong presence in health care.

CONCLUSION

The dynamic interplay of partnerships and interdependence between advanced practice and other team roles in health care is a professional opportunity. Working with and through others is the cornerstone of the successful engagement of the health-care team and endorses the presence of advanced practice over time.

Competency
in Advanced Practice

13

Evidence-Based Practice

Deborah C. Messecar and Christine A. Tanner

Learning Outcomes

Learning outcomes expected as a result of this chapter:

- Describe the relationship between clinical judgment and using the best evidence to make decisions.
- Identify and analyze the elements of research methodology that are critical in providing evidence for practice settings.
- Discuss the advantages and limitations of various types of knowledge.
- Demonstrate the ability to access information and evaluate the quality of evidence relevant to practice settings.
- Describe tools and strategies for finding the best and most appropriate evidence to improve practice.
- Communicate search strategy to others.
- Identify forces (i.e., ethical, legal, political, cultural, logistical, and economic) that influence research methodology and interpretation of findings in clinical settings.

INTRODUCTION

Translating evidence into practice is a key skill for advanced practice nurses (APNs). The increasing interest in knowledge translation, the process of moving research into practice and putting knowledge into action, coincides with the growing engagement in the evidence-based practice (EBP) approach in which practitioners make practice decisions based on the integration of the research evidence with clinical expertise and the patient's unique values and circumstances (Straus, Glasziou, Richardson, & Haynes, 2011). EBP builds on the process of using knowledge gleaned from systematic reviews and the results of individual studies, but includes much more such as evidence from opinion leaders, the products of reasoning, clinical knowledge from practice experience, and patient preferences, to name a few (Melnyk &

Fineout-Overholt, 2014; Melnyk, Fineout-Overholt, Gallagher-Ford, & Kaplan, 2012). The importance of teaching critical appraisal of evidence and knowledge translation skills has only intensified in APN programs for several reasons. First, EBP is often not the standard of care. In many cases patients fail to receive recommended standards of care or are receiving potentially harmful or unproven treatment (Fink, Thompson, & Bonnes, 2005; McGlynn, Asch, & Adams, 2003; Melnyk, Grossman, et al, 2012; Sung et al, 2003). A second major impetus for the movement to EBP is the growth of scientific evidence supporting high-value health care and the development of methods for integrating the available evidence expeditiously into guidelines for practice (Arnoff, 2011). Information technology has also greatly augmented our ability to access this information. A third factor is that media dissemination of information has made patients increasingly savvy about different available treatments, enabling them to ask more informed questions about their illnesses and care (Amante, Hogan, Pagoto, English, & Lapane, 2015; Cohen & Adams, 2011). Fourth, the urgency of using evidence to improve clinical care has been highlighted by the Institute of Medicine (IOM) reports on the future of nursing (IOM, 2011) and finding and knowing what works in health care (IOM, 2008, 2011) as well as prior reports on quality and safety (IOM, 2001, 2004). Robust EBP skills applied with expert clinical judgment can help APNs narrow the gap between research and practice and improve the quality and safety of care.

The objective of this chapter is to present a view of clinical judgment and the different patterns of clinical reasoning and their relationship to translating evidence into practice. The importance of fostering clinical judgment and critical thinking in APN education was emphasized in the Carnegie Report (Benner, Sutphen, Leonard, & Day, 2010). The emphasis on clinical judgment in APN education is consistent with recognizing that knowledge translation should include the complex process of applying the general facts derived from research in a particular situation, given the patient's circumstances and preferences (Tanner, 2009). Research on clinical judgment is presented to illustrate how nurses use reasoning patterns as they assess patients, selectively attend to clinical cues, interpret these data, and respond or intervene, and how evidence translation fits into this process. The role of context, the knowledge and experience background of the nurse, and the effect of knowing the

patient on these reasoning processes is also described. A research-based model of clinical judgment (Benner, Tanner, & Chesla, 2009; Tanner, 2006) is presented to provide a framework for understanding how the APN can draw on clinical decision-making skills developed over time in practice along with new skills in transforming evidence into knowledge to continuously improve the methods of care being employed. This model helps guide judgments about what scientific literature and guidelines are relevant for the questions at hand and whether the evidence the APN has to support the assessments, interpretations, and actions has the utility and relevance to be applied to their clinical decision making. In addition, tips on how to access and evaluate research evidence to improve the quality of the APN's point of care decisions are provided.

EVOLUTION OF EVIDENCE-BASED PRACTICE AND KNOWLEDGE TRANSLATION

Historically, EBP was presented as a new paradigm in health professions practice (Tanner, 1999). This approach devalued intuition, the use of clinical opinion based on experience, and basic scientific rationale as sufficient grounds for clinical decision making and instead stressed the examination of evidence solely from clinical research (Bergus & Hamm, 1995). The aim of EBP defined in this manner is to reduce wider variations in individual clinicians' practices, eliminating worst practices and enhancing best practices, thereby reducing costs and improving quality. This goal and the assumptions underlying what counts as evidence were troubling to many clinicians (Dearlove, Rogers, & Sharples, 1996; Mitchell, 1999; Rycroft-Malone et al, 2004; Smith, 1996). Their concern was that expert clinical judgment would be replaced by a cookbook approach to decision making. In response to this criticism, the definition of evidence-based medicine was revised to be more comprehensive in its view of what counts as evidence and what should figure into decisions regarding patient care. Evidence-based medicine is the use of the best research evidence in making decisions about the care of individual patients. To practice evidence-based medicine, clinicians must integrate their personal clinical expertise with the best available evidence from systematic research, the local context of care and the internal evidence generated there such as patient assessment, outcomes management, and quality improvement data and apply this within the context of their patient's unique values and circumstances (Melnyk, Gallagher-Ford, Long, & Fineout-Overholt, 2014; Rycroft-Malone et al, 2004; Sackett, Rosenberg, Gray, Haynes, & Richardson, 1996; Straus, Glasziou, Richardson, & Haynes, 2011).

This revised and updated view recognized individual clinical expertise, which is defined as the proficiency and judgment that individual clinicians acquire through clinical experience and clinical practice as a valid source of evidence. Increased expertise not only includes more effective and efficient diagnosis but also more thoughtful identification and compassionate use of individual patients' predicaments, rights, and preferences in making clinical decisions about their care (Sackett et al, 1996; Straus et al, 2011). Best available external clinical evidence was defined as clinically relevant research, which may include basic sciences research but was preferentially from patient-centered clinical research that focused on the accuracy and precision of diagnostic tests (including the clinical examination), the power of prognostic markers, and the efficacy and safety of interventions. Use of external clinical evidence should invalidate previously accepted diagnostic tests and treatments and replace them with new ones that are more powerful, more accurate, more efficacious, and safer. External clinical evidence can inform, but can never replace, individual clinical expertise; this expertise allows a clinician to decide whether the external evidence applies to the individual patient at all, and if so how it should be integrated into a clinical decision. In contrast, internal evidence is typically generated through practice initiatives such as outcomes management or quality improvement projects undertaken for the purpose of improving clinical care in the setting in which it is produced (Melnyk, Gallagher-Ford, et al, 2014).

The terms *EBP* and *knowledge translation* are related and sometimes used interchangeably. However, knowledge translation is a larger, more inclusive concept than EBP and is defined as a process that includes knowledge synthesis and the tailored dissemination of knowledge inquiry to improve health and provide more efficient and effective health services (Straus, Tetroe, & Graham, 2009). Knowledge translation includes all steps between the creation of new knowledge and its application. It includes evaluating practice-based evidence, facilitating EBP, and engaging in collaborative practice inquiry. The discussion of EBP in this chapter is focused on the search for, synthesis of, and implementation of research findings in practice and how this links with use of the APN's clinical judgment. EBP in this view includes decision making about and implementation of care practices based on several kinds of evidence such as findings from the literature, local practice data, national standards or opinions of recognized experts, and information on patient preferences. APNs are expected to integrate their clinical experience with conscientious, explicit, and judicious use of research evidence to inform their clinical judgment and make decisions that maximize the well-being of their patients.

RESEARCH ON CLINICAL JUDGMENT AND THE RELATIONSHIP TO EVIDENCE-BASED PRACTICE

What is clinical judgment? Almost all health professionals view clinical judgment as an essential skill. In nursing, the terms *clinical decision making* or *problem solving* and more recently *critical thinking* have been used interchangeably to refer to the same phenomenon, which has been viewed as a disengaged, analytical, and objective process directed toward resolution of problems and achievement of clearly defined ends. However, research on expert practice suggests that clinical judgment is far more complex (Benner, Tanner, & Chesla, 2009; Tanner, 2006) and incorporates skills that look more like engaged practical reasoning. Engaged practical reasoning occurs when the nurse recognizes a pattern by being attuned to subtle changes in the patient's clinical state and other salient information and then forms an intuitive clinical grasp of the situation without evident forethought (Benner, Tanner, & Chesla, 2009; Tanner, Benner, Chesla, & Gordon, 1993). This flexible and nuanced ability to read the clinical situation is key to interpreting what is going on and responding appropriately. Knowledge of the illness experience for both the patient and the family as well as their physical, social, and emotional strengths and weaknesses are just as important as clinical features of the disease.

Clinical judgment is thus defined as an understanding or inference about a patient's needs, concerns, or health problems, followed by the decision to act (or not act), to use or modify standard approaches, or to improvise new ones as deemed appropriate by the patient's response (Benner, Tanner, & Chesla, 2009; Tanner, 2006). *Clinical reasoning,* in contrast to clinical judgment, is the thinking process by which clinicians make their judgments and includes the process of generating alternatives, weighing them against the evidence, and choosing the most appropriate course of action (Benner, Tanner, & Chesla, 2009; Tanner, 2006).

Clinical judgment has been studied from different theoretical perspectives (Benner, Tanner, & Chesla, 2009; Brannon & Carson, 2003; Kosowski & Roberts, 2003; Ritter, 2003; Simmons, Lanuza, Fonteyn, Hicks, & Holm, 2003; White, 2003), with different clinical foci (McCarthy, 2003), and with different research methods (Benner et al, 2009; Kosowski & Roberts, 2003; McDonald, Frakes, Apostolidis, Armstrong, Goldblatt, & Bernardo, 2003; Ritter, 2003; Simmons et al, 2003; White, 2003). From this historical body of literature on clinical judgment, several general conclusions were drawn.

The Clinician's Background Is More Influential Than Objective Data on Clinical Judgment

The clinician's background influences his or her clinical judgment in a given clinical situation more than the objective data at hand. Clinical judgment requires knowledge, which is abstract, generalizable, and applicable in many situations. Knowledge required for clinical judgment is derived from science and theory and grows with experience as scientific abstractions are filled out in practice. This knowledge is often tacit and is an important factor in aiding clinicians to recognize clinical states instantaneously.

The clinician's background includes experiential learning, particularly that gleaned from personal clinical experience. Three types of knowledge play a part in the clinician's perception of a given situation: theoretical knowledge, practical knowledge, and research-based knowledge. Theoretical knowledge, which is acquired through understanding of scientifically derived knowledge and theory, is used in a particular situation as a specific application of an abstract rule or principle. The description of techniques for examining the thorax and lungs in a physical assessment text is an example of theoretical knowledge that may be applied by the clinician to individual patients. Practical knowledge, also known as knowledge from clinical experience, is acquired through working with many patients. Adapting or revising one's examination of the thorax and lung

techniques for a patient who cannot sit up based on one's past experience or the experience of others is an example of practical knowledge. Knowledge, both theoretical and practical, often determines what stands out as important in a particular situation. Research-based knowledge can contribute to the clinician's overall knowledge base for assessing risks. Knowledge helps the clinician observe selectively. Research directed toward describing phenomena of concern to the nurse helps provide information about what cues are highly associated with particular problems. This allows the nurse, using this knowledge base, to select data relevant to determining the problems the patient may be experiencing. Knowledge also guides action and contributes to the clinician's repertoire of interventions.

An additional essential component of the knowledge required for clinical judgment is the importance of knowing the individual patient and being able to draw on this understanding to better predict and anticipate individual patient responses (Benner et al, 2009; Peden-McAlpine & Clark, 2002). Clinicians come to clinical situations with their own perspectives on what is good and right and these values profoundly influence what they attend to, the options they consider using, and ultimately what they decide to do (Benner et al, 2009; Ellefsen, 2004). The clinician's outlook is not determined by individual notions of right and wrong but rather is developed through interaction with others in the practice discipline. For example, the ethic for disclosure to patients and families or the importance of comfort in the face of impending death sets up what will be noticed in a given clinical exchange and will shape the way in which the clinician responds. Stereotypes and biases also affect perception.

Good Clinical Judgment Requires Knowing the Patient and Responding to His or Her Concerns

In addition to theoretical and practical knowledge, knowledge of the particular patient, both knowing the patient's typical responses and knowing the patient as a person, is central to good clinical judgment (Haynes, Sackett, Guyatt, & Tugwell, 2006; Tanner et al, 1993). When the clinician knows the typical patterns of responses, certain aspects of the situation stand out as salient and others recede in importance. Comparing the current picture to the patient's typical picture allows the clinician to make important qualitative distinctions about how a patient's condition has or has not changed. Knowing the patient facilitates the provision of individualized care.

Knowing patients is defined as a taken-for-granted understanding of patients that comes from working with them, listening to their accounts of their experiences with illness, watching them closely, and understanding how they typically respond (Tanner et al, 1993). This tacit knowledge, which the clinician may not be able to fully describe to an outside observer, is more than what can be obtained in formal assessments. Knowing the typical pattern of responses, certain aspects of a patient's situation stand out as salient, and other aspects of that same patient situation may recede in importance. Understanding how this patient responds under these circumstances forms the basis for the individualized care called for by the IOM's report (2001) on quality.

The level of involvement with the patient influences the way the clinician engages in problem solving, the outcome of the process, and the sense of satisfaction on the part of the clinician (Benner et al, 2009). Central to sound clinical decision making is a concern for revealing and responding to patients as persons, respecting their dignity, and caring for them in ways that preserve their personhood. Developing a sense about the right level of involvement is a skill learned through experience. The skilled clinician has a good clinical grasp, recognizing both familiar and individual patterns. The patient's responses to the nurse's actions are observed and the nurse's reactions are then modified according to how the patient is responding (Benner et al, 2009; Tanner, 2006). Clinical grasp and clinical response are therefore inextricably linked.

Clinical Judgment Is Influenced by the Context in Which Care Occurs

Neither context nor emotions have typically been accounted for in most models of rational decision making. Models of decision making that ignore context, emotion, and the individual's experience eliminate the possibility of seeing these as important in clinical judgment. However, from the work of Benner and colleagues (2009), we know that judgment occurs in the context of a particular situation, when the nurse is emotionally attuned to the situation, meaningful aspects simply stand out as important, and the choice of responses is guided by the nurse's interpretation

of the particular situation. The context for practice that influences decisions to test and treat can include political and social milieu (Benner et al, 2009; Tanner, 2006) as well as patient factors such as socioeconomic status (Scott, Schiell, & King, 1996). Another view is that social judgment or moral evaluation of patients is socially embedded, independent of patient characteristics, and a function of the pervasive norms and attitudes of the clinicians in a given setting (McDonald et al, 2003).

For clinician providers, health care is increasingly practiced in a context of heightened accountability (Klardie, Johnson, McNaughton, & Meyers, 2004; Vincent, Hastings-Tolsma, Gephart, & Alfonzo, 2015). APNs are expected to demonstrate that they can provide care that is both clinically and cost effective (DeBourgh, 2001; Facchiano & Snyder, 2013; Vincent et al, 2015; Youngblut & Brooten, 2001). The struggle for the APN in this environment is to deliver high-quality cost-effective care while still incorporating the needs and preferences of the individual patient (Klardie et al, 2004).

Clinicians Use a Variety of Clinical Reasoning Patterns Alone or in Combination

Work in the art of medical decision making has illustrated that the essence of clinical reasoning eludes understanding (Sox, Blatt, Higgins, & Marton, 2007). The results of studies conducted with nurses during the past 20 years suggest that nurses use a variety of reasoning patterns alone or in combination (Benner et al, 2009; Tanner, 2006). The pattern of reasoning used depends on the demands of the situation, the goals of the practice, the clinician's experience with similar situations, and the perception of what makes excellent practice. The reasoning patterns used are influenced by the nurse's knowledge, biases, and values; the relationship with the patient; and other factors in the clinical situation.

Analytic Processes

An analytic reasoning pattern is characteristic of a beginner's performance or a more experienced clinician when stumped. Analytic reasoning is characterized by deliberate, rational thought that includes the generation of alternatives, weighing against evidence, and evaluating possible courses of action. Analytic reasoning can be influenced by biases and stereotypes. Diagnostic reasoning is an example of analytic thinking. This is a process in which the clinician attends to presenting signs and symptoms (cues), generates alternative explanations for the cues (diagnostic hypotheses), collects additional data to help rule in or rule out possible explanations, systematically evaluates each explanation in light of the data, and arrives at a diagnosis or inference about the patient's health status. Once sufficient data are gathered, the process of evaluating hypotheses begins.

Intuition

Intuition is characterized by immediate grasping of a clinical situation and is a function of familiarity with similar experiences (Benner et al, 2009). Intuition is a judgment without a rationale. Researchers speculate that intuition is a form of pattern recognition in which the practitioner picks up on cues that are perceived as a whole and are not arrived at through conscious or linear analytic processes. Experienced clinicians develop a sense of salience in which important aspects of a given clinical situation stand out because of past experience with similar situations. Rational calculation is not required to make use of this form of reasoning; however, deliberative rationality may be used to check out the soundness of conclusions derived from intuition. The role and desirability of intuitive reasoning patterns continues to be controversial within the nursing literature.

Intuition has been decried as a poor substitute for science. In this view, intuition is minimized as nothing more than a special case of inference, drawing on rational processes that are unconscious and inaccessible (Crow & Spicer, 1995; English, 1993). Studies in primary care and the application of EBP indicate, however, that intuition is a highly valued form of reasoning and plays a vital role in clinical decision making (Tracy, Dantas, & Upshur, 2003).

Narrative Thinking

Evidence suggests that narratives are an important part of clinical reasoning (Bruner, 1986; Kleinman, 1988). Patient narratives provide us with access to understanding the experience of health and illness. Bruner claims that human motives, intents, and meanings are understood through narrative thinking, which he contrasts with paradigmatic thinking that conforms to the rules of logic. Paradigmatic thinking is thinking through propositional argument. Narrative thinking is thinking through telling and interpreting stories. The difference between these two types of thinking involves how humans make sense of and explain what they see. Propositional argument is making sense of a particular by seeing it as an instance of a general type. Narrative thinking is trying to understand the particular case. It allows us to acknowledge individuals' values and personal experiences as important sources of knowledge that inform the evidence base (Rycroft-Malone et al, 2004). Kleinman has identified the importance of understanding the narrative component of illness, claiming that patient narratives may help clinicians direct their attention not only to the biological world of disease but also to the human world of meanings, values, and concerns.

Hence, patient narratives help clinicians to focus their attention not only on the patient's disease problems but also on the meaning of that illness for the particular patient and on the effect that disease will have on the patient's lifestyle and ways of coping. Hearing the account of an experience with an illness not only improves the understanding of the patient's overall situation, it helps identify problem-solving priorities that cannot be made explicit through disengaged analytical reasoning. Past studies of physicians (Borges & Waitzkin, 1995; Hunter, 1991) and nurses (Benner et al, 2009; Zerwekh, 1992) have suggested that narrative reasoning creates deep background understanding of the patient as a person; consequently, clinicians' judgments can be understood only against this background.

Clinical narratives are a way of teaching and learning from other care providers and a way of reflecting on and understanding one's own practice. Dialoguing with others who have different vantage points will produce knowledge about clinical situations that helps to limit tunnel vision and snap judgments. Using narrative as a way of communicating with other health providers leads to learning how to better identify signs and symptoms in particular patient populations, knowing specific patients and learning to recognize how these patients respond, and identifying clinical experts with whom you can consult (Benner et al, 2009). Discussing your observations and data with more experienced clinicians enhances clinical judgment. Even as an experienced nurse, you consult with colleagues, draw on their perspectives, and benefit from the pooled experience of other clinicians. Clinical narratives and the multiple perspectives of skilled clinicians work together with science and technology to create knowledge that is both cumulative and reliable.

Clinical reasoning can also include processes that might be characterized as engaged practical reasoning. Engaged practical reasoning includes recognition of a pattern, an intuitive clinical grasp, or a response without evident forethought. Conditions of uncertainty are what prompt the seeking, appraising, and implementation of new knowledge by clinicians. Uncertainty occurs when the best course of action to take, or best decision, is not readily apparent. The openness to accept that there may be different, and possibly more effective, methods of care other than those that are currently employed acts as the impetus to weighing evidence against expectations, norms, or standards.

Reflection on Practice Is Often Triggered by a Breakdown in Clinical Judgment

Reflection is defined as a process of thinking about and exploring an issue of concern triggered by an experience. For example, clinicians are often troubled by a patient encounter that did not go well. Reflecting on the meaning of an experience, making sense of it, and incorporating it into one's view of self and the world is part of everyday life. Reflection prompts the clinician to identify new information or alternative perspectives that can be helpful in future encounters. To engage in reflection, the clinician has to be able to connect the patient's response and outcomes with specific clinical actions. Narrative is an important tool of reflection; having and telling stories of one's experience as a clinician helps turn experience into practical knowledge (Aström, Norberg, Hallberg, & Jansson, 1995;

Benner et al, 2009; Rycroft-Malone et al, 2004). Use of reflection is a habit and a skill that can be cultivated and developed over time. Through the introspective process of connecting one's actions to patient outcomes, reflection has the potential for generating new knowledge (Kuiper & Pesut, 2004; Ruth-Sahd, 2003).

Model of Clinical Judgment

A research-based model of clinical judgment developed by Tanner in 1998 and revised in 2006 is presented in **Figure 13.1.** There are four key phases in the model. The first is "noticing," in which the clinician develops a perceptual grasp of the situation at hand. In this phase the clinician's expectations of the situation are formed because of his or her knowledge of the patient; clinical or practical knowledge of similar patients; and textbook and research-based knowledge. The context of the clinical situation will further influence the initial grasp of the situation. The second phase depicted in the model is "interpreting." In this phase the clinician forms an understanding of the situation by using one or more reasoning patterns. Assessments and additional data collection may be conducted to rule out hypotheses until the clinician reaches an interpretation that supports an appropriate response. During the "responding" phase, the clinician may act or choose not to act depending on the situation. "Reflecting" occurs when the clinician observes the patient's responses to the action taken. *Reflection-in-action* refers to the clinician's ability to see how the patient is responding

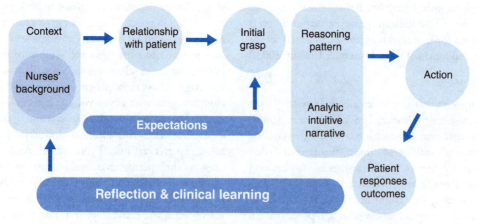

FIGURE 13.1 A model of clinical judgment.

to the action—and adjust the treatment based on that assessment. Much of this reflection-in-action is tacit and not obvious. Reflection-in-action with its subsequent clinical learning completes the cycle, showing that what clinicians gain from their experience contributes to their ongoing clinical knowledge development and their capacity for clinical judgment in future situations.

Summary

The model of clinical judgment presented provides a framework for improving the quality of the clinical judgment used by the APN. First, the model illustrates where in the process of clinical reasoning the knowledge that might be obtained by external evidence can be applied. Second, the model recognizes the value of clinical expertise initially not accounted for by the original proponents of EBP. Third, because the model recognizes a broader range of contextual factors that could affect the patient's responses, it is more inclusive in the types of research that are viewed as valid. Fourth, because the model incorporates the value of knowing the patient in the clinical reasoning process, it supports a model of patient-centered care (IOM, 2001).

ACCESSING AND EVALUATING RESEARCH EVIDENCE TO IMPROVE CLINICAL JUDGMENTS

Several problems exist with using the research literature for evidence-based primary care and hospital practice (Gorman, 2001; Melnyk & Fineout-Overholt, 2014; Shapiro, 2007, 2010). Clinicians are under increasing pressure to keep up-to-date and to base their practice more firmly on evidence, but few feel that they have the necessary time or skills to do this (Melnyk & Fineout-Overholt, 2014; Melnyk et al, 2012; Melnyk, Gallagher-Ford, et al, 2014) or that they work in organizational cultures that support it (Melnyk, Gallagher-Ford, et al, 2014).

Historically, only a small fraction of the total research literature included efficacy studies of clinical practice that form the basis for evidence-based medicine (Haynes, 1993; Shapiro, 2010). Few if any studies addressed appropriateness, meaningfulness, and feasibility of health-care innovations (Shapiro, 2010). Barriers to using research evidence cited in a recent study included the lack of usable information from this source (Melnyk et al, 2012). This has contributed to the complaint of many clinicians that the research literature has limited applicability to clinical practice (McAlister, Graham, Karr, & Laupacis, 1999; Melnyk et al, 2012; Rycroft-Malone et al, 2004).

In the past, most clinicians considered the research literature to be unmanageable (Gorman, 2001; Melnyk et al, 2012; Melnyk & Fineout-Overholt, 2014; Rycroft-Malone et al, 2004; Shapiro, 2007, 2010; Williamson, German, Weiss, Skinner, & Bowes III, 1989). On top of this difficulty, many clinicians do not know how to interpret the statistical results of the studies they do locate (Melnyk et al, 2012; Rycroft-Malone et al, 2004; Windish, Huot, & Green, 2007). If clinical research is to improve clinical care, it must be relevant, of high quality, and accessible, and clinicians must have the skills they need to use it. To address these difficulties, APNs need to build skills sharpening their focus on the outcomes of care, forming clear and researchable questions, accessing the literature and developing strategies for maintaining currency in the research literature, and interpreting its relevance.

To access the best possible evidence at the point of clinical contact, the clinician should work on the development of several competencies that support EBP.

Competencies That Support Evidence-Based Practice

Focusing on Outcomes and Context

Evidence-based medicine has been widely promoted as a means of improving clinical outcomes. To focus on outcomes in medical decision making, Bergus and Hamm (1995) and Sox and colleagues (2007) suggest that clinicians use the following four-step process. First, the clinician forms an internal mental framework for the decision task, sketching out the potential treatment options and outcomes. Next, the variations among the different outcomes are estimated. In collaboration with the patient and family, the values of the potential outcomes are considered. The course of action that, on average, will result in the best outcome is then chosen. The scientific evidence—base rate information, sensitivity, specificity, positive predictive value of a positive test result, and proportion of the population positively affected by certain interventions—is the information needed for estimating the likelihood of achieving different outcomes with different courses of action.

Straus, Glasziou, Richardson, and Haynes (2011), in their guidebook on the practice and teaching of evidence-based medicine, define the best research evidence as patient-centered clinical research into the accuracy and precision of diagnostic tests, prognostic markers, and interventions. These elements of evidence used for predicting outcomes are defined and described in **Table 13.1**. Several practical implications can be drawn from review of the definitions of

TABLE 13.1		
Information Needed for Estimating the Likelihood of Achieving Different Outcomes With Different Courses of Action		
Core Concept	**Definition**	**Features**
Base rate information: prevalence	The proportion of persons in a given population who have a particular disease at a point or interval of time	Useful for health services planning. May be the only rates available. Prevalence studies are particularly useful in guiding decisions about diagnosis and treatment. Knowing that a patient has a given probability of having a disease influences the use and interpretation of diagnostic tests.
Base rate information: incidence	New cases in a specified period	Use incidence rates when (a) you are comparing the development of disease in different population groups; (b) you are attempting to determine whether a relationship exists between a possible causal factor and a disease. Allows you to determine whether the probability of developing a disease differs in different populations or periods in relationship to specific causal factors.
Sensitivity	Proportion of people with the disease who have a positive test	Determines the ability of the test to identify correctly those who have the disease. The more sensitive a test, the more certain you can be that a negative test rules out disease.
Specificity	Proportion of people without the disease who have a negative test	Determines the ability of the test to identify correctly those who do not have the disease. The more specific a test, the more certain you can be that a positive test rules in disease.
Positive predictive value of positive tests	Probability of disease, given the results of a positive test	Sensitivity and specificity are characteristics of the test itself; however, predictive values are influenced by how common the disease is. For diseases of low prevalence, the predictive value of a positive test goes down sharply.
Absolute risk reduction	Difference in adverse event rates between the control and experimental group	Is used to help determine the clinical significance of a treatment—needed to calculate NNT[*]
Number needed to treat	Number of patients needed to treat to prevent one additional bad outcome	Calculated by dividing 1 by the absolute risk reduction. NNT indicates clinical impact of a treatment.
Confidence interval	Range of values on either side	A 99% confidence interval is interpreted of an estimate as the range of values within which one can be 99% sure that the population value lies.
P value	Measure of statistical significance	Specifies the strength of the evidence.

[*]*NNT*, number needed to treat.

the core concepts in the table. For example, to determine the predictive value of a test, clinicians need good estimates of the prevalence or probability of disease in a patient.

A limitation of this approach to best evidence is nursing's interest in questions beyond diagnostic tests and interventions (Jennings, 2000) to include important issues surrounding the context of care (Rycroft-Malone et al, 2004). Although evidence from qualitative exploratory studies is not usually included in texts on evidence-based medicine, these studies are helpful for guiding advanced practice decision making. Appropriateness and meaningfulness, according to Evans (2003) and the Joanna Briggs Institute (2008), addresses the psychosocial aspects of care relating to the patients' experiences, their understanding of health and illness, and the outcomes they hope to achieve from their health-care encounter. These dimensions of care are best addressed with nonexperimental research designs, including both quantitative and qualitative methods (Shapiro, 2010). Change in health-care delivery environments is difficult and evidence of effectiveness and appropriateness may not be enough to overcome problems that surface with change. In addition to the usual sources of high-level evidence, such as randomized controlled trials (RCTs), systematic reviews, observational studies, and interpretive studies may yield good evidence, especially related to aspects of organizational culture that could both affect the ease of acceptance of the new practice and help determine how best to implement it (Evans, 2003). These studies inform our decision making by helping us better understand patient responses. Understanding patient responses is a critical condition for using reflection to engage in clinical learning.

Asking Answerable Questions

The inability to ask a focused and precise clinical question can be a major impediment to EBP. To build skill in asking focused clinical questions, it helps to categorize questions according to their level of specificity and according to whom the question applies, the intervention being considered, and the outcomes of interest.

Clinical questions can be categorized into needs for background and foreground knowledge (Melnyk & Fineout-Overholt, 2014; Straus et al, 2011). Background knowledge is needed when our experience with a condition or problem is limited. Background questions ask *who, what, for whom, why, where, when,* and *how well?* Framing a background question is relatively easy because the question is usually asking in general about a disorder. Finding information to answer background questions is also relatively easy. Sources of information likely to provide answers to these questions include textbooks, drug guides or other reference books, and narrative review articles— summaries of an area or topic written by an expert in the field (McKibbon & Marks, 2001).

As clinicians grow in experience, they have increasing numbers of questions about the foreground of managing patients. Foreground questions are prompted by a precise need for information about a specific clinical situation. This skill of framing foreground questions can be improved by breaking the question down into its component parts. Think about the subjects or groups involved, what intervention is being used, and what the outcomes of interest are. The four key elements of foreground questions are the patient or problem, the intervention or treatment, the comparison intervention or treatment, and the outcome of interest (Melnyk & Fineout-Overholt, 2014; Straus et al, 2011). Foreground questions typically require more information sources to adequately supply the answers (McKibbon & Marks, 2001). For example, questions about treatment effectiveness are best addressed by evidence from an RCT design, whereas questions about patients' feelings and perceptions about their illness experiences are better addressed in studies that use a qualitative design.

Using the Clinical Literature

The clinical literature can be used for regular surveillance or keeping up-to-date and for problem-oriented searches. To conduct searches on a regular basis, clinicians need effective searching skills and easy access to bibliographic databases. After the answerable question has been identified, use the population/problem, intervention, comparison, outcome, time (PICOT) format to help frame the literature search **(Box 13.1)**. The PICOT format is a particularly useful framework to help novice searchers organize their electronic database searches (Craig & Smyth, 2007; Melnyk & Fineout-Overholt, 2014; Shapiro, 2007, 2010; Shapiro & Donaldson, 2008).

Two types of electronic databases are available. The first type is bibliographic and permits users to identify relevant citations in the clinical literature. MEDLINE and the *Cumulative Index to Nursing and Allied Health Literature* are examples of this first sort of database. Google Scholar (http://scholar.google.com) is a new database

---

Box 13.1

PICOT Format

P   Population or problem of interest
I   Intervention or practice of interest
C   Comparison intervention or practice—usually what is currently done
O   Outcome of the intervention or practice
T   Time frame in which outcome is expected

Box 13.2

Appraising Therapy Articles

Critical appraisal questions used to evaluate a therapy article:

Is the study valid?
Was there a clearly defined research question?
Was the assignment of patients to treatments randomized and was the randomization list concealed?
Were all patients accounted for at its conclusion? Was there an "intention-to-treat" analysis?
Were research participants "blinded"?
Were the groups treated equally throughout?
Did randomization produce comparable groups at the start of the trial?
Are the results important?
How large is the treatment effect?
How precise is the finding from the trial?

---

that is also becoming more popular. The second type of database focuses on evidence summaries and takes the user directly to primary or secondary publications of the relevant clinical evidence. Examples of this second type of database include the *Cochrane Database of Systematic Reviews* and the American College of Physicians (ACP) Journal Club, a publication of the ACPs–American Society of Internal Medicine, which abstracts articles on diagnosis, prognosis, treatment, quality of care, and medical economics. The ACP database has been formatted to make clinician searching for answers to clinical questions easier and to help focus searches on the highest rated and most accessed articles (Haynes, 2008, 2009). These databases are available online from libraries and from the organizations themselves via the Internet.

Several tactics can be used to maintain currency in the research and clinical literature (Vincent, Hastings-Tolsma, Gephart, & Alfonzo, 2015). With many journals and library databases, it is possible to set up regular alert notifications when a new article or summary appears on an identified topic or author. It is also possible to get table of content notifications from selected journals. Real Simple Syndication (RSS) feeds are files that Web sites update with their newest content and are used by many databases like PubMed and Web of Science, as well as several journals and news sites. RSS feed aggregators allow you to open an RSS reader app like Feedly and Feedburner and see what is new at many sites all in one location. Another good option is to use Listservs like those offered by the several institutes at the National Institutes of Health. Several mobile apps are available to organize and store PDFs and bibliographic references. Mendeley is a free application that can store references and articles and then be retrieved and be accessible by many different types of

devices. Clinicians should also seek out subscriptions to electronic practice newsletters.

Appraising Evidence From Studies

After evidence has been retrieved, the next step is to evaluate, or appraise, the evidence for its validity and clinical usefulness. Appraisal is crucial because it lets the clinician decide whether the retrieved research literature is reliable enough to give useful guidance. Because several published reports lack sufficient methodological rigor to be reliable enough for answering clinical questions, guidelines for evaluating literature have been developed to assist clinicians without extensive research expertise to evaluate clinical articles.

Box 13.2 shows a typical set of critical appraisal questions for evaluating articles about therapy. These questions were synthesized from several sources (EBP HealthLinks and CEBM Web site; Badenoch & Heneghan, 2006; Straus et al, 2011). Although the questions seem to reflect common sense, they are not entirely self-explanatory. Some assistance is required to help clinicians apply them to specific articles and individual patients. The *Evidence-Based Medicine Toolkit* (Badenoch & Heneghan, 2006) provides guidance on how to answer the appraisal questions that they specifically recommend. For example, on the question

"Were research participants 'blinded'?" the text gives the clinician a definition of the term *blinding* and then might provide an example that would help the clinician decide whether the studies he or she was evaluating met this criteria. In addition to providing a guide for evaluating therapy articles, the *Evidence-Based Medicine Toolkit* has questions for appraising articles on diagnosis, prognosis, and harm (risks for certain diseases or conditions). The *Evidence-Based Medicine Toolkit* is a great resource for beginners. As with any other skill, expertise and speed come with practice. The evidence does not automatically dictate patient care, but it does provide the factual basis on which decisions can be made.

As APNs begin to build their literature critical appraisal skills, several Web sites can be accessed to further refine these skills. The library guide in EBP (http://guides.lib.uw.edu/friendly.php?s=hsl/ebp) at the University of Washington includes an EBP section that contains numerous resources for finding, evaluating, and rating the literature. In addition to this site, the Center for Evidence-Based Medicine (CEBM) has the CATmaker critical appraisal tool (http://www.cebm.net/index.aspx?o=1157), which can be downloaded to help the APN create Critically Appraised Topics (CATs) for the key articles he or she encounters about therapy, diagnosis, prognosis, etiology/harm, and systematic reviews of therapy.

Sources of Primary Clinical and Research Literature

MEDLINE is provided free on the Internet from many sites and at least one of these, PubMed (http://www.ncbi.nlm.nih.gov/pubmed), also includes restored search strategies that are designed to select studies most likely to be relevant and valid for clinical practice. MEDLINE is produced by the National Library of Medicine in Bethesda, Maryland, and is the best-known bibliographic database of indexed medical literature. MEDLINE is searchable by medical subject headings and subheadings, as well as by author, journal, title, and keyword. The journals covered by MEDLINE are noted for their overall reliability and quality; however, the articles still must be scrutinized carefully for their validity and quality as evidence. A hand search of current journals is still one of the best ways to find newly published information. However, this is one of the most time-consuming and labor-intensive approaches

to retrieving evidence. Use of an e-mail alert for the latest table of contents from selected journals can make this strategy less time consuming and more effective.

Using Appraising Summaries

Meta-analysis uses statistical techniques to combine results across studies. Integrative reviews rely on summaries, logical synthesis, and narrative to characterize findings. Research-based guidelines center on care of a particular patient population and specify processes of care associated with good outcomes. Both HealthLinks and the CEBM Web sites have links to several sources of summaries. UpToDate at www.uptodate.com is updated daily and has summaries on many clinical topics. BMJ Clinical Evidence at www.clinicalevidence.com is regularly updated and has clearly outlined explicit review criteria posted.

Meta-Analysis

Meta-analysis requires enough studies with sufficient commonality to provide a valid conclusion. In other words, studies have to be looking more or less at the same outcome and the same intervention. Meta-analysis is often used when several studies have been conducted but findings were inconclusive. Meta-analyses combine the statistical results from several studies into one statistic that can be used to gauge the size of the treatment's impact on the outcome of interest. To do this, first an effect size is calculated for each finding of interest in the studies being reviewed. Then a pooled effect size is calculated for all findings together.

There is controversy about the statistical techniques and assumptions of meta-analysis. Bias in the combined analysis is possible if the selection of studies was flawed or the elimination of methodologically poor studies was not done using an objective process. There are also inherent problems with data pooling, especially if the studies are not similar enough in design, sample size, outcome types, and forms of the independent variables used. Identifying weaknesses in this kind of systematic review can be done by using the guidelines in the *Evidence-Based Medicine Toolkit* (Badenoch & Heneghan, 2006) or by using a similar guide on the HealthLinks or CEBM sites. Once you have examined the major components of the review, you can make a judgment about whether you think it is a high-quality review and whether the findings are valid.

Integrative Research Review

Integrative research reviews do not use statistical techniques to summarize results across studies. Rather, they rely on the logical comparison and synthesis of the reviewer. The integrative research review method is the research synthesis approach used by most review articles in clinical care journals. The quality of these reviews and their resulting conclusions are even more dependent on the reviewer's skill in critical appraisal. High-quality reviews make explicit how studies were selected for review and the rules that were used to judge the overall evidence. The reviewer should state whether some studies were weighted more heavily than others and should provide a rationale for doing so. If some studies were discounted, this also should be described. At present, integrative research review is the only mechanism available for looking at qualitative studies that address the same topic.

Practice Guidelines

Practice guidelines can include formal clinical protocols put forth by a professional organization, clinical paths formed by a practice group, and research-based recommendations that translate conclusions of a meta-analysis or an integrative research review into clinical practice conclusions. A practice guideline should clearly state what the guideline does and does not cover, for what patient group it was designed, the options at each decision point, the actions recommended, and the outcomes associated with each course of action. There should be a clear description of the supporting evidence and how it was gathered and evaluated. Because the literature is always evolving, practice guidelines should be explicit about how current they are. The comprehensiveness of the guideline should also be described. On the HealthLinks site, there is a link to the EBM toolkit that has a practice guidelines appraisal tool.

Locating Sources of Summaries

Ovid (www.ovid.com) has released an integrated literature service called Evidence-Based Medicine Reviews (EBMR). This Web-based service includes the *Cochrane Database of Systematic Reviews, Best Evidence,* MEDLINE, and full-text journals. This resource contains full-text reviews of clinically relevant articles from throughout the medical literature published in EBMR and ACP Journal Club and full-text topic overviews published in the *Cochrane Database of Systematic Reviews,* which is published by the

Cochrane Collaboration. Links between the Ovid databases and EBMR allow users to link from a citation to a review to the full text of that reviewed article and then to other readings referenced in the article.

The *British Medical Journal* (BMJ) publishing group and the ACPs–American Society of Internal Medicine have created *Clinical Evidence,* the first major attempt to provide an up-to-date, evidence-based textbook (www .clinicalevidence.com). Subscribers can choose between receiving the service online via a handbook titled the *Clinical Evidence Handbook* or a combination of the handbook plus online, as well as via PDA, resources. A free trial is permitted to allow potential users the opportunity to explore the usefulness of the service.

The Agency for Healthcare Research and Quality (AHRQ) National Guidelines Clearinghouse provides evidence-based information on health-care outcomes; quality; and cost, use, and access. In examining what works and does not work in health care, AHRQ's mission includes both translating research findings into better patient care and providing policy makers and other health-care leaders with information needed to make critical health-care decisions. Reports compiled by EBP centers are available on a range of topics and can cover several therapies for a given condition. By using your browser's "Find" feature, you can quickly locate a given topic.

The Cochrane Collaboration produces a structured database of high-quality systematic reviews of RCTs. Originally established in Britain, it is presently composed of numerous centers in several countries. Reviews involve exhaustive searches for all RCTs, both published and unpublished, on a particular topic. One limitation of the database is that the reviews focus mainly on therapies, although an increasing number of reviews on diagnostic topics are being developed. The studies are analyzed using standardized methodology and meta-analysis. The Cochrane Library, now managed by Wiley, contains high-quality, independent evidence to inform health-care decision making. It includes reliable evidence from Cochrane and other systematic reviews, clinical trials, and more. Cochrane reviews bring you the combined results of the world's best medical research studies and are recognized as the gold standard in evidence-based health care.

Nursing-specific resources for evidence reviews have also been developed. The Joanna Briggs Institute (JBI; at www.joannabriggs.org), based in Australia, is committed

Box 13.3

Clinical Significance Appraisal Process: Questions to Guide Thinking

To determine applicability to practice, answer the following questions:

Were the subjects similar to patients for whom you might provide care now or in the future?

Could you base an intervention on the findings of this external evidence?

Would any intervention you might identify be within your scope of practice?

What does the body of evidence say about the general question that motivated the inquiry?

What actions does the body of evidence warrant?

to evidence translation and use worldwide. JBI produces evidence summaries and provides guidelines on evidence application to practice. The *Online Journal of Knowledge Synthesis for Nursing* is a peer-reviewed online journal dedicated to the scientific advancement of EBP in health care. The journal presents current scientific evidence to inform clinical decisions and ongoing discussions on issues, methods, clinical practice, and teaching strategies for evidence-based practice. Each article is written as a synthesis of research studies on a single topic and concludes with practice implications.

Clinical Significance and Appraisal Process

Having identified evidence that is both valid and relevant, the next step in using the evidence is to make a judgment about applying the evidence with your patient in your setting. **Box 13.3** provides a list of questions that clinicians can use to make a judgment about the clinical application of the research findings. You must determine whether your patient is sufficiently similar to the study participants for the results to be applicable. Critical factors that can affect generalizability include demographics such as race, age, and gender. Other factors to consider relate to the feasibility of implementation of the proposed intervention, diagnostic

test, and so on. Once the clinician has weighed the clinical use of the evidence and determined that implementation is feasible or desirable, he or she can either implement it directly in a patient's care or use it to develop protocols and guidelines.

EVIDENCE-BASED PRACTICE AND ATTITUDE

This chapter should not be considered a stand-alone resource for learning the principles of EBP. It is almost impossible to learn how to search effectively and appraise efficiently without the help of others and without good resources. Working in groups is the best method to master these skills. Share the task of searching and appraising with others. Use secondary publications such as the *Best Evidence* text developed by the BMJ publishing group. Develop a system for storing work and sharing it with others. Electronic information storage and retrieval systems are evolving rapidly, so continued updates in the available technology are necessary. When evidence is used to inform clinical judgment, the APN can take advantage of new knowledge developments so that care can be more individualized, effective, streamlined, and dynamic.

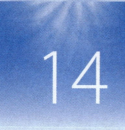

Advocacy and the Advanced Practice Registered Nurse

Andrea Brassard

Learning Outcomes

Learning outcomes expected as a result of this chapter:

- Demonstrate skills needed to advocate for consumers, families, and public policy change.
- Present health and wellness coaching as a model of advocacy.
- Identify examples of advanced practice registered nurse (APRN) advocacy.

INTRODUCTION

The health-care delivery system is a complicated maze of services with many gates and gatekeepers. Not surprisingly, consumers often need help navigating their way through this intimidating maze. The advanced practice registered nurse (APRN) is well positioned to advocate for individual consumers and families who confront barriers to getting the health-care services they need. APRNs can also advocate for systemic changes to remove the barriers. It takes education, sophistication, and determination to advocate at both of these levels. This chapter provides the context for advocacy and advocacy education. Advocacy and health coaching are described as well as examples of individual,

family, and consumer-driven systems-level advocacy. Nurse advocates in each of the four APRN roles are highlighted. Web-based resources for APRN advocacy are provided.

CONTEXT FOR ADVOCACY

Nursing leaders Florence Nightingale, Sojourner Truth, Lillian Wald, and Margaret Sanger are testaments to the nursing profession's historic roots in championing improved health care, especially for the most vulnerable among us (Mason, Gardner, Outlaw, & O'Grady, 2016). These pioneers advanced human rights, compassionate care, and lasting societal changes.

Advocacy is derived from the Latin *advocatus,* which means one who summons to give evidence (Gates, 1995). *Advocate* is a noun and a verb—to act for, speak for, plead for, or defend. *Advocacy* has been described as informing, advising, or counseling (Gadow, 1980, 1989; Kohnke, 1982; Mitchell & Bournes, 2000).

The American Nurses Association (ANA) *Guide to the Code of Ethics for Nurses* 2015 defines advocacy as "the act or process of pleading for, supporting, or recommending a cause or course of action. Advocacy may be for persons . . . or for an issue" (ANA, 2015, p. 37). The ANA *Code of Ethics* calls on nurses to promote, advocate for, and protect patients' rights, health, and safety. Advocacy is based in the fundamental principles of respect for human dignity, the right to self-determination, and primacy of the patient's interests (ANA, 2015).

Nurse leaders, researchers, and educators have described philosophical foundations for advocacy (Curtain, 1979), required skills (Connolly, 1999), and curricula (Jones, 1982). Advocacy is highly desirable, an indicator of excellence in practice, and a domain in advanced practice nursing (Benner, 1984; Gadow, 1980; Millette, 1993). Nurses occupy a middle ground between the consumer and the health-care system, an optimal place to mediate (Bishop & Scudder, 1990; Stein, Watts, & Howell, 1990).

Historically, advocacy has been linked to the potential powerlessness of a patient, although the rising power of the consumer affects our definitions of advocacy (Hewitt, 2002). Advocacy must be distinguished from paternalism and consumerism (Schroeder & Gadow, 2000). Paternalism is the commitment to making decisions for the client because the professional is obligated to impose expertise on behalf of the person in need. Professionals often presume that a person in need is incapable of rational judgment. In contrast, consumerism includes the commitment to remain uninvolved in client decisions. Persons in need are presumed to be capable of rational judgment and their right to self-determination must be respected (Schroeder & Gadow, 2000).

ADVOCACY AND COACHING

A newer model of patient advocacy is health and wellness coaching. Eileen O'Grady, APRN and wellness coach, empowers clients to take an active role in their own health (Gardner, 2014). Coaching involves teaching clients to advocate for themselves for self-care and within the complicated health-care system. It is a natural extension of nursing practice (Hess, Dossey, Southard, Luck, Schaub, Bark, 2013). Health coaching goes beyond patient education; coaches empower clients to set and keep wellness goals (Swarbrick et al, 2011). Health coaches acknowledge clients as experts in their own care (Hess, Dossey, Southard, Luck, Schaub, Bark, 2013). Health coaches and advocates recognize what an individual is striving for, identify goals and values, and respect the person's choices (Thrasher, 2002). Health coaches increase the options that are available to clients in order to allow them to exercise control over their lives. Health coaches are often care coordinators who use their advocacy skills to help clients negotiate the complex health-care system.

LEVELS OF ADVOCACY

Definitions of advocacy focus on the individual and family or public policy, suggesting two levels of advocacy for APRNs. Client-focused definitions of advocacy emphasize enhancing client autonomy and assisting clients in voicing their values (Connolly, 1999). At the individual and family client level, the APRN uses a set of skills to help people identify their needs and obtain services and provides coaching to meet those needs. Public policy-focused advocacy aims to influence legislators and policy makers to change laws or policies with the ultimate goal of improving public health (Taylor, 2016). At the public policy level of advocacy, the APRN uses many of the same skills needed at the individual/family level—and some new ones—to advocate for changes in the health-care delivery system itself.

Advocacy at the Individual and Family Levels

The client-focused definition of advocacy speaks to patient advocacy, which focuses on individual patients and their families. The most dominant model for patient advocacy comes from the counseling paradigm. Burgeoning during the civil rights and women's movements of the 1960s and 1970s, nurses were moving past previous modes of subservience to physicians and institutions to a direct relationship with the patient. Inherent in that relationship is the recognition that the nurse has the authority that comes with a claim to a scientific body of knowledge that is not fully accessible to the lay person (Abbot, 1988). The nurse's ethical responsibility is to transfer as much of that knowledge as possible to the patient and support that person in making informed choices. Patient advocacy becomes teaching, nonjudgmental support of the person's choices and assistance in acting on those choices (Hanks, 2010).

The counseling model is the mainstay of advanced practice nursing at the individual and family levels. The more contemporary "consumer empowerment" model reminds us that most people do not want or need continual counseling by professionals. Consumers are breaking away from the medical model orientation that assumes that health professionals know what is best to "protect" patients. Nurses who define advocacy primarily as protecting patients (Foley, Minick, & McKee, 2002) may have difficulty with the contemporary principles of consumer self-advocacy. Consumers do not seek paternalistic protection. They do seek professionals who can help them navigate the system, a high priority for consumers and families who define advocacy as "a go-between who knows the system and will advise you" (Connolly, 1999, p. 390).

The skills and competencies needed by APRN patient advocates include empathetic listening, self-confidence, assertiveness, negotiation, collaboration, communication, physical assessment, mental status assessment, crisis intervention, case management, change agency, and teaching (Connolly, 1999). Clearly all these skills are within the scope and education of APRNs. However, paramount to the success of the patient advocate is a philosophical foundation that individuals, particularly those who are vulnerable and suffer from any disease or impairment, are unique human beings who deserve and require respect, dignity, and the right to make decisions concerning their lives. Advocacy for patients and families is a fundamental part of the nursing process.

Advocacy Exemplar: Individual and Family Level

There are many ways that APRNs can advocate at the individual and family level. The case example that follows provides one exemplar.

The complex issues of removing children from their families and placing them with adoption services while negotiating a difficult, fragmented child protection system provides fertile ground and many opportunities for APRNs to demonstrate their role as advocates. The overburdened,

disjointed systems make it difficult for members of a care team to understand the complexities of an individual seeking to regain custody of his or her children. In many ways, the individual is alone, pitted against a group of professionals representing the children—professionals who barely have time to communicate. Negotiating the system is a complex, difficult endeavor.

Individual and family advocacy can be valuable to individuals attempting to navigate these systems. Vulnerable populations such as the poor and uninsured, victims of abuse, single mothers, and individuals with developmental disabilities or mental illness are in particular need of advocacy services. These individuals are often prohibited from participating in decisions regarding health care (Schroeder & Gadow, 2000). Professionals identify themselves as the expert authority, thereby disempowering the individuals and destroying the possibility of an equal (or mutual) relationship between an individual and professional. APRN advocates can counter the effects of this paternalistic system by enhancing personal autonomy and participating with individuals in determining their needs (Schroeder & Gadow, 2000).

The Case of Maria

This case study describes Maria and her involvement in the family court system and illustrates how an APRN can identify barriers within a multifaceted system; plan, coordinate, and monitor services; and follow up with other advocates within the system.

Maria is a 30-year-old, single mother of four. Her involvement with the court began several years ago when her estranged husband abused their oldest daughter. Maria herself had also been the victim of his abuse. Although she left her husband shortly after her daughter's abuse, three of her four children were placed in foster care. The fourth child resided with Maria's mother and Maria participated fully in this daughter's daily life. Maria enjoyed a close and loving relationship with her intact family, which included a sister.

Maria was referred to a psychiatric-mental health APRN by a family court as part of a child welfare mediation process of planning for the future of the three children in foster care. Concurrently, the APRN collaborated with a university law school, a court-appointed mediator, various child protection case managers, and Maria's attorney. The APRN provided strength-based case management services (Sullivan, 1991), counseling, and support to Maria during court-mediated meetings, as well as links to services identified by the client and nurse.

In addition to attending monthly mediation hearings over a 6-month period, the APRN met with Maria weekly. Maria was a quiet, shy young woman who exhibited developmental and speech delays. Her affect was depressed and she expressed feelings of hopelessness and despair. The legal system had, in fact, determined that three of her four children would be placed for adoption. Maria, on the other hand, expressed a strong desire to be reunited with her family. In particular, Maria wanted to regain custody of her oldest daughter.

The APRN used the strengths-based case management model (Sullivan, 1991) in her assessment. Maria had several strengths. She was young, relatively healthy, and able to identify solid family supports. She expressed a fervent desire to care for her children and demonstrated a willingness to discuss difficult, painful issues. She expressed a strong desire to follow the recommendations of the court, although she sometimes found it difficult to do so. In addition to reuniting her family, her personal goals were to obtain a high school diploma and get a driver's license and a car. The ocean was less than an hour away and she dreamed of driving to the beach with her children to see the ocean for the first time.

Initially, Maria did not make eye contact with the APRN and answered questions only after careful thought. The nurse construed this to mean that Maria was searching for the answer she thought the nurse wanted to hear. Her feelings of powerlessness and hopelessness were highlighted during the first mediation meeting when the nurse noted that no one in the room spoke to Maria. They spoke about and around her. For her part, Maria sat quietly listening to the discussion about the future of her family.

Victims of abuse require empowerment and advocacy (Shea, Mahoney, & Lacey, 1997). Creating and sustaining a therapeutic caring relationship, encouraging self-determination, and supporting patient decisions are essential (Shea, Mahoney, &

Lacey, 1997). The APRN needs to communicate a sense of hope while establishing realistic expectations for success to promote client empowerment and independence.

In order to break the coercive control that abusers have over their victims, nurses need to avoid using interventions that represent further control of the victim, thereby perpetuating the cycle of abuse (Shea, Mahoney, & Lacey, 1997). Advocates must be wary and avoid paternalistic relationships, exercising care in understanding the needs and desires of those in need of their services (Mitchell & Bournes, 2000).

The primary issue preventing Maria from regaining custody of her children was their safety. Maria's estranged husband had continued to contact her despite the fact that there was a restraining order against all contact with her or the children. Maria felt powerless and clearly did not know how to react when this occurred. The APRN and university law school advocates discovered that Maria had never been provided with a copy of the restraining order. The university law school advocates obtained a copy of the order and gave Maria clear, concise instructions regarding its implementation. In addition, they arranged for Maria to receive a free cell phone from a battered women's shelter, enabling her to call 911 in the event of an emergency. For additional security, the APRN and Maria located a safe house and developed an escape plan.

Several other issues were apparent to the APRN nurse and university law school advocates in this case. First, before the nurse and law school involvement, Maria's only advocate throughout the process had been a very caring but overburdened court-appointed attorney. Although he did everything he could to assist Maria, time constraints and the inability to assess Maria's cognitive deficits limited his ability to assist her. On the other hand, the children had individual case managers, the Department of Youth and Family Services, the assistant attorney general, child advocates, individual therapists, and numerous others working on their behalf. It was easy to understand why the court and mediation process were intimidating to Maria and how they contributed to her feelings of hopelessness and powerlessness. A second issue that affected

Maria's need for advocacy was that many individuals involved in her case scheduled her appointments at overlapping times without consideration for the time or money required to keep them. In addition, Maria had difficulty reading, a fact that was unknown to any of the individuals involved in her case.

The APRN needed to help overcome all these barriers. Reinforcing her strengths, she helped Maria find hope tempered with realistic expectations. In addition to arming her with the restraining order, cell phone, and escape plan, the APRN helped her obtain a city bus pass and a color-coded calendar she could read to help her keep her appointments. She also helped her enroll in high school general equivalency diploma classes. This set of advocacy interventions helped set in motion immediate and long-term forces of self-empowerment for Maria.

In the end, the court changed its position and granted Maria custody of her oldest daughter. The two younger children were placed for adoption in the foster home they had resided in for several years. Although Maria was distraught over the loss, she was able to meet the family, who invited her to remain involved in the children's lives.

In this case study, the APRN used Sullivan's strength-based case management model to guide her advocacy efforts. She identified strengths as well as gaps in the system and applied practical solutions to overlooked troubles. The interventions built on Maria's strengths, supported her autonomy, and ultimately enhanced her self-esteem. Collaborating with child protective services and others involved in the case created an environment wherein the advocates identified an opportunity to propose meaningful interventions and broaden the range of options to Maria that had long been overlooked by the team.

Systems-Level Advocacy

Systems-level advocacy is nursing practice at the population or community level. Public health nurses think of it as "upstream thinking." For example, an APRN can treat a child with lead poisoning and help navigate the child and his family through specialty clinics and lead abatement programs case by case. However, a more upstream advocacy approach would be to prevent lead poisoning through strict preventive policies and programs for abating all houses with lead paint. Consumers need both levels and APRNs can be engaged in both levels with different intensity. Although not all APRNs desire a policy-level advocacy role, they can support policies and programs that their nursing colleagues are advancing on behalf of consumers.

The advocacy skills that APRNs need to successfully advocate for individuals and families are foundational for systems-level advocacy. Advocacy at this level usually involves developing new policies, programs, or regulations, or at least changing the old way of doing things enough to make a difference for the people that nurses serve. Communication skills are crucial. Active listening skills are as important as verbal skills; indeed, more insight is gained from listening than from speaking. Insight into the problem leads to more creative problem solving and ideas for negotiating system solutions. Negotiation is more complex at the systems level than at the individual and family levels because generally there are more stakeholders involved when advocating policies and programs. The APRN needs to be assertive enough to overcome resistance to change and collaborative enough to create or join with others who can help advance the advocacy goal.

To be most effective at the systems level, APRNs need to understand program and policy development. The stage-sequential model described by Hanley (2002) can guide this process. The first stage is identifying a policy problem and getting that problem placed on the policy discussion and action agendas in the appropriate forum (i.e., state or federal legislature, administrative agencies, funding organizations, and the like). Developing policy options with supporting budget, infrastructures, and regulations follows. Program implementation and evaluation are the final stages. Moving through these stages requires an understanding of the change process in general with skill development in creating and sustaining a vision for change, anticipating and dealing with resistance to change, developing a broad base of support, and understanding the art of compromise. Systems-level advocacy requires determination and persistence.

Few APRNs will choose to lead this kind of systems advocacy. But many will choose to support or resist it. At a minimum, APRNs need to understand systems advocacy. Systems advocacy involves citizenship and a call for participation in the decisions that affect our lives and the lives of those we serve (Joel, 1998; Paquin, 2011).

Consumer-Driven Systems-Level Advocacy

Nurses can lead systems advocacy efforts both as professionals and as consumers. One case example comes from AARP (formerly the American Association of Retired Persons). This exemplar is driven by nurses and nurse advocates working in a consumer organization and illustrates several of the themes in the literature on advocacy, including the following:

- Advocacy is an activity that is not owned by one sector of health care.
- The consumer is an expert.
- Advocacy is a partnership between consumers and professionals.
- Advocacy calls for the development of creative strategies.

Advocacy Exemplar: CARE Act

Most family caregivers perform complex medical/nursing tasks with very little guidance, according to a groundbreaking study by the AARP Public Policy Institute and the United Hospital Fund entitled *Home Alone: Family Caregivers Providing Complex Chronic Care* (Reinhard, Levine, & Samis, 2012). AARP surveyed family caregivers across the country to get a look at the type of help they were providing and found that they were providing much more complex care than many had thought:

- Nearly half were performing some kind of medical/nursing tasks or medication management.
- Most did not get any training to perform these tasks.
- Most care recipients did not have home visits by a health-care professional.
- Understandably, family caregivers performing medical/nursing tasks were most likely to report feeling stressed and worried about making a mistake.
- More than half reported feeling down, depressed, or hopeless in the last 2 weeks, and more than a third reported fair or poor health. These negative impacts increased with the number of the care recipients' chronic conditions (Reinhard, Levine, & Samis, 2012).

Family caregivers reported receiving little formal training in medical/nursing tasks such as managing medications, performing wound care, or operating medical equipment, despite patients' frequent hospitalizations. When nurses in selected hospitals, nursing homes, and home care agencies were surveyed about how well they trained family caregivers, most were very positive. Family caregivers of patients who had been discharged from the same settings did not agree (Levine, Halper, Rutberg, & Gould, 2013). "Staff may have indeed given family caregivers . . . information, but not in a way that those family caregivers understood and could use" (Levine et al, 2013, p. 20).

In response to the *Home Alone* report, AARP developed model legislation to help family caregivers get the recognition, information, and instruction they needed to perform the complex medical/nursing tasks that they were often expected to perform. The Caregiver Advise, Record, Enable (CARE) Act required hospitals to ask patients to designate a caregiver, to notify the caregiver before discharge, and to educate the caregiver in medical/nursing tasks they will be expected to perform ("New state law to help family caregivers"). Educating caregivers on medical/nursing tasks included providing training and the opportunity for return demonstration of procedures.

Implementing the CARE Act in hospital settings has been uneven. Although hospitals may identify the family caregivers on admission paperwork, especially if they are the next of kin, other aspects of the CARE Act such as timely notification of discharge are more difficult to enforce. Educating caregivers on medical/nursing tasks may only consist of "telling." Many hospitals do not allow anyone other than a hospital employee to perform medical/nursing tasks on a hospital patient, so there is no opportunity for return demonstrations. APRNs in hospital settings have needed to advocate for institutional policy changes to allow caregivers to perform procedures such as insulin administration or tracheostomy suctioning to their hospitalized loved one (Personal communication, Sincere McMillan, June 7, 2016).

ADVOCACY TO REMOVE BARRIERS TO APRN PRACTICE AND CARE

Chapter 6, "Advanced Practice Nurses and Prescriptive Authority," describes statutory and regulatory barriers to APRN practice and care (Towers, 2017). Recall from

Chapter 6 that the first recommendation of the landmark 2011 Institute of Medicine (IOM) report, *The Future of Nursing: Leading Change, Advancing Health,* is to remove scope-of-practice barriers to enable APRNs to practice to the full extent of their education and training (IOM, 2011). Since the report was released, significant progress has been made in removing state and federal barriers to APRN practice and care.

The *Campaign for Action* is coordinated through the Center to Champion Nursing in America, an initiative of AARP Foundation, AARP, and the Robert Wood Johnson Foundation (RWJF). AARP leads the *Campaign's* advocacy efforts. Several years ago AARP endorsed the major recommendations of *The Future of Nursing* report and changed its policy book to recommend that states should "amend current . . . licensing laws to allow APRNs to perform duties for which they have been educated and certified" (AARP Policy Book, 2016). The *Campaign for Action* Web site details progress that has been made in removing state and federal barriers to APRN practice and care through the efforts of APRNs, AARP state offices, and other advocates.

HOW NURSES LEARN ADVOCACY

Whether advocating for individuals and families or advocating for system changes that will support them better, APRNs need to develop advocacy skills. Developing these skills takes practice. The expert nurse learns the advocacy role through regular dialogue with other members of the nursing community, the patient, the patient's family, and other clinicians (Benner, 1991). New APRNs need nurturing and administrative support to take on this role (Foley et al, 2002).

Fundamental to nursing is the understanding of each individual as a unique human being and of the needs created by their illness or condition. This knowledge is acquired through the nurse-patient relationship and therefore is distinctly nursing knowledge. Recognition that it is the individual, not the professional, who can make decisions for himself or herself calls for a synthesis of this knowledge and an understanding that "freedom, respect and integrity are essential to our full development as a person" (Foley et al, 2002, p. 3).

Application of this philosophy may be more deeply rooted in a value system than in a learning process (Foley et al, 2002). In their study, Foley and colleagues found that advocating for others was a natural and important aspect of practice rather than a learned process. The value of advocacy stems from family and community experience and is integral to their (nurses') being as persons. Although the value of advocacy cannot be taught, faculty "may need to define advocacy in relationship to patient care" (Foley et al, 2002, p. 185).

Nurses can learn how to advocate by watching other nurses interact with patients and providers and by working with mentors (Foley et al, 2002). Role modeling and dialogue provide opportunities for positive learning experiences. Expert APRNs are positioned to provide examples and communication strategies necessary for developing advocacy. Throughout the process of role modeling and mentoring, validation and a supportive environment are necessary if nurses are to gain the confidence required to advocate for patients (Foley et al, 2002). New APRNs require corroboration that their practice and judgment are correct. Experienced APRN preceptors who recognize the risk taken by new APRNs in revealing their knowledge deficits create positive learning experiences and support a foundation for the development of advocacy practice. One-to-one mentoring can help new APRNs consciously learn how to advocate (Foley et al, 2002).

ADVOCACY IS AN ESSENTIAL COMPONENT OF MASTER'S EDUCATION

Advocacy is one of the American Association of Colleges of Nursing (AACN) Essentials of Master's Education. Master's education prepares the APRN to advocate for "policies that improve the health of the public and the profession of nursing" (AACN, 2011, p. 21). Learning strategies include analyzing roles, empowerment, and values clarification needed to be an effective advocate. Additional learning strategies include preparing a position paper on a policy issue that advocates for a solution that is politically feasible and economically viable. As more APRNs are educated at the doctoral level, formal education in advocacy will increase. Doctor of nursing practice (DNP) graduates are able to "design, implement and advocate for health policy that addresses issues of social justice and equity in health care" (AACN, 2006, p. 13). Additionally, DNP graduates are educated to engage in systems-level advocacy by engaging in political action (AACN, 2006). See **Boxes 14.1** and **14.2** for examples of APRN roles and resources.

Box 14.1

Advocacy Examples in APRN Roles

Family Nurse Practitioner Advocates to Decrease Childhood Obesity in North Carolina

Sandy Blizzard Tripp, DNP, FNP-BC, provides pediatric primary care in eastern North Carolina. Dr. Tripp advocates to reduce the high rates of childhood obesity by collaborating with political leaders, school officials, child nutrition directors, and farmers to offer healthier options for school meals. Dr. Tripp also advocates for children and their parents through motivational interviewing and health coaching (Reardon, 2015).

Clinical Nurse Specialist Advocates to Increase Advance Directives

Meehan (2009) describes the efforts of a clinical nurse specialist (CNS) on a cardiac surgery unit to advocate for institutional change in the advance directive process. CNSs are expert communicators with patients and families, role models and educators, and leaders of change in health organizations. The CNS improved the advance directive process in the patient, nursing, and system spheres (Meehan, 2009).

Certified Nurse-Midwives Advocate for Women

Certified nurse-midwives (CNMs) have been described as equal parts nurse, coach, and advocate (Cleveland Clinic, 2014). Callister and Freeborn (2007) interviewed 10 CNMs practicing in Utah who described their advocacy for women in direct care (micro level) and in complex health-care systems (macro level). Advocacy is essential to increasing access to certified nurse-midwifery care, which has been shown to improve pregnancy outcomes (ACNM, 2012).

Certified Registered Nurse Anesthetist Advocates for Interventional Pain Management

W. Keith Barnhill, CRNA, PhD, ARNP, received the 2015 Ira P. Gunn for Outstanding Professional Advocacy from the American Association of Nurse Anesthetists. Dr. Gunn is a crusader for CRNAs administering pain management. "His everyday life is a lesson in advocating effectively" for his profession (AANA, 2015 i).

Box 14.2

Advocacy Resources for APRNs

- American Association of Colleges of Nursing
  - AACN's Advocacy at Work for You **http://www.aacn.nche.edu/government-affairs/AACN-Advocacy-Brochure.pdf**
  - APRN Advocacy **http://www.aacn.nche.edu/government-affairs/aprn-scope-of-practice**
  - State Advocacy **http://www.aacn.nche.edu/government-affairs/state-advocacy**
- American Association of Critical-Care Nurses–Advocacy 101 Tool Kit **https://innovations.ahrq.gov/qualitytools/implementing-abcde-bundle-bedside**
- American Association of Nurse Anesthetists–Advocacy **http://www.aana.com/advocacy/Pages/default.aspx**
- American Association of Nurse Practitioners–Advocacy Center **https://www.aanp.org/legislation-regulation/advocacy-center**
- American College of Nurse Midwives–Advocacy **http://www.acnm.org/Advocacy**
- American Nurses Association
  - Policy and Advocacy **http://nursingworld.org/MainMenuCategories/Policy-Advocacy**
  - Advanced Practice Nurses **http://nursingworld.org/EspeciallyForYou/AdvancedPracticeNurses**
- Future of Nursing: *Campaign for Action*
  - Lessons Learned: Gaining Full Practice Authority in Nebraska http://campaignforaction.org/resource/lessons-learned-gaining-full-practice-authority-nebraska/

Box 14.2

Advocacy Resources for APRNs (*Continued*)

- Lobbying Basics **http://campaignforaction.org/resource/lobbying-basics/**
- Lobbying for Action Coalitions **http://campaignforaction.org/resource/lobbying-considerations-action-coalitions/**
- The Evidence Shows: Better Laws Mean Better, More Accessible Care **http://campaignforaction.org/resource/evidence-shows-better-laws-mean-better-accessible-care/**
- National Association of Clinical Nurse Specialists–Advocacy and Policy **http://nacns.org/professional-resources/toolkits-and-reports/**
- National Association of Pediatric Nurse Practitioners –Advocacy **https://www.napnap.org/advocacy**

CONCLUSION

Advocacy is an essential APRN role. APRN educators and preceptors are responsible for teaching APRN students how to advocate. APRN organizations advocate to remove state and federal barriers to APRN practice and care. APRNs in all roles and settings have the opportunity and responsibility to advocate on behalf of their clients, their profession, and the public. Advocacy is key.

15

Case Management and Advanced Practice Nursing

Denise Fessler* and Irene McEachen*

HISTORICAL BACKGROUND

Case management and advanced practice nursing share a long history in the United States. Although these concepts have been coined in nursing literature only for the last two decades (Tahan, 1998), their roots can be found in nursing history as early as the 1860s (Kersbergen, 1996). Reading between the lines of health-care and nursing history, it is possible to witness the evolution of the process of nurses with expert clinical knowledge who manage care. With the passage of the Patient Protection and Affordable Care Act of 2010 (PPACA) the evolution continues, and at a more accelerated pace.

---

* Earlier versions of this chapter were authored by Patricia M. Haynor and Marylou Yam with Denise Fessler and Irene McEachen.

The case management process was used in the 1860s in early settlement houses for immigrants and the poor. Information was collected on family needs, required services were identified and delivered, and a system of follow-up was designed to ensure appropriateness and continuity (Reynolds & Smeltzer, 1997). In 1901, Mary Richmond, a social services pioneer, published a model of case coordination with the client as the core concern. Richmond's concern for her clients revolved around the lack of communication and coordination that frequently resulted in the duplication of services as clients moved through the system (Weil & Karls, 1985).

U.S. public health nursing was founded toward the end of the 19th century by Lillian Wald (Dock, 1937). The work of the public health nurse was to respond to the needs of the populations at greatest risk in society (i.e., new immigrants living in tenement housing) and to provide ways to reduce illness and promote health (Wald, 1915). Wald was considered a visionary not only for her pioneering work in public health but also for the establishment of a nationwide system of insurance for home-based care and the recognition of the independence and accomplishments of public health nurses. Interestingly, the public health nurses in the early 1900s were not subject to physician orders and established themselves as health educators and promoters of wellness (Frachel, 1988). The following quote from an editorial in *The Public Health Nurse,* although written in 1919 about public health nurses, could easily appear in today's literature referring to the advanced practice nurse (APN) (Profession of Promoting Health, 1919, p. 12):

> Why not come boldly forth, one and all, and claim the right to exercise the promotion of health as a profession? The best-educated nurses spend as many years in training to exercise their profession as physicians to prepare themselves for the care and scientific prevention of disease.

These public health nurses were perceived as the elite in nursing because they practiced autonomously and creatively (Reverby, 1987). The clinical expertise of these nurses is explained historically by the presentation of practice stories using an approach that seeks to understand the narrative without preconceived expectations or judgment (Palmer, 1969). Several competencies of the public health nurse were readily elicited from historical anecdotes: public health nurses' activities included "making inquiries,

shrewd identification of evidence, steady plodding, helping others to help themselves, teaching, explanation and demonstration, and organizing a household to knit the family" (Zerwekh, 1992, p. 85). In short, this could be a description of today's APN. Wald's (1915) early experiments in community-based care left a rich legacy that is still pertinent in today's health-care environment. Her work suggested that we (a) create a mix of public and private programs that link effectively with health-care institutions as "value-added" or complementary to client needs, (b) use evidence-based practice as a counterbalance to document cost versus effectiveness, (c) institute sufficient control over practice to produce desired outcomes, and (d) have expert practitioners with sufficient education and abilities to manage complex care (Buhler-Wilkerson, 1993).

Wald's legacy is similar to the interdisciplinary definition of case management that was developed by the Case Management Society of America (CMSA), defining case management as "a collaborative process of assessment, planning, facilitation and advocacy for options and services to meet an individual's and family's health needs through *comprehensive* communication and available resources to promote quality cost effective outcomes" (CMSA, 2016, p. 8). The historical anecdotes of Wald's public health nurses demonstrated the work of an expert nurse who managed care for individuals and populations. These nurses practiced the core functions of case management: assessment, planning, linking, monitoring, advocacy, and outreach.

In the early 1900s, as an expansion of the role of the community-based public health nurse caring for individuals, the federal government mandated the United States Public Health Service to develop a system of case management with the community as the client. Their initial charge was to coordinate larger environmental problems such as sanitation and the prevention and control of epidemics. The 1920s saw the development of the Community Chest Movement and other social planning agencies (excluding nursing) to deal with coordinating care for families in distress and abused children. Within this same period, child guidance centers were created that experimented with multidisciplinary team planning (including nursing) to avoid duplication or fragmentation of services (Kersbergen, 1996). The thrust to address individual needs through the United States Public Health Service did not occur until passage of the Social Security Act in 1935, which provided funds to support these activities (Shonick, 1988).

After World War II, the Veterans Administration established a center in Los Angeles for veterans' benefits, which was its first model for "one-stop" health care. This was the inception of its ongoing model for a continuum of care (Weil & Karls, 1985).

The 1960s and 1970s witnessed a proliferation of human services because of the Civil Rights Movement and President Johnson's "War on Poverty" (Weil & Karls, 1985). This proliferation of newly developed programs resulted in fragmented, duplicative, and uncoordinated services that were difficult for the public to navigate. Case management enabled the consumer to become an active participant in services provided. Additional programs for the mentally ill and mentally challenged, and legislation for health services to the military, continued to encourage integration of services and the development of a continuum of care. Demonstration projects in the 1970s created the role of "systems agent," a person charged with coordinating system resources for clients and accountability for success of this movement (Intagliata, 1982).

In the 1980s, with the initiation of the prospective payment system that included reimbursement based on diagnosis-related groups (DRGs), case management services moved beyond public health and the mentally ill and veterans' administration services into the acute-care hospitals. At the same time health insurance companies initiated case management to shorten hospital stays and coordinate and manage services for participants with high costs or catastrophic illnesses (Brault & Kissinger, 1991; Mollica & Gillespie, 2003). The entrance of health maintenance organizations (HMOs) and preferred provider organizations (PPOs) as insurance products for prepaid health-care delivery added to the frenzy to control costs while delivering quality care. The efforts to coordinate services and control costs affected the majority of health-care consumers by the late 1980s as prepaid or per-case payment systems became the norm in both private and public sectors. At the start of the 21st century HMOs and PPOs are giving way to accountable care organizations (ACOs) and medical homes (Watson, 2011). Controlling costs remains the mainstay for fiscal viability and nurse case management continues to play a pivotal role in this arena.

On March 23, 2010, President Obama signed into law the PPACA (CMS.gov). The intent of this act was to ensure access to high-quality, affordable health-care coverage for 93% of all Americans. Its goal was to contain costs while delivering this comprehensive care. The act is complex and has been constitutionally challenged by several states. On June 28, 2012, the United States Supreme Court released its ruling, finding PPACA to be constitutional. In the majority opinion, the constitutionality of the individual mandate section of the PPACA—the centerpiece of the case—was upheld. This individual mandate requires all Americans to buy insurance or pay a fine. The concept of a fine was seen as unconstitutional and subsequently redefined as a tax that the government has the constitutional power to impose; the PPACA survived on that basis. The future of PPACA is currently in question with a new president who is not supportive of this legislation. Repeal or significant reform of PPACA could be a possibility, if the Congress aligns itself with the president's sentiments.

Within the Centers for Medicare and Medicaid Services (CMS), provisions of the PPACA create ACOs. An ACO is a network of professional care providers and settings for care, including hospitals. Each network will address the needs of a minimum of 5,000 patients (kaiserhealthnews.org). An ACO is not a place but a concept contained within a corporate structure. ACO professionals include physicians, nurse practitioners (NPs), physician assistants (PAs), and clinical nurse specialists (CNSs) (HealthCare.gov, 2012).

An example of PPACA affecting the role of NPs is contained in Section 5501 (PPACA, 2010, p. 534), which "provided a 10 percent (10%) bonus payment under Medicare for fiscal years 2011 through 2016 to primary care practitioners (including nurse practitioners, clinical nurse specialists, and physicians assistants) and general surgeons practicing in health professional shortage areas." The act also turns the spotlight on medical homes. The concept of a medical home grew from a 2002 Future of Family Medicine project that recommended that every American have a "personal medical home" through which to receive comprehensive health-care services. The Medical Home model is designed to improve the delivery of patient-centered health care. Similar to an ACO, the Medical Home is not a place but a concept that organizes primary care to meet a patient's physical and emotional needs utilizing the entire team of providers. Additionally, the interdisciplinary team works with the family and other home care providers to deliver comprehensive and coordinated health care that includes education to the whole person.

DIFFERENTIATING THE LEVELS OF NURSE CASE MANAGEMENT PRACTICE

Historically discussion has centered on the use of nurse case managers prepared at the baccalaureate versus the advanced practice level (Cesta & Tahan, 2003; Connors, 1993; Mahn & Spross, 1996; Tahan & Treiger, 2017). The American Nurses Association (ANA, 1992) asserts that minimum preparation for a nurse case manager is a bachelor's degree with 3 years of relevant experience. However, in practice nurses functioning in case management positions have differing clinical and educational backgrounds, including, in some settings, registered nurses (RNs) without a master's degree or even a bachelor of science in nursing (BSN) degree. Their roles and responsibilities are also quite varied and defined in different ways, depending on the clinical site. The Tahan and Huber study (2006) provides an analysis of changes that occurred in the practice of case management over the 5-year period between the mid-1990s and early 2000s and highlights the activities, relationships, knowledge, and skills most required in recent years.

Connors (1993) suggested that because case managers serve clients with varying levels of care across the continuum, not every client who is case managed is complex or catastrophic. He pointed out that even though the nurses with master's degrees may be best suited to fill case management positions, this may not always be possible given the practice demands. One approach would be to have baccalaureate-prepared nurses manage the more routine clients and have APNs manage those cases with more complex needs. In other words, the nurse's expertise "should be matched with the complexity of the situation and amount of autonomy required to fulfill the role" (Connors, 1993, p. 196).

Support for the APN case management role, particularly with high-risk or high-cost client populations, has been documented in the literature (Connors, 1993; Cronin & Maklebust, 1989; Hamric, 1992; Krichbaum, 1999; Naylor et al, 2010). The APN has expert knowledge regarding the clinical population for which standards and pathways are written, sees the whole client, and understands his or her needs on a continuum-of-care basis. Moreover, the APN has the additional requirement of outcome accountability (Krichbaum, 1999).

An expanding use of APNs is in the case management of patients with chronic diseases. Because of their education and clinical skills, APNs are able to focus on the multidimensional nature of chronic illness. A group of hospital-based clinics called on APNs to join a team effort that successfully improved clinical outcomes for patients with diabetes (Boville, Saran, Salem, & Clough, 2007). Bodenheimer and Bauer see NPs as underutilized. Economic and clinical gains could result by allowing NPs to practice independently and as team leaders for a large number of services across settings (2016).

Similarly, Mahn and Zazworsky (2000) pointed out that APNs are well suited to perform case management for complex client populations because of their advanced education, autonomy, ability to conduct extensive assessments, and ability to initiate and modify treatment regimens. These authors cited the work of Connors (1993), Hamric (1992), Lamb (1992), and Mahn and Spross (1996) to describe how the competencies of the APN role mirror those of the nurse case manager. Umbrell (2006) and Curtis, Lien, Chan, Grove, and Morris (2002) demonstrated the effectiveness of the APN in trauma management. The APN possesses specialized knowledge in providing "direct care, consultation, research utilization/continuous quality improvement, collaboration, data analysis and information management, change agency, ethical decision making and expert guidance and coaching" for a specific client population (Mahn & Zazworsky, 2000, p. 568). Such competencies are all congruent to those of nurse case managers.

To a lesser extent, arguments have also been presented for separate graduate programs in case management versus increasing case management content in existing advanced practice master's programs (Falter, Cesta, Concert, & Mason, 1999; Sowell & Young, 1997). One argument is that NPs and CNSs who are prepared at the master's level have the advanced clinical knowledge needed to care for clients with complex health-care needs and these nurses can effectively work with high-risk clinical populations. On the other hand, graduates who are master's prepared in case management have in-depth knowledge and skill in case management models, systems, and tools; health-care financing; reimbursement; and community resource use. These nurses can provide case management services and provide the leadership to design systems of care coordination and quality management in health-care organizations. Graduates from both types of master's programs can make a significant contribution to case management practice,

Box 15.1

Differentiating Between the Nurse Case Manager With a Baccalaureate Degree or Master's Degree as an APN and a Nurse With Specific Master's Preparation in Case Management

Levels of Case Management

Baccalaureate registered nurse (RN) case managers have foundational theoretical and clinical knowledge in nursing. These nurses are able to manage the care of patients who are less complex and more predictable, often with the assistance of critical paths. These nurses may work in collaboration with an APN case manager prepared at the master's level or a nurse case manager prepared at the master's level.

Master's–APN case managers have clinical expertise and advanced knowledge in health and wellness promotion and illness intervention models for specific patient populations. These nurses can manage patients with complex health needs, such as those in high-risk, vulnerable populations and those who require high resource consumption. In addition, these nurses are expected to conduct research related to case management practice, disease management, and clinical outcomes.

Nurses with master's level preparation specifically for the functional role of case manager possess expert knowledge and skill in case management models, processes and tools, health-care financing, reimbursement, outcome monitoring, and measurement. These nurses are able to design and monitor systems of care coordination and deliver case management services and are expected to conduct research related to case management practice and clinical outcomes.

administration, education, and research (Cesta & Tahan, 2003, Tahan & Treiger, 2017). More research demonstrating the effectiveness of nurses who have baccalaureate and master's degrees is needed. Moreover, it is important that a distinction be made among nurses prepared at the baccalaureate, master's–advanced practice (NP or CNS),

and master's–case management levels. See **Box 15.1** for a description of the levels of nurse case management practice.

EDUCATION FOR NURSE CASE MANAGEMENT PRACTICE

Outside academic settings, education on case management can occur via continuing education courses, institutes, and on-the-job training. Within academic settings, case management concepts may be integrated into baccalaureate- and master's-level curricula or taught in required or elective courses. Also, at the graduate level there are master's programs in case management. Another model is to offer case management as a concentration in which students take a required number of courses in addition to training in a clinical specialty or administration.

On-the-job training or short training courses are not likely to be adequate because offering content solely in these formats cannot expose all nurses to essential knowledge bases necessary to assume case management functions. To best prepare nurses for case management practice within a managed care environment, it is recommended that educators adopt a systematic approach to the integration of case management in nursing curricula. Approaches to incorporating such content are described elsewhere (Mundt, 1996; Powell & Tahan, 2008; Sinnen & Schifalaqua, 1996; Sowell & Young, 1997).

At the baccalaureate level, case management should be considered a core curriculum concept and threaded throughout the undergraduate program. At the graduate level, in addition to core graduate and specialty content, advanced practice curricula should contain theory and clinical experiences related to case management, care coordination across the continuum, community resource use, and managed care concepts including reimbursement and health-care financing. Because nurse case managers look to the skills of other health-care professionals in their care planning, an interdisciplinary course would also prove invaluable.

The curriculum sponsored by the CMSA notes that there are essential elements of study. These include managed care, use management, and legal and ethical issues, among others. It is also noted that change is constant and case managers must keep up with the changes in the health-care system (Powell & Ignatavicius, 2001).

Finally, there is a need for graduate programs to prepare nurse case management specialists. Master's programs in case management should include core graduate content as well as specialized content related to case management models, strategies, tools, quality management, health-care financing and reimbursement systems, managed care, health-care outcomes, client education, community resources, clinical practice in case management, and role development. Course work and clinical experiences with specific aggregate populations is highly recommended. Moreover, such curricula need to prepare graduates who can practice case management in both inpatient and outpatient settings and organizational venues, such as insurance companies. Offering master's programs in case management and integrating case management content at the master's level for APNs will produce practitioners who can deliver nursing case management services, create systems of care coordination, and institute policy that will reflect quality outcomes.

The newer terminal degree offering for APNs, the doctor of nursing practice (DNP), offers many new avenues of knowledge and skills to further enhance the case management role of the APN. The integration of nursing science with advanced levels of systems thinking and accountability in designing, delivering, and evaluating evidence-based practice to improve quality, safety, and outcomes should add significantly to the patient experience and decrease cost. New leadership skills directed at the development and implementation of patient-driven health policy and effective collaboration with nursing and other disciplines to promote cultural competence in response to health-care needs has the potential to engage patients as active participants in improving their health status.

CASE MANAGER RESPONSIBILITIES AND SKILLS

Quality of care and efficient use of limited resources have been *the* hallmarks of case management since the 1860s, with the intervening influence of early settlement houses, public health nursing, federal and state legislation, and managed care. Regardless of who drives the process (e.g., provider, insurance company, employer, federal government, or private entrepreneur), the outcome expectations are similar. The definitions of quality and efficiency may differ by source but all models require a skill and knowledge set of their case

managers. The setting in which the case manager practices, the model design, and the patient population dictate the overall knowledge base and clinical expertise required. The national quality agenda will be supported by the involvement of nurse case managers. Case managers in all settings are alert to the importance of evaluation of quality and the appropriateness of care delivered to patients (White, 2004).

Successful nurse case management mandates a wide variety of both management and clinical skills. Some of the most typical management skills include delegation, conflict resolution, collaboration, crisis intervention, coordination, direction, consultation, and fiscal accountability. Clinical skill requirements vary from model to model and may include nurses educated from the diploma/associate degree to master's level. The suggested practice areas for differing levels of education (baccalaureate to master's) are also discussed in this chapter. Nurses educated at the diploma/associate degree level frequently find themselves in positions in nurse case management similar to the baccalaureate RN case manager described in Box 15.1. A summary of the most common skills and competencies of nurse case managers is found in **Table 15.1.** This table is not meant to be an exhaustive listing of skills and competencies but rather a snapshot view of what is needed by nurse case managers in varying situations.

Nurse case management continues to be a hybrid within nursing and has led many to examine the issue of "clinical expertise" as listed in the job descriptions of case managers. Calkin (1984), in attempting to differentiate between the expertise of a nurse case manager and an APN case manager, defined the former as experts by experience and the latter as prepared by a combination of clinical experience and education. The advanced practice case managers retain their use of experience-based intuition but use their additional academic and clinical preparation to manage more highly complex and unpredictable individuals and populations. Although the focus of advanced practice case managers is still on providing direct patient care, they also make significant contributions toward coordination of multidisciplinary care. This advanced practitioner in a case manager role can continue to monitor, advocate, and coordinate care for patients across the continuum and can develop programs and systems to support both community-based and private-practice-based care (Erickson, 1997).

TABLE 15.1

Skills and Competencies of the Nurse Case Manager

Skill or Competency	Goal
Patient advocacy	Assist patient in achieving autonomy and self-determination
Guardian of confidentiality	Preserve dignity and privacy
Case selection expert	Identify recipients of case management
Care coordinator	Procure and broker services; seamless continuum
Assessment and reassessment	Problem identification and resolution; monitor outcomes
Discharge planner	Facilitate movement in care continuum
Follow-through	Optimum care within resources available
Use management	Use resources appropriately
Knowledge of insurance structures and benefits	Interpret resources available to the patient
Cost-benefit analysis (fiscal advocacy)	Demonstrate case management effect on care, usually monetary
Negotiation	Procure what the patient requires for health purposes
Clinical expertise*	Intervene appropriately, improve outcomes
Critical thinking	Think out of the box to find creative solutions and increase case manager autonomy
Competent professional (includes accountability, knowledge of standards of practice, legal issues, and research ability)	Do the right thing at the right time for the right reason
Outcomes management	Evaluate and manage outcomes
Interpersonal (communication, assertiveness, collaboration, and tact or diplomacy)	Gather information and channel to appropriate sources
Organizational (time management, marketing or networking, prioritization, and report writer)	Use time and people resources wisely

*Depends on case management model and setting.
Sources: More, P. K., & Mandell, S. (1997). *Nursing case management: An evolving practice.* New York, NY: McGraw-Hill; and Powell, S. K. (2000). *Case management: A practice guide to success in managed care.* Philadelphia, PA: Lippincott Williams & Wilkins.

Not all case managers practice the duties and responsibilities of managing patient care at the same advanced level. As nurse case managers become involved in more complex cases, the need for advanced education becomes apparent. This growth in complexity has resulted in the need for APNs to join the ranks of case managers (Stanton, Swanson, Sherrod, & Packa, 2005).

TOOLS AND STRATEGIES

Through the development of clinical expertise, knowledge of research processes, communication skills, critical thinking, decision making, and leadership skills, the APN is uniquely qualified to influence case management and chronic care management in a variety of health-care environments. The strategic use of APNs in the case management role to improve communication and collaboration with the treatment team is an effective tool given the importance of primary care practitioner involvement in the success of case and chronic care management interventions. Evidence-based interventions and standardized outcome measures are important strategies used in chronic care management programs to improve the quality of health-care services. In an effort to assist case managers and program designers to identify effective tools and evidence-based guidelines for case management and to standardize the evaluation of the outcomes of case management interventions, the CMSA created the Council for Case Management Accountability (CCMA) in 1996 (CMSA, 2002). Through the use of expert case management researchers and practitioners, the CCMA identified five care domains and outcomes in which case management has been shown or believed to have an effect:

- *Patient knowledge:* Case management patients need adequate knowledge on several fronts, including knowledge about health benefits and services, knowledge about their health conditions, and knowledge about their treatment plans. Successful case management results in improved patient knowledge.
- *Patient involvement in care:* Health care is a cooperative endeavor; patients play a key role in high-quality, cost-effective care. Successful case management involves clients in the decisions and actions of self-care.
- *Patient empowerment:* Case management should help patients build a sense of self-efficacy regarding their ability to manage their own health, as well as an ability to negotiate the care system successfully.
- *Patient adherence:* Cost-effective health care is predicated on patients' consistent adherence to their treatment programs. Successful case management results in higher rates of patient adherence.
- *Coordination of care:* Case managers provide consistency of care across the continuum while eliminating redundancy and waste (CMSA, 2002).

These domains continue to be relevant, particularly the emphasis of patient and family engagement in health care. Use of assessment tools such as the Patient Activation Measure, PAM* (Hibbard, Stockard, Mahoney, & Tusler, 2004) have been increasingly effective in assisting APNs and others to understand the importance of their patients' activation level and to tailor case management interventions accordingly.

Little is known to date regarding the amount or type of nursing (or "dose of nursing") needed to affect patient outcomes. This knowledge is necessary in applying case and chronic care management interventions (Brooten & Naylor, 1995). For example, there have been several published studies highlighting the effectiveness of APNs as case managers for Medicare-aged members with heart failure. The question becomes, is it necessary for the APN to have direct patient interaction or contact at the primary care office or clinic or in the home, or is it just as effective to use telemedicine approaches with this population? Should the use of the APN be applied to high-risk chronic care management, or should APNs be included in health education and promotion strategies? What interventions provide the most effective quality of care, satisfaction, and financial outcomes? The continued evaluation and support of new payment and delivery models is beginning to shed light on the amount and timing of nursing "doses."

Another strategy used to ensure high-quality, effective case management processes and outcomes is the development of electronic medical records and database systems with care management assessment, planning, and outcomes tracking capabilities. Systems that alert the treatment team to gaps in care—for example, abnormal biometric data and non–evidence-based treatment regimens—improve patient outcomes as well. Sharing data between disparate systems has become a major emphasis for health-care providers and payers as they assume accountability for population health management and financial outcomes in value-based purchasing agreements with CMS.

Finally, and most important, tools used to identify those individuals who can most benefit from exceptional case management services and interventions that focus on communication and relationship building are critical. Predictive models and algorithms that produce registries of the chronically ill high-risk patients have become important tools in identifying the 5% of the population that can account for 50% of the medical costs—these are the individuals who can benefit most from case management services (Forman & Kelliher, 1999). Additional training and development in techniques such as motivational interviewing and intrinsic coaching increases the case manager's ability to improve a person's ability to make choices and to seek relevance and value in making health changes that directly relate to his or her life goals (Miller & Rollnick, 2002).

NURSE CASE MANAGEMENT MODELS

A review of the literature provides many types of case management models and differentiates the contributions each makes within a designated field. The common aspects of these models are advocacy, services brokering, risk management, care coordination, and a process designed to accomplish these objectives (Huber, 2000). Knollmueller (1989) identified seven models of case management: (a) social, (b) primary care, (c) medical/social, (d) HMO, (e) independent, (f) insurance, and (g) in-house. Stempel, Doerge, Van Mie, and Combs (1997) describe four types of nurse case management: (a) clinical case management, (b) payer-based case management, (c) program case management, and (d) community case management. More recently Daniels and Ramsey (2005) proposed the use of five main models of case management that they have observed: (a) clinical case management, (b) collaborative practice models, (c) populations models, (d) functional models, and (e) clinical resource management models. In commenting on these models, Zander (2008) noted that some hospitals are using APNs to fill the case management functions alone or working with other case management personnel. A multidisciplinary team at the Johns Hopkins Bloomberg School of Public Health designed the Guided Care Model for the better care of older people with chronic conditions. In this model, a primary care RN prepared in chronic care works with two to five physicians and members of the care team to provide patient-centered, coordinated, and cost-effective care. Their research demonstrated that the Guided Care Model improved the self-reports of chronic health care for multiple-morbid older persons (Boyd et al, 2009).

The literature on nurse case manager practice within the different models reflects some dilemmas regarding the purpose, scope, and functions of the nurse case manager role. Although there is a large body of anecdotal stories, research in the field is still working to control the effect of extraneous variables in studies and developing nursing-sensitive outcomes. Qualitative descriptions of nurse case management practice have pointed to some common themes across all nurse case management practice. They include (a) working with individuals, families, and populations at risk; (b) applying the nursing process to enhance quality and cost outcomes; (c) accessing individuals and families in more than one setting; and (d) coordination and advocacy integrated throughout (Lamb, 1995).

Hellwig, Yam, and DiGiulio (2003) proposed an advocacy model for nurse case management practice. In the authors' qualitative study, hospital-based nurse case managers described that their advocacy was based on the needs of the patient and the patient's family, payer issues, and obstacles and opportunities for advocacy. Participants indicated that obstacles included time constraints, and examples of opportunities were physician support, rapport with insurance companies, and use of a team approach (Hellwig et al, 2003).

The nurse case management models used in practice today are as rich and diverse as the individuals, families, and populations they serve. Current practice within hospital-based models in many organizations has moved from a primarily clinical case manager role to one of an intense discharge planning model. Conversely, the hospital-to-community-based and community-based models have experienced an increasing need for a high level of clinical expertise in their case managers, as well as the traditional knowledge of community resources and health-care reimbursement methodologies. As models continue to evolve in response to practice needs and environmental changes, the models for the 21st century must continue to include and enhance the role APNs can and do play in community-based practice models. According to Zander (2008), case management models that are reviewed at the executive level in hospitals are considered very expensive. In light of this we need more cost-benefit research on case management efforts and models.

The CMS has created The Innovation Center Home that "develops new payment and service delivery models . . . in accordance with the Social Security Act." The Affordable Care Act (ACA) and additional legislation was also included. CMS has organized their models into seven categories:

1. Accountable Care Organizations
2. Episode-Based Payment Initiatives
3. Primary Care Transformation/Medical Homes
4. Initiatives Focused on the Medicaid and CHIP population
5. Initiatives Focused on the Medicare-Medicaid Enrollees
6. Initiatives to Accelerate the Development and Testing of New Payment and Service Delivery Models
7. Initiatives to Speed the Best Practice

Individual case management models are too numerous to detail here but early on they were categorized into "within the walls" and "beyond the walls." In devising their own case management models today health-care providers consider the factors that impact models of case management such as those proposed by Tahan. These are the context of the care setting (acute, long term, etc.), the patient population served, the reimbursement method, and the care providers needed (Tahan & Campagna, 2010). Other models include the AIDS Institute Models of Case Management described as comprehensive case management and supportive case management (health.ny.gov/diseases).

Case management or care coordination models evolve over time. For patients with complex needs we are seeing more models that focus on care transitions. This Transition Model has improved care for older adults at risk for readmission within the 30-day postdischarge window. Some variations on this model use geriatric NPs to manage care from inpatient to home or long-term care facilities (Hirschman, Shaide, Pauly, & Naylor, 2015). Under the ACA "a variety of transitional care programs and services have been established to improve quality and reduce costs" (Naylor, Aiken, Kurtzman, Olds, & Hirschman, 2011).

The TCM and the Patient-Centered Medical Home (PCMH) focus on the health-care needs of older adults with those models incorporating integrated, multidisciplinary teams along with the patient and family caregivers. The creation of these models finds support in the Institute of Medicine (IOM) report *The Future of Nursing: Leading Change, Advancing Health* that addresses the importance of efforts of nurses to lead change. Most TCM models are nurse-led and always include interdisciplinary coordination. Social workers are key players in the success of case/care management models and in some health-care facilities take the lead role in newly designed models of care.

CHRONIC CARE MANAGEMENT AND THE ROLE OF THE ADVANCED PRACTICE NURSE

APNs have played an active role in both acute and chronic care management, particularly as a case manager within the acute and community care settings. Research has found many benefits of using APNs in the case management role, in particular qualities such as clinical expertise and improved access and communication with treating physicians in the community. This improved access and communication, along with the expert clinical knowledge regarding a particular disease state, can result in observable improved outcomes for individual patients receiving treatment for these targeted conditions within disease management programs.

According to Watts and colleagues (2009), the skills of the APN in case management led multidisciplinary teams to achieve significant gains in patient self-management, decision support, and delivery system design. Because APNs are trained to think holistically, to foster team building (a factor in implementing planned care), and to educate and motivate patients, they are particularly needed in multidisciplinary/group-based practices such as the PCMH or the ACO that strive to address the needs of chronically ill members (Dancer & Courtney, 2010; Naylor & Kurtzman, 2010; Watts et al, 2009).

Some research has been conducted on the cost effectiveness of APN management of patients with chronic illness. Paez and Allen (2006) evaluated the cost effectiveness of APN case management to lower blood lipids in patients with coronary heart disease. Their findings "suggest that case management by an APN is a cost-efficient and therapeutically effective strategy in managed care, to improve the care of patients with cardiovascular disease" (p. 439) (Boville et al, 2007).

The Advanced Practice Nurse: Chronic Care Management Examples

Example 1: The Advanced Practice Nurse in the Program Development Role in a Managed Care Setting

K is a typical APN care manager within the managed care setting. She has a strong clinical background in oncology. As part of her role in the medical management department, K was recently asked to participate in the strategic planning for the development of a new care management program.

Expert clinical knowledge and an ability to apply this knowledge are critical in the development of successful care management interventions for managed care. Knowledge of a particular disease process is essential to identify the applicability of disease management interventions. For example, many conditions are considered to be potential targets for disease management primarily because of a high prevalence or high costs of preventable complications associated with the particular disease. However, not all diseases can effectively be managed using disease management program principles. The hallmark of these programs is coordination of health-care services and improving self-care measures. The APNs' expert clinical knowledge of a particular disease state and their knowledge of the care provided within the health-care system can identify critical junctures at which disease management interventions can be the most effective.

Cancer is prevalent among commercial populations and is also a high-cost disease state; it is also considered to be a difficult disease to manage. K noted that many individuals with cancer are admitted to the hospital because of the side effects of chemotherapeutic agents. With education and improved self-care measures, could these admissions be avoided? Could this be the critical juncture in managing avoidable costs? K used both her clinical knowledge and her knowledge of the care provided within the health-care system in her evaluation of cancer as a potential target for disease management. She then proceeded to recommend the design of an education packet and telephonic outreach protocol focusing on prehydration for members undergoing chemotherapy to prevent dehydration admissions and dietary considerations in the prevention of anemia. She designed an educational packet to include reputable Web sites for lay review of the national cancer treatment protocols and several community resources and support groups. Through her knowledge of the disease process and an opportunity for improved care, K identified a key juncture for focused disease management intervention. The rate of admissions for the complications of chemotherapy—specifically dehydration and anemia—are the clinical outcome measures that will determine the success of this program.

In addition, collaboration with the treating oncologist to support the physician's treatment plan and encourage patient participation in the program is critical. The APN, working with the health plan's medical director, can assist in meeting this goal.

Example 2: The Advanced Practice Nurse's Role in Quality and Performance Improvement

M is an APN with extensive experience in hospice care. Many cancer patients are successfully treated; however, many other cancers result in terminal conditions. The average length of stay in hospice care was 2 weeks or less and many patients with terminal conditions did not receive the benefits of hospice care. M, as a newly hired APN in the hospital's new population health program, has noted this trend and has suggested that there be an evaluation of end-of-life care for disease management. Improvements in the quality of care provided in these circumstances may result in the reduction of acute service admissions and improved quality of life, particularly through early advanced care planning, pain management, and support of individuals and families through dying and death experience. This example demonstrates the need to have APNs in the population health-care development process consistently in search of areas for improvement and disease management intervention. With frequent review of the literature and observation of trends, the APN frequently identifies, plans, and implements care management solutions. Rather than reacting to market forces and trends, the APN, as a member of the new population health management team, consistently seeks areas for continued improvement and service to clients. The health system that uses this intellectual capital is provided with care solutions that not only provide value to its customers facing escalating health-care costs and the challenges of variability in the quality of care received, but also can differentiate itself from reactionary competitors.

Example 3: The Advanced Practice Nurse's Role in High Risk Population Management Within the Patient-Centered Medical Home

J is an APN specializing in family medicine within a primary care practice that uses a patient-centered medical home model. The practice had agreed to participate in an ACO agreement and as such agreed last year to provide primary care services for a distinct population of fee-for-service Medicare beneficiaries. Part of the agreement provides for shared savings in the event that certain quality, satisfaction, and cost measures are met. Early results showed that the practice was not meeting targets for clinical quality and cost measures along with a poor completion rate of annual wellness visits by the population. Therefore, the primary care practice lead assigned J to evaluate and make practice changes to improve the outcomes for this population.

In evaluating the population, J noted that a small percentage (5%) of the population was driving the costs for the group. In further analysis of the top 5%, the members of this cohort had similar profiles—chronic illness with frequent exacerbations and high reliance on acute care services, poor completion rate of annual wellness examinations, and end-of-life care without benefit of advance care planning. Behavioral health issues were also evident among the population. In general, this population of patients was seen in the office, which was in rural Pennsylvania, episodically—only when there were issues or need for medication changes.

The APN was newly hired, along with a physician who had experience with population health and medical home principles. Together they devised a system by which the high-risk population that was frequently admitted to the hospital (more than 2x/year) would be encouraged to be seen at the primary care office by the APN as often as necessary or desired. J established an open access schedule, ensuring that time would be blocked in her daily schedule to accommodate last minute visits. Each of these patients would be encouraged by the APN as well as the office staff to schedule an annual wellness visit at each in-person or telephonic encounter. J also worked with patients and their families to establish their wishes as they related to end-of-life care with the goal of establishing advance directives for all patients in this cohort population. Total admissions to the hospital, annual wellness assessment completion rates, percentage of advance directives, satisfaction, and total costs of care were calculated by J. This population was called the "frequent flyer club," given how frequently they utilized the hospital as their point of care. With increased access to primary care, hospitalization rates were decreased and annual wellness visits and presence of advanced directives were increased substantially (greater than 50%) within a short period of time (6 months). Quality and cost metric improvements were realized after 1 year for the entire population at risk.

The addition of an APN in the primary care practice served two goals: increased access to primary care services along with improved population management. The goal of patient-centered medical home care is for the patient and family to seek care coordination and support for improved self-care at the primary care site. More frequent visits by the APN with the population increased the health-care literacy level as well as the trust and self-care capabilities of these patients and families. The APN also knew these patients and families well and developed a strong trusting, therapeutic relationship. By knowing the patient, the APN was better equipped to provide care. By knowing the APN, the patient was better equipped to care for himself or herself as well as use the health-care system effectively.

REIMBURSEMENT AND MARKETING OF CASE MANAGEMENT PRACTICE

Physicians' current procedural terminology (CPT) codes are available for the reimbursement of case management services in a fee-for-service environment. Therefore, clinicians who normally bill for services using the CPT coding system, such as physicians and APNs, can bill for time used to deliver case management services in the outpatient setting. CMS and managed care organizations have also begun to pay for improvement to establish ACOs and ACAs with primary care practices providing shared savings and/or pay for improvement opportunities focusing on quality of chronic care management, transitions in care, patient access, and cost effectiveness. As more physician groups enter shared-savings, ACOs, ACAs, and pay-for-performance arrangements, predictive modeling and case management services (many monikers such as nurse navigation, care coordination, community care management, etc.) have become the solution to managing the health risk of the small percentage of individuals who drive the large percentage of health-care expenditures. In addition, it is not uncommon for case management to be a revenue-generating option/service line for hospitals and managed care organizations affected or motivated by health-care reform and new reimbursement models. Case management services and the systems or tools used to support these activities are in high demand. Consequently, APNs with exceptional case management skills and experience are valuable.

A downside to the popularity and use of case management solutions across the continuum of care has been the lack of coordination of case management services. For example, it is not uncommon for a patient at the time of discharge from the hospital to have a case manager in the hospital, a disease state case manager (usually an NP) specific for their condition, and a community-based case manager all provided by the hospital (particularly if the hospital health system has assumed risk for the patient's care outcomes as part of an ACO) along with a nurse navigator at the hospital-owned PCP office. If the patient is discharged to a post-acute care provider such as a skilled nursing facility or a home health provider, these settings typically will deploy a case manager. It is ironic that the role of the case manager was established to reduce fragmentation and improve coordination of care. Multiple case managers, with multiple titles and educational backgrounds and experiences, not only have led to patient confusion but have also contributed to increased duplication resulting in higher administrative costs of care. Care management role definitions and delineations are therefore a critical consideration in effective population care management models and solutions.

CONCLUSION

This chapter has explored the historical roots of the case manager role; levels of practice for nurse case managers; various case management models; case management roles and skills; tools and strategies, including chronic care management for APNs; and issues such as reimbursement, marketing, and education for practice. This is an exciting and challenging time to be an APN within a case management practice environment. Those who successfully grasp the role and function will be the pacesetters for tomorrow's health-care challenges. This will also ensure a place at the table for nursing as it grows and develops and provides the nation with innovative care models.

16

The Advanced Practice Nurse and Research

Beth Quatrara and Dale Shaw

Learning Outcomes

Learning outcomes expected as a result of this chapter:

- Integrate research as a role component of advanced practice.
- Describe the phases of research competency development.
- Demonstrate outcome expectations in education and practice.
- Clarify outcomes measurement.
- Support the benefits of collaborative research.
- Adopt research practices that are feasible within the clinical setting.
- Instill research mentorship.
- Solidify a culture of clinical research.
- Establish resources and structures that support clinical research.
- Identify elements that contribute to a successful clinical research study.

INTRODUCTION

The advanced practice nurse (APN) is a consumer, facilitator, collaborator, and leader in research. The APN is expected to develop a research attitude in others and foster evidence-based practice (EBP) through the integration of research findings into clinical practice. The APN applies the scientific method to clinical problem solving and provides

leadership in the use and conduct of research. Although for many years the concept of "conducting research" was not considered to be a dominant APN competency, the attitude toward this has changed. This chapter discusses APN research competencies and behaviors and practical methods to successfully integrate research activities into practice. Buy-in and barriers to the APN research role are discussed in addition to strategies for success. Most importantly, the chapter discusses how the APN develops a practice milieu that embraces evidence and considers research "part of what we do every day."

RESEARCH AS AN APN ROLE COMPONENT

The APN, a practice-based clinician with graduate education, is educated to contribute to nursing knowledge. APNs' education and clinical expertise contribute to their unique potential to be consumers of research while understanding the nuances of applying the new knowledge to patient-specific situations and unique practice settings. They translate research into practice and pragmatically implement the findings to provide high-quality care. By promoting EBP through knowledge and skill acquisition, APNs help to reduce barriers to the theory-research-practice transition gap that plagues the clinical environment (Melnyk, Fineout-Overholt, Gallagher-Ford, & Kaplan, 2012). Research is a long-standing core competency of the APN role that continues to be emphasized as a central component regardless of the practice setting or specific role function (American Association of Colleges of Nursing [AACN], 1995, 2011; American Nurses Association [ANA], 2010; Hamric, Hanson, Tracy, & O'Grady, 2014). It is not limited to a few clinicians practicing in a defined area.

Today, the role of the APN as a researcher is stressed as an essential element of APN education and practice. The *Essentials of Master's Education in Nursing* requires that APNs graduate with the knowledge and skill to translate and integrate scholarship into practice (AACN, 2011). Schools of nursing that graduate master's-prepared nurses are required to demonstrate that APNs are trained to apply research outcomes within practice settings, resolve practice problems, work as change agents, and disseminate results (AACN, 2011). Similarly, the doctorate of nursing practice degree (DNP) emphasizes that the APN is expected to maintain a scholarly practice by focusing on practice improvement and innovation as well as testing care delivery models (AACN, 2006). The DNP is delineated as different from the PhD with a focus on practice, stating that DNPs are "prepared to generate new knowledge through innovation of practice change, the translation of evidence and the implementation of quality improvement (QI) processes in specific practice settings, systems or with specific populations to improve

health or health outcomes" (AACN, 2015, p. 2). The APN role in research is further endorsed in the ANA's *Scope and Standards of Practice* (2015), noting that APNs integrate research findings into practice in addition to demonstrating competency behaviors that require APNs to "contribute to nursing knowledge by conducting or synthesizing research and other evidence that discovers, examines and evaluates current practice, knowledge, theories, criteria, and creative approaches to improve healthcare practice" as well as "promote . . . clinical inquiry" and to "disseminate research findings through activities such as presentations, publications, consultations and journal clubs" (ANA, 2010, p. 58). These educational requirements and practice statements clarify and reinforce the APN practice role in research. APNs' unique contributions as consumers of and contributors to research are recognized on many levels.

APN RESEARCH COMPETENCIES

Similar to other APN core competencies, research is a skill that builds and strengthens over time (Hamric, Hanson, Tracy, & O'Grady, 2014). As the APN advances in the research role, she or he moves through three competency phases (De Palma, 2009). The first phase focuses on interpreting and implementing research outcomes (De Palma, 2009). During this time, the APN gains research confidence and proficiency by introducing EBP. The APN facilitates the application of research by introducing both clinicians, including registered nurses, and administrators to EBP. When responding to clinical questions, the APN directs others to the literature and teaches them how to critique research and adapt their practice as appropriate to the findings. Effectively integrating research into practice with attention to the patient, nurse, and the science is a key attribute that the APN brings to the practice setting. Taking into consideration readiness for change, resource requirements, and educational needs, the APN uses training, experience, and clinical authority to lead EBP changes and influence quality of care. The APN uses a variety of forums to demonstrate this competency, including role modeling, journal clubs, grand rounds, and clinical practice meetings.

In the second research competency phase, the APN begins to evaluate practice (De Palma, 2009). Using outcomes research, the clinician examines the effect of applying EBP guidelines to patient care or explores the impact of using research findings to improve quality indicators (De Palma, 2009). At this competency level, the APN begins to define measurement criteria and evaluate interventions in terms of documented outcomes. Measuring outcomes to determine the effectiveness of change is essential to the research role. Outcome results are used to make a final decision about sustaining the change versus placing the intervention on hold and reevaluating the process. Defining outcome measures before implementing change is required to obtain maximum effectiveness. Determining specific measurements, the method of data collection, and the party responsible for the data collection facilitates the evaluation process. Evaluation points, although specific to the exact intervention, can include a variety of indices such as clinical outcomes, satisfaction, time, and money. Several outcome tools already exist, and resources such as the *APN Data Collection Toolkit* may assist clinicians in the evaluation process (Vohra & Bryant-Lukosius, 2009).

In addition to clinical practice evaluation, APNs are also obligated to examine their own practice by evaluating the effect of their role. APN-specific outcomes, which can be similar to practice outcomes, are measured to showcase role efficacy, demonstrate research role competency, and validate APNs' unique contributions to patient care. Collecting APN role-specific outcome measures is an important aspect of practice that cannot be overlooked (Bryant-Lukosius et al, 2016).

The third research competency incorporates the collaborative generation of new knowledge (De Palma, 2009). At this final stage of research competency, APNs are working with interprofessional team members to design and implement studies that have implications for nursing practice. The benefits of collaborative APN research include shared expertise, academic influence, access to clinical populations, efficient data collection, improved research relevance, and the creation of an environment that promotes the application of scholarship in patient care (Burman, Hart, & McCabe, 2005; Mercer, 2008; Schramp, Holtcamp, Phillips, Johnson, & Hoff, 2010; Hutchinson, East, Stasa, & Jackson, 2014).

There are also benefits to collaborative research with APN peers. For example, a collaborative APN research network founded by six university schools of nursing (APRNet) and supported by the Agency for Healthcare Research and Quality united research among primary care practice APNs (Deshefy-Longhi, Swartz, & Grey, 2002).

Through this network, currently known as NetHaven, APNs across participating states are sharing data and designing studies to meet their clinical needs and enhance nursing knowledge. Since 2000, this APN practice-based research network has contributed to the development of several APN practice-focused studies (Deshefy-Longhi, Swartz, & Grey, 2008; McCloskey, Grey, Deshefy-Longhi, & Grey, 2003; Olsen, Dixon, Grey, Deshefy-Longhi, & Demarest, 2005). Today, its efforts are continuing to expand through examining care needs such as treatments for childhood obesity and smoking in young adults (Yale Center for Clinical Investigation [YCCI], 2015). APNs benefit from collaboration in the research process and dissemination efforts such as publication and presentations (Christenbery, 2011). Partnering with colleagues to build skills in manuscript preparation and response to editor requests contributes to the APN's professional growth in the research role. Working with peer groups provides support and encouragement.

De Palma (2009) suggests that APNs operationalize the three research competencies at two levels. At the fundamental level, the APN learns and applies these skills in graduate school. At the expanded level, the APN builds on these skills through actual research involvement. It is undoubtedly difficult for the beginning APN to readily implement classroom research skills; however, practical investigative experience can be achieved through a variety of activities such as clinical problem solving, presenting research findings, participating in QI projects, conducting product evaluations, and examining practice protocols for evidence of needed change. As the APN progresses from a facilitator of research to a conductor of research, the APN's competency in this role component is developed. Early research experience as a team member helps to build skills as a team leader. Acquiring skills in the research process, including protocol testing and publication writing, result from active participation, mentored guidance, and teamwork.

FROM APPLICATION TO CONDUCTION OF RESEARCH: STEPS ALONG THE WAY

As described, the APN's academic preparation includes how to evaluate and conduct research, yet few practicing APNs feel adequately prepared to lead a research project in their practice arena immediately following graduation.

Clinicians may find that many of the principles learned in school seem less applicable when trialed in the clinical setting. However, there are practical steps for successful integration of APN research competencies. For the research gap to narrow so that an evidence-based scientific approach to care is embraced by nursing staff, the APN must develop a milieu that promotes such a philosophy (Burns, 2010; Kleinpell, 2008; Melnyk, Fineout-Overholt, Gallagher-Ford, & Kaplan, 2012). To successfully engineer a scientific milieu in a clinical setting, the APN must use selected behaviors such as problem solving, change agency, mentoring, leadership, and collaborating with an interprofessional team.

Problem Solving and Applying the Evidence to Practice

The APN is often called on to propose solutions for clinical problems. The imperative for success is improving outcomes. Oddly enough, even when strong evidence exists, practice changes may occur slowly or not at all. An example is the ubiquitous practice of instilling normal saline into endotracheal tubes before suctioning. Though evidence continues to strongly suggest that the practice is both ineffective and potentially harmful, it has continued to be a common practice for decades (Makic & Rauen, 2016). Thus, the ability to use a logical yet creative approach to applying evidence or conducting clinical research serves to support the reality that research must be an integral and important part of everyday practice.

The APN begins by helping staff nurses to understand the meaning of EBP. The clinician must first be aware of the evidence that exists for a practice and the strength of that evidence. Professional and regulatory agencies often perform systematic reviews to determine the existing evidence for selected practices, especially high-risk procedures or practices. Practice guidelines are developed from these reviews and generally identify the level of scientific evidence for each recommendation from the lowest (i.e., consensus statements by professional organizations) to the highest (i.e., meta-analyses of randomized controlled trials [RCTs]). The decision to implement the guidelines is made by considering the relevancy of the practice change to the specific population of interest and by considering the potential for "unintended consequences" that may ensue. EBP changes may also be required by regulatory agencies, in which case the hospital must comply. APNs are often the individuals charged with implementation. An example is the use of restraints. Health-care agencies must ensure that they are used judiciously, applied appropriately, and that use is monitored rigorously. Another example is the implementation of a new technique that could potentially affect the rate of central line-associated bloodstream infections. Noting that the new technique may trigger either a reduction in infections or potentially development of sepsis, the APN requires a process of rigorous identification of barriers, follow-up evaluation, or outcomes tracking following implementation. The risk of a significant adverse outcome raises the intensity of the evaluation process. In contrast, implementation of a low-risk intervention such as the use of "bagged baths" in the place of traditional options may require only periodic audits of clinicians using the products and oversight by seasoned clinicians or certified wound, ostomy, and continence nurses.

When authoritative guidelines do not exist to help with EBP changes, consensus statements by professional organizations may be available and are quite helpful. These statements are based on systematic reviews of the available evidence. Similar to guidelines, the statements help the user understand the level of evidence so that careful application may occur. Other similar resources that may also be referenced are clinical updates or practice alerts. These tend to be published by professional organizations and are generally narrowly focused on a specific practice such as avoiding the use of blue food coloring in tube feedings or incorporating chlorhexidine bathing into preoperative care plans. Finally, a literature review on the topic of interest will help the APN guide clinicians in determining the need for a practice change or for a clinical study to answer the question.

Although some EBP changes may be initiated using existing research, the vast majority of existing practice traditions have little science to validate their efficacy. For example, although the Centers for Disease Control and Prevention (CDC) and the Infusion Nursing Society both recommend specific timing related to the use of selected site dressings used to cover and secure central venous (CV) catheter lines, they do not direct the clinician to any of the many commercially available products. Related questions, such as how long the dressings adhere, which are best for the skin, and which dressings work best with specific catheters, remain unanswered. In these cases the design and conduct of a clinical study to determine the answer is a reasonable and expected part of the APN's role.

APNs integrate evidence from many realms and also blend experiential knowledge of the culture and support systems to shape recommendations for clinical practice changes (Profetto-McGrath et al, 2007). If the APN determines that a clinical study is necessary to answer a practice question, it is essential to determine the project feasibility. A well-thought-out, narrowly focused, well-designed study is essential for clinician buy-in. In fact, selection of projects, especially first-time projects, should be carefully done to ensure a "quick win." More difficult projects can follow as clinicians and the APN become more sophisticated in the conduct of clinical studies and more confident in each other's capabilities. The following questions are helpful to determine the potential feasibility and subsequent success of conducting a clinical study:

1. *Is the proposed study a topic of interest to the clinicians?* Without clinician interest in the topic, the study is unlikely to move forward. In fact, it may be seen as the "APN's project" versus one owned by the unit or clinicians.

2. *Can it be done in a reasonable amount of time?* This is especially important for first-time projects. The project should be able to be completed in a couple of months or interest and enthusiasm will diminish. In a study by Winfield, Davis, Schwaner, Conaway, and Burns (2007), clinicians in a postanesthesia care unit questioned the best method for securing peripheral intravenous (PIV) lines. Because they were able to estimate the number of PIVs placed in a month, they were able to complete their study in approximately 3 months. With the relatively short data collection period, interest in the study stayed high throughout.

3. *Can the data be collected in the course of a clinical day?* Although qualitative studies are important to practice and are attractive to nurses, they are time consuming and difficult to accomplish in a clinical setting. Quantitative studies, on the other hand, are easier to accomplish. Nurses are used to collecting data. If the study is focused on a clinical problem, such as the PIV study noted previously, much of the data collection can be accomplished in the course of providing patient care. In addition, data that are routinely collected may also

contribute to evaluating nursing interventions; when aggregated and analyzed, they can help establish best practices (Resnick, 2006). Utilizing the electronic medical record can help to facilitate data collection in a timely manner because most elements of patient care are already documented and can be integrated into reports for analysis (Clark & Normile, 2012).

4. *Will the study require informed consent?* Studies that measure the effect of an intervention or practice or that challenge a "policy" or established practice standard require informed consent. From a practical perspective, it is desirable, especially for beginning clinical researchers, to design studies that do not require consent. The time that practicing clinicians must spend to obtain consent is often beyond that reasonably taken from normal care responsibilities and may be especially complicated if the patient is unable to give consent and the family must be approached.

   Studies that do not require informed consent are relatively common and are better choices for beginning researchers. For example, in the PIV study noted previously, four different PIV-securing methods were compared and assigned randomly. Consent was waived because no standard of care was breached (there was no existing standard securing method).

5. *Will the study require funding?* Many clinical projects such as the PIV example do not require a funding source. Supplies are often those used in the course of patient care and complex analyses are rarely necessary. However, some may require financial support and this should be considered before beginning. If an institutional or unit budget is not available for such support, other avenues may be explored.

   Small amounts of money are fairly easy to obtain, but they require time and energy to acquire. Examples include funding sources such as institutional quality assurance grants or small project monies ($100 to $500) provided by professional organizations. Another source may be unit funds; the manager or administrator should be consulted ahead of time to determine if this is a viable solution. Another option is to collaborate with an academic colleague or a statistician from the beginning so that person is part of the project team. Regardless of the source, to be feasible funding for selected elements of the project should be considered early in the project's development and design. It is desirable to have an infrastructure in place that ensures support for statistical analyses so that each project does not require a unique solution.

6. *Are there barriers to evidence use?* Some cultures resist the APN's efforts to implement practice changes. It may be useful to develop a strategy for delivering the findings in a less formal manner. Staff members often prefer one-on-one coaching, in-services, staff meetings, and learning methods that are not intimidating. Involving others from the start helps reinforce the premise that the work does not belong solely to the APN. Regardless, not everyone is successful in implementing research findings. The process requires strong critical thinking and facilitation skills. APNs can enhance the growth of clinicians in these areas by meeting their learning needs early on, exchanging expertise, and stimulating participation throughout the study (Burns, 2010; Ferguson, Milner, & Snelgrove-Clarke, 2004; Kennel, Burns, & Horn, 2009). These and other successful strategies are discussed later in this chapter.

Mentoring and Leadership

To encourage staff to accept the philosophy that research is a necessary part of their daily work, the APN's ability to mentor goes a long way. Although this statement seems somewhat obvious, it is far from being so. Many individuals are good at envisioning projects and some may even inspire others to participate. Unfortunately, a less appreciated behavior linked with success is the APN's ability to ensure that all steps of the project are fully completed in the predetermined manner. This is hard work and often requires dedicated determination to support, lead, and mentor others throughout the course of the project. Past performance speaks to this ability and it is essential that the APN be able to realistically assess his or her previous experience in completing projects and mentoring others. An APN who is working with clinicians on a clinical or service line project, for example, should not assume that participating individuals can independently accomplish the assigned tasks. Clinicians working on the project may have selected a project to learn how to do clinical research. However, they may lack experience in some of the steps of the process such as how to accomplish a literature review. The APN needs to anticipate this and help the individual accomplish the review. This one-on-one teaching is

important to demystify the process, eliminate barriers, move the process along, and ensure success. The support and teaching provided by the APN also helps with his or her credibility and ensures the development of others.

The APN's enthusiastic leadership goes a long way to making others excited about the process. This leadership extends to all aspects of the clinical project from problem identification to application. Most important, the project should be fun. As noted previously, many bedside clinicians feel that research is for others (e.g., those with doctorates) and they are fearful of embarking on any project that remotely looks similar to a study. A sense of humor, as in all aspects of nursing practice, goes a long way toward eliminating the fear of doing research and making it fun to accomplish.

Change Agency and a Systems Approach

Perhaps one of the most important behaviors of the APN is the ability to navigate the environment in which he or she practices. This understanding of the system is essential if appropriate changes are to be implemented. The APN must be able to identify the need to change an existing practice and the effect of this practice change. The APN's clinical knowledge and understanding of how to get something done in a clinical environment helps ensure that high quality is maintained. To that end, the APN has a responsibility to the institution to evaluate clinical and system-focused initiatives. In fact, these initiatives may be another way of demonstrating that "research is part of what we do" and are essential to the development of a widespread scientific approach to practice. An example might be an initiative to implement a specific care protocol derived from a published RCT. The protocol may well be evidence-based and warranted; however, implementation without careful consideration of existing processes of care and barriers to change could result in negative unanticipated outcomes. The APN's knowledge of the processes of care and understanding of how best to apply and monitor adherence to the new protocol is essential to evaluate its effect on the outcome of interest. This kind of scientific approach to the problem proactively avoids variations in practice that negatively affect clinical and financial metrics.

In some cases, data do not exist to guide system changes. The role of the APN is to help evaluate the outcomes associated with the system change so that the initiatives can be adapted as needed or to maintain and sustain positive outcomes. These kinds of projects often fall under the title of QI. Although slightly different from research studies in that they are rarely as rigorous in design or methods for conduction, they can be popular projects for clinician participation. An example is a project designed to determine if the implementation of an enhanced recovery (ER) protocol improved the outcomes of patients undergoing elective colorectal surgery. Clinicians and the institution were interested in the project because of the desire to improve clinical and financial outcomes for this patient population. A multidisciplinary team implemented an ER protocol that included preoperative counseling with patient participation, analgesia with the avoidance of intravenous opioids, specific intraoperative fluid management, a preoperative carbohydrate loading diet, and immediate postoperative ambulation (Theile et al, 2015). The project resulted in the improvement desired—patient satisfaction and reductions in length of stay, complications, and cost for elective colorectal patients at the institution. Because of this project the institution adopted the protocol as the standard of care and there is incentive to replicate it in other surgical populations.

The behaviors discussed previously, in addition to the attributes of the APN, determine the effectiveness of the APN in making research come to life in a clinical setting. However, barriers to success do exist (Higgins et al, 2010; Poghosyan et al, 2013). The most commonly cited barriers to the development of a research milieu include clinical access to patient populations, "buy-in" from clinicians, administrative support, attaining resources (i.e., time and money), and completing and publishing the results. Barriers and potential solutions are addressed in the following section.

Removing Barriers to APN Research Activities

Although the application of evidence to practice has been an expectation of the APN role in the past, the actual conduction of clinical research has not been strongly emphasized. This is changing as regulatory agencies, such as The Joint Commission, and professional groups, such as the American Nurses Credentialing Center (ANCC) Magnet Recognition and the American Association of

Critical-Care Nurses (AACN) Beacon awards that reward hospitals for demonstrating an evidence-based nursing practice, include the conduction of research as part of their expectation for recognition. These organizations have identified that clinical outcomes improve when nursing care is evidence based (AACN, 2011; ANCC, 2011; Steele-Moses, 2010). In addition, the presence of an active formal nursing research program demonstrates the hospital's commitment and support.

Clinical research and APN involvement are critical to the profession. To that end a variety of methods are necessary to remove barriers and facilitate the role of the APN in conducting clinically relevant research activities.

Clinical Access and Clinician Buy-In

Selecting a patient population to study is not generally difficult; the choice is driven by the question and the practice or service setting in which the APN works. It is important to remember that for clinical research to become a useful and real part of everyday practice the research must be relevant. Greater buy-in is achieved when there is harmony or mutual interest of the involved participants. APNs can foster a spirit of inquiry and reinforce the idea that research is a journey. The APN acts as a clinical intermediary to influence practice changes by sharing evidence through clinical rounds, in staff education, and by demonstrating practice changes. In this way APNs can bridge the gap between theory and clinical practice (Hutchinson et al, 2014).

Clinical access may be denied (or even covertly discouraged) if the research is not seen as important to the clinical practice. When clinicians are involved and buy-in is high, access to patients is rarely an issue. Unfortunately, APNs who seek to pursue only their own research interests will quickly find that clinicians may not be supportive.

Strategies that have been suggested to encourage a research philosophy and buy-in include traditional solutions such as the establishment of journal clubs. In reality, journal clubs tend to last only for a few meetings, may be poorly attended because they are often held away from the clinical setting, and are often less than inspiring. Although they may be one way of infusing a research focus into practice, they are rarely the complete answer. Instead, the evaluation of scientific articles may be more acceptable and interesting if used in conjunction with a clinical question that emerges from a practice committee meeting or clinical dilemma.

As previously noted, clinicians are interested in research that has direct application to their practice (Chulay, 2006; Gawlinski & Miller, 2011). An evaluation done by staff nurses in a cardiothoracic intensive care unit on the implementation of unit-based research teams revealed value in contributing to nursing research and improving patient outcomes (Gawlinski & Miller, 2011). The clinicians recognized the importance their research had on their clinical practice.

Administrative Support

Administrative support for clinical projects (especially those requiring clinician time or money) heavily hinges on the APN's previous accomplishments. Generally, many of the same attributes (e.g., perseverance, follow-through, and attention to detail) are required for any project to be successful. In addition, communication is essential for a true partnership built on trust and mutual respect between the administrator and the APN. Updates on the project's progress, identification of barriers to the process, and plans for dissemination of the results help ensure administrative understanding and future support.

It is helpful for the APN and administrator to have a discussion early in the partnership about goals for developing a research-based practice. Through the conversation a logical and sequential set of steps can be designed to ensure the APN's success. It is important as well that the APN and administrator agree on the program philosophy and define the boundaries for the program (e.g., support of various aspects such as meeting times, statistical analyses, and financial or educational support for clinicians who present study results outside of the institution).

Fueled in part by the growth in the Magnet Recognition Program, more organizations are establishing dedicated clinical nursing research roles. A more formal framework for research enhances the APN's opportunity to lead or participate in some aspect of clinical research. This may also take the form of including research as an element in the performance appraisal for staff at designated points in a clinical ladder.

Time and Money

In today's practice environment, it is sometimes difficult to believe that there is also time to do research or even to evaluate existing research to determine whether practice changes should be implemented. The refrains "We're too busy" or "We'll do it when we have more time" are common.

The APN's ability to demonstrate how research activities can be accomplished as part of a normal clinical day is essential to ensuring success. In fact, as discussed previously, when considering the feasibility of a research project or EBP change, a realistic assessment of the clinical environment should be accomplished first. Feasibility includes the cost of the project and potential financial outcomes associated with it. Both feasibility and financial solutions were addressed previously in this chapter.

COMPLETING THE RESEARCH ("CLOSING THE LOOP"): ADVANCED PRACTICE NURSE SCHOLARSHIP

A mark of true scholarship is to "close the loop" by presenting the outcomes of the research project to key stakeholders. In some cases this means providing an update in the form of a study summary at the unit level or, if generalizable, to other patient care areas. The outcomes may also be presented at local or national meetings and may be published as well. Unfortunately, many APNs accomplish wonderful research-based practice changes or research studies but they do not disseminate the results.

Learning how to present the material is an important skill that improves with practice. Initially, the APN should seek a mentor who is experienced in presenting and publishing. Although writing and presenting skills may be difficult for the beginning APN, the importance of working to improve the skills cannot be understated. Institutions interested in presentation and publication of APN-related research activities are wise to consider built-in supports such as individuals who have publication experience to help the clinicians learn how to present and publish their work. This specific kind of mentoring is helpful to teach APNs these scholarly activities. In addition, such a supportive commitment is a practical means of ensuring that the work is disseminated and that the APN and institution are recognized for these contributions to nursing knowledge.

AN APPROACH TO CLINICAL RESEARCH: THE EXPERIENCE OF TWO INSTITUTIONS

As discussed throughout this chapter, the APN's level of development largely determines the scope of the clinical research that is attempted. It is essential to start slow and small; the unit level is appropriate at the early stages. Subsequent projects may be attempted at a service line level or with more than one unit. Finally, institutional research projects can be initiated. Regardless of the level, the support of the institution is essential and good communication and a team approach are required. Two institutions' experiences are described to illustrate key components of a successful clinical research program.

Unit Based Research Teams—A Nursing Research Program

A research institute was developed at the Ronald Reagan University of California at Los Angeles (UCLA) Medical Center with an emphasis on mentoring staff nurses to work on unit-based research teams (Gawlinski & Miller, 2011). The staff nurses work collaboratively with APNs called research team leaders. In a competitive process, the research institute recruits one to five research teams. Each team consists of four to five staff nurses and one research team leader. The director of the institute is a doctorally prepared researcher who oversees the institute and is research mentor (RM) to the staff nurses and team leaders. Teams meet twice a month to address aspects of their project and the research process, including choosing the research question, developing the proposal, synthesizing the literature, and analyzing the data. Research results have been shared internally and externally on a national level.

Feedback from participants in the research institute reported it to be an excellent experience. All participants have stated that they would recommend the experience to their colleagues. The program supports and promotes nurses' participation in the development of nursing research.

A Professional Nursing Staff Organization Research Program

At the University of Virginia, the Professional Nursing Staff Organization (PNSO) set a goal of establishing a program of clinical nursing research that is productive, widely disseminated within the hospital, and sustainable.

To accomplish this goal, the PNSO sought the help of one of the hospital's APNs who had a background in clinical unit-based research (Burns, 2010).

The philosophy of the program is that clinical research is a necessary part of nursing practice and clinicians at all levels should be included. To that end the infusion of an institution-wide research milieu is essential. A formal institutional research program designed for professional nurses is a key component.

To ensure that the PNSO research program is successful and sustainable, the focus of the program is the development of bedside clinician researchers. The program director's role is to teach research, one step at a time, to selected clinicians. This oversight is time and effort intensive because the director provides formal classes to teach aspects of research and subsequently helps the clinicians as needed to develop studies with their teams.

The clinician researchers are carefully selected. They are called RMs for two reasons. First, the clinicians are taught by the director how to guide and mentor their teams through all aspects of conducting a project. The mentoring skills that the RMs learn are transferable to other aspects of leadership and are at the core of the APN role. Second, one of the major objectives of the program is to develop a *sustainable* program. Following the completion of the RMs' first study, they are expected to develop second-generation projects with *less* need for intensive oversight and guidance from the director. The RM program is one of the best ways to build research capacity and create a sustainable structure for the organization and conduct of research.

This successful model is popular and more than 400 bedside clinicians are currently involved in research projects of some type (Burns, 2010). The study topics vary widely, but all are fairly narrowly focused to ensure completion. Three examples are described in the following sections to illustrate this concept.

Comparing Adenosine Triphosphate (ATP) Results in Disposable ECG Cables Versus Nondisposable ECG Cables in the Postoperative TCV Pediatric Patient

Mediastinal infection rates were above the target goal in the Pediatric Intensive Care Unit (PICU). The clinicians in this unit were interested in exploring potential risks and implementing strategies to reduce infections. The clinicians understood that contaminated ECG leads posed a potential threat to the cleanliness of the mediastinal surgical site and designed a study to examine the ATP levels on ECG leads.

The purpose of the study was to collect ATP levels on disposable and nondisposable ECG leads from postoperative cardiovascular patients in the PICU (Addison et al, 2014). They designed a study in which patients were randomized to nondisposable ECG leads or disposable ECG leads. The study demonstrated a statistically significant reduction in ATP counts with the disposable ECG lead wires as compared with the nondisposable lead wires in the early postoperative period after pediatric cardiac surgery. Because of this study, the institution removed nondisposable leads from inpatient settings and the outpatient ambulatory surgery center and replaced them with disposable leads. The results were presented in a variety of professional forums and published in a peer-reviewed journal.

Do Nurse-Driven Strategies Improve Pneumococcal Vaccination Rates in Adults Cared for in a Heart and Vascular Clinic?

Nurses in the heart and vascular center were concerned about a lower than desired rate of adherence to recommended pneumococcal vaccination guidelines. Each clinic nurse evaluated his or her own barriers to vaccination using a previously established research tool. After a review of the results, the nurses noted several barriers to vaccination. They questioned whether or not the implementation of a multifaceted intervention program would increase vaccination rates among eligible patients (Turner et al, 2014). The study revealed that implementation of the intervention program was effective in improving vaccination rates. The research team concluded that all ambulatory nurses should integrate assessment, advising and administering the vaccine into their daily practice, and become the standard of care. Because of this work the health system established a task force to develop strategies to improve vaccination rates across the institution. The findings of this study were shared at numerous professional conferences and published in a journal.

What Factors Are Associated With the Development of Pressure Ulcers in a Medical Intensive Care Unit?

Pressure ulcers (PU) contribute to adverse outcomes in patients including pain and discomfort, increased risk of infection, increased cost, and length of stay. The nurses in the Medical Intensive Care Unit (MICU) realized that tools used to assess risk of PU development do not differentiate between adult patients in an intensive care setting versus those in an acute care setting (Lahmann et al, 2012). The research team sought to identify factors that were associated with PU development in a MICU setting. They conducted a 15-month retrospective chart review of patients with PU in the MICU. The results revealed that the presence of hemodynamic support with vasopressor administration and length of stay were the most significant factors of PU development in this population. The findings suggest that instruments specific to the intensive care population are necessary and should include characteristics unique to this population. This study was shared through professional forums and peer-reviewed journals.

Research Program Outcomes

This clinical research program has accomplished the goals set for the first 5 years of program development (Burns, 2010). Selected examples appear in the list that follows by program objective:

- *To develop a research-based nursing* **culture** *by training selected clinicians.* More than 52 clinicians have been trained and more than 400 nurses from 32 practice units or settings are involved in team projects led by the program clinician researchers. The program accepts new applicants yearly via a competitive process and interest and enthusiasm are high.

- *Development of an* **infrastructure** *that supports the evolution and growth of a nursing research program and nurses who do clinical research.* The PNSO research program director and assistant are on the organizational chart and their roles are clear and visible. Administrative and clerical support is present and financial support for research activities is available.

- *To improve nursing practice by* **disseminating the results** *of the studies.* Application of study findings occurs as appropriate within the institution via the nursing institutional practice committee mechanism. Many presentations have been given locally, regionally, or nationally. Sixteen manuscripts are published or in press (many more have been submitted and are in review).

- **To recognize and celebrate** *the accomplishments of the nursing research.* The program and program outcomes have been recognized both directly and indirectly via mechanisms such as the Magnet and Beacon awards, as well as media recognition (local TV station video pieces on the nursing studies, Web postings, and even news articles [e.g., *New York Times*]). Plus the program outcomes and the research projects are recognized at our annual EBP Day and with internal awards for the projects.

CONCLUSION

Excellence in advanced practice depends on creating sustainable and active EBP. For the APN to guide and shape practice, research must be integrated. Whether we serve as consumers of research by reading and applying results of scientific reports or actually conduct studies to determine the answer to a clinical question, research must be evident as an important element of everyday practice. The role of the APN as a RM and leader is essential to ensure that EBP is integrated and widespread. Only then will research truly be "part of what we do."

17

The Advanced Practice Nurse
Holism and Complementary and Integrative Health Approaches

Carole Ann Drick

Learning Outcomes

Learning outcomes expected as a result of this chapter:

- Discuss the implications of renaming the National Center for Complementary and Alternative Medicine (NCCAM) as the National Center for Complementary and Integrative Health (NCCIH).
- Illustrate the holistic framework as an expanded theoretical base for advanced practice nursing.
- Evaluate progress in the development of complementary and integrative health (CIH).
- Explain the NCCIH categorization of holistic approaches.
- Discuss the effect of health-care reform on the future of holistic nursing.
- Explain nurse coaching as an adjunct to advanced practice nursing.
- Support the need for expanding research on CIH.
- Demonstrate the relationship between advanced practice holistic nursing and CIH.
- Distinguish the advanced practice nursing practice issues and CIH.
- Discuss ethical issues in holistic nursing.

INTRODUCTION

Increasing interest in "natural remedies" and Eastern and indigenous healing in the last 35 years has become more evident as consumers are more knowledgeable in accessing health and illness information from the Internet. The field known historically as *alternative medicine* has slowly evolved into *complementary-alternative medicine (CAM).* "Now realizing the recent change in name of the National Center for Complementary and Alternative Medicine (NCCAM) to the National Center for Complementary and Integrative Health (NCCIH), nurses as patient advocates need to be familiar with the emerging terminology to support health literate decisions by patients. NCCIH defines 'complementary' as a practice used **together with** conventional medicine, while 'alternative' refers to a non-mainstream practice used **in place of** conventional medicine. 'Integrative' health care involves the coordination of conventional and complementary approaches. The change from a focus on alternative medicine to integrative health further supports the role of holistic nurses, who have long been champions of integrative health" (American Holistic Nurses Association [AHNA], 2016). The NCCIH in turn has developed more concise types of complementary health approaches. See **Table 17.1.**

For advanced nursing, the terms *complementary* and *holistic* are preferable because both imply a philosophical framework that is greater than the modality. For the larger picture of health care, the term *integrative health* is more appropriate. Because some of the data presented in this chapter reflects practice and research literature before the name change and redefinitions, the term *CAM* will occasionally be used. Note, however, that CAM implies an emphasis on modality rather than on a philosophical approach. In this chapter the terms *CAM, complementary,* and *holism* will reflect "the integrative nature of nursing practice with the term *integrative health* reflecting the inclusion of complementary modalities into the biomedical model of care." The term *approach* now replaces modalities, treatments, or therapies. Hopefully this is the first step in the transformation of the Western biomedical health-care system changing its philosophical base to one grounded in holistic, caring philosophy.

Historically, nurses have been at the forefront of developing holistic care and complementary and integrative health (CIH) modalities. Florence Nightingale's (1859/1969) early statistical and clinical work taught the health-care community about the importance of environment and spirituality on health and healing. Nightingale believed that nurses put the patients in the best condition for nature to act on them and that all disease is essentially a "reparative process." She argued for a comprehensive approach that emphasized cleanliness, fresh air, color, fresh food, and the presence of pets to aid healing in the sick and injured. She also emphasized spirituality.

The holistic, bio-psycho-social-spiritual-cultural model has been introduced in fundamental nursing texts. Nurses value the role of the interpersonal relationships in their healing work and incorporate the role of environmental influences and culture. Nurses have been pioneers in the integration of comfort-enhancing mind-body approaches such as prepared childbirth education, preparation for surgery programs, and

TABLE 17.1		
Terms Associated With CIHA and Holistic Nursing		
Term	**Definition**	**Source**
Holistic care	Refers to approaches and interventions that address the needs of the whole person: body, mind, emotion, and spirit.	AHNA Position on the Role of Nurses in the Practice of Complementary and Integrative Health Approaches (CIHA) 2016
Complementary approaches	As a practice, used *together with* conventional medicine.	National Center for Complementary and Integrative Health
Alternative approaches	Refers to a nonmainstream practice used *in place of* conventional medicine.	National Center for Complementary and Integrative Health
Integrative health care	Involves the coordination of conventional and complementary approaches	National Center for Complementary and Integrative Health

the use of gentle massage. Relaxation, imagery, fostering a therapeutic relationship and communication, and the development of therapeutic touch (TT) and healing touch (HT) have been part of our holistic nursing lexicon for decades. To promote comfort and enhance healing nurses in many hospitals and outpatient settings now practice Reiki, another "subtle energy" approach. However, the holistic nursing foundation that formally began in 1981 has waxed and waned throughout our development as a profession. As the nurse practitioner (NP) movement developed in the late 1960s nurses became more "medicalized" and specialized in both focus and practice. Consequently, many nurses may be marginally prepared or unprepared to meet their patients' holistic needs. Advanced practice nurses (APNs), aware that they are focusing exclusively on the medical aspects of their practice, may re-discover the richness of more holistic approaches that also promote more job satisfaction and less burnout.

As NPs became more specialized in developing group-specific knowledge and skills (i.e., children, women, and mental health clients), they became preoccupied with *parts* of the person or group but not the integral whole (Erickson, 2007). In response, Kubsch and colleagues (2007) advocated for a paradigm shift from a reductionist frame of reference (i.e., characteristic of our current allopathic health-care system and some NP programs) to one that reflects a holistic philosophy that includes complementary approaches. In such a shift, health is synonymous with well-being. Tension, however, continues to exist between physicians, nurses, and consumers as this paradigm shift is occurring. The tension is further accentuated in the attempt to balance client satisfaction with the demands for cost containment and institutional practitioner productivity quotas.

HOLISM AND HOLISTIC NURSING

Many nurses who identify themselves as "holistic" incorporate complementary and integrative health approaches (CIHA). According to the American Holistic Nurses Association (AHNA), holistic nurses recognize two views of holism: (a) identifying the interrelationships of the bio-psycho-social-spiritual dimensions of the person; that is, recognizing that the whole is greater than the sum of its parts; and (b) understanding the individual as a unitary whole in mutual process with the environment. Both views are valued, and the goals of nursing can be achieved within either framework (AHNA, 2013). Either holistic philosophy is congruent with the theoretical base for advanced nursing practice of CIHA and a holistic nursing practice. This holistic emphasis is the framework for this chapter. An approach (complementary or conventional), therefore, is less important than the holistic intent of the practitioner. A danger for APNs lies in placing too great an emphasis on the approach rather than the theoretical and philosophical foundations for practice. These foundations can also be seen as the science and art of holistic nursing.

Healing is basic to nursing practice and is a term often used in conjunction with holistic nursing and complementary modalities. It is a process rather than an endpoint. Holism may include cure, but it implies recovery from a state of feeling shattered or fragmented into one of new or restored wholeness. The person becomes aware of a shift in his or her perception of a life experience, finds new meaning, and often develops new behaviors (Zahourek, 2009).

At the First American Samueli Symposium (2002, consortium of academic health centers with a focus on integrative medicine), a panel that included six nurse leaders grappled with issues of definition and research in healing. They discussed the process and potential outcomes of a "healing relationship" as the basis for both research and practice (Quinn et al, 2003). This relationship is the "quality and characteristics of interactions between healer and healee that facilitate healing" and includes "empathy, caring, love, warmth, trust, confidence, credibility, honesty, expectation, courtesy, respect, and communication" (Dossey, 2003, p. A11). During that period Donnelly (2006) explained that "holistic nursing interventions have always originated from the perspective of the person, community or family" (p. 215) and suggests that holistic nursing can help transform today's health-care system. Holistic nursing is "all nursing practice that has healing the whole person as its goal" (AHNA, 1998). Holistic nurses become "therapeutic partners" to strengthen human responses by facilitating the healing process and promoting wholeness (Mariano, 2007, p. 166).

About the American Holistic Nurses Association

Holistic nursing focuses on integrating traditional, complementary, and holistic approaches to improve the physical, mental, emotional, and relational health of the whole person. It fosters the nurse's self-care, self-reflection, and presence to enhance quality person-centered care.

At its founding in 1981, the AHNA adopted as its primary mission the advancement of holistic health care by increasing awareness and promoting education as well as personal community-building among nurses, other health-care professionals, and the public. This professional specialty nursing membership organization is becoming the definitive voice for holistic nursing for registered nurses (RNs) and other holistic health-care professionals around the world.

In 2007 the AHNA was recognized by the ANA as a specialty with its own *Scope and Standards of Practice* (AHNA & ANA, 2007; Mariano, 2007). The AHNA *Scope and Standards of Practice* was revised in 2013 (AHNA & ANA, 2013) and a third edition will be available in 2018.

As a specialty, holistic nursing is based on "a philosophy, a body of knowledge, and an advanced set of nursing skills applied to practice that recognize the totality of the human being, the interconnectedness of body, mind, spirit, energy, social/cultural relationship context, and environment. Philosophically it is a world view, and not just a modality" (Mariano, 2007, p. 166). This clear and concise summary statement still holds true today. Practice is drawn from various healing systems, incorporates CIHA, and through "unconditional presence and intention" creates healing environments; self-care and self-responsibility are essential components. Holistic nursing approaches may be integrated into any conventional practice.

For decades before 1985, nurses used holistic approaches that are presently clearly defined by the now renamed NCCIH. Some of these include relaxation, art, guided imagery, movement, massage, meditation, music, sound therapy, and prayer. Nurses incorporate subtle energy therapies such as TT, HT, aromatherapy, and Reiki in their work in various clinical settings (Dossey & Keegan, 2016).

MILESTONES IN THE DEVELOPMENT OF COMPLEMENTARY AND INTEGRATIVE HEALTH

The research base for complementary health approaches continues to grow. NCCIH was founded at the National Institutes for Health (NIH) in 1999 as an outgrowth of the Office of Alternative Medicine. Its mission is to define,

through rigorous scientific investigation, the usefulness and safety of CIH interventions and their roles in improving health and health care (NCCIH, 2016a).

The most current (2012) National Health Interview Survey (NHIS) and continuing studies support that approximately 33.2% of adult Americans use complementary health approaches (NCCIH, 2016b). NCCIH funds research in more than 260 institutions and supplies information for practitioners, researchers, and consumers, including Internet-accessible information sheets; up-to-date research compilations on approaches and supplements; research blogs; entries on Facebook, Twitter, and YouTube; and continuing education series and outreach to health-care providers through a dedicated portal.

NCCIH recently (2016a) changed its categorization of CIHA from categories of natural products, mind-body approaches, manipulative body-based practices, whole system approaches, and other to two subgroups of *natural products* and *body-mind practices* plus an *other* for approaches that do not fit exclusively into one of the two larger subgroups. This change will probably not satisfy many nurses who practice TT, HT, Reiki, or other energy therapies because they have been omitted in the examples. Likewise, the term *energy therapies* has been omitted. See **Box 17.1.**

According to the old Web site (NCCAM), "some CAM practices involve manipulation of various *energy* fields to affect health. Such fields may be characterized as veritable (measurable) or putative (yet to be measured)." Practices based on veritable forms of energy include those involving electromagnetic fields (e.g., *magnet therapy* and *light therapy*). Practices based on putative energy fields (also called biofields) generally reflect the concept that human beings are infused with subtle forms of energy. Such interventions include Qigong, Reiki, TT, and HT. In these modalities practitioners use intent in transmitting a universal energy to a person, either from a distance or by placing their hands on or near that person. Unfortunately this extensive explanation is no longer available on the Web site as of 2016. However, there is now a much more extensive in-depth research and publication listing. What was once in need of explanation is now becoming more commonplace and accepted.

Many complementary health approaches involve personal or self-care activities (e.g., exercise, meditation, and prayer), natural and herbal products (e.g., over-the-counter

Box 17.1

National Center for Complementary and Integrative Health Classification System

Most complementary health approaches fall into one of two subgroups—natural products or mind and body practices.

Natural Products

This group includes a variety of products, such as herbs (also known as botanicals), vitamins and minerals, and probiotics. They are widely marketed, readily available to consumers, and often sold as dietary supplements.

Mind and Body Practices

Mind and body practices include a large and diverse group of procedures or techniques administered or taught by a trained practitioner or teacher. The 2012 NHIS showed that yoga, chiropractic and osteopathic manipulation, meditation, and massage therapy are among the most popular mind and body practices used by adults. The popularity of yoga has grown dramatically in recent years, with almost twice as many U.S. adults practicing yoga in 2012 as in 2002.

Other mind and body practices include acupuncture, relaxation techniques (such as breathing exercises, guided imagery, and progressive muscle relaxation), TaiChi, Qigong, HT, hypnotherapy, and movement therapies (such as Feldenkrais method, Alexander technique, Pilates, Rolfing Structural Integration, and Trager psychophysical integration).

The amount of research on mind and body approaches varies widely depending on the practice. For example, researchers have done many studies on acupuncture, yoga, spinal manipulation, and meditation, but there have been fewer studies on some other practices.

Other Complementary Health Approaches

The two broad areas discussed previously—natural products and mind and body practices—capture most complementary health approaches. However, some approaches may not neatly fit into either of these groups—for example, the practices of traditional healers, Ayurvedic medicine, traditional Chinese medicine, homeopathy, and naturopathy.

Adapted from National Center for Complementary and Integrative Health. Retrieved from nccih.nih.gov.

nonregulated dietary supplements, herbs, megavitamins, and probiotics), or treatments given by specialized practitioners (e.g., acupuncturists, chiropractors, and doctors of oriental medicine). Some practices are grounded in culture and tradition (Ayurveda) and others are original nursing interventions (TT and HT). Modalities considered to be complementary health approaches continue to change as a specific practice becomes more standardized because research supports its mechanism, efficacy, or safety. Acupuncture, acupressure, aromatherapy, biofeedback, chiropractic care, diet, exercise, guided imagery, some herbal medicine, some homeopathy, humor, hypnosis, magnets, massage, meditation, music, prayer, and relaxation techniques all currently enjoy a substantial research base; reports of these modalities can be found on the NCCIH Web site (http://nccih.nih.gov/health). See **Box 17.2** for the variety of materials available through NCCIH.

NCCIH 2016 Strategic Plan

In February 2016, NCCIH released its strategic plan, *Exploring the Science of Complementary and Integrative Health: Fourth Strategic Plan 2016–2020*. The plan outlines goals and objectives and takes into account scientific gaps and opportunities under three scientific and two cross-cutting objectives. Note that the scientific objectives within the plan are aligned with those of the *NIH-Wide Strategic Plan, Fiscal Years 2016–2020: Turning Discovery Into Health* (https://www.nih.gov/about-nih/nih-wide-strategic-plan).

Within this strategic plan are five goals with two to three strategic objectives underneath each one. Three overarching goals have relevance for APNs:

1. Advance fundamental science and methods development
2. Improve care for hard-to-manage symptoms
3. Foster health promotion and disease prevention

Resources Available at National Center for Complementary and Integrative Health

The NCCIH Web site includes a broad range of information in the public domain and encourages duplication and dissemination.

- Complementary, Alternative, and Integrative Health: What's in a Name?
- Dietary and Herbal Supplements
- Herbs at a Glance
- Statistics on Use
- Safety Information
- Health Topics A–Z or Health Information: Most frequently viewed health topics: acupuncture, arthritis, black cohosh, cancer, chelation, chiropractic, dietary supplements, depression, Echinacea, ephedra, gingko, ginseng, glucosamine, homeopathy, herbs at a glance, meditation, menopause, and St. John's wort

- Clinical Trials and Research
- Grants and Funding
- NCCIH Clearing House—information about NCCIH or any complementary health approach. Phone: 888-644-6226, FAX: 866-464-3616, e-mail: info@nccih.nih.gov; Written: NCCIH Clearinghouse, PO Box 7923, Gaithersburg, MD, 20898-7923
- Connect With Us: E-mail, Updates, Follow on Social Media, Live Chats With Experts, or Subscribe to a Variety of E-mail Updates
- Treatment Information: Relabeled and available under Health Topics A-Z and listed as Condition. Available at https://nccih.nih.gov/health/atoz.htm
- National Institute of Health Consensus Development Program: In 2013 the Office of Disease Prevention formally retired this program.

Adapted from National Center for Complementary and Integrative Health Web site: nccih.nih.gov.

Goal 1: Advance Fundamental Science and Methods Development

People commonly use complementary health approaches to manage symptoms of diseases and conditions that are difficult to treat such as back or neck pain, arthritic or other musculoskeletal pain, and insomnia. Recent evidence suggests that some complementary health approaches help to mitigate these symptoms; in some cases, they engage innate biological processes involved in pain and emotion management. More research is needed to understand whether and how such interventions augment existing approaches and to identify the related biological mechanisms.

Goal 2: Improve Care for Hard-to-Manage Symptoms

Many advanced practice practitioners use complementary health approaches such as aromatherapy, meditation, relaxation, movement therapies, or yoga to help motivate people to adopt and sustain healthier lifestyles. Natural products such as dietary supplements or herbs are also used to promote better health. The evidence supports the idea that those who use complementary health approaches may have better health-seeking behaviors.

Goal 3: Foster Health Promotion and Disease Prevention

NCCIH continues to fully support research that addresses promotion and prevention and provides evidence-based information on the complementary health approaches that support this for both the professional and lay public. A continued realization and emphasis in the 2016 plan is for research that is applicable to, and generated from, the "real world" of clinical practice. Basic research to study biological processes associated with complementary health approaches will continue. Outcomes research and effectiveness of complementary health approaches in practice is a welcomed and pertinent addition.

HEALTH-CARE REFORM IN 2011

After 4 years implementing many aspects of the Affordable Care Act (ACA) and an estimated 48.6 million people originally uninsured eligible to join, many provisions still remain that have implications for APRNs, including an emphasis on health maintenance, prevention, and better management of chronic disease and related symptoms. For example, combating the high percentage of obesity in Americans, particularly in children, provides opportunities for APRNs using a variety of approaches including complementary health approaches. These health-care challenges often respond well to complementary health approaches.

Although APNs are ready and very capable of practicing within their scope and standards of practice, there continues to be a shortage of both nurses and physicians, presenting a huge challenge to an already overtaxed health-care system. Equally important is the issue of nurses being able to practice to the full extent of their license. The Institute of Medicine (IOM) report that follows sheds further light on this situation.

THE 2010 INSTITUTE OF MEDICINE REPORT ON THE FUTURE OF NURSING AND PROGRESS REPORT ON NURSING GOALS 2020

The IOM report on *The Future of Nursing* (2010) saw the United States transforming its health-care system to provide high-quality care leading to improved health outcomes with nurses playing a significant role. Although the APN's expanded role has been under scrutiny, this role in primary care was seen as important in providing wellness and prevention services, as well as diagnosis and management of many uncomplicated common illnesses and the management of chronic illness. The conflicts between what APRNs could do based on their education and training and what they may do according to state and federal regulations needed to be resolved so that they would be better able to provide seamless, affordable, and high-quality care (Fairman, Rowe, Hassmiller, & Shalala, 2011). Scope-of-practice regulations in all states needed to reflect the full extent not only of nurses' but of each profession's education and training. Elimination of barriers for all professions with a focus on collaborative teamwork would maximize and improve care throughout the nation.

The IOM report, NCCIH's 2010 strategic plan, and the tenets of the ACA all contended that prevention, management of chronic illness, and the promotion of comfort at all stages of life are goals to which our society must aspire. These tenets resonate with many complementary health approaches that focus on noninvasive, more natural interventions to promote healthy lifestyles and the management of chronic conditions that do not seem to respond well to conventional medical practices.

In 2015 the IOM came out with a progress report on nursing goals for 2020 (Lynch, 2015). Specific recommendations were in the areas of removing barriers to practice and care, transforming education, collaborating and leading, promoting diversity, and improving data. The committee concluded with, "no single profession, working alone, can meet the complex needs of patients and communities. Nurses should continue to develop skills and competencies in leadership and innovation and collaborate with other professionals in health-care delivery and health system redesign. To continue progress on the implementation of *The Future of Nursing* recommendations and to effect change in an evolving health-care landscape, the nursing community, including the campaign, must build and strengthen coalitions with stakeholders both within and outside of nursing."

In the last 5 years the following progress has been made:

- Many nurses are returning to school for higher education; many institutions and communities and some states have reached or will reach the goal of 80% of nurses having a baccalaureate degree.
- Physicians continue to pose barriers to modernizing scope of practice legislation . . . working to improve our collaboration with physicians, consumers, and others, advance practice nurses will be recognized and accessed to their full scope of practice.
- Now nurses speak in terms of "we" and "us," rather than "they" and "their," . . . finding new ways of re-engaging ourselves and creating new opportunities to build a culture of health in our communities through collaboration with others.
- Campaign fostering nursing leadership; 21 organizations are working jointly to have 10,000 nurses on various organizational boards by 2020 including public health, philanthropic, corporate, and governmental boards.

THE COACHING MOVEMENT

Since the mid 1990s health, wellness, and life coaching roles have been growing in numbers across disciplines. Part of health-care reform is to establish a *medical home.*

The term was originally used for primary care physicians in 1967 by the Academy of Pediatrics. The medical home was conceived to be the "home base" for health care. Currently, it is conceived to be a multidisciplinary team whose emphasis is prevention of illness and wellness maintenance in primary care. The health coach is considered part of wellness initiatives (Jonas, 2009).

Concurrently, the International Council of Nurses with Sigma Theta Tau created the document *Coaching in Nursing* (Donner & Wheeler, 2009), which established its own scope and competencies and described a relationship between health and wellness coaching and nursing. When coaching was first being developed, the word *competencies* rather than *standards* as written by ANA was chosen to avoid any confusion.

Hess (2011) defines *holistic* coaching as "skilled purposeful results-oriented and structured relationship-centered interactions with clients by registered nurses for the purpose of promoting the health and well-being of the whole person" (p. 16). It is not therapy or counseling. The goal is to create healthy behaviors and lifestyle changes, and the relationship offers the opportunity to use numerous complementary health approaches as appropriate. The nuances and diversity of nurse coaching can be seen as it is being brought to a cardiovascular health clinic (Stuart-Mullen et al, 2015) considering it through the theory of Integrative Nurse Coaching (Dossey & Luck, 2015) or Transpersonal Coaching (Schaub & White, 2015) and Cultural Diversity in Coaching (Southard, 2015).

National Certification as a Nurse Coach

The American Holistic Nurses Credentialing Corporation (AHNCC) is committed to values that enhance professional practice and contribute to competency for practicing nurse coaches. In this capacity, nurse coaches do the following:

- Facilitate individuals to make healthy choices resulting in long-term sustainable lifestyle changes that improve health, wellness, and well-being.
- Respect the client's worldview, culture, and priorities.
- Create an interactive partnership that challenges perceptions and examines barriers.
- Support self-identified goal selection and journey.

As health care moves toward a focus of health, wellness, and well-being, it is essential that APRNs provide leadership in this arena. Holistic nursing, which is based on facilitating an individual's greatest state of wellness and quality of life, regardless of the population or setting, is best achieved by nursing leaders who are certified in holistic nursing, advanced practice holistic nursing, or nurse coaching. The AHNCC Nurse Coach certification examination is given yearly in the spring and fall (www.ahncc.org).

RESEARCH ON COMPLEMENTARY AND INTEGRATIVE HEALTH USE

Over the last 25 years numerous national surveys have demonstrated a consistent increase in the use of CAM. The most recent survey by NCCIH, released in December 2012, revealed that about 33.2% of U.S. adults aged 18 years and older and 11.6% of children use some form of CAM (NCCIH, 2016b). The first landmark utilization survey (Eisenberg et al, 1993) established that approximately 33% of individuals in the United States had used one or more unconventional therapies during the preceding year. In a follow-up study, Eisenberg and colleagues (1998) found an increased use—42.1% of Americans had used one or more CAM approaches. The NCCIH report released in May 2004 of the largest survey of Americans to date was conducted with the National Center for Health Statistics (NCHS) in the Centers for Disease Control and Prevention (CDC). The study surveyed 31,044 adults and found that 55% believed CAM was beneficial, particularly when combined with conventional approaches; 36% used some form of CAM, and when prayer was included as a modality, up to 62% used CAM. When prayer was included, the mind-body domain was most commonly used; when prayer was excluded, biologically based approaches (22%) were most common (mind-body therapies: 17%). Prayer and seeking spiritual guidance continued to be the most commonly used approach for specific health problems. According to all the epidemiological studies, in addition to prayer, the most commonly used approaches include mind-body interventions, herbs, supplements, homeopathy, acupuncture, massage, chiropractic, stress management procedures, and energy work such as Reiki and TT (NCCAM, 2008).

Compare the previous report to the NCCIH 2012 report with its newly developed subgroups of natural products, mind and body practices, and other complementary approaches. This report overview states the following.

- The most commonly used complementary approach was use of natural products (dietary supplements other than vitamins and minerals). Per the research, 17.7% of adults and 4.9% of children age 4 to 17 used natural products.
- Pain—a condition for which people often use complementary health approaches—is common in U.S. adults. More than half had some pain during the 3 months before the survey.
- U.S. adults who take natural products (dietary supplements other than vitamins and minerals) or who practice yoga were more likely to do so for wellness reasons than for treating a specific health condition. In contrast, people who use spinal manipulation more often do so for treatment reasons than wellness.
- Around 60% of NHIS respondents who used chiropractic care had at least some insurance coverage for it, but rates were much lower for acupuncture (25%) and massage (15%).
- About 59 million Americans spend money out-of-pocket on complementary health approaches, and their total spending adds up to $30.2 billion a year.

Interestingly, this report on the amount of money spent on CIHA is less than the Eisenberg et al (1998) estimate of $36 to $46 billion. Continued research may show that the reasons and purposes for complementary health approaches are as diverse as the consumers who use them.

Consumers incorporate complementary approaches in designing their own integrative health plans. Success of these plans is demonstrated by the findings that 79% of respondents using both CAM therapies and traditional medicine "perceived the combination to be superior to either one alone" (Eisenberg et al, 2001, p. 1). Jonas (1997) concluded that consumers' complementary therapy use does not always mean dissatisfaction with conventional medicine (p. 34). One might speculate, however, from simply listening to the evening news that in the years since his article, dissatisfaction with health-care accessibility, expense, and quality has continued. Newer statistics on CAM use are not currently available.

One most revealing finding from all the different surveys is that greater than half of the respondents do *not* share their use of CAM practices with their health-care provider. Reasons for this nondisclosure ranged from feeling that it was not important for the provider to know, the provider did not ask, the patient thought it was none of the provider's business, or the provider would not understand. It is important to note that in 1998 primary care providers were mandated to question patients about the use of complementary health approaches and record the information in their permanent records (United States Department of Health and Human Services [USDHHS], 1998).

National Center for Complementary and Integrative Health as a Resource

NCCIH is a vitally important link for health-care professionals and consumers in providing information about the research status of CAM therapies (see Box 17.2). Resources are now easily available through direct download or by signing up online for their updates or to access your subscriber preferences.

Evidence-based research is becoming more prominent and also easily accessible on the NCCIH Web site. Listing of both their conducted and sponsored research is readily available along with highlights of recently published studies funded by NCCIH (nccih.nih.gov).

It is more and more evident that consumers are engaging in complementary health approaches whether the health-care professional guides them or not. Consumers want to be in charge of their health and are taking more responsibility for their well-being. As APNs we must be knowledgeable about the safety and efficacy of complementary therapies to assist clients to choose the best modalities.

COMPLEMENTARY AND INTEGRATIVE HEALTH AND ADVANCED PRACTICE HOLISTIC NURSING

One of the important roles of the advanced practice holistic nursing (APHN) is to support patients in their choice of complementary health approaches, make recommendations, and deliver safe and effective complementary approaches when appropriate. Being able to see the whole person, the person's values, and what is important in his or her life is an important part of effective quality care.

Examples of Complementary and Integrative Health Approaches (CIHA) in the Literature

Several years before the landmark Eisenberg and colleagues study (1993), nurses were practicing and publishing about CAM approaches. Snyder (1985) completed a book titled *Independent Nursing Interventions* that included CAM approaches (e.g., relaxation, imagery, massage). Clark (1986) wrote *Wellness Nursing*, and Dossey and Keegan's *Holistic Nursing: A Handbook for Practice* was first published in 1988. Clements and Martin wrote *Nursing and Holistic Wellness* (1990). Zahourek authored early papers on the use of hypnosis with pain (1982a, 1982b) and two clinically based books: *Clinical Hypnosis and Therapeutic Suggestion in Nursing* (1985) and *Relaxation and Imagery* for nurses (1988). Delmar published *The Nurse as Healer,* a series of small books edited by Keegan on such topics as *Creative Imagery in Nursing* (Shames, 1996) and *Awareness in Healing* (Rew, 1996).

It is also paradoxical that McCloskey and Bulechek (1992) classified several of these same therapies as nursing interventions in the year before Eisenberg's report (1993). Their 7-year research project funded by the National Institute of Nursing culminated in the publication of the *Nursing Interventions Classification* (NIC). This comprehensive standardized classification of research-based nursing interventions (McCloskey & Bulechek, 2000) included "simple guided imagery" (p. 595), "simple massage" (p. 596), and "simple relaxation therapy" (p. 598). The literature since then has blossomed and articles now appear with some regularity on holistic approaches and nurses' involvement with CAM.

General practice journals such as *American Nurse* and *American Journal of Nursing,* as well as specialty journals (e.g., *Journal of the American Psychiatric Nurses Association*), theoretical journals such as *Nursing Science Quarterly,* and research journals such as *Nursing Research* and *The Journal of Holistic Nursing,* all publish articles related to CAM practice. In addition, the seventh edition of *Holistic Nursing: A Handbook for Practice* was published in 2016 by editors Barbara Dossey and Lynn Keegan. These publications are valuable resources for holistic nursing theory development and for providing the newest research and thinking on numerous CIHA practiced by holistic nurses.

Natural Products

The NCCIH recognizes that most complementary health approaches fall into one of two subgroups. The following sections will also recognize the subgroups of natural products and mind and body practices.

The natural products subgroup includes herbs, also known as botanicals, vitamins and minerals, and probiotics. Although widely marketed and readily available to consumers, they are often sold as dietary supplements. The 2012 NHIS included a comprehensive survey on the use of complementary health approaches by Americans, finding 17.7% of American adults using a dietary supplement other than vitamins and minerals during the past year. The most commonly used natural product was fish oil.

Although natural products are not regulated, the Food and Drug Administration (FDA) is currently developing good manufacturing practices (GMPs) for dietary supplements. Newly marketed products are not subject to pre-market approval or surveillance. Americans use supplements and herbs to promote overall health, to improve performance and energy, to treat depression, and to treat and prevent such illnesses as colds and flu. Because new research changes our knowledge base, readers are referred to the NCCIH and Cochrane Review Web sites where updated research results from large national studies and systematic reviews on natural products can be found (nccih.nih.gov)(http://www.cochrane.org).

The journal *Holistic Nursing Practice* has a regular column on herbs and supplements. Regular articles in *Holistic Nursing Practice* by Stephanie Ross include arnica gel for osteoarthritis (2008) and herbal medicine in women's health (2011). Topics have included the use of cranberry for urinary tract infections, chocolate for cardiovascular health, valerian for sleep, and St. John's wort for mild to moderate depression. The *American Nurse Today* (Fitzgerald, 2007) published a continuing education article on the use of herbs that included descriptions of six herbs (feverfew, gingko biloba, red yeast rice, saw palmetto, St. John's wort, and valerian) and their potential drug-herb interactions. Rosenfeld (2008), in the popular magazine *Parade,* reviewed the safety and effectiveness of ginseng, garlic, Echinacea, chamomile, St. John's wort, ginkgo biloba, valerian, ginger, saw palmetto, hawthorn, black cohosh, and feverfew. His information coincided with the office of dietary supplements fact sheets, which review the research, uses, and side effects of these and other herbs and supplements. Currently, more studies are being conducted on black cohosh for menopausal symptoms and vitamin D for bone health. Health effects of Omega-3 fatty acids for people with depression and B vitamins and berries in age-related neurodegenerative diseases are also being reported on the NCCIH and Cochrane Review Web sites. NCCIH has several Web pages devoted to herbs and supplements. The page "Herbs at a Glance" lists 42 popular herbs that can be accessed, including black cohosh, cranberry, ephedra, ginger, gingko biloba, kava, milk thistle, and green tea. Consult the NCCIH Web site for the most current information on their effectiveness, as well as drug-herb-supplement interactions.

Because many patients may use supplements without knowledge of their dosages, effects, or potential side effects, APNs—and particularly those with prescriptive authority—need to know how to access accurate information on herbal remedies and supplements. Used for centuries and in many cultures, herbs can be as effective as our manufactured medications; therefore, some of the same cautions exist. Cautions for herbs and supplements listed by NCCIH include being aware of the following:

- Whether a person has substituted an herb or supplement for a conventional medication
- The potential impact of the supplement on the client's overall condition
- Potential interactions between the supplement or herb and other medications
- Particular risks for people with diabetes, hypertension, or mental health problems such as depression and for people facing invasive procedures
- If a woman is pregnant or if treating children

Because many studies indicate that patients do not tell their health-care providers what supplements or herbs they are taking, it is vital to ask patients what they taking, even if the substances are "over the counter," are "natural," or seem benign. A practitioner well educated in supplements and herbs can be a useful resource to the clients served.

Aromatherapy

As a popular natural product aromatherapy is grounded in a holistic philosophy of treating the whole person (Smith & Kyle, 2008). Jane Buckle, PhD, RN, introduced aromatherapy to nursing in 1995. Basically, essential oils derived from plants (common herbs) are either placed on cotton near a person or in a steam distiller. Aromatherapy is often used in conjunction with conventional therapies for pain, anxiety, spasms, insomnia, and infection (Buckle, 2015, 2016). As with herbs and supplements, the practitioner needs to be aware of potential side effects and interactions (Tisserand & Young, 2014). These oils should never be used internally because they are many times stronger than the herb itself (Buckle, 2016).

Aromatherapy research began with anecdotal reports describing positive effects in nursing homes, hospitals, and emergency rooms (Garner, 2007). Now, because of much more sophisticated research, aromatherapy is proving to be an exciting addition to the health care of clients. For example, Canella et al (2012) clearly demonstrated that the use of peppermint aromatherapy can be advantageous in treating nausea in women post C-section. Aromatherapy has been documented to help in a wide variety of diverse conditions including Eucalyptus and Tea Tree as alternatives for treating methicillin-resistant *Staphylococcus aureus* (MRSA) and tuberculosis (Sherry & Warnke, 2002), behavior problems in dementia (Fung et al, 2012), renal colic (Ayan et al, 2013), and wound healing (Chin & Cordell, 2013).

Mind and Body Approaches and Advanced Practice Nursing

It is interesting to note that this section is titled "Mind and Body," not "Body and Mind," which is an indication that the NCCIH recognizes the power of the mind over the body. Knowing that they choose their words very carefully, this is no mistake. It is exciting to see this beginning shift in awareness away from the predominantly biomedical model of health.

According to the 2012 NHIS the 10 most common complementary health approaches were as follows: Natural Products 17%; Deep Breathing 10.9%; Yoga, TaiChi, or Qigong 10.1%; Chiropractic or Osteopathic Manipulation 8.4%; Meditation 8.0%; Massage 6.9%; Special Diets 3.0%; Homeopathy 2.2%; Progressive Relaxation 2.1% and Guided Imagery 1.7%. Note that half of the top

10, or 50% (Deep Breathing; Yoga, TaiChi, or Qigong; Meditation; Progressive Relaxation; and Guided Imagery), are approaches that holistic nurses are aware of, are practiced by many themselves, and are often incorporated into care plans based upon the clients' interest.

With the current concern regarding the increased overuse of narcotics, it comes as no surprise that there is budding research to provide evidence for alternatives. Breathing, meditation, relaxation, and imagery have become standard approaches to assist in pain relief. The NIH News in Health (2013) reports that researchers are exploring relaxation techniques and the effects of stress and often combine breathing and focused attention to calm the mind and body. Relaxation techniques include progressive relaxation, biofeedback, guided imagery, self-hypnosis, and deep-breathing exercises. Holistically, they work even better when combined with good nutrition, regular exercise, and a strong social support system.

Kitko (2007) describes rhythmic breathing as an intervention for pain reduction that is easy to learn. The nurse helps the patient focus on an activity (e.g., purposeful breath), enhancing the relaxation response. Busch et al (2012) advanced the knowledge around deep breathing by simultaneously studying the effects of deep and slow breathing (DSB) on pain perception, autonomic activity, and mood processing with attentive DSB and relaxing DSB as additional variables. Their results suggest that the way of breathing decisively influences autonomic and pain processing. Further, they identified DSB together with relaxation as the essential feature in the modulation of sympathetic arousal and pain perception.

Good and colleagues (2010) used a set relaxation process of jaw and mouth relaxation, slow breathing, and stopping thinking in words. This set was compared with music, as well as music combined with these relaxation techniques, in patients following abdominal surgery. All three groups were compared with a control group. Immediate effects of pain reduction on day one and day two were found with the relaxation and music group. Similar results were obtained by Sand-Jecklin and Emerson (2010) in their exploratory study on the impact of live music with patients who had an unplanned/emergent admission to an acute-care hospital. It was assumed that these patients would have a high level of muscle tension, pain, and anxiety. Participants in this study reported significant reduction in pain, anxiety, and muscle tension and rated the live music as highly helpful

with these symptoms. There were also significant reductions in systolic blood pressure and respirations but not in the diastolic or pulse rate.

Probably the most common types of meditation are guided meditation and now, most popular, mindfulness meditation. Melville et al (2012) compared the effects of a guided meditation practice with acute (15 min) yoga posture performed seated in a typical office workspace on physiological and psychological markers of stress. For the 20 participants the yoga postures or meditation performed in the office acutely improved several physiological and psychological markers of stress. The physiological adaptations generally regressed toward baseline postintervention. Zeidan et al (2016) addressed mindfulness meditation, pain relief, and endogenous opioids. The subjects were 78 healthy adults who were either meditating or not meditating while receiving painful heat stimuli and intravenous administration of either an opioid antagonist or a saline placebo. The findings demonstrate that mindfulness meditation reduces pain independently of opioid neurotransmitter mechanisms. The results suggest that combining mindfulness-based and pharmacological/nonpharmacological pain-relieving approaches that rely on opioid signaling may be particularly effective in treating pain.

NCCIH reviewed studies on mind-body interventions with cancer patients and found evidence that these interventions aid in improving mood, coping, and quality of life, as well as ameliorating chemotherapy-induced nausea, vomiting, and pain. According to this report, strong evidence exists that these techniques also are effective in the treatment of coronary artery disease and enhance cardiac rehabilitation. Several systematic reviews are available through the Internet site Google Scholar (scholar.google.com). Most of these reviews were completed before 2012 and most are for specific conditions such as fibromyalgia, cancer pain, and lifestyle change and management.

Placebo Effect

The *placebo effect* is an unexpected beneficial mind-body response that results from a person's anticipation that an intervention—pill, procedure, or injection—will help. A clinician's style in interacting, certain symbols such as the stethoscope, and certain rituals also may bring about a positive response that is independent of any specific treatment and are easily and consciously used during an interaction.

A major report on the mechanism and value of the placebo as a mind-body response can be found in the *CAM at the NIH Newsletter* (2007). In this newsletter, the placebo effect is treated as a potentially positive therapeutic tool rather than a research problem. Using positive suggestions, no matter what the modality, has a greater chance of success than if communication is negative or fosters a poor response to an intervention. Saying "this will hurt" (negative) or "this may cause some brief discomfort but is so powerful we know it can make you better" (positive) may both set off a "placebo" response but in opposite directions.

According to a study by Kaptchuk and colleagues (2010), placebos given without deception improved symptoms of irritable bowel syndrome (IBS). However, Kahn and colleagues (2014) demonstrated with deception that elastic compression stockings as compared with placebo stockings did not prevent postthrombotic syndrome after a first proximal deep venous thrombosis. The findings did not support routine wearing of elastic compression stockings after deep venous thrombosis. Perhaps the effectiveness of the placebo is dependent on more factors than simply with deception or without deception.

Guided Imagery

Human imagery is a holistic phenomenon described as a "multidimensional mental representation of reality and fantasy that includes not only visual pictures but also remembrance of situations and experiences such as sound, smell, touch, movement and taste" (Zahourek, 2002, p. 113). Imagery is part of the multilayered process of hypnosis that also includes relaxation techniques and suggestion (Jackson, 2016, p. 833). There are many different forms of imagery, including imagery for behavioral rehearsal, impromptu imagery, biologically based imagery, and symbolic and metaphoric imagery (Schaub & Dossey, 2009). Ashen (1977) developed a still relevant theory of imagery: Images are stored in the mind as an experiential unit that includes the image, somatic response, and its meaning. In this context, imagery is used as a therapeutic tool for aiding anxiety, pain, and behavioral rehearsal for change.

Imagery is used in healing trauma and posttraumatic stress disorder, often combined with cognitive-behavioral therapy. It is used to treat numerous acute problems such as preparation for childbirth and for surgery, as well as augmenting and minimizing side effects from medications

and treatments. Grief resolution is, in part, an imagery process because people can be guided to imagine their loss and themselves as strong and coping, and subsequently find meaning in their experience. Reed (2007) describes several uses of imagery in clinical practice in which the study groups who received the imagery intervention had significantly more pain relief and required less pain medication. Eslinger (2000a, 2000b) encourages nurse anesthetists to incorporate some of the techniques to "greatly enhance patient comfort and satisfaction" (2000a, p. 159). Eslinger (2000b) also presents case studies of hypnosis combined with guided imagery to help patients with hemophilia and migraine headaches.

Recent studies from Belgium (Macrae, 2011) have documented the positive effects of hypnosis on women with breast cancer recovering from surgery. Menzies and Jallo (2011) reviewed eight studies in which guided imagery as a dependent variable was used to treat fatigue. In this meta-analysis, 25% demonstrated a significant reduction of fatigue after using guided imagery. Although this study was small, it is reflective of the dearth of research evidence as to the effectiveness of guided imagery, whereas anecdotal reports document the effectiveness of this strategy (Jackson, 2016, p. 833).

Energy Approaches and Holistic Nursing Practice

The human energy field is the basis for practice of holistic nurses and other health practitioners including those practicing yoga, acupuncture, TaiChi, acupressure, Reiki, HT, TT, and many others. "Imbalance in the Energy Field" is the nursing diagnosis when an assessment reveals that realignment is needed to the body for a higher level of functioning (NANDA, 2005). Energy therapies include both nontouching and hands-on therapies that work in the person's biofield of energy. Energy therapies most often used by nurses include TT, HT, and Reiki. They are purported to facilitate both a person's physical and energetic balance, as well as reduce symptoms of disease and the disease itself. Energy approaches are currently taught in continuing education and in holistic nursing programs and courses. Denner (2009) discusses the science of energy therapies as "communication networks," relating them to concepts from quantum physics, as well as ancient Eastern and Shamanic healing practices. Being centered, focused, meditative, and intentional are foundations for these practices. Generally, the practitioner holds an intention for the greatest good for the person rather than for a specific outcome. The practitioner's qualitative sensations of energy flow and balance are the cornerstones of these therapies.

Research on energetic modalities has been difficult in both nursing and in CIHA. Engebretson and Wardell (2007) discussed in detail the methodological issues and problems for these approaches that apply to research. Reviewing published research related to Reiki, TT, and HT used in oncology nursing, Coakley and Barron (2012) found growing evidence that energy therapies have a positive effect on symptoms associated with cancer and for oncology nurses providing integrated nursing care to alleviate suffering and symptom distress of patients with cancer. Floriana (2016) reports the positive effects of energy therapies at the end of life, whereas Hart (2016) adds effects with chronic pain and addiction. Research continues to support that these energetic approaches produce comfort and relaxation and do not cause harm unless an important conventional treatment is avoided.

Anderson and Taylor (2011) discussed biofield therapies on cardiovascular disease management and reviewed studies on HT, TT, and Reiki. They concluded that the primary benefit is using these interventions as adjuncts to standard treatment because they enhance relaxation and enhance the body's own healing capacity. They also recommend continued rigorous study of these interventions with specific populations.

Therapeutic Touch, Healing Touch, and Reiki

In the early 1970s, nurse Dolores Krieger and healer Dora Kunz developed TT to help people with comfort and healing. According to meta-analyses of studies on the effects of TT (including quantitative, qualitative, and mixed-methods research), TT is useful in decreasing anxiety and promoting comfort (Peters, 1999; Winstead-Fry & Wijeck, 1999). Madrid et al (2010) looked at the feasibility of introducing TT into the operative environment with patients undergoing cerebral angiography. Although the protocol was successful, the therapeutic impact of TT was not statistically significant, possibly because of the small sample size. However, TT does show potential to contribute to a positive patient experience in an operative setting. Some studies have also been conducted on the

effect of TT on wound healing, but these effects have been inconsistent.

HT, a biofield energy modality, evolved from TT in the early 1980s and was more extensively developed as a training program by Janet Mentgen in 2002. Similar to TT, HT incorporates other theories and practices and is based on the idea that the body is a complex energy system that can be influenced by another's intention for healing and well-being. In a review of over 30 studies on HT, Wardell and Weymouth (2004) found that the studies reported positive results in reducing stress, anxiety, and pain, and enhancing healing time and quality of life. However, the quality of the research was such that the results could not be generalized. Wardell compiled an annotated bibliography that is available on the Healing Touch International Web site (http://healingtouch.net).

HT research continues to blossom. Tang et al (2010) concluded that training nurse leaders in an academic health center in HT is associated with significant improvements in subjective and objective measures of stress. Decker et al (2012) used HT as an intervention in older adults with persistent pain and with interesting findings: Groups in both studies showed improvement in pain scores, which had implications for both HT and nursing care for the elderly with pain. Wake Forest Medical Center evaluated the impact of HT on nurses beginning their training and reported significant improvement in their stress, depression, anxiety, relaxation, well-being, and sleep (Kemper, 2016).

Originally practiced outside of conventional health care, the Japanese spiritual practice of Reiki is an increasingly popular modality. Reiki is an energy-based therapy in which the practitioner's vibrational energy is connected to a universal source (e.g., chi, qi, prana) and is transferred to a recipient for healing (Miles & True, 2003). Additional nursing reports discuss reducing anxiety and pain after abdominal hysterectomy (Vitale & O'Conner, 2006), self-care for nurses (Vitale, 2009), and orthopedic pain (DiNucci, 2005).

Reiki is similar to HT and TT, but these modalities have had substantially more research and are grounded in nursing theory and practice. Baldwin and colleagues (2010) assembled three teams to collect and systematically review the research on Reiki. In meta-analysis, 26 Reiki articles have been reviewed for strengths and weaknesses. Their results and a database that continues to grow are accessible on the Web site www.centerforreikiresearch .org. Only 12 articles were based on robust experimental design and used adequate outcome measures.

In a review by Janin and Mills (2010) researchers used a best evidence synthesis approach to evaluate 66 studies on TT, Qigong, Reiki, HT, Johari, and other techniques using a specific critical review checklist. Most of the studies were of average to minimum quality for randomization, use of control, and statistical methods. The outcome measures were pain related. Strong evidence was found that pain intensity was reduced and general functioning increased. Related disorders of anxiety and depression and long-term benefits were equivocal. Fazzino and colleagues (2010) completed another review of literature on energy healing and pain from 1980 to 2008. Reiki, HT, and TT were included. Although they made recommendations for future research on these modalities, they concluded that studies which included anxiety and pain found some reduction, and that the amount and frequency of pain medication were reduced.

Emotional Freedom Technique

Emotional Freedom Technique (EFT) was initiated by Gary Craig in the 1990s and is a form of psychological acupressure. It's based on the same energy meridians used in traditional acupuncture to treat physical and emotional ailments for more than 5,000 years, but without the invasiveness of needles. Instead, simple tapping with the fingertips is used to input kinetic energy onto specific meridians on the head and chest while the patient thinks about his or her specific problem—whether it is a traumatic event, an addiction, pain, and so on—and voice positive affirmations.

This combination of tapping the energy meridians and voicing positive affirmation works to clear the "short circuit"—the emotional block—from the body's bioenergy system. This restores the mind and body's balance, which is essential for optimal health and the healing of physical disease. EFT is based on the electromagnetic energy that flows through the body and regulates our health. This is only recently becoming recognized in the West.

Because the techniques are so simple, they can be used effectively as a self-help tool, which empowers people to actively contribute to their own healing and development process. This facilitates a much faster relief process previously believed impossible by health-care professionals who advocated lengthy (and often painful) hours in psychotherapeutic or medical care, often with limited results. These techniques do not discredit the medical and psychotherapeutic professions, but rather serve to contribute to a holistic healing process.

The previous statements are adapted from http://eft .mercola.com.

In relation to phobia-related anxiety, Salas et al (2011) found a significant reduction in phobia-related anxiety and ability to approach a feared stimulus after using EFT. Church et al's (2012) work with depression in college students resulted in determining that EFT has a clinical usefulness as a brief, cost-effective, and efficacious treatment. In treating PTSD, Dawson et al (2013) concurred with other published reports that EFT is efficacious in treating PTSD and comorbid symptoms and its long-term effects. EFT has many therapeutic uses, can be easily taught, and is very useful as a self-help tool for nurses as well as the patient's family, clients, and community.

Quantum Physics

For more than a century the field of quantum physics has been studied among physicists. This brief discussion is meant to awaken awareness for further exploration and the possibilities for quantum physics as a next step in health and healing. Although it appears that the leap between what is occurring on the quantum level and the cellular level could be quantified, what is changing for certain is the gap in our level of understanding.

Heisenberg was the first to publish the idea that the objective reality of Newtonian Physics working does not exist (Heisenberg, 1958). In other words, quantum physics has made the notion of only solid matter or "stuff" incomplete. Quantum's theory of nonlocality suggests a connection between objects that are synchronized, connected, and without distance being part of the equation. This theory of action at a distance demonstrates how objects communicate faster than the speed of light (Shields & Wilson, 2016). Further, these ideas suggest a universal connectedness wherein one can act instantaneously on another regardless of distance.

Today consciousness has many descriptions, such as the awareness of the world. One view by Watts (1960) suggested consciousness was similar to an individual "looking out" from inside a physical body and as a function of the brain. Compare that with quantum physics, which proposes we are more than benign viewers of what is outside ourselves in the world. Think of consciousness as an assortment of subatomic packets of information, moving in a distinct way, interacting with matter. In contrast, traditional Newtonian physics explains the world as matter separated by a void of nothing (Shields & Wilson, 2016).

The psychologist Carl Jung and the physicist Wolfgang Pauli together proposed that the concept of synchronicity might build the connection between the hard science and the subjective experience. They saw synchronicity as "happenings" that seem unrelated but to which people attribute meaning. Further, synchronicity reveals an underlying pattern to the universe as a connectedness that does not seem to be influenced by the distance between coincidental events. Consequently, the world is not a series of random events. Rather, the universe has a deep sense of order (Shields & Wilson, 2016).

It is important to note that there is currently no agreement on the theoretical concepts of quantum physics and its relevance to healing. Some ascertain that the minute layers of waves are too small and cannot have an effect on the larger macro world. However, substantiation is building. Consider that in the 1800s, before Semmelweis's germ theory was accepted, the "modern scientific minds" of the day declared things such as, "It's too small to have an effect" or "Nothing too small for the human eye to see could cause disease; therefore hand washing is a superstitious ritual" (Thompson, 1949). Then the microscope was developed and corroborated germ theory.

Here we are again at the edge of a potential breakthrough in our understanding and thinking—a quantum shift in consciousness, if you will. Perhaps we need a new microscope to unmistakably display this subatomic world and its impact on living things.

Spirituality

One of the most frequently reported components of CIHA is prayer and spirituality. Because the efficacy studies on prayer are contradictory, the controversy most likely will continue. However, dealing with patients' spiritual needs, and our own, is important. For many, coping with this rapidly changing and increasingly technological world is causing existential crises of disconnectedness and a sense of alienation. Threats of devastation from global warming, wars, and financial crises dominate the news,

compounding the anxiety with futility. When illness or injury occurs, or when a loved one dies, the need for solace and a sense of connection, purpose, and meaning become even greater.

The North American Nursing Diagnosis Association (NANDA) recognizes spiritual distress as a diagnosis and the ANA's Code of Ethics (2015) states that nurses must consider a person's value system and religious beliefs. Burkhardt and Nagai-Jacobson (2002) did early work on spirituality in nursing. Spirituality is different from religion; it is the "essence of our being . . . it permeates our living in relationships and infuses our unfolding awareness of who and what we are, our purpose in being, and our inner resources" (Burkhardt & Nagai-Jacobson, 2015, p. 135).

In practice, spirituality is related to active intentional listening and presence. It may involve helping others to find meaning in suffering. Being present with a patient, creating a healing environment, and "inviting reflections" as stories from patients may ameliorate suffering (Deal, 2011). Older adults, for example, derive a sense of meaning from reminiscing and telling their life story to someone who is genuinely interested. Spiritual practices, such as performing mindfulness meditation, centering, practicing yoga, and developing the capacity to be present, are useful for nurses themselves to prevent burnout and create a sense of purpose and meaning in busy and demanding practices.

Baldacchino and Draper (2001) reviewed the literature from 1975 related to spiritual coping (187 articles) and concluded that illness often rendered feelings of a loss of control. Support of spiritual coping strategies in holistic care seemed to enhance self-empowerment, leading to a sense of purpose and meaning. Nurses need to know how to address patients' spiritual needs as they arise. Eldridge (2007) lists nine spiritual interventions: be there, listen actively, use touch, reflect and remember, laugh, share the experience, pray or encourage the patient to pray, use inspirational words or music, and evaluate spiritual needs. Nurses do not force their own beliefs on others; they need to remember the difference between spirituality and religion and respect the religious beliefs and practices, or lack thereof, in those for whom they care.

Tate (2011) performed a systematic-integrated review to provide a comprehensive understanding of the importance of spirituality for African American women during diagnosis and treatment of breast cancer. The foundational theme was a strong belief in and reliance on God. Minden (2013) developed an education approach called Bearing Witness to teach nursing undergraduates soft skills to use with patients living with physical or mental health challenges. Studying acute care nurses' spiritual care practices, Gallison et al's (2013) findings included nurses needing to be in tune with their own spiritual needs in order to be effective in meeting the patients' needs.

Describing spirituality as a personal experience of presence not delineated by religion, Drick (2015) explains that in presence all our senses become involved and we become alert and aware of an essence that is greater than our mind. Presence is an integral part of the holistic healing relationship. Burkhardt and Nagai-Jacobson (2015) view spiritual caregiving as grounded in attentiveness in connection with self, others, nature, and the sacred, whereas Schultz and Loen (2015) reflected on a personal pilgrimage as a sacred journey. The journey is as important as the destination. It is engaging in a journey of physical challenge and self-reflection.

ADVANCED PRACTICE NURSING AND THE AGING POPULATION

The number of Americans age 65 and older will double to more than 72 million, or one in five, by 2030. It is clear we have inadequate facilities and infrastructure to serve the needs of older adults who are dying or living with debilitating chronic disease. Furthermore, the majority of our health-care providers, physicians and nurses, are not trained nor comfortable with dealing with the dying let alone their own mortality. The costs of caring for these individuals are spiraling out of control with the majority of Medicare funds spent on the last month of life (Keegan & Drick, 2011). The perfect storm of dying in America is growing closer and we need to act now (www.GoldenRoomAdvocates.org).

An APN must not only be skilled with "care of the elderly" but also comfortable with his or her own mortality. This seems to be a tall order; however, we cannot give what we do not have. Our compassion can only go as far as we are comfortable. With an understanding of this, Keegan and Drick (2013) wrote a second book for the lay public (*The Golden Room: A Practical Guide for Death With Dignity*) to assist them in beginning the discussion with themselves, their families, and their friends.

Death and dying is a subject that most adults find difficult to talk about in specific and often prefer to change the topic unless it is forced upon them. APNs have an opportunity to lead the way to assist patients to speak about this difficult but critically important topic and to gently use the words *death, dying,* and *end of life.*

On the national level, the Coalition to Transform Advanced Care (C-TAC) was established in 2011 as the largest and most diverse coalition of its kind with more than 110 members. They are dedicated to transforming the care delivery system for those with advanced illness in America. *Advanced illness* and *advanced care* are their words for end of life and dying. They bring together national experts to identify best practices models of care. They use this information to establish effective community-health system partnerships. Then, they disseminate findings to improve the U.S. advanced care laws and policies. In 2015 C-TAC published *A Roadmap for Success: Transforming Advanced Illness Care in America.* This is indeed a road map as it looks at the big picture, the key elements of reform, and action steps for taking this forward. C-TAC is located in Washington, DC, and is one of the more progressive and active end-of-life organizations.

In September 2014, the IOM released a new report, *Dying in America: Improving Quality and Honoring Individual Preferences Near the End of Life.* The report concluded, "a patient-centered, family oriented, approach to care near the end of life should be a high national priority and that compassion, affordable, and effective care for these patients is an achievable goal."

NURSE SELF-CARE IN THE HEALTH-CARE ENVIRONMENT

Nurses must nurture their own spirits by pausing and reflecting about what is going on around them and how that feels inside. Realizing when they are uncomfortable with the situation is the first step to staying in balance. This pausing to reflect and then setting one's intention to be in this moment and bring comfort to the client assists some to relax and become present with the patient. Nurses often find that stopping at the door before entering the room and taking three to four slow, easy breaths to focus on their breathing assists them in entering the room with their attention completely on this patient and his or her needs. This breathing, refocusing, and setting intention can also occur when one washes his or her hands between patients. Frequent self-reflection, centering, and setting intention may be a way to relax and prevent burnout, as well as focus attention more completely on the patient and the tasks at hand. These are simple first steps that can immediately be implemented and that require no extra time. Rather, they are included in the day and what we are already doing.

The American Nurses Association (ANA) focused on 2016 as the yearlong Culture of Safety Campaign, Safety 360. This is part of the ANA's Healthy Nurse, Healthy Nation 2020 initiative. Although we can and do create a culture of safety for our patients, it is also important to create a culture of safety for ourselves—the caregivers. As nurses we often forget this part. The ANA's (2015) *Code of Ethics for Nurses With Interpretive Statements* fully supports both safety for the patients and for the nurses. One of the important ways to create this culture of safety is to be attentive and mindful. When the nurse is fully present, alert, and aware, decisions are not only precise but also appropriate as they affect human lives (Drick, 2016a).

Self-care appears challenging in today's complex fast moving society and equally demanding health-care environment. Drick (2016b) proposes simple effective ways to integrate self-care into our busy professional lives without adding extra time. Nurses need to find creative solutions to promote their own self-care and healing because the current health-care system currently does not provide any assistance.

Creating a Healing Environment

Modern health-care facilities are more aware of the need to create healing environments. Newer hospitals have largely private rooms that are bright with pleasant views. More space is provided in patient rooms to allow for families. The impact of noise and aromas are considered. The old locker room for the staff is being replaced in some forward-thinking institutions with stress reducing, peaceful spaces with recliners, soft lighting, and music where staff can rest.

Healing gardens, meditation areas, animal and fish tanks, and attention to color and use of space to create calm and rest is becoming the norm. McCaffery (2007) compared the effect on mildly depressed older adults of participation in different environmental strategies: walking in a beautiful Japanese garden, a walk with guided imagery, and art therapy. Using focus groups, she determined that all three groups' symptoms improved. McCaffrey et al (2010) described the effects of garden walking and reflective journaling for adults ages 65 and older with depression and showed significant reduction in depressive symptoms and feeling. Matuszek's (2010) comprehensive literature review examines how health care has used animal-facilitated therapy in general and how nursing practice has done so in particular. Consistent with a holistic nursing model, animal-facilitated therapy has been shown to be beneficial, although it is not part of most nursing education.

Realizing the importance of healing environments, the AHNA devoted the December 2015 *Beginnings* to Nurses Go Green: Greener Places Mean Wellness Spaces. Koenig (2015) advocated for nurses as stewards and advocates for our health and food systems and embracing our connection to nature through connecting to the Earth and our food sources. Shields (2015) reflected upon opening our eyes to what is happening to our planet even if it breaks our hearts. We then realize our true heart size, for when our heart breaks open it will hold the entire universe. Case (2015) made the illustration for imagining what nurses could do to enrich their patients' well-being if they took time to tune into nature and had healthy environments. Reid (2015) described the Five Principles of Reiki from Usuri, its founder, as they related to holistic nursing and beekeeping. Bennett (2015) reframed climate change conversations within the context of resilience—disabling obstructions, planning for the future, and maintaining openness to change so we can live sustainably.

PRACTICE ISSUES FOR APNS AND CIHA

The APN's responsibility to society's changing health-care needs can be interpreted through the ANA's *Social Policy Statement* (2010). In this document, *expansion* "refers to the acquisition of new practice knowledge and skills and legitimizing role autonomy within areas of practice that overlap traditional boundaries of medical practice." Expansion includes specialization and "is characterized by the integration of theoretical, research-based, and practical knowledge (as part of graduate education)" (p. 4). New practice knowledge and skills related to holism and complementary approaches for APNs may include CIHA science, nursing science, research-based nursing interventions, and guidelines for integrative or holistic practice.

Activities for the RNs and for APNs are outlined in the *Holistic Nursing: Scope and Standards of Practice* (AHNA/ANA, 2013; currently being revised). Each of the 16 Holistic Nursing Standards delineate additional competencies for the graduate level prepared holistic nurse and the APN. Two of the standards are specific to the APN:

- STANDARD 5C: CONSULTATION provides for only the APN to "provide consultation to influence the identified plan, enhance the abilities of others and effect change" (p. 62).
- STANDARD 5D: PRESCRIPTIVE AUTHORITY AND TREATMENT provides for only the APN to "use prescriptive authority, procedures, referrals, treatments, and therapies in accordance with state and federal laws and regulations" (p. 63).

The Consensus Model and Implications for APNs

Since approximately 2005, major changes in society shifted the focus of credentialing from validation of expertise to requirement for leadership roles in the transformation of health care. Nursing's response was to develop the Consensus Model, designed to standardize graduate nursing, provide a framework for legislating graduate nursing practice, and provide standardized educational guidelines.

The AHNCC recognized the need to create a structure for graduate nursing that would guide legislation and education. AHNCC also recognized that health-care reform calls for nurses expert in knowledge and skills of holistic healing. They recognize the client as the expert in their own care and the use of self as an instrument of healing. Certified graduate holistic nurses are uniquely prepared to assume national leadership roles. The AHNCC, with the endorsement of the AHNA, has taken a proactive position: Advanced holistic nursing, both with and without prescriptive authority, should be included in the Consensus Model. Several position statements (2005–2013) distinguishing the philosophy, knowledge, and skills of the holistic nursing model from the biomedical model of nursing and requesting inclusion in the Consensus Model were drafted, disseminated, and posted on the AHNCC Web site. A major White Paper defining the unique roles of certified advanced holistic nurses (AHN-BC) and certified advanced practice holistic nurses (APHN-BC), declaring intent to pursue recognition of the AHN-BC and APHN-BC and to draft the Essentials of Graduate Level Holistic Nursing education, was disseminated in November 2015. All documents are available on the AHNCC Web site (ahncc.org).

Educational Considerations for Holistic Nursing Plus CIHA

Preparing APNs with the education and experiences to support patients in their plans to use complementary and integrative approaches and to deliver safe and effective holistic nursing care is a challenge for nurse educators, continuing education providers, administrators, and accrediting agencies. Although holism plus complementary and integrative health approaches have been included in medical education, they are much more frequently presented in nursing undergraduate and graduate programs. The inclusion of holistic nursing and complementary and integrative approaches in graduate and undergraduate nursing curricula is vital for all nurses to be current and knowledgeable in their practice. According to Burman (2003), most NP programs include some CAM education. Sok, Erlen, and Kim (2004) evaluated the integration of CAM material into nursing education and advanced practice programs and suggested that graduate programs develop a recognized course of CAM study. They proposed a 2-year program for NPs that included content on the basics of CIHA CAM the first year followed by a second year of intensive specialization. Fenton and Morris (2003) completed an electronic Web survey of deans of schools of nursing to determine the degree of integration of CAM into their curricula. They concluded from a sample of 125 schools that 60% used the definition of holistic nursing practice in their curricula and 84.8% included complementary modalities.

For more than three decades members of AHNA have been committed to developing resources for nurses seeking to expand their practice. The AHNA has an active and well-developed education committee that addresses curriculum development in formal education. It also monitors and endorses continuing education programs in holistic nursing and CIHA. Currently 11 educational programs are endorsed by the AHNA. Endorsement only comes after a rigorous peer-review process and approval by the ANHA Board of Directors. See **Box 17.3.**

Box 17.3

American Holistic Nurses Association Certificate Programs August 2016

- Certificate in Holistic and Integrative Health
- Certificate in Spirituality, Health, and Healing
- Clinical Aromatherapy for Health Professionals
- Great River Craniosacral Therapy Institute Training Program
- HTI—Healing Touch Certification Program
- Healing Touch Program (HIP)
- Holistic Coach Training for Health Professionals
- Integrative Aromatherapy Certificate Program
- Integrative Reflexology Program
- RN Patient Advocates Learning Intensive
- Whole Health Education Certificate

Box 17.4

American Holistic Nurses Association Resources

- *Holistic Nursing: Scope and Standards of Practice* (American Holistic Nurses Association and American Nurses Association)
- *Holistic Nursing: A Handbook for Practice* (Dossey and Keegan)
- *Core Curriculum for Holistic Nursing* (Helming, Barrere, Avino, and Shields)
- *Journal of Holistic Nursing,* the official journal of the American Holistic Nurses Association (AHNA), published by Sage Publications
- *Beginnings,* the newsletter published by AHNA
- *Monthly eNews*
- AHNA Web site: www.ahna.org
- Certificates of continuing education programs approved by the AHNA

Educational opportunities and online modules such as Foundations of Holistic Nursing and Gerontology Modules are available on the AHNA Web site (ahna.org). Continuing educational opportunities include monthly webinars on current topics, articles in the bimonthly journal *Beginnings,* and articles in the quarterly referred research *Journal of Holistic Nursing.* Current resources for accessing the scope of knowledge such as the *Holistic Nursing: Scope and Standards of Practice* and the Core Curriculum in holistic nursing are available from the office for a fee. See **Box 17.4.**

American Holistic Nursing Certification Corporation

National certification is an important and valued process that many AHNs choose to undertake. The AHNCC offers two types of AHN examinations. The first is for nurses who meet graduate level requirements for advanced holistic nursing; the second is for AHNs who wish to practice at the prescriptive level. Both groups of nurses are required to master core graduate competencies; the second group is also required to master graduate competencies for prescriptive practice. The national credential for the first is AHN-BC; the second is APHN-BC. National certification for AHNs requires graduation from a nationally accredited, graduate nursing program; 48 continuing education hours of holistic nursing; and 300 hours practice in advanced holistic nursing. See their site for more information (www.ahncc.org).

National certification is pursued for both individual and professional reasons: Personal reasons include a desire to grow and learn across the life span, affirmation of achievements, and personal empowerment related to professional achievement. Professionally, certification validates possession of the knowledge and set of skills required to practice a unique role; demonstrates acquired expertise to one's community and stakeholders; meets basic requirements for professional advancement such as increase in salary and job promotion; and facilitates assumption of national leadership roles. Professional reasons for national certification have become a primary focus of AHNCC over the past several years.

AHNCC School Endorsement Program

In 2000, the AHNCC designed a school endorsement program to facilitate the advancement of holistic nursing through nursing education. The AHNCC endorses university-based academic undergraduate and graduate nursing programs that have curricula grounded in holistic nursing philosophy, theory, and concepts consistent with the AHNA *Holistic Nursing: Scope and Standards of Practice*

TABLE 17.2

American Holistic Nurses' Certification Corporation, Endorsed Programs, August, 2016

University/College	Location	Program(s)
Capital University	Columbus, OH	Baccalaureate, Accelerated, Bachelor of Science Completion, and Master of Science in Nursing Programs
Eastern University College of Nursing	Richmond, KY	Baccalaureate, Accelerated BSN, Entry Level Master's, Graduate, DNP
Florida Atlantic University	Boca Raton, FL	BSN, Accelerated BSN, RN-BSN Programs, MSN, PhD, and DNP
Metropolitan State University	St. Paul, MN	RN-BSN Program, Entry-Level Master of Science
MGH Institute of Health Professionals	Charleston, MA	Postgraduate: Certificate of Advanced Mind Body Spirit, Nursing Certificate of Completion in Mind Body Spirit Nursing
Northern New Mexico College	Espanola, NM	RN to BSN Program
New York University, Department of Nursing	New York, NY	Holistic Nurse Practitioner
Quinnipiac University	Camden, CT	Baccalaureate and Master's Programs
The University of Texas at Brownsville	Brownsville, TX	Baccalaureate Program
The University of Texas Medical Branch	Galveston, TX	Baccalaureate Program, Generic and Flexible Option Program
Western Michigan University Bronson School of Nursing	Kalamazoo, MI	Baccalaureate Program
Xavier University	Cincinnati, OH	Baccalaureate, RN to MSN, and MIDAS Programs

(AHNA & ANA, 2013). AHNCC's intent and goal are to support and facilitate curriculum development that advances holistic nursing consistent with the current and future health-care trends. Endorsement of these programs identifies universities that are graduating nurses as transformational leaders that are focused on changing the health-care paradigm from one of illness and disease to health promotion, wellness, and well-being. Graduates of these programs are eligible for certification in holistic nursing after passing the NCLEX and obtaining their RN license. See **Table 17.2.**

Holistic Nursing and CIHA in Regulated Nursing Practice

Requirements for education and training, licensure, and reimbursement for CIHA practitioners and APNs are regulated by each individual state. Understanding the qualifications and practice domains of nurses and other practitioners is the foundation for holistic nursing and integrative health approaches. Because holistic nursing is an ANA recognized specialty, similar to pediatrics or medical-surgical, every state board of nursing (BON) is obligated to recognize holistic nursing although they may choose to limit their practice.

Sparber (2001) surveyed state BONs to identify policies regarding RNs' use of complementary therapies. At that time "47% of the BONs had taken positions that permitted nurses to practice a range of complementary therapies; 13% were in the process of discussing this matter; and 40%, although they had not formally addressed the topic, did not necessarily discourage these practices" (p. 1). In 1991, the Arizona BON was one of the first to issue a formal advisory on CAM. Kentucky, Massachusetts, and Pennsylvania followed by recognizing energy therapies of TT, HT, and massage therapies (now recognized in 25 states and under consideration in an additional seven). Annually the AHNA prepares a Nurse Practice Act (NPA) analysis report for each U.S. state BON on holistic nursing and CIHA performed by nurses in the respective state plus the board's contact information. The 2015 report is available on the AHNA Web site (ahna.org/Resources /Publications/State-Practice-Acts). Highlights of changes since the NPA analysis in 2014 include:

- The Massachusetts BON was the only state to make major updates. This occurred in September of 2015 when the Massachusetts BON revised and retitled their advisory opinion "Holistic Nursing and Complementary Integrative Health Approaches" and expanded the scope of practice for RNs and LPNs in the state regarding the incorporation of CIHA and what is considered CIHA.
- Four states have direct references in their respective NPA that mention holism or that recognize holistic nursing as a specialty (IL, NV, OR, TX).
- Seventeen states incorporated references or position statements from their NPA on holism or holistic approaches or CIHA. Not all BONs are authorized to adopt position statements.

The following is a summary of AHNA's findings for the 17 states that incorporated holistic-related references:

- All CIHA modalities (AR, FL, MN, NC, CA, ND, NY, TX, VT)

Box 17.5

Legal Questions for APNs

1. Is the approach within the scope of practicing nursing or is it practicing medicine without a license? This is a particular problem as APN practice begins to look similar to medical practice with overlapping roles and functions. Here a firm grounding in nursing theory and diagnosis will add clarity.
2. Standards of care for complementary and integrative health approaches may be less clear than for conventional practice. Consider risk management guidelines of the institution and state NPAs.
3. Is the approach in concert with the guidelines of the NPA in the state in which the nurse practices?
4. Has the approach been limited to another discipline? Some disciplines have their own licensure (e.g., chiropractic might limit the nurse's practice of craniosacral therapy).
5. Nurses traditionally counsel clients regarding nutrition and supplements. Does the state in which the nurse practices limit that counseling or prohibit prescribing over-the-counter herbs and supplements? Most often APNs with prescriptive authority are the only nurses qualified to prescribe such substances.

- Hypnotherapy, dietary supplements, food additives, homeopathic remedies, or massage (AK, MA, VT)
- The role of nurses in businesses offering CIHA or holistic practices (KY, LA, MA, NH, NV, PA, TX, VT)

Sparber's previously mentioned 2001 report has not been updated. More recently Denner (2007) and Radzyminski (2007) reviewed the legal parameters of nurses and CIHA. There are five legal questions APNs can use to assist them in considering the appropriate use of a CIHA. See **Box 17.5.**

Kranlich (2014) reflects that with the increasing use of CIHA, patients and families are bringing these approaches into the acute health setting. Nurses, and especially APNs, are both trusted and in a unique position to advocate for their patients while promoting safe incorporation of the approaches into the patient's plan of care. A Legal FAQ for Holistic Nurses is maintained on the AHNA Web site that has application to all APNs that use CIHA.

The APN, Holistic Nursing Research, and CIHA

The holistic nursing and CIHA research base has grown substantially in recent years. Graduate nursing programs have supported research focused on both theory development and the evaluation of modalities. Enzham-Hagedorn and Zahourek (2007) provide both a theoretical model and an extensive chart of studies on all aspects of holistic nursing. Updating this review, in 2016 the AHNA Research Committee completed a 5-year review with annotated bibliography of all aspects of holistic nursing as part of the background data and information for the third edition of the *Holistic Nursing: Scope and Standards* that is due out in 2018.

It is imperative that APNs become aware of the evidence and precautions derived from various research approaches to make informed choices about using any modality or encouraging their clients to do the same. The AHNA Web site has an ever-growing research section that includes articles, a Web library, a glossary of terms, and many other resources for those wishing to do holistic nursing research (www.AHNA.org/research). For specific case studies, refer to the bibliography located online.

Role Development With Avenues and Models for APNs as Holistic and CIHA Practitioners

Nontraditional, holistic interventions are common APN practices. More nurses are becoming independent CIHA or holistic practitioners. The June (2016) *Beginnings* focused on advanced practice holistic nursing with topics including creating a holistic graduate nursing curriculum (Shields & Weaver, 2016); leaders in implementing core values (Rosa & Lubansky, 2016); the emerging role of AHNs (Hines, 2016); increasing patient health outcomes (Wylie, 2016); envisioning the future of advanced practice (Hines & McCaffrey, 2016); advanced holistic nursing certification (Erickson & Sandor, 2016); and nurse coaching for APNs (McElligott, 2016). The August 2013 issue of *Beginnings* was devoted to integrative health care.

Even health coaching has become a role with a scope and standards of practice for the holistic nurse, with the 2011 and August 2015 *Beginnings* devoted to holistic health coaching. In February 2013, *Beginnings* was focused on *Healthy People 2020*. A 2008 issue described various practice settings including an herbal practice, home care, and hospice providing bedside music, aromatherapy, palliative care, and private practice. Numerous reports exist about nurses integrating relaxation, imagery, and music. A 2006 issue of *Beginnings* was devoted to holistic nurses developing private practices. Nurses described practices that include HT, massage, counseling, a radio show, work in cardiology, and integrating aromatherapy, HT, and Reiki into conventional practice in hospitals, offices, and community settings.

APNs interested in developing CIHA practices or delivering holistic nursing interventions must take responsibility for obtaining the necessary education, experience, and (when appropriate) certification. *Beginnings* is an exceptional resource to assist the APN to become more current on CIH approaches and to keep current on changing and developing issues.

APNs may be involved in situations where patients have a choice between a conventional and a holistic or CIHA practitioner. If APNs recommend CIHA they need to be informed about which approaches are safe and effective for a specific patient's plan of care, yet remain cognizant about the patient's condition. **Box 17.6** contains questions that APNs can use as a guide to recommend CIHA. Many approaches are elective and can be integrated into conventional care to assist the patient and family to increase comfort and a sense of mastery over their situation. **Box 17.7** describes the elements that an APN will need to do to assist in integrating CIHA into conventional health care.

The NCCIH home page offers guidance on multiple topics in the section "Health Information." This includes such issues as "How to Find a Practitioner," "Health Topics A to Z," and "Be an Informed Consumer." NCCIH and the Office of Dietary Supplements continue to be valuable resources for updated reviews and meta-analyses of research. Sufficient understanding of both the patient's disease process and the specific therapy are mandatory requirements before referral to a specific complementary practitioner is made. Ongoing collaboration with the CIHA practitioner is useful in providing comprehensive care.

Box 17.6

Question Guide for APNs Recommending CIHA

- Has the approach been used to manage the symptom or initial treatment?
- Is there research evidence that the approach is safe and effective?
- Is the approach appropriate for the patient?
- Does the patient want or expect the approach to work?
- Are there providers who are skilled in providing the approach?
- Has the patient had prior or current experience with complementary approaches?
- What approach does the patient's cultural group tend to use most frequently?
- When you refer a patient to a CIH-care provider, do you know the provider's credentials and licensing requirements, the qualifications of the practitioner, and some evidence of competence?
- Counseling patients in their decision to use complementary approaches also includes consideration for the cost of the treatments. Although insurance companies cover some complementary approaches (e.g., chiropractic, hypnosis, and massage), most approaches are paid for out of pocket and are often quite expensive.
- Counsel patients about access to herbs and supplements on the Internet. Which are legitimate and is the cost reasonable?

Box 17.7

Expanding and Advancing CIHA in Conventional Health Care

To integrate CIHA into conventional health care and enable clients to benefit from the best of all approaches available, the APN will need to include the following elements:

- Acquire and maintain current knowledge and competency in holistic nursing practice, including CIHA and approaches integrated within holistic nursing practice.
- Provide care and guidance to persons through nursing interventions and approaches consistent with research findings and other sound evidence.
- Adhere to a professional code of ethics and healing that seeks to preserve wholeness and dignity of self and others.
- Recognize each person as a whole: body-mind-spirit in an ever-changing environment.
- Assess patients holistically, using appropriate conventional and holistic approaches.
- Create a plan of care in collaboration with the patients and their significant others, if they wish, consistent with cultural background, health beliefs, sexual orientation, values, and preferences that focuses on health promotion, recovery or restoration, or peaceful dying so that the person is as independent as possible.

Based on American Holistic Nurses Association. (2016). *AHNA: Position on the role of nurses in the practice of complementary and integrative health approaches (CIHA)*. Prepublication copy from Holistic Nursing: Scope and Standards of Practice (2018).

Holistic Ethical Considerations

The APN is obligated to foster patients' choices about the care they receive and must function within the *ANA Code of Ethics for Nurses With Interpretative Statements* (ANA, 2015). The AHNA also has a Position Statement on Holistic Nursing Ethics located in Appendix D of the *Holistic Nursing: Scope and Standards of Practice* (AHNA/ANA, 2013) that outlines the holistic nurse's ethical responsibilities. In order to provide services to others, a holistic nurse has a responsibility to self, the client, coworkers, nursing practice, the profession of nursing, society, and the environment as abbreviated here:

- *Nurses and self:* . . . a responsibility to model health-care behaviors and achieve harmony in their own lives and assist others striving to do the same.
- *Nurses and the client:* . . . primary responsibility is to the client needing nursing care . . . seeing the client whole and providing care that is professionally appropriate and

culturally consonant . . . confidentially . . . relationship guided by mutual respect. . . .

- *Nurses and coworkers:* maintains cooperative relationships . . . responsible to nurture each other and assist as team . . . if career endangered by coworker . . . take appropriate actions.
- *Nurses and nursing practice:* . . . personal responsibility for practice and maintaining continued competence . . . right to use all appropriate nursing interventions . . . obligation to determine efficacy and safety of all nursing actions . . . as applicable use research findings in directing practice.
- *Nurses and the profession:* . . . play a role in determining and implementing desirable standards of nursing practice, education, and research . . . assume leadership position to guide the profession toward a holistic philosophy of practices . . . support nursing research and development of holistically oriented nursing theories . . . participate in establishing and maintaining equitable social and economic working conditions (pp. 178–179).
- *Nurses and society:* . . . along with other citizens . . . responsibility . . . initiating and supporting actions to meet health and social needs of all society.
- *Nurses and the environment:* strive to create client environment . . . peace, harmony, and nurturance so that healing may take place. . . . Considers ecosystem health in relation to the need for health, safety, and peace of all persons (pp. 177–179).

In essence, holistic nurses further recognize and honor the ethic that the person is the authority on his or her own health experience. The holistic nurse is an "option giver" who helps the person develop an understanding of alternatives and implications of various health and treatment options. Holistic nurses embrace a professional ethic of caring and healing. It is an ethic that seeks to preserve the dignity and wholeness of themselves and others (AHNA/ANA, 2013, pp. 10–11).

Within holistic ethics there is a basic underlying concept of unity and the integral wholeness of all people and of all nature. This integral wholeness is identified and pursued by finding unity and wholeness within the self and within humanity. It is very important to note "acts are not performed for the sake of law, precedent, or social norms, but rather from a desire to do good freely in order to witness, identify and contribute to unity" (AHNA/ANA, 2013, p. 89).

CONCLUSION

Holistic philosophy, evidence-based nursing science, and experience-based learning facilitate the systematic development of integrative health care. Holism recognizes the innate wholeness of each person as he or she interacts with, and reacts to, his or her personal inner environment and increasingly larger outer environment. In today's hurried world the challenge remains to keep the holistic focus for both nurses and patients. Maintaining healthy wholeness for the nurse is an important part of this holistic balance. Nurses must take care of themselves in order to give authentic heartfelt care to others. For example, without regular and sufficient sleep, no matter how much coffee one consumes, all energy goes to keeping the body awake and functioning. There is little if any extra energy available to extend to another. This is known to be true. One can fool himself or herself into thinking he or she can function well, but patients and others can readily see and feel the difference.

As role models for other nurses and health professionals, APNs can affect the entire health-care system. Because of nursing's legacy in holistic philosophy, APNs have much to offer in the fields of holistic nursing and CIHA. Although modalities, treatments, and therapies, now known as health approaches, are important, they become more powerful for patients and the nurse's own well-being when grounded in a strong commitment to holism. With this commitment to practice, nurses can participate in creating a future that expands to enrich themselves, patients, the families, the local community, and even the global community.

18

Basic Skills for Teaching and the Advanced Practice Registered Nurse

Valerie Sabol, Benjamin A. Smallheer, and Marilyn H. Oermann

Learning Outcomes

Learning outcomes expected as a result of this chapter:

- Define learning and teaching.
- Contrast the relationship between teaching and learning.
- Describe the educational process from assessment through evaluation.
- List areas to assess before beginning instruction.
- Illustrate strategies for assessment, such as questions, pretests, and others.
- Demonstrate domains of learning, taxonomies, and writing objectives.
- Develop a plan for instruction.
- Select appropriate teaching methods.
- Evaluate learning outcomes and evaluation methods.
- Explain the role of the APRN as educator.

INTRODUCTION

In today's health-care environment, the advanced practice registered nurse (APRN) serves a critical role in educating patients, students, staff, and other learners. The extensive knowledge base, clinical competencies, and communication skills of the APRN prepare the nurse for carrying out this role across practice settings. Patient education is an important part of managing the patient's care to achieve optimal outcomes. Through this education, patients gain an understanding of their health problems and treatments, how to care for themselves at home, and health-promoting behaviors. By learning about their conditions and treatment options, patients can participate more fully in health-care decisions.

Teaching patients and their families, however, is only one educational role of the APRN. In many settings the APRN also teaches staff, assisting them in developing the knowledge and skills essential for providing care, keeping them up-to-date with advances in clinical practice, and mentoring nurses in the practice setting, ultimately improving the quality of patient care. For some APRNs the educator role extends to nursing students with the APRN serving as a preceptor to nursing students, guiding their learning in the practice setting and teaching students in schools of nursing.

The purpose of this chapter is to describe the qualities of an effective teacher in nursing, the educational process from assessment through evaluation, strategies for teaching, and the role of the APRN as educator. The chapter provides an overview of these topics as a way of preparing the APRN for teaching patients, staff, students, and others.

FRAMEWORK FOR TEACHING

Every APRN needs an understanding of the concepts of learning and teaching. These concepts provide a framework for the APRN to use when making educational decisions.

Learning

Learning is a process of gaining new knowledge and skills because of experiences in which the learner engages. These experiences may be planned activities intended to guide the learner in acquiring this knowledge and these skills or they may be unplanned experiences that lead to a new understanding. Learning may result in an overt and measurable change in behavior, such as patients' ability to perform a procedure after teaching by the APRN, or the outcomes of learning may not be readily apparent, such as gaining a new perspective on a chronic illness or insight about one's own condition. Although learning has occurred, it may be more difficult to assess those outcomes.

Teaching

Teaching is a series of planned actions by the APRN to facilitate learning. Teaching is not merely giving information, although that might be included in the process. Instead, teaching is identifying individual needs, setting goals in collaboration with the learner, planning experiences that guide the learner toward meeting those goals, and monitoring the learner's progression and determining where further learning is indicated (Gaberson, Oermann, & Shellenbarger, 2015). Teaching is facilitating learning through experiences that actively involve the learner. Rather than telling a nurse what care to provide, the APRN asks higher level questions about the patient to guide the nurse in thinking through possible options.

Supportive Environment for Learning

The relationship between teacher and learner is critical to the educational process. Learning is facilitated in a supportive environment in which there is mutual trust and respect (Gaberson, Oermann, & Shellenbarger, 2015). Establishing this environment is particularly important when working with new graduates and students in the clinical setting. Clinical practice is stressful for new graduates (Gardiner & Sheen, 2016) and students (Galbraith & Brown, 2011; Hensel & Laux, 2014).

Although education is a shared experience between the APRN and learners, the APRN has the ultimate responsibility for establishing a supportive learning environment. When working with new graduates and students, the APRN should remember that they are beginning practitioners and have varying levels of clinical knowledge and competencies. The expectations set by the APRN for these learners should be realistic considering their background and prior experiences.

TABLE 18.1

The Five Predominant Qualities of Effective Teaching

Quality	Details
Expert knowledge	Has expertise in content area to be taught Is up-to-date with interventions and new developments in that area Is aware of and able to translate current research findings and evidence into clinical practice
Clinical competence	Knows how to care for patients Uses sound clinical judgments Has advanced clinical skills in area of practice and can guide learners in developing these skills
Teaching skills	Knows how to teach and has the ability to use those principles in teaching Assesses learning needs and plans instruction that meets those needs Explains ideas clearly at a level each learner can understand Asks thought-provoking questions that promote critical thinking and clinical judgment Effectively demonstrates procedures and technical skills Evaluates learners fairly, corrects mistakes without embarrassing them and decreasing their self-confidence, and gives immediate, specific, and instructional feedback
Positive relationships	Has strong interpersonal skills and an understanding of the importance of communication in the student–teacher relationship Provides support for students Communicates clearly
Personal characteristics	Includes enthusiasm for teaching, patience, a sense of humor, friendliness, and willingness to admit mistakes

Qualities of Effective Teachers in Nursing

Research conducted over the years has established the qualities of an effective teacher in nursing, particularly for teaching in the clinical setting. The findings of this research are significant because they guide the APRN in developing skills that promote learning and avoiding behaviors that might impede learning. There are five predominant qualities of effective teaching: (a) expert knowledge, (b) clinical competence, (c) teaching skills, (d) positive relationships, and (e) personal characteristics. **Table 18.1** describes these qualities in more detail.

ASSESSMENT OF LEARNER

The teaching process begins with an assessment of learning needs and other determinants of learning and progresses through planning, implementation, and evaluation. The process, however, is not linear; teaching does not necessarily start with assessment and end with evaluation.

For example, the APRN may plan a program for staff education following a needs assessment, but he or she may realize at the start of the program that most of the nurses lack the knowledge base for understanding the new content. This in turn suggests that different content should be presented to assist staff in gaining the prerequisite knowledge.

Assessment of Learning Needs

Assessment is the first step in the teaching process because it determines the learner's present knowledge and skills and examines other characteristics, such as readiness to learn and health status, which may influence achieving the objectives. The goal of assessment is to identify the knowledge and skills the learner has already acquired and the needs for learning. Assessment reveals gaps in learning to be met through education. Questions that guide assessment of learning needs are highlighted in **Box 18.1.**

Box 18.1

Questions That Guide Assessment of Learning Needs

What does the learner already know about the content?

What competencies does the learner already have?

Is this knowledge and are those competencies sufficient to learn the new content?

Based on this information and the goals or objectives to be achieved, what should be taught?

Learners frequently have more needs than the time and resources for teaching allow. Therefore, the APRN prioritizes the learning needs, focusing the instruction on the essential knowledge and skills for self-care if teaching patients and for safe, effective practice if teaching staff. For example, the mother of a toddler recently diagnosed with asthma needs to know the warning signs of an asthma episode and how to manage them, her child's asthma medications, the correct use of inhalers, asthma triggers for her child and how to prevent them, and when to seek treatment. These are immediate learning needs and should be the priorities for teaching by the APRN. Although the mother may ask about the relationship between asthma and participating in organized sports, this information is not essential and is a low priority for teaching.

There also is limited time for staff education, and the APRN needs to focus the instruction on knowledge and skills essential for safe and competent practice. What are the most common practice problems new graduates and nursing staff are likely to encounter? What content must be learned to understand those problems and provide effective nursing care? What knowledge and competencies are required for safe care of patients? Once these essential learning needs are met, the APRN can extend the instruction to other areas of learning.

Assessment of Readiness to Learn

A second area to assess is the learner's readiness to learn. Readiness is the point in time when the learner demonstrates an interest in learning and is able to participate in the teaching process (Bastable, 2014). The learner must be ready physically, psychologically, and cognitively to engage in learning; otherwise, learning will not occur regardless of the importance of the content and skills.

In assessing *physical readiness,* the APRN focuses on whether the learner has the physical ability to learn the skill. For example, a patient must have a certain degree of strength to learn to transfer from the bed to a wheelchair. Health status also affects physical readiness because it often influences the energy the learner has to engage in learning and degree of comfort. A patient experiencing acute pain following a surgical procedure or who is fatigued because of a treatment may not have the energy to learn and may be too uncomfortable to participate. Teaching the family or planning instruction for the follow-up visit may be more appropriate.

Psychological readiness includes the degree of anxiety and stress experienced by the learner, motivation to learn, and developmental stage. The learner needs to be able to focus on learning and be actively involved in it. The stress associated with the diagnosis of a serious health problem, fear of losing one's job because of illness, and concern about not being successful in an educational program, to name a few, may influence readiness to learn. In assessing psychological readiness, it is important for the APRN to get a sense of the learner's state of mind and determine whether the learner is emotionally ready to engage in learning.

Motivation is the desire of an individual to learn—the drive to gain new knowledge and skills or to change a behavior. Differences among staff and students in their motivation to learn are often apparent in the effort they give to learning, their desire to achieve at a high level of performance rather than meet minimal expectations, and their willingness to engage in remedial learning and practice. Motivation may change over time and with different learning situations. Strategies for motivating learners as part of the teaching process are presented in **Box 18.2.**

Readiness to learn also is determined by the learner's developmental stage. Pediatric nurses are well aware of differences in how children learn based on their ages and development. Knowledge of growth and development guides the APRN in determining the complexity and outcomes of learning and the types of teaching strategies that are appropriate.

Cognitive readiness relates to the knowledge base of the learner—whether the learner has the prerequisite knowledge and skills for beginning the instruction. This is a critical area of assessment, particularly for content and skills that

---

> ## Box 18.2
> ### Strategies for Motivating Learners as Part of Teaching
>
> Teach *for* the learner based on the learner's needs, not the educator's needs.
>
> Teach when ready to learn or develop alternate strategies, such as teaching family members and planning instruction for follow-up visits.
>
> Set small and attainable goals so learners can meet them.
>
> Focus the learner's attention on what needs to be learned.
>
> Explain why this content and these skills are important.
>
> Divide information to be learned into small segments, organize them logically, and teach only the amount learners can retain at a time.
>
> Provide frequent and positive reinforcement (e.g., praise, for correct answers and accurate performance of skills).
>
> Give immediate feedback at the time of learning, clarifying incorrect responses and errors in performance and reteaching as needed.
>
> Allow for practice so the learner develops skill and confidence in abilities.
>
> Review essential content and skills over a period of time to improve retention.

build on one another. When lacking the prerequisites, it is up to the APRN to fill in these gaps and guide learners to resources and experiences they can complete on their own. Assessment of cognitive readiness also allows the APRN to determine if the learner has already mastered the objectives and is ready to progress to a new area of learning.

Other Assessment Areas

Other areas to assess depend on the educational situation and type of learner. In teaching patients and families, the APRN should be aware of their culture and how that might influence the education and methods selected for teaching. The patient's cultural values, health practices, and literacy are important to assess before teaching (Ashton & Oermann, 2014; McCleary-Jones, 2016; Sidhu et al, 2015).

Cultural differences also may exist when teaching staff and students and should be assessed by the APRN. The educational level of learners is often an important area for assessment, although the highest grade achieved in school does not necessarily indicate the learner's knowledge of a health problem or how that person will respond to the instruction.

Strategies for Assessment

Questioning Learners

One of the most effective strategies for assessment is questioning learners about their understanding of the content and what they believe are their educational needs. For patient education, it is valuable to develop a list of questions about the conditions and treatments commonly found in the APRN's practice; a standardized list of questions facilitates assessment and enables the APRN to document the learning needs, instruction provided to patients and family, and outcomes. These questions can be asked in a structured interview or they can be integrated in the interactions between the APRN and learner for a more informal means of assessing needs.

Questions for assessment need to be open ended and probing to be effective. Asking patients, "Do you have any questions about your asthma?" is of limited value in assessing their understanding of asthma and self-care. A more effective line of questioning is, "Tell me about the medications you are taking for your asthma and whether they are helping. What problems are you still having and what are you doing about them?" Using open-ended and higher-level questions is particularly important when assessing the learning needs of staff and students. Learners may be able to answer questions that ask for recall of facts and specific information but be unable to answer those that require application to new situations, analytical thinking, and clinical judgment. By asking different levels of questions, the APRN can identify more clearly the actual learning needs.

Questionnaires

A second strategy for assessment is to develop a questionnaire that lists content areas and asks learners to identify where they need further instruction. One problem with questionnaires, however, is that learners rate their own instructional needs, which may not reflect an accurate assessment. A second problem when used for staff development is the length of time between conducting the assessment and planning and implementing the educational program. In that period, the learning needs of staff may change significantly.

Pretests

Written tests given before the instruction provide a reliable and valid means of assessing learning needs. By using pretest results, the APRN can determine the content already mastered and identify gaps in learning that become the focus of the instruction. An advantage of using written tests is the opportunity to administer both a pretest and posttest as a means of evaluating the effectiveness of the instruction and educational programs offered by a facility. Although staff and students are conditioned to testing as a way of measuring learning, patients may be uncomfortable with written tests and care should be used to write questions at a level patients can understand.

Observations

There is no better means of assessing psychomotor and technical skills than by observing the learner performing them. Ideally, the APRN should observe performance more than once.

Development of Objectives

Assessment reveals the knowledge and skills that the learner needs to acquire to meet the educational goals and the characteristics that might influence the learning process. From these needs the APRN specifies the objectives to be met by the learner. These objectives reflect the outcomes of learning—the cognitive, affective, and psychomotor skills and values to be attained by the learner. The objectives also guide the selection of content and teaching strategies; assessment determines the extent to which learners have achieved the objectives and where further learning is indicated (Oermann & Gaberson, 2017). The planning phase of the teaching process includes the development of objectives and the selection of content, teaching methods, and learning activities.

Objectives specify who the learners are and what they will know or be able to do at the end of the instruction. For example: "The staff nurse identifies nursing interventions with supporting evidence for care of patients in heart failure." Objectives should be clear, measurable, and attainable, considering the level of the learner and time frame allotted for the instruction. Behaviors such as list, identify, apply, and compare are measurable in contrast to terms such as *know* and *understand*. The time frame for teaching also dictates the number of objectives and their complexity.

Taxonomies of Objectives

There are three domains or areas of learning: cognitive, psychomotor, and affective. Objectives may be written in each of these domains and leveled using the taxonomies, which are classification systems for objectives.

Cognitive Domain Learning in the cognitive domain relates to the acquisition of knowledge and development of intellectual skills such as problem solving and clinical reasoning. In many teaching situations, the outcome of learning is memorizing facts and specific information; however, at other times, the goals are learning to apply concepts to new situations, analyze complex data about patients, arrive at decisions about patient problems and alternative possibilities that exist, and make decisions about the most appropriate course of action.

The taxonomy of the cognitive domain enables the teacher to organize the learning outcomes in a logical way from memorization to increasingly more complex cognitive skills. There are six levels in the cognitive taxonomy, beginning with recall of specific facts and information (the lowest) and progressing through comprehension, application, analysis, synthesis, and evaluation (Bloom, Englehart, Furst, Hill, & Krathwohl, 1956). Anderson and Krathwohl (2001) updated the taxonomy, rewording the categories as verbs (e.g., remembering instead of knowledge) and reordering synthesis and evaluation. The highest level of learning in the adapted taxonomy is creating—synthesizing elements to form a new or different product. A definition and sample objective for each of the six levels of the revised cognitive taxonomy are found in **Table 18.2.**

Psychomotor Domain Psychomotor learning results in the development of motor skills, ability to perform technical procedures, and other competencies that involve physical coordination. In developing psychomotor skills, learners progress through different phases: cognitive (learning about the skill and how to perform it), associative (refining movements until they become more consistent),

TABLE 18.2	
Cognitive Taxonomy and Sample Objectives	
Levels of Cognitive Taxonomy	**Sample Objective**
Remembering: Ability to recall facts and specific information	The patient identifies side effects of medications.
Understanding: Ability to understand and explain information	The nurse explains the underlying pathophysiology of the patient's condition.
Applying: Ability to use knowledge in a new situation and apply concepts and theories to practice	The student plans interventions for critically ill patients that are based on current evidence.
Analyzing: Ability to identify relevant parts and their relationships	The manager analyzes the outcomes of the new staffing pattern on patients and nursing staff.
Evaluating: Ability to arrive at judgments based on internal and external criteria	The student evaluates research studies on the use of relaxation for adults with chronic pain.
Creating: Ability to develop a new product	The nurse designs a protocol for pain management.

and autonomous (practicing the skill until it can be performed automatically without thinking about each step) (Oermann, Muckler, & Morgan, 2016; Schmidt & Lee, 2005). In teaching skills these phases are important to keep in mind. In the cognitive phase learners are attempting to understand the skill and how to accurately perform it. In this phase questions from the teacher about the rationale for the skill and its underlying principles are appropriate. However, in the other phases in which learners are developing and refining their performance of the skill itself, the teacher should not ask questions about the "why" of the skill. When learning to drive a car, the instructor does not ask how the engine works. Similarly, as the patient is learning to draw up the insulin or the student is setting up an infusion pump, the focus of the teacher and any questions asked should be on guiding performance, not on the underlying principles of the skill.

Progressing through these phases of learning and developing motor skills requires deliberate practice. Practicing a skill one time is generally not sufficient. Learners need an opportunity to practice a skill multiple times with specific feedback from the teacher on their performance and how to improve it (McGaghie, Issenberg, Petrusa, & Scalese, 2010; Oermann, Molloy, & Vaughn, 2015; Oermann, Muckler, & Morgan, 2016; Ross, Bruderle, & Meakim, 2015). Feedback should focus on the motor components of the skill. Although objectives can be written

for psychomotor learning, similar to the cognitive domain, in most situations skills are taught using a checklist of the steps of the procedure.

Affective Domain   In some educational situations, the APRN assists learners in developing values important in professional practice. Value development in this context builds on an understanding of the values and beliefs that are essential to practice as a professional, such as confidentiality and privacy. From this knowledge base, learners need to then accept these values and beliefs as their own and internalize them as a basis for their own professional practice (Oermann & Gaberson, 2017). In most teaching situations, the APRN would not specify values to be taught to patients and other learners in the form of objectives but would be aware of these outcomes when planning the instruction.

DEVELOPMENT OF A TEACHING PLAN

The objectives represent the outcomes of learning based on the APRN's assessment and form the basis for the teaching plan. The aim of the teaching plan is to guide learners to achieve the objectives while considering other characteristics of the learner also examined during the assessment. The APRN plans and organizes content related to the objectives, selects teaching methods, and plans learning activities, all with the intent of assisting the learner in meeting the objectives or outcomes of learning.

In developing the teaching plan, the APRN should consider the level of learning to be achieved because of the instruction. If the outcome of learning is to recall facts, the teaching methods could be lecture, discussion, and readings. When the objective is to *use* the knowledge gained from the instruction to decide on the most effective nursing interventions for a patient (applying) or to determine the priority problem (analyzing), the teaching strategies need to extend beyond lecture and discussion. For example, with those outcomes of learning, the APRN might develop a short case in which the learner applies the concepts to a patient scenario or have a discussion with staff about how to manage a patient's care, considering the evidence on interventions that might be used.

Although teaching often occurs without a written plan or by using or adapting a standardized plan, having a teaching plan is useful because it specifies the intended learning outcomes or competencies to be developed, content, teaching methods, time allotted for the instruction, and strategies for assessing if learning occurred. When offering an educational program for a group of learners, a written plan guides the teacher in the depth of content to present and types of teaching methods that can be used within the time frame. For programs that provide contact hours for continuing education, written plans are required and the organization offering the contact hours specifies the form to be used.

There are many formats for developing written plans for teaching and educational programs. Generally, they include at least six components that relate to one another: (a) purpose of the education, (b) objectives or outcomes to be met, (c) outline of the content, (d) teaching methods for presenting the content and guiding learners in meeting the objectives, (e) time frame for the instruction, and (f) evaluation methods. **Figure 18.1** provides a sample teaching plan developed for a continuing education program; this can be used as a template for the development of teaching plans by the APRN.

The content is organized logically from simple to complex, with prerequisite content presented first. The extent of content to include depends on the objectives and the amount of time allotted for the instruction. If there is only a limited time available, the goal is to present the content

that is critical to foster achievement of the outcomes. The content is usually listed on the teaching plan in outline format with sufficient detail for other educators to know what to teach and in what order. If only a brief outline is required in the setting, the APRN can develop a more detailed one for personal use in delivering the instruction.

The next component of the plan is a list of the teaching methods, the strategies the APRN will use to help learners achieve the outcomes and gain the knowledge and skills they need. Methods should be appropriate for the content to be presented and for achieving the objectives. The type of learner—patients, students, new graduates, or experienced staff; size of the group; and time frame also influence the selection of teaching methods.

For patient education, discussion, handouts, visual aids, and demonstration are effective because they lend themselves to individualized instruction and allow the APRN to individualize the teaching to the particular needs of the patient. With students and staff, there are many teaching methods from which to choose, but some, such as written assignments, are more appropriate for students than staff.

The group size is significant in that some methods, such as discussion and demonstration, are best used for individual instruction and with small groups, whereas others, such as lecture, are useful for larger groups. Along the same line, some strategies are more time consuming to implement. For example, small group activities add time to the instruction compared with presenting content in a lecture format, but activities such as these might be critical considering the outcomes to be met and learner needs.

The next component of the teaching plan specifies the time frame for the instruction. The time allotted for teaching determines the depth and complexity of the content and also influences the selection of teaching strategies. The APRN should carefully plan the content to avoid running out of time and to include essential information that the learner needs. It is less of a problem when the instruction is completed early because the APRN can review the content, ask questions to ensure learner understanding, and provide additional practice for skill learning.

The last component of the teaching plan is the evaluation method used to measure achievement of the outcomes. Evaluation may be formative, providing feedback to learners on their progress in meeting the objectives, or summative, measuring achievement of the outcomes of learning. Evaluation methods are described later in this chapter.

Sample Teaching Plan
Continuing Education Offering Documentation Form
Title of Activity: Clinical Teaching and Evaluation
Purpose: Examine a variety of clinical teaching and evaluation methods for use in nursing education.

Objectives	Content	Time Frame	Teaching Methods	Evaluation Methods
1. Examine varied clinical teaching methods and related evidence.	I. Lack of evidence base for clinical teaching II. Guidelines for good clinical teaching III. Clinical teaching methods A. Patient assignment B. Higher level questions and what research shows C. Case method D. Unfolding cases E. Short papers for clinical courses and why use them F. Conferences G. Media clips H. Others	1 hour	Lecture, discussion, PowerPoint, handouts, examples, small group work: develop each clinical teaching method and share with large group	Questioning, review of clinical teaching methods
2. Describe clinical evaluation methods and principles for assessing clinical performance in nursing.	I. Framework for evaluating clinical performance II. Methods for assessing clinical competencies A. Observation of performance and need for recording observations B. Problems with observations C. Rating forms 1. Types 2. Validity, reliability, and other standards D. Preparing teachers to rate performance: What can be done? E. Multiple assessment methods III. Summary and evaluation	1 hour	Lecture, discussion, PowerPoint, handouts role-play (teacher observing student performance and giving feedback on it), video clips: observe performance and rate using forms	Questioning, feedback during discussions of video clips, self-assessment

FIGURE 18.1 Sample teaching plan.

Teaching Methods

Many teaching methods are available for use by the APRN in educating patients, students, and staff. This section presents several of these methods. The goal is to choose methods that facilitate achievement of the objectives and are appropriate for the learner. The APRN should be aware of different teaching methods that can be used and the evidence on their effectiveness (Oermann, 2015).

Lecture

Lecture is a structured means of presenting information to a group. In recent years with the focus on higher level thinking, there has been a shift from lecturing, in which students are usually passive participants, to more active learning methods. However, a lecture that synthesizes from multiple sources, is well organized, is delivered with skill, and allows for questions and open discussion is an effective method for presenting a large body of content in a short period. Lectures can be efficient in that the teacher can emphasize key points to learn and can integrate different sources of information not available to the learners. To promote thinking and higher level learning, the teacher can include examples that apply content from the lecture to clinical situations and can ask questions about alternative perspectives and different possibilities (Oermann & Gaberson, 2017). By adapting the traditional lecture with minimal learner involvement to an interactive format with open-ended questions and discussion, lecture can be used for higher level learning.

A lecture begins with an introduction that presents the objectives to be met, an overview of the content, and why this information is important. The content presented during the lecture should reflect a synthesis from multiple sources of information rather than repeating what could be read in an article or a textbook. The intent of the lecture is to synthesize from resources not available to learners. Content should be clear and organized logically, beginning with simple concepts and progressing to more complex ones, consistent with the outline in the teaching plan. Questions and clinical examples integrated throughout allow for higher level learning and actively involve the participants. Small group activities within the lecture or at the end serve a similar purpose, as well as encourage collaborative learning. The lecture ends with a summary that reviews the main points, and for students and staff their relevance to clinical practice.

The use of video clips and other types of multimedia in the lecture provides for visualization of the content, allows the teacher to highlight key points as the lecture progresses, and adds variety to the presentation. Although in some nursing programs there has been a transition from the use of PowerPoint presentations in class to more active learning methods, such as flipped classrooms in which students complete preclass activities and then engage in problem-based learning in class, APRNs still need to have skill in lecturing. Even in a flipped classroom model, the preclass learning activities typically include viewing recorded lectures with PowerPoint. Some important principles for developing presentations are shown in **Box 18.3.** In addition, there are many online tutorials that prepare teachers for developing quality multimedia for their lectures and other types of presentations. Other guidelines for presenting an effective lecture or speech are also found in Box 18.3.

Inexperienced teachers should practice their lectures and presentations and video-record them for self-assessment or critique by a colleague.

Discussion

Discussion is an exchange of ideas between teacher and learner to meet an educational goal (Gaberson, Oermann, & Shellenbarger, 2017). Although the teacher often plans the topic, the intent of the discussion is for learners to express their views, not to provide a forum for teachers to express their own. Both teacher and learner should actively participate.

Discussions are particularly valuable for students and staff to express their feelings and beliefs about a situation, examine values that influence patient care and their interactions with others, and explore ethical issues. Discussions also are effective for encouraging higher level thinking and development of clinical judgment because the teacher can ask the "right" questions—open-ended questions that ask learners to think beyond the obvious, consider alternative perspectives, and examine different options (Alfaro-LeFevre, 2017; Oermann & Gaberson, 2017).

The cognitive taxonomy described previously in the chapter is a valuable tool to guide the level of questions asked in a discussion. The APRN can begin with recall questions that assess the learners' knowledge of facts and can then progress toward higher level questions. **Table 18.3** illustrates questions at each level of the taxonomy. It is important to ask questions at higher levels because these encourage learners to think critically.

A discussion can occur on a one-to-one basis with a learner or in a small group. Gaberson, Oermann, and Shellenbarger (2015, 4th edition) recommended limiting small group discussions to 10 people to provide an opportunity for everyone to talk. Learners need to know that their views and opinions in a discussion are accepted even if different from the teacher's. The following are guidelines for conducting an effective discussion:

- Focus the discussion on the outcomes to be met.
- Encourage the participation of each learner, but do not force a learner to participate.
- Actively participate as a means of guiding the discussion toward the outcomes but do not dominate the discussion.
- Ask open-ended questions that cannot be answered with a "yes-no" response.
- Sequence questions from low to high level; the taxonomy is useful for this purpose.

Box 18.3

Guidelines for Presentations (Lectures, Speeches, and Other Types)

Identify Learners and Objectives

Know your learners and their background.

If presenting to learners about whom you have limited information, review materials that describe the educational program and ask program planners about learners.

Review objectives for presentation.

Plan Presentation

Plan content to meet objectives, considering learners and time allotted.

Do not develop content from one article or textbook; synthesize literature and resources not available to learners.

Develop a list of topics and subtopics to be presented or use outline format.

Prepare an introduction that includes objectives to be met, an overview of content, and why the information is important.

Do not write out presentations in sentence form to avoid reading to the group; use short phrases.

Next to the list of topics or outline, include sample questions to ask learners.

Develop clinical scenarios and examples of how content applies to practice; integrate these throughout the presentation, use for small group work, or save for the end of the presentation if the presentation is finished early.

Underline or highlight with color key points to make during the presentation so they are easy to see in notes.

List key points to include in the summary.

Develop Media

Develop media, such as a PowerPoint presentation, that emphasize major points.

When using PowerPoint:

Check that each slide presents one idea and begins with a clear title.

Use key words and short phrases rather than sentences and keep to a minimum so the slide is not too "busy."

Make sure the font is large enough, at least 24-point or larger, for everyone to read.

Choose contrasting colors for the text and background so the text is easy to read.

Avoid changing the format, such as adding underlining, bold, *italics;* changing font size; or using different fonts on the same slide.

Combine uppercase and lowercase letters instead of all uppercase.

Avoid varying transitions between slides to avoid distracting the learner from content.

Mark on the list of topics or outline when to change slides or introduce new media.

Integrate other multimedia in the presentation to illustrate content and engage learners.

Deliver Presentation

Practice your presentation and consider video-recording it to assess style and gauge time.

Open with an interesting anecdote, question, photo, humor, or another statement to get the learners' attention.

During the presentation, repeat and emphasize important points.

Include transitions between the different content areas. Be enthusiastic.

Speak clearly, loud enough for everyone to hear, and at an appropriate speed.

Scan learners as you speak to gauge their attentiveness.

Never tell learners you "ran out of time"; if you finish early, move to your clinical scenarios and extra learning activities, then summarize the content.

TABLE 18.3

Levels of Questions for Discussion

Level	Sample Questions
Remembering: Questions that ask for recall of facts and specific information	What is this type of breath sound called? Define peak expiratory flow rate.
Understanding: Questions that explore understanding of content	What is the difference between emphysema and chronic bronchitis? Give an example of a short-acting bronchodilator.
Applying: Questions that examine the ability of learners to relate content to a new or different situation	How do your patient's symptoms compare with what you read about chronic obstructive pulmonary disease? Why is it important to monitor these symptoms?
Analyzing: Questions about analyzing data and relationships	What data support your diagnosis, and why are these data relevant? What are alternative interventions that might work in this situation and why?
Evaluating: Higher level questions that ask for judgments, critical thinking	Are your interventions effective, and how can you determine that? Your patient is still coughing. What changes can be made in the plan of care, and why would these be appropriate?
Creating: Questions that ask for development of new ideas and plans	How would you modify this teaching plan to better meet your patient's needs? Tell me about two new interventions that would be effective in your patient's care, their evidence base, and how you would decide whether to use them.

- Do not accept the first answer to a question, even if correct; explore other possibilities and ask for a rationale.
- Prevent side-tracking of ideas and help learners return to the topic.
- Summarize what was learned and how it relates to the objectives set for the discussion (Gaberson, Oermann, & Shellenbarger, 2015).

Clinical Conference

Clinical conferences are specific types of discussions held with students and staff in the clinical setting. They can precede the clinical experience to ensure that learners have the prerequisite knowledge and skills to provide patient care and engage in other learning activities planned by the teacher. Often the APRN can use these conferences to explain patient problems, interventions, and underlying rationales to learners if they lack the knowledge base to care for those particular patients.

Conferences held after the clinical experiences provide an opportunity to review patient care; discuss patient problems, interventions, and other possible approaches; apply concepts to clinical practice; and explore issues in practice. Conferences also provide a forum for learners to reflect on their experiences in clinical practice. In clinical conferences, similar to other types of discussions with staff and students, the APRN should ask open-ended and probing questions that encourage learners to think about alternative ways of addressing clinical problems and new evidence that might influence decisions about interventions. The need for these questions and examples of them were described previously. The APRN should be creative in planning conferences to provide variety and maintain learner interest, particularly at the end of a tiring clinical day.

Clinical Case

Clinical cases are actual or simulated scenarios for analysis. This method is effective for learning how to apply content to clinical practice and gaining skill in analyzing data, identifying problems, and deciding on possible solutions (Gaberson, Oermann, & Shellenbarger, 2015). The value of cases for analysis is that they provide experience for learners in thinking through clinical decisions before they are faced with those decisions in actual practice.

With this strategy, the APRN develops a case followed by open-ended and higher level questions about it. The cases should be short, a few sentences to a paragraph, and present only essential information. Questions can be directed toward assessment, focusing on missing data in the case and what additional information is needed for decision making. They also can be geared to identifying problems in the case, interventions for immediate action and for planning care, their evidence base, alternative decisions and consequences, and how concepts and theories can be used as a framework for understanding the case and answering the questions.

The questions focus on the objectives to be met by analyzing the case. For example, if the outcome is to select appropriate nursing interventions for a patient with delirium, the APRN could ask learners about guidelines to use, early recognition, and how they would manage the patient's care. In analyzing a case, learners should describe the thought process they used and the rationale for their answers. Because the cases are short, they can be integrated easily within a lecture, used at the end of a class as small group work, discussed in clinical conferences, and explored on a one-to-one basis with the learner. Examples are provided in **Box 18.4.**

Case Study

A case study provides an in-depth description of a patient, family, or community, including background information. Case studies can be developed based on actual or simulated clinical situations, similar to shorter cases. Questioning strategies can include asking learners to differentiate significant from nonsignificant information in the case and examine the effect of the patient's background on current problems and situations. A sample case study is presented in Box 18.4.

Unfolding Cases

An unfolding case represents a simulated clinical situation that changes or evolves over time in a manner that is intentionally unpredictable to the learner (Smallheer, 2016). With this teaching method, the case or clinical scenario is presented first, followed by questions for learners. After they analyze the scenario and answer the questions, the case unfolds with more information such as new laboratory or diagnostic findings or changes in the patient's health status. Learners critique the new scenario and again answer questions about it. Smallheer (2016) described the reverse case study, which incorporates students into the development of the scenario. In this method, students identify information relevant to a clinical situation and analyze content to create details of the case.

Grand Rounds

One other teaching method that also revolves around analysis of a case is grand rounds. In grand rounds the teacher presents an update on a clinical topic or care of a patient with a particular diagnosis or treatment. Observation and assessment of the patient, typical patient problems encountered, interventions, and evaluation of outcomes are often described. In some settings the grand rounds presentations are video recorded and available on the Web for nurses and other health providers to view at a time and place convenient for them. Many of the programs are offered for continuing education contact hours. Nursing grand rounds also can be conducted in the clinical setting with observation of the patient and discussion about care.

Multimedia

Multimedia provide for multisensory learning. Depending on the type of media, different sensory modes are used. In many teaching situations, it is easier to learn when more senses are involved in communicating the message. Learners can see a patient on video rather than imagining what the patient looks like or how the intervention should be implemented from the verbal description by the APRN or from their readings. Multimedia are useful for demonstrating procedures and technological skills, from gathering the equipment through each step to follow. As learners practice their skills, they can record their performance and replay the video-recording when questions arise or they are unsure about their performance.

Multimedia also are valuable for exploring ethical issues and values. For example, a short segment from a video can be used to present clinical situations for learners to examine their values and beliefs and consider how they would respond in those situations. Scenarios can be used to present ethical dilemmas for individuals and groups of students and staff to analyze; small group activities accompanying the media can teach valuable lessons in analyzing and resolving ethical issues.

Box 18.4

Examples of Clinical Cases and Case Study

Examples of Clinical Cases

Mrs. B, a 46-year-old, is brought to the clinic by her husband with complaints of weakness of the left arm and difficulty "getting her thoughts." The husband tells you that his wife was treated a few months ago for a cerebral aneurysm but has been fine since then. Mrs. B's blood pressure is 210/90. She slowly answers your questions with long pauses in between sentences.

1. What information would you collect from the husband as a priority? Provide a rationale why this information is critical to deciding on the diagnosis and actions to take.
2. What are possible problems that Mrs. B might be encountering? Describe why each of these is a possibility.

You are working in home health care and have a new patient with edema of both legs and extreme fatigue. The patient has no family in the area.

1. What additional data would you collect in your first home visit? Why is this important?
2. Summarize the information you might obtain in the home visit and identify a priority problem. What resources are needed for this patient's care?

You believe your patient may be experiencing side effects from her medication, but your preceptor does not agree and tells you to give the medication to the patient.

1. What are two possible approaches you could take in this situation?
2. What are the advantages and disadvantages of those options?
3. What would you do? Why?

Your patient who is increasingly restless pulls out her endotracheal tube. What should you do first? Include evidence to support this action.

You are working in the emergency department when a young man is admitted following a motor vehicle accident. His larynx appears to be fractured and there are many facial cuts and bruises. You suction him only to find large amounts of blood; you determine that the only way to keep the airway clear is by suctioning.

1. What are your options for managing his airway?
2. What observations would you make and what other data would you collect that might affect your decision about how to manage his airway?
3. How would you manage this patient's airway? Provide a rationale.

Example of Case Study

Sally is a 6-year-old who has been complaining of pain in her abdomen off and on for the last week. Two weeks ago, she was seen by the pediatrician for a respiratory flu. Sally's current symptoms are two episodes of vomiting this morning, abdominal cramps, no appetite, and a rash on her back. Vital signs, blood pressure, height, and weight are normal. Sally is holding her abdomen and tells you it hurts. When you palpate her abdomen, you find diffuse tenderness without any rebound. There are no masses that you can detect. Sally's past medical history is unremarkable. She has never had any serious illnesses and has never been hospitalized. Her mother tells you that there are no changes in the family or home situation; they recently returned from a camping trip that Sally enjoyed.

1. What laboratory tests would you expect to be ordered? Explain each test and its relationship to this case.
2. What is the significance of "diffuse tenderness without any rebound"?
3. Name all possible problems Sally might have and why.
4. If Sally asks you what's wrong, how would you respond? Provide a rationale based on her age and development.

Distance Education

Distance education is defined as a learning environment where teacher and student are at different locations. In some instances the entire course or instruction is online, and in other situations a hybrid or blended model is used with part of the learning online and part face-to-face. Distance education is continuing to expand in nursing with many programs offered completely online.

The qualities of effective teachers identified earlier in the chapter are essential whether teaching in-person or online. However, in online courses some additional practices are critical to develop a community of learners and keep them engaged in learning in the online environment. Dreon (2013) applied Chickering and Gamson's (1987) seven principles for good instructional practices to teaching online. These are: (1) encourage contact between students and faculty; (2) develop collaboration and cooperation among students; (3) encourage active learning; (4) give prompt feedback to students; (5) emphasize to students that learning takes time and they need to devote sufficient time to learning the content; (6) develop high expectations and clearly communicate them to students; and (7) respect diverse ways of learning and skills, integrating varied multimedia to deliver content to students and assess their outcomes.

Technologies for Teaching

The growth of online courses and programs in nursing has led to many new technological innovations for teaching in nursing. Foronda (2014) described the use of VoiceThread, a blog center, and a chat room instead of discussion boards for creating a sense of community in an online course. As learning activities, students can develop Web sites, infographics, YouTube videos, educational videos for patient education, and many other types of products using technology. A growing number of courses integrate virtual simulations and interactive case studies, and new technologies using virtual reality and augmented reality are developing at a fast pace. Other technology-based strategies such as electronic concept mapping, electronic case histories, and digital storytelling can be used to facilitate clinical reasoning skills (Shellenbarger & Robb, 2015). It is beyond the scope of this chapter to examine the multiple types of technology available for teaching in nursing, but the APRN should keep current with the development of these technologies and their use in nursing education.

Selecting Media and Technologies for Teaching Considering the variety of multimedia available for teaching, the APRN first needs to evaluate the quality of any multimedia program or Web-based method under consideration. Not every teaching situation needs the addition of multimedia or technologies. The goal is to use media when they clarify the content better than an explanation alone, such as a video clip to depict a patient with the condition being discussed or demonstrate a procedure. Multimedia should be selected based on the outcomes to be achieved and individual learner needs. In addition to evaluating the quality of the multimedia as a basis for their selection, the second area of concern is their appropriateness for the intended learners.

The following are questions the APRN can use to guide this evaluation:

1. Is the content presented in the multimedia accurate?
2. Is the content up-to-date?
3. Is the content organized effectively and presented clearly?
4. Are procedures, techniques, and equipment illustrated consistent with current practice in the setting or can they be adapted easily?
5. Are the multimedia of high technical quality (e.g., graphics, sound, interaction with learner, feedback mechanism, etc.)?
6. Are the multimedia appropriate for the outcomes to be met and will they meet the learner's needs?
7. Are the multimedia appropriate for the learning situation (e.g., patient versus student education, setting for the education, time frame, etc.)?

Readability One additional consideration in evaluating print materials and Web sites for use in patient education is their readability. The reading level of patient education materials should be no higher than the sixth- to seventh-grade level (Badarudeen & Sabharwal, 2010; Hutchinson, Baird, & Garg, 2016; National Institutes of Health [NIH], 2016); however, most educational materials for patients are written above this level. This discrepancy inhibits many patients and families from understanding the information in written materials, including important documents such as consent forms, medication package inserts, educational pamphlets, handouts, and discharge instructions, among others.

Early research on readability focused on print materials, but patients accessing health information on the

Internet also need to understand what they are reading and health Web sites need to present accurate and complete information. Studies have examined the readability of Web sites for patients, revealing that much of the health information on the Web is at too high a reading level for many consumers (Diamantouros, Bartle, & Geerts, 2013; Eltorai et al, 2016; Joury et al, 2016). Hutchinson et al (2016) assessed the readability of online health information for nine common internal medicine diagnoses. The lowest reading level content was available on the NIH, WebMD, and Mayo Clinic Web sites. However, even the reading grade level of those sites ranged from 10.7 (NIH) to 11.3 (Mayo Clinic), higher than recommended. In another study Diamantouros et al (2013) evaluated the accuracy and completeness of content and the reading level of patient education sheets on warfarin distributed by pharmacies in Canada. Only 63% of the educational sheets for patients had essential information, and the reading level was grade 8.

There are different readability formulas for assessing patient education materials. These include the Flesch Reading Ease (FRE) score, which ranges from 0 (unreadable) to 100 (most readable) based on the average number of syllables per word and length of the sentences; the Flesch-Kincaid grade uses the score to determine a grade level. Another readability formula is the Fry Readability Graph. This formula assesses readability based on the average word length but requires only three 100-word samples from the document rather than the full text (Badarudeen & Sabharwal, 2010). Another readability formula is the Simple Measure of Gobbledygook (SMOG). This measure is determined based on the number of words with more than two syllables: a grade of 7 means the patient education materials could be understood by individuals with a seventh-grade reading ability. Developed specifically for assessing the readability of patient education materials, the New Dale-Chall Readability formula is based on sentence structure and the number of unfamiliar words in the text (Badarudeen & Sabharwal, 2010). Badarudeen and Sabharwal reported that the New Dale-Chall Readability formula had the highest validity among these formulas (p. 2574). In a study of online patient education resources found on National Cancer Institute-Designated Cancer Center Web sites, Rosenberg et al (2016) used these formulas and others to assess readability. The mean readability score of patient education materials at these Web sites was 12.46 (college level), too high for most patients and families.

One easy way of estimating readability is by using the spelling and grammar function in Microsoft Word. The first step is to generate a Word file of the materials to be assessed; documents from Web sites can be copied and pasted as plain text (without the HTML tags), deleting information not relevant to the content such as the citations and copyright statement. In the Word file to be checked, the APRN should omit the headings, tables, figures, and illustrations. To check readability, these steps can be followed:

1. Click File, then Options, and then Proofing.
2. In the section, "When correcting spelling and grammar in Word," select the check boxes "Check grammar with spelling" and "Show readability statistics," and click OK.
3. Perform a spelling and grammar check.
4. When completed, a pop-up screen will appear with the readability scores.

The APRN has an important role in assessing the readability of patient education materials, discharge instructions, and documents given to patients. Before recommending health Web sites to patients, the quality of those sites including readability should be evaluated first. When teaching patients and families who lack the ability to read and understand the information, the APRN should focus on key concepts to be learned, use easy-to-understand words, and use varied teaching strategies that rely on visuals. Use simple words and find alternate words for medical terms; ask patients and families to repeat back the information in their own words. Remember to evaluate the English proficiency of the patient, and if this is an impediment use one of the many translating devices available and required by law in most health-care settings.

Self-Directed Instructional Methods

Self-directed instructional methods are completed by learners on their own to meet remedial needs, acquire prerequisite knowledge and skills, and fulfill personal interests. These methods include online modules, independent study, multimedia programs, and a wide range of instructional technologies that learners complete independently. Self-directed methods are well suited for learners who are motivated, committed, and independent because they can be completed at a time and in a setting of the learner's choice.

A major advantage from an educational point of view is the ability of learners to progress through the instruction at their own rates of learning. This affords learners the opportunity to repeat the instruction when unsure or until competent and to omit content areas already mastered.

Although self-directed methods may be planned for all students, the advantages they offer in terms of individualizing the instruction make them a better resource for meeting remedial needs and gaining prerequisite knowledge and skills. That way, learners who have already met the objectives and can demonstrate the competencies can progress to new areas of learning. Self-directed learning places the responsibility for achieving the competencies on the learner rather than the teacher. The teacher, however, might establish time frames for completion for certain activities and monitor learner progress by asking for a self-assessment or by periodic quizzing.

Demonstration

Demonstration is the presentation of how to perform a procedure or skill with the intent for learners to model that performance and implement the skill on their own. Before demonstrating the procedure, the APRN should explain its purpose, equipment to gather, and steps to follow. Any explanation of the principles underlying the skill and discussion about its use in clinical practice should occur at this point in the instruction. As learners practice, feedback from the APRN should focus on the performance itself. Because psychomotor learning is egocentric, learners need to focus on manipulating the equipment and refining their skill.

All learners must be able to see each step to be performed and hear any explanations. By observing the demonstration, learners develop an image of what the skill looks like and how to perform it, which then guides their practice of the skill. The return demonstration is when the learner performs the skill and the APRN gives specific, instructional feedback to improve the performance. Once competent, learners can practice skills on their own. Practice is critical to refine performance, become more consistent, and develop the ability to carry out the skill in a reasonable period of time. Practice also is essential to retain the skill over time. With human patient simulators, students and nurses can practice and develop competency in the skill before performing it in the clinical setting.

Simulations

With simulations learners have an opportunity to develop their decision-making and clinical judgment skills, learn to communicate with others and work as a team, and practice psychomotor and technical skills in a safe environment. With high fidelity simulation, they can analyze scenarios, conduct assessments, make decisions and view the outcomes of those decisions, and develop their ability to think critically and act quickly before caring for a real patient. With procedures and technologies that require costly equipment and supplies, learners need an opportunity to practice those procedures in a controlled environment before trying them with patients in the clinical setting. Simulations are also useful for assessment of clinical performance.

The use of simulation in nursing has expanded rapidly. Some of this growth relates to the lack of clinical sites available for student experiences and the realization that simulation can serve as an adjunct or replacement for traditional clinical experiences. Simulation exposes learners to clinical situations and technologies not available to all students in the clinical setting. The complexity of health care and increasing presence of technology create the need for more in-depth learning and deliberate practice to develop and maintain skills, which can be met with simulation.

There are varied types of simulations, and the APRN should consider these carefully when planning the instruction. Simulations differ based on fidelity or the realism of the simulation. Manikins that are life-sized with technology to mimic changes in physiology are called high fidelity simulators (Jeffries et al, 2015). They create a realistic patient situation and respond to student actions in real time. Moderate fidelity simulators are typically life-sized manikins that only mimic some physiological changes (e.g., the learner may hear heart and lung sounds but without chest movement of the manikin). Low fidelity simulators are task trainers for practicing skills, such as a gel pad for practicing intramuscular injections. Simulations are used frequently for developing skills in teamwork and collaboration and for interprofessional education.

Standardized patients represent another type of simulation that can be used for teaching students and staff. Standardized patients are individuals who are trained to portray a patient with a diagnosis or health problem for learners to collect a health history, practice a physical examination, interact with the patient, and develop other skills. Standardized patients are effective for assessment of learner competencies because the actors recreate the same patient situation with all students (Oermann & Gaberson, 2017).

With simulations, learners should have an opportunity to reflect on their experiences and decisions; this occurs in the debriefing session after the simulation. During debriefing, the teacher guides learners to reflect and discuss what went well, where improvements are needed, and what they would do differently next time. This is where much of the learning occurs. The debriefing provides an opportunity for students to share their reflections and perceptions with peers and the teacher. The discussion also may include how their personal values influenced their decisions. In developing values, learners need to experience situations to determine how they will respond to them; simulations provide this type of experience and help learners develop a sensitivity to how others may feel in a situation.

Evaluation of Learning

Evaluation is an integral part of any teaching situation and serves different roles. In working with patients, students, and staff, individually and in small groups, the APRN continually assesses how well learners are acquiring an understanding of the content and developing the ability to perform skills. Using this information, the APRN modifies the teaching, perhaps explaining the content again and in a different way, adding multimedia, suggesting remedial instruction, and allowing the individual more practice time for skills. This type of evaluation is diagnostic; it represents feedback to the learner about progress in meeting the objectives and provides the basis for developing a plan for improvement (Oermann & Gaberson, 2017). This is referred to as formative evaluation.

A second type of evaluation is summative. As the name suggests, this type of evaluation summarizes what has been learned rather than providing feedback to learners. Examples of summative evaluation are final examinations in a course and annual performance evaluations.

With both formative and summative evaluation, the objectives to be met or competencies to be developed serve as the framework for evaluation. The evaluation determines the progress of learners in meeting the objectives and developing clinical competencies or for summative evaluation if they have achieved them.

There are many methods for evaluating learning. The APRN selects methods that provide information on the outcomes to be assessed and are appropriate for the learner. Evaluation methods include the following:

- *Questioning:* Questions are asked to assess the extent of learning.
- *Observation of performance:* Learners are observed while performing procedures, providing care, and carrying out interventions in clinical practice. Often a summary of the observations is recorded in a narrative note or on a checklist of performance.
- *Rating scale:* Performance of competencies is rated on a scale.
- *Checklist:* Steps in a procedure or skill are checked off as the learner performs them.
- *Test:* The learner is asked to answer a set of written questions about the content.
- *Written assignment:* Students complete papers of varying length.

ROLE OF ADVANCED PRACTICE NURSE AS EDUCATOR

Providing education to patients, students, and staff is an integral part of the APRN role. The APRN has a critical role in teaching patients about their illness and preventing further complications, treatments and medications, how to provide self-care, and the importance of follow-up care. In many settings it is up to the APRN to prepare the patient for discharge and managing his or her own care at home.

Teaching about the illness and self-care is only one of the areas of education provided by the APRN. The APRN also teaches patients and families about preventing illness and staying healthy. Without education by the APRN, few patients would be informed about their health and how to maintain it. APRNs are well suited to provide health-related patient education because they understand interventions for both health and illness.

In some settings, the APRN also may be involved in teaching graduate and undergraduate nursing students. The APRN may serve as a preceptor for students or guide student learning for individual clinical experiences. Because of their extensive clinical knowledge and skills, APRNs may participate in classroom teaching and give lectures and speeches in their area of expertise.

Another component of the APRN role is to educate nursing staff and health providers. This education may be informal, teaching in the clinical setting as the need arises and through formal continuing education programs. As APRNs become known for their particular areas of expertise, they are often asked to organize and present continuing education programs.

CONCLUSION

The APRN has an important role in educating patients, students, and staff. The teaching process described in this chapter—assessing learner needs, planning instruction, selecting varied teaching methods, and evaluating learning—provides a framework for teaching any of these groups of learners. Nurses in advanced practice are well prepared for their role as educator with their extensive knowledge base, expert clinical skills, and strong communication skills. The knowledge and expertise of the APRN combined with an understanding of the educational process prepare the APRN to meet the learning needs of patients, families, students, and staff regardless of the setting in which the nurse chooses to practice.

19

Culture as a Variable in Practice

Mary Masterson Germain

Learning Outcomes

Learning outcomes expected as a result of this chapter:

- Discuss the relationships between race, ethnicity, poverty, and health disparities.
- Evaluate your level of cultural and linguistic proficiency in caring for culturally diverse patient populations.
- Identify areas of knowledge and skill that would make you a more culturally proficient caregiver.
- Analyze the extent to which your current practice meets the legal and regulatory requirements established for the delivery of culturally competent care.
- Identify resources that you and your professional colleagues can utilize to promote culturally proficient care in your practice setting.
- Integrate the new knowledge that you gain from this chapter into your practice.

This chapter is an invitation to step into other worlds—worlds where experiences may be quite different from your own. You will be asked to reflect on the beliefs and values that make you who you are and to examine how they affect you as a healer and caregiver. As an advanced practice nurse (APN) you play a pivotal role in shaping the quality of care that patients receive, both directly and indirectly. You are privileged to share in some of your patients' most profound and intimate experiences. Your challenge is to provide comprehensive, culturally

competent care to populations and in practice settings that are increasingly diverse.

To fully enter into the patient's experience and to provide comprehensive care that is respectful of the patient's cultural beliefs and practices, nurses need to find ways to bridge the linguistic and cultural challenges that are inherent in caring for increasingly diverse populations. It is uncomfortable to stretch our ethnocentric boundaries; it is much easier to care for replicas of ourselves. However, if you are open to learning from your patients, the transient discomfort that you experience from having your time-honored interventions and teaching strategies tested and found wanting by patients with different cultural perspectives will be rewarded by gaining rich insights into cultural beliefs and practices that will inform your practice for years to come. Let us begin the journey.

SCOPE OF THE NEED

Every 10 years, the U.S. Department of Health and Human Services (USDHHS) produces a comprehensive assessment of the health of Americans and sets goals and objectives for improving their health and well-being over the next decade. (See *Healthy People 2010* and *Healthy People 2020*). *Healthy People 2010,* published in 2000, established two overarching goals for improving the health of U.S. residents and communities in the first decade of the 21st century: (1) increase quality and years of healthy life and (2) eliminate health disparities.

These two goals representing 28 focus areas and 467 measurable objectives had a single, overarching purpose of promoting health and preventing illness, disability, and premature death, and a unifying vision: healthy people living in healthy communities (USDHHS, 2000). Note that goal 2 does not say *reduce.* It says *eliminate;* a lofty goal. In December of 2010, the USDHHS released the next decennial document: *Healthy People 2020.* It identified the following four critical goals encompassing 42 topic areas and identified approximately 1,200 objectives to be tracked over the next decade:

- Attain high-quality, longer lives free of preventable disease, disability, injury, and premature death.
- Achieve health equity, eliminate disparities, and improve the health of all groups.
- Create social and physical environments that promote good health for all.
- Promote quality of life, healthy development, and healthy behaviors across all life stages (USDHHS, 2010).

As with *Healthy People 2010,* the goals are uncompromising; disparities in access and quality of health care are to be eliminated and equity becomes a key goal. It is also critical to note that ethnicity and the social determinants of health care are inextricably linked in the discussion of the disparities in health status and access and use of health-care services presented in both *Healthy People 2010* and *Healthy People 2020* and in the Center for Medicare and Medicaid Services (CMS) 2016 Quality Strategy (AHRQ, 2007; CMS, 2016b).

This chapter will approach cultural competence in advanced practice nursing from a similar frame of reference and will begin by examining key characteristics of the American population and how much progress has been made in achieving the goals of *Healthy People 2020.*

WHO ARE WE CARING FOR?

As of December 1, 2016, the estimated number of people living in the United States was 325,032,763 (U.S. Census Bureau, 2016b). A large number of U.S. residents were born elsewhere, as shown by the following:

- More than 41 million immigrants lived in the United States in 2013 (Pew Research Center, 2015) compared with 19.8 million in 1990. Gibson & Lennon, 1999, p. 65).
- Around 13.1% of the U.S. population were foreign born in 2013 (Pew Research Center, 2015, p. 65).
- Immigration to the United States represents 29% of the growth in the U.S. population since 2000 (Pew Research Center, 2015, p. 65).
- The majority of the current immigrant population comes from Latin America or South or East Asia, in contrast to immigrants in the 1960s and 1970s who came mostly from Europe (Pew Research Center, 2015, p. 65).
- The five states with the greatest percentage of immigrants relative to the state's total population were California (10.5 million; 27%); New York (4.5 million; 23%); New Jersey (2 million; 22%); Florida (4 million; 20%); and Nevada (no number reported; 19%) (U.S. Census Bureau, 2016a).
- The five states with the largest percentage of immigrant children under 18 living with their parents, relative to the state's total number of children, were California (49%); Nevada (38%); New Jersey (37%); New York (36%); and Texas (35%) (Zong & Batalova, 2016).

In addition, the following population changes are expected in the coming years:

- By 2030, one in five Americans will be 65 or older (Colby & Ortman, 2015, p. 1).
- By 2044, more than half the population of the United States will be members of a minority group (Colby & Ortman, 2015, p. 1).
- By 2051, the population of the United States is expected to reach 400 million people (Colby & Ortman, 2015, p. 1).

Because the demographic data previously discussed represent nationwide statistics, they do not capture the complexity of delivering culturally competent care, especially in urban settings that traditionally have large immigrant populations. The data on racial origin are associated with significant differences in health status and disease, condition-specific morbidity and mortality, and socioeconomic status. In order to effectively measure and address disparities in access and quality of care in the United States, several critical federal initiatives should be noted.

In 1997, President Clinton appointed a Presidential Advisory Commission on Consumer Protection and Quality in the Health Care Industry. On March 12, 1998, the Commission completed its final report to the president, "Quality First: Better Health Care for All Americans" (Agency for Healthcare Research and Quality [AHRQ], 1998). The report called for the president to take a leadership role in developing a broad national consensus on the need to improve the quality of health care. The Commission recommended six national goals and the development of measurable objectives for each goal. It also recommended the development of core sets of quality measures that should be standardized and utilized across the entire health-care industry. The national goals and objectives were to be revised as improvement was documented and new areas of need arose.

The AHRQ has played a pivotal role in implementing the recommendations of the Commission. Since 2003, the AHRQ, on behalf of the secretary of Health and Human Services, has led an Interagency Work Group, with guidance from the AHRQ National Advisory Council and the Institute of Medicine (IOM), recently renamed the National Academy of Medicine, effective July 1, 2015 (National Academy of Sciences, 2015), that has produced two annual comprehensive reports:

the National Healthcare Quality Report (NHQR) and the National Healthcare Disparities Report (NHDR). After generating the fifth set of reports in 2007 the AHRQ asked the former IOM for recommendations as to how the reports could be improved. The IOM formed a Consensus Committee to study the reports, headed by Sheila Burke, MPA, RN, former chief of staff to Senator Robert Dole and currently a Faculty Research Fellow at the Malcolm Weiner Center for Social Policy and an adjunct lecturer at the John F. Kennedy School of Government, Harvard University. The Committee's report, titled *Future Directions for the National Healthcare Quality and Disparities Reports,* was released by the IOM on April 14, 2010. The report acknowledged the need to continuously assess quality and equity in health care on an ongoing basis and commended the AHRQ for developing the annual set of reports. The Committee also made recommendations as to how the reports could be made more effective in promoting the reduction of disparities and improving the quality of health care. The Report Brief summarized the recommendations of the IOM's authoring committee as follows:

- Select measures that reflect health-care attributes or processes that are deemed to have the greatest impact on population health.
- Affirm that achieving equity is an essential part of quality improvement.
- Increase the reach and usefulness of AHRQ's family of report-related products.
- Analyze and present data in ways that will inform policy and promote best-in-class achievement for all actors.
- Identify measures and data needs to set a research and data collection agenda (IOM, 2011).

The Patient Protection and Affordable Care Act (P.L. 111-48), commonly referred to as the Affordable Care Act (ACA), passed by the 111th Congress and signed into law by President Obama on March 23, 2010, mandated the development of a National Quality Strategy (NQS). With input from more than 300 organizations, individuals, representatives of the health-care industry, the public, and other stakeholders, the NQS established three comprehensive goals (better care, healthy people/healthy communities, and affordable care), coupled with six priorities representing the major health issues confronting Americans (i.e., care coordination and patient-provider communication, patients and families as full partners in their care, and so on). The six priorities were aligned with nine levels (e.g., payment, health information technology, and so on) that would help health-care businesses and organizations to maximize their potential to address the six priorities (AHRQ, 2011).

In 2014, acting on the recommendations in *Future Directions for the National Healthcare Quality and Disparities Reports,* as well as input from end product users and other federal agencies conducting health-related research, particularly the NQS implementation staff, the AHRQ made a major change in the documents. The previously separate NHQR and NHDR were combined into a single document, entitled the *National Healthcare Quality and Disparities Report (QDR).* In addition, instead of presenting extensive data for each of the priority populations and measurement parameters in the integrated report, individual Chartbooks were created for key areas requiring individual analysis (e.g., priority populations such as Hispanic and black populations, women's health, rural health, and so on). The Chartbooks for each year become available on a rolling basis as data analysis is completed. The *QDR(s)* and Chartbooks may be accessed at www.ahrq.gov/research/findings/nhqrdr/index.html. In 2015, data synthesis took another big step forward as the annual NQS Update was integrated into the 2015 *National Health Care QDR.* For the first time, information on the status of health-care quality, access, and disparities was available in a single document (AHRQ, 2016b, pp. vii & 5). You can access the integrated document at http://www.ahrq.gov/sites/default/files/wysiwyg/research/findings/nhqrdr/nhqdr15/2015nhqdr.pdf.

The 2014 *National Healthcare QDR* makes it clear that 14 years after the publication of *Healthy People 2010,* disparities persist. ". . . As noted above, disparities in quality and outcomes by income and race and ethnicity are large and persistent, and were not, through 2012, improving substantially" (AHRQ, 2015b, p. 2). Two examples of disparities are the following:

- In 2010, the infant mortality rate per 1,000 live births was worse for non-Hispanic black (10.3 per 1,000) and total non-Hispanic (5.8) compared with non-Hispanic white infants (4.7) (AHRQ, 2015c, p. 33).

- In 2013, Asian women were less likely than white women to have received a Pap smear in the last 3 years regardless of educational level. About half of Asian women with less than a high school education (49.8%) received a Pap smear compared with 69.5% of white women. For those with any college, the percentages were 76.3% for Asian women and 86.5% for white women (AHRQ, 2015c, p. 36).

Access to health care, as defined in the 2016 *National Healthcare QDR* Chartbook on Access to Health Care, uses the 1993 IOM definition: "the timely use of personal health services to achieve the best health outcomes" (AHRQ, 2016a, p. 3). The 2016 Chartbook on Access identifies four factors that impact access: health insurance, having a usual source of care, timeliness (the ability to access care when needed), and infrastructure (a competent workforce equipped with effective health information technology). Using these four criteria, the 2016 Chartbook on Access and the 2015 *QDR* found several disparities, which are listed in **Box 19.1.**

Clearly racial origin alone does not account for these disparities in health and health outcomes. Health status is influenced by a multiplicity of factors, as reflected in **Figure 19.1.** Key determinants associated with poor health status and outcomes also tend to reflect such factors as economic status and household composition (DeNavas-Walt, Proctor, & Smith, 2011), as well as English language proficiency and insurance status. The following statements further illustrate disparities in health and health outcomes:

- *Overall rate:* In 2013, the overall percentage of people unable to get or delayed in getting needed medical care, dental care, or prescription medicines in the last 12 months was 11.7% (AHRQ, 2016a, p. 8).

- In all quarters, people in poor and near-poor households were more likely to be uninsured than people in households that were not poor (AHRQ, 2016a, p. 6).

- From January 2010 to September 2015, the percentage of people under age 65 who were uninsured at the time of interview decreased from 17.5% to 10.8%. Adults ages 18 to 29 experienced the largest declines (AHRQ, 2016a, p. 4).

- From 2002 to 2013, there were no statistically significant changes by insurance in the percentage of adults needing urgent care who sometimes or never got care as soon as wanted. In 2013, the percentages were 32.8% for uninsured people, 23.1% for those with public

Box 19.1

2015 National Healthcare Quality and Disparities Report, National Quality Strategy (NQS) and 2016 Chartbook on Access to Care Data

- In all years, from 2010 to the first half of 2015, blacks and Hispanics were less likely than whites to have a usual place to go for medical care (AHRQ, 2016a, p. 7).
- People in poor households had worse access to care than people in high-income households on all access measures (AHRQ, 2016a, p. 2).
- Hispanics had worse access to care than whites for more than two-thirds of access measures (AHRQ, 2016a, p. 2).
- Blacks had worse access to care than whites for about half of the access measures (AHRQ, 2016a, p. 2).
- Asians had worse access to care than whites for about one-third of access measures, and American Indians and Alaska Natives had worse access to care than whites for about one-quarter of access measures (AHRQ, 2016a, p. 2).
- From 2002 to 2013, Hispanic children were more likely than non-Hispanic white children to sometimes or never get care as soon as wanted (AHRQ, 2016a, p. 12).

- People in poor households received worse care than people in high-income households for about 60% of quality measures (AHRQ, 2016b, p. 11).
- Blacks, Hispanics, and American Indians and Alaska Natives received worse care than whites for about 40% of quality measures (AHRQ, 2016b, p. 11).
- Asians received worse care than whites for about 20% of quality measures (AHRQ, 2016b, p. 11).
- For each group, disparities in quality of care are similar to disparities in access to care, although disparities in access tend to be more common than disparities in quality (AHRQ, 2016b, p. 11).
- Disparities also varied across NQS priorities.
  - Disparities were more common among measures of person-centered care and care coordination, involving about 60% of comparisons (AHRQ, 2016b, p. 11).
  - Disparities were less common among measures of patient safety, effective treatment, and healthy living, involving about 30% of comparisons (AHRQ, 2016b, p. 11).

insurance, and 12.5% for those with private insurance (AHRQ, 2016a, p. 11).

"In 2014, there were 46.7 million people in poverty, for an official poverty rate of 14.8 percent. Neither the poverty rate nor the number of people in poverty were statistically different from the 2013 estimates. The 2014 poverty rate was 2.3 percentage points higher than in 2007, the year before the most recent recession (DeNavas-Walt & Proctor, 2015, p. 12). The 2014 poverty rate increased for two groups: people aged 25 and older with at least a bachelor's degree and married-couple families" (DeNavas-Walt & Proctor, 2015, p. 2).

- Poverty rates in 2014 by age and race are listed in **Boxes 19.2** and **19.3.**

Having examined some of the major social determinants of health and access to health-care services, let's return to a major goal for the next decade, set by *Healthy People 2010,*

that 100% of Americans would have health insurance. A major provision of the ACA was federal support for expansion of states' Medicaid programs and their eligibility requirements. Approximately 20 million persons acquired health insurance between 2010 and 2016 because of provisions included in the ACA. By March 2016, 30 states had expanded their Medicaid programs; 20 had not. Under the provisions of the ACA, beginning January 1, 2014, the majority of non-elderly adults with incomes at or below 138% of the Federal Poverty Level (FPL) became eligible for Medicaid in the states that expanded their Medicaid programs. The law provided for full federal funding of the Medicaid expansion in participating states in 2016, with funding decreasing to 90% of the expansion costs in 2020. In 2015, the FPL was set at $27,724 for a family of three (Garfield & Damico, 2016). Contrast this with the median income of a Medicaid eligible family of three in 19 of the states choosing to not expand their Medicaid

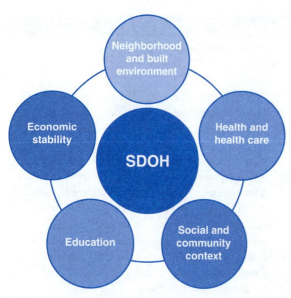

FIGURE 19.1 *Healthy People 2020* approach to social determinants of health. (Retrieved from www.healthypeople.gov/2020/topics-objectives/topic/social-determinants-of-health)

programs: $8,840 (44% of the FPL). In addition, most of the 19 states do not offer Medicaid coverage to childless adults. Economically challenged persons in non-Medicaid expansion states have a significant barrier to accessing timely,

---

Box 19.2

Poverty Rates in 2014 by Age

Children under age 18: 21.1%, 15.5 million (p. 12)
People aged 18 to 64: 13.5%, 26.5 million (p. 14)
People aged 65 and older: 10.0%, 4.6 million (p. 14)

(DeNavas-Walt & Proctor, 2015, pp. 12, 14)

Box 19.3

Poverty Rates in 2014 by Racial Grouping

- Non-Hispanic whites: 10.1%, 19.7 million (p. 12)
- Blacks: 26.2%, 10.8 million (p. 14)
- Asians: 12.0%, 2.1 million (p. 14)
- Hispanics: 23.6%, 13.1 million (p. 14)

(DeNavas-Walt & Proctor, 2015)

---

high-quality health care (Garfield & Damico, January 2016). The following have occurred because of the ACA:

- Racial disparities in insurance coverage diminished from October 2013 to the beginning of 2016. Approximately 3 million black, non-Hispanic adults acquired coverage, dropping the uninsured rate by more than 50%, from 22.4% to 10.6%. In addition, about 4 million non-elderly Hispanic adults acquired coverage, reducing the uninsured rate from 41.8% to 30.5%, a 27% decline (Uberoi, Finegold, & Gee, 2016, p. 2).
- Through the ACA's provisions 6.1 million young adults have gained insurance coverage: 2.3 million ages 19 to 25 were allowed to remain covered under their parents' health insurance plans until age 26 and another 3.8 million joined from the start of open enrollment in the health insurance marketplaces in October 2013 through the beginning of 2016 (Uberoi, Finegold, & Gee, 2016, p. 2).

It is estimated that some 1.9 million (2014 data) uninsured persons with mental health or substance abuse disorders resided in the 20 states that opted out of expanding their Medicaid programs and had incomes that would make them eligible for care under an expanded Medicaid program. The 1.9 million persons represented 28% of the low income, uninsured populations in these 20 states (Dey et al, 2016, p. 1).

ETHICAL MANDATE

APNs frequently face a dual challenge: to provide high-quality, evidence-based care to culturally diverse populations and to do so in communities that are often socially and economically disadvantaged. Our profession's response to this challenge is found in the American Nurses Association's (ANA's) *Code of Ethics for Nurses With Interpretive Statements,* particularly Provisions 1 and 8 (ANA, 2015a, p. 31).

Central to the concept of ethical practice is the principle of justice: fair and equitable access to high-quality health-care services. That this access is not available for many Americans is indisputable and has served as the focal point for the debate over whether health care is a right or a privilege. The late Dr. Martin Luther King Jr. addressed the inherent injustice in disparities in health care by saying, "Of all the forms of inequality, injustice in health is the most shocking and inhumane" (Changing the Present, 2012). The racial, ethnic, and social factors creating existing disparities in health and access to health-care services create a moral imperative for APNs to integrate cultural competence into all their direct and indirect care roles. Cultural competence demands not only incorporation of the patient's cultural beliefs and practices into our caregiving but also broader application of the principles of cultural competence in the management of clinical services, resource allocation, and professional activities such as the formulation of health policy. It is inadequate for APNs to simply do no harm. APNs represent the majority of our profession's most highly educated nurses. It is their responsibility to do more than just render high-quality care on a one-to-one basis with their patients. They are also accountable for continually improving the systems within which that care occurs.

WALK A MILE IN SOMEONE ELSE'S SHOES

Imagine that you are an elderly U.S. tourist participating in an elder hostel tour abroad. This is the first time that you have ever been out of the United States. You have a history of hypertension and coronary artery disease as well as myopia and moderate, bilateral hearing loss. While abroad, you experience recurrent chest pain. The tour guide tries unsuccessfully to locate an English-speaking physician, so you are brought to the local hospital where you are admitted for observation. After your glasses and clothing are removed, you are placed on bedrest and receive nitroglycerin intravenously and oxygen by nasal cannula. You are unable to reach the bedside table and you cannot see the other patients or the staff in the ward clearly. You are unable to speak or understand the language, so you have no idea of the severity of your condition or its treatment. The tour guide, who initially served as your interpreter, has had to return to the group that is departing for the next tour destination in the morning.

If this were you, how would you feel? Vulnerable? Frightened? At the mercy of a health-care system and care providers whose language, and perhaps beliefs and practices, are totally unfamiliar to you? Now imagine that you and your family recently immigrated to the United States. You may or may not speak and read English. The health-care beliefs and practices of your culture may differ significantly from those of Western medicine. You may be an undocumented immigrant, fearful of detection and reticent to seek care. Superimposed on your ethnic and racial status may be the social implications of coming from a culture of poverty.

In short, you would be a prototype for many of the patients cared for by APNs. How would you want to be treated if the roles were reversed and you were the patient?

THEORETICAL BASIS FOR CULTURAL COMPETENCE IN ADVANCED NURSING PRACTICE

Madeleine Leininger's (2001) pioneering work in transcultural nursing and the development of her Culture Care Theory provides a framework for the practice of APNs who care for culturally diverse populations. Care and caring, distinguishing characteristics of professional practice to which APNs lay particular claim, are central to her theory: "Care is the essence of nursing and the central, dominant and unifying focus of nursing" (p. 35). Leininger holds that for too long caring has been the "covert, unknown, and almost invisible aspect of nursing and health services" (p. 32).

Leininger's commitment to the development of a theoretical framework that would assist nurses and other health-care providers to deliver culturally congruent care to patients from diverse populations evolved from a commitment to improve the health of clients, families, and cultural groups; to better help patients from diverse cultural groups to maintain or regain their health; or to experience death in a manner compatible with their cultural beliefs and practices. Leininger's theory of culture care acknowledges both universal and culture-specific care patterns. For instance, although beliefs and expressions associated with caring may vary widely from one cultural group to another, human care practices have been documented from the beginning of recorded history.

Formulated from an anthropological perspective, the theory questions nursing's traditional reliance on the concepts of person, health, and the environment. Leininger (2001) notes that, in many non-Western cultures, family and social institutions are primary and that the language may not even have a word for person. She also notes that although nurses and nursing exert significant influence over individual and societal health and the environment, these concepts are hardly unique to our profession or its practice. In place of these generic concepts, Leininger proposes that care and caring are the central core of nursing, stating, "Care is the nurse's way of being with and helping people" (p. 40).

Leininger's theory and the Sunrise Model in **Figure 19.2,** which depicts both the universality and diversity of cultural care, provide a framework for the APN to examine the dynamic interplay of the many forces that influence the delivery of care. The Culture Care Theory incorporates three

major approaches to the delivery of culturally congruent nursing assessment, decision making, and interventions. Leininger defines these modalities as the following:

1. *Cultural care preservation and maintenance:* "Professional actions and decisions that help people of a particular culture to retain and/or preserve relevant care values so that they can maintain their well being, recover from illness, or face handicaps and/or death" (p. 48).

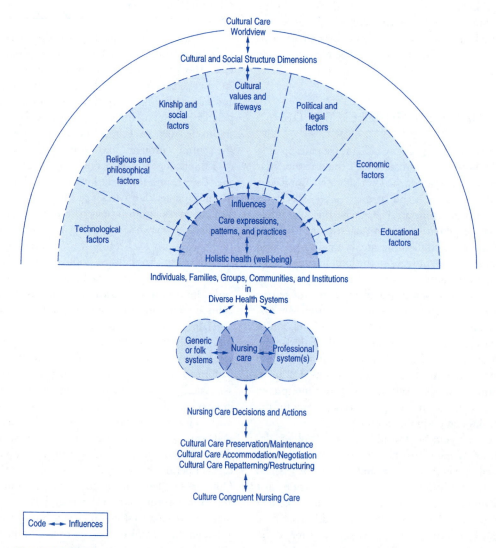

FIGURE 19.2 Leininger's Sunrise Model to depict the theory of cultural care diversity and universality. *(Source: Leininger, 1991, p. 43, with permission of the National League for Nursing.)*

2. *Cultural care accommodation and negotiation:* "Creative professional actions and decisions that help people of a designated culture to adapt to, or to negotiate with others for a beneficial or satisfying health outcome with professional care providers" (p. 48).
3. *Cultural care repatterning or restructuring:* "Professional actions and decisions that help a client(s) reorder, change, or greatly modify their lifeways for new, different, and beneficial health-care patterns while respecting the client(s) cultural values and beliefs and still providing a beneficial or healthier lifeway than before the changes were co-established with the client(s)" (p. 49).

Inherent in each of these modalities are three of the core values that underlie all advanced practice nursing: respect, advocacy, and partnership. The culturally competent APN is knowledgeable and respectful of diverse cultural beliefs and practices, partners with the patient to develop a care regimen that produces the desired health outcomes within the context of the patient's cultural values, and advocates for the development of culturally appropriate patient care services.

APNs who apply these modalities in their care of patients provide what Leininger (2001) terms *culturally congruent (nursing) care.* Leininger (2001, p. 49) states that this term:

refers to those cognitively based assistive, supportive, facilitative, or enabling acts or decisions that are tailor made to fit with individual, group or institutional cultural values, beliefs, and lifeways in order to provide or support meaningful, beneficial, and satisfying health care, or well-being services.

MOVING FROM THEORY INTO PRACTICE

The year 1985 was transformative for American health care. On October 16, 1985, Margaret M. Heckler, the former secretary of HHS, released *The Report of the Secretary's Task Force on Black and Minority Health* (Heckler Report). The task force was composed of senior officials and scientists from governmental agencies and civilian organizations with leadership responsibilities in health care. In a little more than a year, the task force, under the chairmanship of Thomas E. Malone, PhD, deputy director of the National Institutes of Health, led an intensive,

in-depth exploration of the health status and disparities in access, quality of care, and outcomes ranging from infant mortality and low birth weight to chemical dependency and cardiovascular and cerebrovascular disease among black and other minority populations in the United States. The report drove the creation of new and aggressive federal initiatives to combat disparities in health care as well as new governmental offices within existing federal agencies specifically commissioned to fight disparities and promote access to high-quality health care for previously underserved populations (Malone, 1985). Thus in 1986, the Office of Minority Health (OMH) was created within the USDHHS. The OMH defines *cultural competence* using the pioneering work conducted by Cross and colleagues (1989) that established cultural competence as an essential component of quality health care. The OMH uses the following definition:

Culturally and linguistically appropriate services are respectful of and responsive to the health beliefs, practices and needs of diverse patients. The percentage of Americans who are racial and ethnic minorities and who speak a primary language other than English continues to grow rapidly. Organizations are looking to meet the challenges of serving diverse communities and provide high quality services and care.

By tailoring services to an individual's culture and language preference, health professionals can help bring about positive health outcomes for diverse populations. (USDHHS, OMH, 2016e) and defines its mission as:

. . . improving the health of racial and ethnic minority populations through the development of health policies and programs that will help eliminate health disparities. (USDHHS, 2016b)

The OMH has been in the forefront of our nation's efforts to identify and eradicate disparities in health and health care. In 1987, the OMH established a Resource Center. The Resource Center houses the largest collection of information in the country on health disparities and its three core services—the Knowledge Center, Capacity Building, and Information Services—make it indispensable to health-care professionals, policy makers, consumers (health literature in more than 35 languages), researchers, organizational representatives, and so on. The OMH's leadership has also played a pivotal role in moving our health-care system and the educational institutions that educate our health professionals to a greater understanding of the importance of addressing the social determinants of health and of the need to move beyond cultural sensitivity to cultural and linguistic competence in health care. To that end, in 1995 the OMH established the Center for Linguistic and Cultural Competency in Health Care (CLCCHC) with the specific focus of working to reduce the barriers to care experienced by persons with limited English proficiency (LEP) (USDHHS, OMH, 2016c). The CLCCHC partners with a wide variety of other federal entities as well as public and private organizations to promote research and demonstration projects, offer direct assistance, and provide e-learning on cultural and linguistic competence to educators and practitioners in the health science. The CLCCHC Web site, Think Cultural Health (TCH) (thinkculturalhealth.hhs.gov), sponsored by the OMH, is a leader in educating healthcare professionals and students in the health professions about cultural and linguistic competency in health care and how to access the resources to improve practice on a personal as well as organizational level. The Web site offers a robust continuing education e-learning program with the goal of equipping individuals in any discipline with the knowledge and skills to promote health and health equity through the delivery of culturally and linguistically appropriate care. Two of the TCH FREE e-learning offerings described in the text that follows warrant your attention. These are "A Physician's Practical Guide to Culturally Competent Care" and "What Is Culturally Competent Nursing Care: A Cornerstone of Caring?" The courses, contact hour information, and accompanying comments on the critical value of these courses to your practice may be accessed at https://www.thinkculturalhealth.hhs.gov. These courses are summarized in **Boxes 19.4** and **19.5**.

ASSESSING AND PROMOTING ORGANIZATIONAL CULTURAL AND LINGUISTIC COMPETENCY

The National Center for Cultural Competence (NCCC) expands on the OMH definition by identifying organizational requirements based on the five essential elements that Cross et al (1989) identify as being necessary for

---

Box 19.4

A Physician's Practical Guide to Culturally Competent Care

This is a self-directed training course designed for physicians, physician assistants, and NPs. With growing concerns about racial and ethnic disparities in health and about the need for health-care systems to accommodate increasingly diverse patient populations, cultural competence has become more and more a matter of national concern. This e-learning program will equip health-care providers with competencies that will enable them to better treat the increasingly diverse U.S. population. The Web site has been updated to include the 2013 CLAS Standards, as well as more case studies, resources, and more interactivity (USDHHS, OMH, 2016a).

The registration process is straightforward and the program was developed to meet the continuing education standards and policies of the American Academy of Nurse Practitioners (AANP): Program ID 1411504.

Upon successful completion of the program, you earn 9.0 contact hours.

It is a win-win-win; you become a better caregiver, your patients or clients receive better care, and you have 9 contact hours to put toward your next re-licensure or recertification! A comment from Dr. Robert C. Like, MD, MS, Director of the Center for Healthy Families and Cultural Diversity, Department of Family Medicine, UMDNJ-Robert Wood Johnson Medical School, is posted next to the "A Physician's Practical Guide to Culturally Competent Care" e-learning program: has "Informative, relevant, and engaging. . . . A marvelous e-learning program that will improve the quality of care provided to all patients. . . . This is likely to be the 'gold standard' in cultural competency training for many years to come!"

Box 19.5

What Is *Culturally Competent Nursing Care: A Cornerstone of Caring?*

Culturally Competent Nursing Care: A Cornerstone of Caring is a free e-learning program from the HHS OMH. It is accredited for up to nine continuing education credits at no cost for nurses and social workers.

This e-learning program is designed to help you deliver culturally and linguistically competent care. Cultural and linguistic competency is the capacity for individuals and organizations to work and communicate effectively in cross-cultural situations. Cultural and linguistic competency can help improve the quality of the care you deliver to patients from diverse cultural backgrounds.

This e-learning program is grounded in the *National Standards for Culturally and Linguistically Appropriate Services (CLAS) in Health and Health Care*. These standards are intended to advance health equity, improve quality, and help eliminate health disparities. The *National CLAS Standards* provide you and other health professionals with a blueprint for increasing cultural and linguistic competency (USDHHS, OMH, 2016f).

In your professional practice, you may have management and leadership responsibilities in addition to your direct provider role. Lead by example by completing one of the two e-learning offerings that best fits your role functions. Then encourage your colleagues to do likewise. Help build a caregiving environment in which all the practitioners demonstrate cultural and linguistic competency. These competencies are even more critical now when patient-provider interaction is often limited. If we are to maximize our effectiveness and patient outcomes in time-limited encounters with increasingly diverse patient populations, we need to be proficient in cultural and linguistic competency.

Becky Patton, former president of the ANA, wrote the following, which is posted by the nursing e-learning offering:

"Providing effective and respectful nursing care to our country's increasingly diverse population is of paramount importance to the ANA. The OMH curriculum offers nurses the most comprehensive program regarding culturally competent nursing care."

Rebecca M. Patton, MSN, RN, CNOR, Past President, American Nurses Association

---

culturally competent organizations. Cultural competence requires that organizations:

- "Have a defined set of values and principles, and demonstrate behaviors, attitudes, policies, and structures that enable them to work effectively cross-culturally.
- Have the capacity to (1) value diversity, (2) conduct self-assessment, (3) manage the dynamics of difference, (4) acquire and institutionalize cultural knowledge, and (5) adapt to diversity and the cultural contexts of the communities they serve.
- Incorporate the above in all aspects of policy making, administration, practice, and service delivery, and systematically involve consumers, key stakeholders, and communities.

Cultural competence is a developmental process that evolves over an extended period. Both individuals and organizations are at various levels of awareness, knowledge, and skills along the cultural competence continuum." (NCCC, 2016; adapted from Cross et al, 1989)

Note that the NCCC definition highlights the developmental nature of cultural competency as applied to individual practitioners and organizations. The development of cultural competency occurs on a continuum, with the ultimate goal of cultural proficiency. The definitions speak to the requirements for achieving organizational as well as individual competence. In an environment in which healthcare delivery systems are increasingly held accountable for continuous quality improvement and cost containment, APNs often straddle dual roles as clinicians and managers of clinical services. Thus, the APN must not only be skilled in the direct delivery of culturally competent care, but also in the implementation of policies and procedures that ensure cultural competence at the organizational level.

Cultural competence is inextricably linked to linguistic competence. The essence of advanced practice nursing is communication. Our ability to engage our patients as true partners in their care, to establish the trust relationship that is essential to building that partnership, requires that we exhibit linguistic competence. Every aspect of our practice, from initial assessment to teaching, counselling, and support, depends on our being linguistically competent. The NCCC (2016a) defines *linguistic competence* as follows:

> The capacity of an organization and its personnel to communicate effectively, and convey information in a manner that is easily understood by diverse groups including persons of limited English proficiency, those who have low literacy skills or are not literate, individuals with disabilities, and those who are deaf or hard of hearing. Linguistic competency requires organizational and provider capacity to respond effectively to the health and mental health literacy needs of populations served. The organization must have policy, structures, practices, procedures, and dedicated resources to support this capacity.

The definition is accompanied by a set of values and guiding principles that lay the foundation for demonstrating linguistic competence at both the individual and organizational levels, including language access. The information available at the NCCC Web site, https://nccc.georgetown.edu/leadership/, provides valuable information to facilitate you in taking a leadership role in promoting linguistic competence within your practice setting.

A very valuable tool for assessing the cultural and linguistic competence of a health-care organization is *Conducting a Cultural Competence Self-Assessment* (Andrulis, Delbanco, Avakian, & Shaw-Taylor, n.d.) The tool outlines a five-step process in which over a period of 3 to 6 weeks, using an interview and questionnaire format for individuals and groups, an organizational task force with diverse membership can complete a comprehensive assessment of its organization's ability to deliver culturally competent care. The data are essential to driving a health-care organization's ongoing initiatives to deliver culturally and linguistically competent care and to meeting the accreditation standards set by The Joint Commission (TJC). Interview data is obtained from multiple sources, including community leaders, professional and support staff, clergy, interpreters, admitting and patient registration staff, union leadership, and so on, as well as the organization's leadership team. The length of the interviews range from 15 to 45 minutes.

Participants are asked to bring and share any relevant materials during the interview session and all information shared is confidential; participants are reassured that the findings of the assessment will be reported in aggregate form. The tool has 17 suggested interview questions designed to elicit information about the strengths and barriers to the organization's ability to provide culturally competent care. The task force members select persons within the organization that in their judgment are most knowledgeable to answer the 62-item questionnaire. The questionnaire is divided into three sections. Section 1 assesses the ethnic and cultural characteristics of the staff and the organization. Section 2 assesses the health-care organization's ability to meet the needs identified in Section 1, including training, human resources, and union presence, if applicable. Section 3 assesses organizational links to the community and diversity initiatives for patients and staff. The questionnaire elicits essential information about what, if any, accommodations (e.g., appointment and testing schedule, dietary needs, discharge planning) are made by the health-care organization to meet the cultural and religious preferences of the population being served. In Section 4 of the questionnaire, Language and Communication Needs of Patients and Staff, the questions elicit in-depth data about the type of interpreter and translation services utilized for the care of LEP persons.

THE AMERICAN HOSPITAL ASSOCIATION AND THE HEALTH RESEARCH AND EDUCATIONAL TRUST

In 2003 the American Hospital Association (AHA) replaced the Patients' Bill of Rights with *The Patient Care Partnership* (AHA, 2003). It is in the form of an easy-to-read brochure that seeks to integrate patients' values and beliefs into their care and describes what patients should expect during their hospitalization with respect to their rights and responsibilities. The brochure is available in eight languages (English, Arabic, traditional and simplified Chinese, Spanish, Russian, Vietnamese, and Tagalog) and may be downloaded in English from the AHA Web site (http://www.aha.org/content/00-10/pcp_english_030730.pdf).

The AHA and its education affiliate, the Health Research and Educational Trust (HRET), have produced multiple products for use by staff and an organization's leadership team to enhance culturally competent care within the United States. The resources in the following list are particularly relevant to the delivery of culturally and linguistically competent care:

- Strategies for Leadership: Does Your Hospital Reflect the Community It Serves? A Diversity and Cultural Proficiency Assessment Tool for Leaders (AHA, NCHL, IFD, & ACHE, 2004), accessible at www.aha.org (enter the title of the document in the Search box to bring up a PDF that can be downloaded) or from http://www.aha.org/content/00-10/diversitytool.pdf)
- The HRET Disparities Toolkit, accessible at http://www.hretdisparities.org (Hasnain-Wynia, Pierce, Haque, HedgesGreising, Prince, & Reiter, 2007)
- Improving Health Equity Through Data Collection and Use: A Guide for Hospital Leaders (Hospitals in Pursuit of Excellence, April 2011), accessible at http://www.hret.org/health-equity/index.shtml
- Bibliography—Cultural Competency. The bibliography contains an extensive list of books, articles, reports, and other resources (AHA, 2011), accessible at http://www.aha.org/content/11/11dispbib-competency.pdf
- Building a Culturally Competent Organization: The Quest for Equity in Health Care (HRET & IFD, 2011), accessible at www.hret.org/cultural-competency
- Becoming a Culturally Competent Health Care Organization (HRET, 2013), accessible at http://www.hpoe.org/becoming-culturally-competent
- Improving Patient Safety Culture Through Teamwork and Communication: TeamSTEPPS (HRET, 2015), accessible at http://www.ahrq.gov/professionals/quality-patient-safety/patient-safety-resources-resources/pstools/index.html

It is important to note that the Diversity and Cultural Proficiency Assessment Tool for Leaders, developed in collaboration with the National Center for Healthcare Leadership, the American College of Healthcare Executives, and the Institute for Diversity in Healthcare, seeks to move the goal of caregiving from *culturally competent* care to *culturally proficient* care (p. 4). The four-part assessment tool is comprehensive, containing not only an evidence-based diversity checklist but also recommended action steps, case studies, and an extensive bibliography.

The HRET Disparities Toolkit is designed for use in a wide variety of settings, ranging from hospitals to private health-care practices and community health centers, and specifically addresses best practices for obtaining accurate race, ethnicity, and primary language data from persons with LEP or visual or hearing deficits. Both of these tools, as well as the other resources listed previously, are invaluable tools for promoting staff and organizational linguistic proficiency.

In addition to creating resources that promote cultural competence in health care, the AHA was instrumental in the development of the Institute for Diversity in Health Management, founded in 1994. The Institute is a nonprofit organization that works with educational institutions and health-care organizations to expand leadership opportunities for ethnic minorities in management of health care. Its Web site is www.DiversityConnection.org.

LEGISLATIVE AND REGULATORY MANDATES AND ACTIONS TAKEN BY THE HEALTH-CARE INDUSTRY

In addition to the professional imperative that APN(s) be culturally and linguistically competent, a variety of federal agencies issue regulations affecting health care and health-care providers. Of most immediate importance are the personal legal implications of failing to practice in a culturally and linguistically appropriate manner. The care that is documented in a patient's clinical record is a direct reflection of your practice. If cultural and linguistic barriers exist between you and your patients and you have not instituted action to address these in your history taking, clinical decision making, and patient education, treatment failure and adverse outcomes may well occur. From a legal perspective, what is not documented has not been done. In our increasingly litigious society, failure to document culturally appropriate care may well serve as an ethical and legal indictment of your practice with very real professional repercussions.

Individual, organizational, and system vulnerability to legal action may also result from failure to comply with the provisions of Section 601 of Title VI of the Civil Rights Act of 1964, as amended, 42 U.S.C. §2000d et seq., which states the following (U.S. Department of Justice [USDOJ], Civil Rights Division, 1998a):

No person in the United States shall, on the ground of race, color, or national origin, be excluded from participation in, be denied the benefits of, or be subjected to discrimination under any program or activity receiving Federal financial assistance.

Previous court decisions involving Title VI have employed the Fourteenth Amendment's standard of proof of intentional discrimination as well as Title VI's requirement for demonstration of "disparate impact." Health-care institutions receiving federal assistance whose programs or policies discriminate against particular cultural groups are liable to be held accountable under the provisions of Title VI. For example, the Supreme Court has held that undocumented immigrants fulfill the definition of "persons" in the context of the Fifth and Fourteenth Amendments to the U.S. Constitution. As such, they are, by extension, included under the protections afforded by Title VI. Keep in mind that federal assistance has been broadly defined as encompassing not only direct financial assistance but also forms of indirect aid such as subsidies, loans, and federal training (USDOJ, Civil Rights Division, 1998b).

On August 11, 2000, Executive Order 13166 was issued: *Improving Access to Services for Persons With Limited English Proficiency.* The executive order required all federal agencies that funded nonfederal program(s) to publish guidance to recipients of such funding as to how they could comply with the provisions of Title VI. To minimize confusion and maximize compliance across all federal agencies, adoption of the uniform criteria established by the USDOJ was encouraged. The current regulatory guidelines of the USDHHS that went into effect in October 2004 define LEP persons as follows (USDHHS, OCR, 2004, pp. 6–7):

Individuals who do not speak English as their primary language and who have a limited ability to read, write, speak, or understand English may be limited English proficient, or "LEP," and may be eligible to receive language assistance with respect to a particular type of service, benefit, or encounter.

The regulations forbid "restrict[ing] an individual in any way in the enjoyment of any advantage or privilege enjoyed by others receiving any service, financial aid, or other benefit under the program" or from "utiliz[ing] criteria or methods of administration which have the effect of subjecting individuals to discrimination because of their race, color, or national origin, or have the effect of defeating or substantially impairing accomplishment

of the objectives of the program as respects individuals of a particular race, color, or national origin" (USDHHS, OCR, 2004, p. 3).

The guidelines identify the types of USDHHS recipients who must comply with the provisions of Title VI, including hospitals and nursing homes, state Medicaid programs, Head Start programs, managed care organizations, and state, county, and local health agencies. They also identify the four criteria that programs and institutions can use to determine the level of resources that must be invested to ensure compliance: (a) the number or proportion of LEP persons eligible to be served or likely to be encountered by the program or grantee; (b) the frequency with which LEP individuals come in contact with the program; (c) the nature and importance of the program, activity, or service provided by the program to people's lives; and (d) the resources available to the grantee or recipient and costs (USDHHS, OCR, 2004, pp. 5–6).

In 2000 the OMH of the USDHHS released the National Standards for Culturally and Linguistically Appropriate Services (CLAS) in Health and Health Care. These standards were developed in response to documented disparities in access to, and quality of, health-related services to an increasingly diverse population. They were designed to help health-care organizations to develop services that would promote culturally competent care with the goal of ultimately eliminating disparities and promoting better health. In 2010, the Office of Civil Rights (OCR) of the USDHHS undertook a comprehensive review of the original CLAS requirements, and in 2013 the OMH of the USDHHS issued a revised, enhanced set of CLAS Standards and a blueprint for effective implementation in 2013. The 15 standards are organized under three themes: (1) Governance, Leadership and Workforce; (2) Communication and Language Assistance; and (3) Engagement, Continuous Improvement and Accountability. The revised 2013 CLAS Standards and the blueprint for implementation may be accessed at https://www.thinkculturalhealth.hhs.gov/pdfs/EnhancedCLASStandardsBlueprint.pdf(USDHHS, OMH, 2013).

The Enhanced CLAS Standards have strengthened the original CLAS 2000 Standards in many ways. The definition of health has been expanded and a new standard on Organizational Governance and Leadership holds an organization's leadership accountable for promoting CLAS and the goal of health equity not only through policy and practices but also by resource allocation. An organization cannot meet Standards 3 and 4, which call for recruiting and supporting a culturally and linguistically diverse workforce at all levels of the organization and ongoing education and training at all levels of the workforce in culturally and linguistically appropriate policies and practices, without providing the necessary funding to do so. It takes resources to "Walk the Talk."

Other notable changes in the Enhanced CLAS Standards (USDHHS, OMH, 2013) are:

- Replacing the terms *patients* and *consumers* with the terms *individuals* and *groups*. The new terms are more inclusive and encompass patients, families, clients, and caregivers (pp. 10–11).
- Beginning each standard with an action word, reinforcing the expectation that the standards are to be actively promoted within each health-care organization (p. 11).
- Using themes in CLAS 2013 that are more dynamic and inclusive (pp. 11–12). Themes from 2000 and 2013 are compared in **Table 19.1.**

It should be noted that Standards 4 to 8, which address the needs of LEP persons, represent standards that are covered by the provisions of Title VI of the Civil Rights Act of 1964 and affect any organization that receives federal funding. These standards are as follows:

STANDARD 4: Educate and train governance, leadership, and workforce in culturally and linguistically appropriate policies and practices on an ongoing basis. (USDHHS, OMH, 2013, p. 66)

STANDARD 5: Offer language assistance to individuals who have limited English proficiency and/or other communication need, at no cost to them, to facilitate timely access to all health care and services. (USDHHS, OMH, 2013, p. 72)

STANDARD 6: Inform all individuals of the availability of language assistance services clearly and in their preferred language, verbally and in writing. (USDHHS, OMH, 2013, p. 79)

STANDARD 7: Ensure the competence of individuals providing language assistance services, recognizing that the use of untrained individuals and/or minors as interpreters should be avoided. (USDHHS, OMH, 2013, p. 85)

STANDARD 8: Provide easy-to-read print and multimedia materials and signage in the languages commonly used by the populations in the service area. (USDHHS, OMH, 2013, p. 93)

TABLE 19.1

Comparison of Selected CLAS Themes; 2000 and 2013

2000 CLAS Themes	2013 CLAS Themes
No Principal Standard	A Principal Standard, Standard 1: Provide effective, equitable, understandable, and respectful quality care and services that are responsive to diverse cultural health beliefs and practices, preferred languages, health literacy, and other communication needs. Standard 1 is only attainable IF the remaining 14 standards are fully and consistently implemented (p. 11).
Culturally Competent Care	Governance, Leadership, and Workforce. (p. 12)
Language Access Services	Communication and Language Assistance (p. 12)
Organizational Supports	Engagement, Continuous Improvement, and Accountability (p. 12)

(USDHHS, OMH, 2013)

A *short* (2 page) overview of how to meet the various federal mandates has been prepared by TJC. It is called Language Access and the Law and covers the institutional requirements of Title VI of the 1964 Civil Rights Act, as well as the requirements of the Americans with Disabilities Act (1990) and the Rehabilitation Act (1973) (TJC, 2008). The document also addresses the needs of the hard of hearing and other groups. It is available at http://www.jointcommission.org/assets/1/6/Lang%20Access%20and%20Law%20Jan%202008%20(17).pdf.

Several states have taken active steps to promote the incorporation of the CLAS Standards within their states. The most frequent (29 states) activity was the development of strategic planning documents and the establishment of partnerships to facilitate the implementation of their recommendations. The next most frequent state activity was wide dissemination of the Enhanced CLAS Standards through a variety of vehicles including newsletters, conferences, toolkits, training, and technical assistance. The OMH has tracked this information and issued a report entitled *National Standards for Culturally and Linguistically Appropriate Services in Health and Health Care: Compendium of State-Sponsored National CLAS Standards Implementation Activities*. The report may be accessed and downloaded at https://www.thinkculturalhealth.hhs.gov/pdfs/CLASCompendium.pdf (USDHHS, OMH, 2016d).

In 2014, TJC produced two critical documents designed to promote health equity and to facilitate their accredited institutions meeting the Enhanced CLAS Standards: These were *A Crosswalk of the National Standards for Culturally and Linguistically Appropriate Services (CLAS) in Health and Health Care to The Joint Commission Hospital Accreditation Standards* (TJC, 2014b) (available at https://www.jointcommission.org/assets/1/6/Crosswalk-_CLAS_-20140718.pdf) and *A Crosswalk of the National Standards for Culturally and Linguistically Appropriate Services (CLAS) in Health and Health Care to The Joint Commission Ambulatory Health Care Accreditation Standards* (TJC, 2014a) (available at https://www.jointcommission.org/assets/1/6/Crosswalk_CLAS_AHC_20141110.pdf).

TJC also took the lead in addressing the health-care needs of lesbian, gay, bisexual, and transgender (LGBT) persons, a population that has long experienced discrimination not only in health and access to quality health-care services but in many other aspects of their lives as well. It had become increasingly clear to TJC that the generic accreditation standards did not adequately address the needs of the LGBT community. With funding from The California Endowment, TJC undertook to work with the LGBT community and an expert advisory panel to create a document that would promote health equity for this underserved population. In 2011, TJC released *Advancing Effective Communication, Cultural Competence, and Patient- and Family-Centered Care for the Lesbian, Gay, Bisexual, and Transgender (LGBT) Community: A Field Guide*. The field guide is organized around five domain areas, each containing strategies and recommendations identified by the LGBT community as being the most in need of action: (1) leadership; (2) provision of care, treatment, and services; (3) workforce; (4) data collection and use; and (5) patient, family and community engagement (TJC, 2011a, p. 4).

Citing disparities such as limited access to insurance and health-care services, diminished overall health status, and increased incidence of mental illnesses such as depression and anxiety, the field guide builds on the work of the 2011 Comprehensive Accreditation Manual for Hospitals (CAMH; TJC, 2011b). Elements of Performance 28 and 29 under RI.01.01.01 in CAMH 2011 prohibit discrimination based on sexual orientation, gender identity, and gender expression and ensure access to a support person of the patient's choice, which are critical issues to the LGBT community. Indeed, although the accreditation standards in CAMH 2011 were not intended to be implemented until January of 2012, these elements of performance had an earlier implementation date of July 1, 2011 (TJC, 2011b, p. 7).

The AHRQ has sought to partner with the nation's hospitals to promote patient safety and positive health outcomes. In 2012 the AHRQ published a monograph entitled "Improving Patient Safety Systems for Patients With Limited English Proficiency: A Guide for Hospitals" (Betancourt et al, 2012). The guide approaches the goal of patient safety holistically, seeking to assist hospitals to create environments and cultures that promote safety for increasingly diverse patient populations. Multiple areas are addressed with particular emphasis on the need for strong collaboration between the staff and leadership of each facility. Everyone is seen as having a vested interest—and responsibility—for achieving a culture of safety that maximizes optimal patient outcomes. The foreword to the guide was written by Rich Umbdenstock, president and

CEO of the AHA, who addresses the importance of the enhanced emphasis on cultural competence as essential to quality patient-centered care. In addition to praising the solid evidence-based research underlying the document, he also praises its vitality, noting that it offers a vast array of strategies; training, documentation, and evaluation tools; and access to materials from a wide array of sources. He identified one of the eight modules in the guide as being particularly valuable to hospitals as they work to maximize the care of their diverse patient populations— the TeamSTEPPS LEP training module, which explores team behaviors and structured communication tools that promote patient safety. The team approach permeates the entire guide (Betancourt et.al, 2012, pp. iii & 31–36). Five nationwide training sites prepare master TeamSTEPPS trainers, who work with individual facilities to train personnel and to plan and implement the interprofessional training. The five regional training sites in the National Implementation of TeamSTEPPS Project are:

- North Shore Long Island Jewish Health System in New Hyde Park, New York (NSLIJ)
- Duke Medical Center, Durham, North Carolina (Duke)
- Tulane University, New Orleans, Louisiana (Tulane)
- University of Minnesota Fairview Medical Center, Minneapolis, Minnesota (UM)
- University of Washington Medicine, Seattle, Washington (UW)

(TeamSTEPPS, 2015)

USE OF INTERPRETER AND TRANSLATOR SERVICES

In 2010 TJC released a new human resources accreditation requirement, HR.01.02.01, specifying staff qualifications for language interpreters and translators:

> EP 1
> The hospital defines staff qualifications specific to their job responsibilities.
> Note 4: Qualifications for language interpreters and translators may be met through language proficiency assessment, education, training, and experience. The use of qualified interpreters and translators is supported by the Americans with Disabilities Act, Section 504

of the Rehabilitation Act of 1973, and Title VI of the Civil Rights Act of 1964. (TJC, 2010, p. 57)

The release of the new requirement was accompanied by a set of self-assessment guidelines to assist the health-care organization with compliance. Components of the guidelines include the following:

- A job description for interpreters includes defined competencies such as language proficiency (in target language and English), skills required, and training needed.
- Human resources files for individuals who are used to interpret include evidence of their competency assessment as outlined in the job description.
- Interviews with individuals used to interpret include discussion about training, experience, and qualifications.
- For contracted interpreter services (either via phone, video, or in person), the hospital receives assurance that the contract includes information about how the service provider defines competencies consistent with your hospital's defined expectations. (Joint Commission Leadership Standard LD.04.03.09 specifically addresses the provision of contracted services within the hospital.)

A 1-year pilot introductory phase began on January 1, 2011, with full compliance as a requirement for accreditation, effective January 1, 2012 (TJC, 2010, p. 58).

As an APN, you know the importance of effective communication to every facet of a person's care, from assessment to adherence to your jointly developed plan of care. With the increasing diversity of the populations for whom we care, access to timely and effective interpreter and translator services is essential to providing high-quality care, achieving good patient outcomes, and avoiding the legal consequences of inadequate care. As an advocate for the quality of your own practice, as well as for your patients, take an active role in assessing the services in the organizations within which you practice. Are the services you need available to you when you need them? What are the qualifications of the interpreters and translators? Are they certified by a major certifying body? Examples of certifying bodies include the National Board for Certification of Medical Interpreters (NBCMI) and the Certification Commission for Healthcare Interpreters (CCHI). Are they required to complete ongoing continuing education? What training do they receive (e.g., HIPAA, medical terminology, cultural competence, ethics, mental health, domestic violence, trauma)? Are the services available in multiple modes—on site, telephonic, interactive video? Video interpreting actively incorporates the interpreter into the caregiving process. A skilled interpreter in an onsite or video encounter will not only facilitate patient-provider communication but can be a valuable asset in picking up nonverbal cues from the patient that lead the provider to seek additional information or clarification. This can be critically important if you practice in a setting where the length of appointments has been shortened and you are trying to record data while you care for your patient, which gives you less opportunity to pick up subtle clues. Skilled interpreters and translators are critical members of the health-care team and should be valued and treated as such.

Two of the major language access service providers are CyraCom and Language Access Network (LAN). If you are thinking of starting your own practice, a very useful resource is "Incorporating Medical Interpretation Into Your Practice." It can be downloaded as a free PDF file from the Family Practice Management Web site at http://www.aafp.org/fpm/2014/0300/p16.pdf (Moch, Nassery, & Fareed, 2014).

HEALTH LITERACY AND NUMERACY: PREVALENCE AND CLINICAL IMPLICATIONS

In 2004 the IOM brought the issue of health literacy to national attention with a comprehensive study of health literacy and its impact on health outcomes, *Health Literacy: A Prescription to End Confusion* (Nielsen-Bohlman, Power, & Kindig, 2004). Key findings can be found in **Box 19.6.** The report brings the impact of deficient health literacy dramatically to light in a case example (Parker, Ratzan, & Lurie, 2003, p. 150):

> A two-year-old is diagnosed with an inner ear infection and prescribed an antibiotic. Her mother understands that her child has an ear infection and knows she should take the prescribed medication twice a day. After looking at the label on the bottle and deciding that it does not tell how to take the medicine, she fills a teaspoon and pours the antibiotic into her daughter's ear.

Cultural competence must be operationalized within the context of health literacy. The definition of health literacy

---

Box 19.6

Institute of Medicine Key Findings

- Finding 3-3: "Adults with limited health literacy, as measured by reading and numeracy skills, have less knowledge of disease management and of health-promoting behaviors, report poorer health status, and are less likely to use preventive services" (Nielsen-Bohlman et al, 2004, p. 8).
- Finding 3-4: "Two recent studies demonstrate a higher rate of hospitalization and use of emergency services among patients with limited literacy. This higher utilization has been associated with higher health-care costs" (Nielsen-Bohlman et al, 2004, p. 9).
- Finding 4-1: "Culture gives meaning to health communication. Health literacy must be understood and addressed in the context of culture and language" (Nielsen-Bohlman et al, 2004, p. 10).
- Finding 6-2: "Health literacy is fundamental to quality care, and relates to three of the six aims of quality improvement described in the IOM Quality Chasm Report: safety, patient-centered care, and equitable treatment. Self-management and health literacy have been identified by IOM as cross-cutting priorities for health-care quality and disease prevention" (Nielsen-Bohlman et al, 2004, p. 12).

---

that was used in the *National Action Plan to Improve Health Literacy* (USDHHS, ODHP, 2010) was presented by the National Library of Medicine (Selden, Zorn, Ratzan, & Parker, 2000) as "the degree to which a person can obtain, process, and understand basic health information and services needed to make appropriate health decisions" (Ratzan & Parker, 2000). The *National Action Plan to Improve Health Literacy* is built upon two principles:

1. Everyone has a right to health information that helps them to make informed decisions.
2. The delivery of health-care services should be done in ways that are understandable and that promote health, longevity, and quality of life (USDHHS, ODHP, 2010, p. 1).

The population data cited in the *National Action Plan to Improve Health Literacy,* and from which this national action initiative was developed, were drawn from the National Assessment of Adult Literacy (NAAL), commissioned by the U.S. Department of Education and conducted in 2003. The NAAL was the last major study of adult literacy to be conducted in the United States; it was the first time that NAAL had included *health* literacy in their data collection (Kutner, Greenberg, Jin, & Paulsen, 2006). Citing findings from *Healthy People 2010,* the action plan starts from the premise that to effectively navigate today's health-care system, and to understand and act on much of the health and disease-related information dispensed today, a person must ideally be *proficient* in health literacy (USDHHS, ODHP, 2010, p. 7). This presents a real challenge to health-care providers, especially APNs, who often care for some of our country's most vulnerable persons.

Key findings from the NAAL cited in the *National Action Plan to Improve Health Literacy* include the following:

- Limited health literacy affected 9 out of 10 Americans surveyed.
- Only 12% of those surveyed demonstrated a *proficient* level of health literacy.
- The subpopulations most likely to have limited health literacy were:
  - Adults older than the age of 65 years
  - Racial and ethnic groups other than white
  - Recent refugees and immigrants
  - People with less than a high school degree or GED
  - People with incomes at or below the poverty level
  - Non-native speakers of English (USDHHS, ODHP, 2010, p. 8)

The NAAL data also suggest that persons with less than basic literacy skills may not even be able to read and understand a chart or simple instructions and that 42% of this same population group describe their health as being poor. The data also suggest that 54 million adults with any type of disability or illness are more likely to have the lowest levels of literacy (USDHHS, ODHP, 2010, p. 9).

In March 2011 the AHRQ released *Health Literacy Interventions and Outcomes: An Updated Systematic Review. Evidence report/technology assessment No. 199* (Berkman et al, 2011). The report used the definition of *health literacy* proposed by Ratzan and Parker (2000) that encompasses oral communication skills and numeracy and was used in *Healthy People 2010* and by the IOM in their 2004 report on health literacy. Review of research studies rated as being

"fair" or "good" demonstrated that lower health literacy was associated with increased hospitalization, increased use of emergency care, lower use of influenza vaccine, and lower use of screening mammography (Berkman et al, 2011, p. ES-4). Two of the studies reviewed suggested that lower numeracy skills mediated the relationship between race and HbA_{1C} values and between gender and self-care management of human immunodeficiency virus (HIV) medication regimens (Berkman et al, 2011, p. ES–6).

Health literacy is directly linked to English language proficiency. Using American Community Survey data from 2009 to 2013, the U.S. Census Bureau compiled detailed tables of the language spoken at home and the ability of persons 5 years of age and older to speak English. Table 1, released in October 2015, reported that 60,361,574 persons 5 years of age and older speak a language other than English at home. The majority, 37,458,624, reported speaking Spanish or Spanish Creole at home. Of the almost 37.5 million persons who reported speaking Spanish at home, 16,344,473 reported that they spoke English less than "very well" (U.S. Census Bureau, 2015). Of those who spoke Spanish or Spanish Creole at home, 24.2% were living below the poverty level (U.S. Census Bureau, 2014). These data paint a picture of millions of potential patients, many of whom are children, who are at high risk for limited access, inadequate care, and inability to acquire the self-care management knowledge and skills essential to maintain health and optimum function. Cultural beliefs and practices, low educational attainment, LEP, and poverty are all barriers to accessing and effectively using health-care resources. When they converge, the negative effects of each individual barrier are magnified.

Low health literacy has a direct impact on the use of emergency departments (ED), especially for pediatric patients. In 2011 to 2012, Morrison and colleagues explored the relationship between the health literacy of caregivers and non-urgent ED visits for children presenting with fever. In the study, 299 caregivers bringing children ranging from 67 days to 12 years of age to the ED for a complaint of fever completed a literacy tool, the Newest Vital Sign (NVS). Only caregivers who spoke either English or Spanish were included in the study, and any child who was in acute distress or had an underlying condition warranting urgent testing—such as sickle cell disease—was excluded from the study. The median age of the children was 2.0 years and 34% of the children had an underlying chronic disease (p. 506). Of the caregivers, 63% demonstrated low health literacy (p. 506). It is interesting to note, however, that in this study a relationship between health literacy and non-urgent ED visits for pediatric patients was found for English- and Spanish-speaking caregivers, not for black caregivers (Morrison et al, 2014).

Multiple tools are available to clinicians to assess the literacy of their patients. As examination of **Table 19.2** reveals, these tools assess the literacy component of health literacy. Although reading comprehension and an understanding of commonly used medical terms are essential components of health literacy, such understanding does not necessarily translate into the ability to navigate the system to obtain the health-care services that promote improved health outcomes. It is important to note, too, that most of the tools used to assess health literacy do not address numeracy; for example, the ability of a person to actually comprehend the meaning of the numerical data with which he or she is presented and to then use that comprehension to carry out the mathematical processes to make informed decisions such as how much of a given food to eat or how many pills to take. Numeracy is critical if Americans are to benefit from the steps being taken by the federal government to provide more information to make informed choices about lifestyle behaviors. On May 20, 2016, the Food and Drug Administration (FDA) finalized the new nutrition facts label for packaged foods. The new labeling requirements are an attempt to combat chronic diseases such as obesity and heart disease by helping consumers to make more informed choices that may result in changes in dietary behaviors. Some of the more important changes are:

- The type size for "calories," "serving size per container," and "serving size" will be increased, and the number of calories and the "serving size" will be bolded.
- The amount (in grams) of "added sugars" and the percent of that amount relative to the 2015 to 2020 Dietary Guidelines for Americans will be included.
- Actual amounts, as well as the percent of daily value, of vitamin D, iron, calcium, and potassium must be listed on the label.

Manufacturers must comply with the new labeling requirements by July 26, 2018. To review the full FDA document, go to http://www.fda.gov/food/guidanceregulation/guidancedocumentsregulatoryinformation/labelingnutrition/ucm385663.htm (USFDA, 2016a).

Another document that may be useful in patient teaching is "How to Understand and Use the Nutrition Facts Label." It can be retrieved from www.fda.gov/food/ingredientspackaginglabeling/labelingnutrition/ucm274593.htm (USFDA, 2016b).

TRANSCREATION

Health literacy is not simply about English proficiency. Even if one is proficient in speaking, reading, and writing English, all individuals process communication with our health-care providers in terms of interpersonal dynamics and through the lens of cultural beliefs and practices. Literal translation of patient education materials, discharge instructions, consent forms, and other written and multimedia patient materials often does not achieve their intended purpose because the content is not presented in a culturally congruent manner. We need to move from *translation* to *transcreation,* which is development of all forms of information within a cultural context.

A driving force for the development of the transcreated educational materials and interactive Web site were findings from a pilot study of Chinese Americans between the ages of 18 and 70 who were diagnosed with diabetes at least 1 year earlier and who were taking either oral agents or insulin. The study, conducted by Hsu and colleagues (2006), consisted of 52 subjects, 91% of whom had type 2 diabetes. Twenty-two of the subjects indicated a preference for English, and 30 indicated Chinese as their preferred language. The Chinese American subjects who indicated a preference for Chinese demonstrated less knowledge about their disease process and had higher hemoglobin A_{1C} levels than did the subjects for whom English was the preferred language. These differences occurred even though the care to all subjects in the study was delivered in culturally competent sites with ready access to translation services. Another interesting finding of the study was that a significantly greater proportion of the English-language preference Chinese immigrant subjects (36.4%) reported diabetes educators as a source of information, compared with Chinese-language preference Chinese immigrant subjects (3.3%). (Hsu et al, 2006).

Asian Americans are the fastest growing population group in the United States, increasing by 43.3% from 2000 to 2010 to 14.7 million, 5% of the total U.S.

TABLE 19.2

Health Literacy Assessment Tools

Name of Tool	Format of the Tool	Test Administration	Approximate Completion Time(s)
Rapid Estimate of Adult Literacy in Medicine (REALM)	A 66-item word recognition test of commonly used medical terms. A visually impaired version uses a font size of 28.	The individual is asked to pronounce words in ascending order of difficulty.	2–6 minutes (Wallace et al, 2006)
Rapid Estimate of Adult Literacy in Medicine–Short Form, revised (REALM-SF)	A seven-item, rapid screening, word recognition test.	The individual is asked to pronounce words in ascending order of difficulty.	Under 2 minutes (Arozullah et al, 2007)
Rapid Estimate of Adolescent Literacy in Medicine: REALM-Teen	A 66-item word recognition test. Appropriate for adolescents ages 10–17. Available only in English.	The individual is asked to pronounce words in ascending order of difficulty.	Under 3 minutes (Davis et al, 2006)
Test of Functional Health Literacy in Adults: original and short versions (TOFHLA and S-TOFHLA)	The original TOFHLA is a 67-item timed test of reading comprehension (50 items) and numerical ability (17 items). Available in both English and Spanish, and in regular (12 pt) and large font (14 pt).	The individual replaces the missing words in paragraphs from four multiple-choice options for each missing word.	22 minutes (TOFHLA); about 7 minutes (S-TOFHLA) (Wallace, 2006)
Short Assessment of Health Literacy for Spanish Adults (SAHLSA-50)	A 50-item tool, based on the REALM, that measures the ability of Spanish-speaking adults to read and understand commonly used medical terms.	Each medical term is followed by two words, one of which is similar in meaning to the medical term; the other is a distracter. The person is asked to read the medical term aloud and to select the word that is similar in meaning.	3–6 minutes (Lee et al, 2006)
Short Assessment of Health Literacy–Spanish & English (SAHL-S&E)	An 18-item tool that tests the ability to pronounce and understand common medical terms.	Each medical term is followed by two words, one of which is similar in meaning to the medical term; the other is a distracter. The person is asked to read the medical term aloud and to select the word that is similar in meaning.	2–3 minutes (Lee et al, 2010)
Newest Vital Sign (NVS)	A six-question tool that tests the ability to read, comprehend, and apply the nutritional information on an ice cream label; tests both reading comprehension and numeracy skills. Available in both English and Spanish.	The person is given the NVS label to read and refer to as needed. The practitioner then asks the six questions.	3 minutes (Weiss et al, 2005)

population (Humes, Jones, & Ramirez, 2010, pp. 3–4). Asians continued to outpace the growth of the Hispanic population from 2012 to 2013, 2.9% vs. 2.1% (Brown, 2014). This population is more at risk for developing type 2 diabetes than non-Hispanic whites even though their body weight is lower. Chinese Americans, 50% of whom self-report being "linguistically isolated," constitute the greatest percentage of Asian Americans. The Joslin Clinic, a teaching affiliate of the Harvard Medical School, took the lead in developing culturally appropriate care sites and educational materials for Asian Americans with, or at risk for, diabetes. All the educational materials, including the Joslin Clinic's clinical guidelines for the prevention, detection, and treatment of diabetes, are available in English, traditional Chinese, and simplified Chinese.

An increasing number of other health-care organizations are developing educational materials and programs that reflect transcreation and are both linguistically and culturally appropriate for the target populations that they serve. Three of the more notable examples are described in the text that follows.

Immigrant Health and Cancer Disparities Service

The Immigrant Health and Cancer Disparities Service (IHCD) has been housed at Memorial Sloan Kettering Cancer Center since 2011 and is directed by Dr. Francesca M. Gany (MSKCC, 2011). It is part of MSK's Department of Psychiatry and Behavioral Sciences and may be accessed at https://www.mskcc.org/departments/psychiatry -behavioral-sciences/immigrant-health/about. It has several programs to tackle some of the most pervasive health problems in immigrants and other medically underserved people. The IHCD Web site identifies some of the immigrant populations for which it has specific programs and outreach efforts:

- *Arab Health Initiative:* Offers patient education and support services to help Arab Americans obtain cancer treatment.
- *South Asian Health Initiative:* Provides health-care services and outreach to the South Asian community in the New York metropolitan area.
- *Ventanillas de Salud (Health Windows) at the Mexican Consulate:* Promotes disease prevention and health awareness for Mexican Americans.

- *Chinese American Cancer Care Access Program:* A research initiative focused on improving support services for Chinese Americans who have cancer.

The service's Web site (https://www.mskcc.org/departments/ psychiatry-behavioral-sciences/immigrant-health) has separate portals for adult, child, and teen; health professionals; and research scientists and provides users with a comprehensive description of the resources available to each group. The Web site also provides access to MSK's virtual library (www.mskcc.org/vp) through which patients and their caregivers can access written professionals.

National Cancer Institute

The National Cancer Institute's (NCI's) Office of Communications and Education maintains a Web site at http:// www.cancer.gov/. Services to consumers and clinicians include a comprehensive list of publications produced by the NCI on a wide variety of subjects (e.g., childhood cancer, coping and support, clinical trials, screening). The publications are available in multiple formats and can be downloaded to a smartphone, tablet, or e-book device, or opened as PDF documents in a browser. There is also an option to order free copies of the publications online. Many of the publications are available in Spanish. One of the NCI's transcreated booklets, *Facing Forward: Life After Cancer Treatment* (NCI, 2014), or its Spanish version, *Siga adelante: la vida después del tratamiento del Cáncer* (NCI, 2012), designed for cancer survivors, is particularly useful in patient education (NCI, 2014).

The staff of NCI's Cancer Information Services (CIS) are available to direct you to sources of information and publications in languages other than English or Spanish. Two of the resources recommended are the National Network of Libraries of Medicine's (NN/LM's) Consumer Health Information in Many Languages Resources page (and the Asian and Pacific Islander Cancer Education Materials Web Tool (APICEM). APICEM is a joint project of the Asian American Network for Cancer Awareness, Research and Training (AANCART) and the American Cancer Society (ACS) and was funded by the NCI. It is designed to help Asians and Pacific Islanders with limited English-speaking abilities gain access to information on cancer by providing links to information that is available in several different languages. The APICEM Web Tool is accessible at http://www.cancer.org/apicem and can be reached by e-mail at APICEM@cancer.org.

NCI's information specialists also provide personalized, confidential cancer and smoking cessation information services by telephone at 1-800-4-CANCER (1-800-422-6237) or through the LiveChat link on NCI's Web site (www.cancer.gov), which will port you to NCI's LiveHelp service. Or you can access NCI's Live Help, available from 8 a.m. to 11 p.m. Eastern Time, Monday through Friday, directly from http://LiveHelp.cancer.gov or http://LiveHelp-es.cancer.gov (Spanish).

NCI's Smoking Quitline: 1-877-44U-QUIT (1-877-448-7848) is available from 8 a.m. to 8 p.m. Eastern Time in both English and Spanish. A very valuable resource to complement the outreach of the Quitline staff is www.Smokefree.gov. This resource is provided jointly by NCI, NIH, and the USDHHS. The free Smokefree apps can be downloaded to patients' smartphones for 24/7 smoking cessation help and support. The two major apps are QuitGuide and quitStart, the latter designed specifically for teens.

Office of Minority Health

The OMH of the USDHHS (http://minorityhealth.hhs.gov/) houses the Center for Linguistic and Cultural Competence in Health (CLCCH). You can join by registering online (https://www.thinkculturalhealth.hhs.gov/) at no cost. Registration provides preferential access to a wide variety of resources, including the quarterly *Think Cultural Health News* which will keep you up-to-date on the latest developments in cultural and linguistic competency and initiatives being undertaken by the OMH and the CLCCH. Both Web sites provide access to the National Standards on CLAS, online training, and continuing education.

PATIENT NAVIGATOR PROGRAM

In addition to empowering patients through the development of transcreated educational materials, vulnerable populations are known to experience significant difficulty in "navigating" the health-care system. The interplay of barriers such as poverty, LEP, and dependence on over-burdened, publicly funded health facilities that often lack

evening and weekend services for non-urgent care leaves many patients feeling overwhelmed by the complexity of the system. Patients' failures to follow through on diagnostic tests and referrals, and to obtain and take their medications as prescribed, are usually ascribed to being "noncompliant." If you dig deeper, often noncompliance represents an inability to access the services necessary to facilitate adherence to their prescribed health-care regimen. In *Crossing the Quality Chasm,* the IOM, quoting the Picker Institute and the AHA, put it bluntly: "It is not surprising, then, that studies of patient experience document that the health system for some is a 'nightmare to navigate'" (IOM, 2001, p. 4).

The potential for wide-scale implementation of patient navigator programs to reduce disparities in health and access to high-quality health-care services has garnered support in Congress. On April 25, 2005, Representative Robert Menendez introduced H.R. 1812, The Patient Navigator, Outreach and Chronic Disease Prevention Act of 2005, to amend the Public Health Service Act. The amendment authorized the secretary of HHS, acting through the administrator of the Health Resources Services Administration (HRSA), to award grants to health-care facilities to develop and implement patient navigator services to reduce barriers to care and to improve health outcomes. Facilities receiving the grants would be required to establish benchmarks and identify outcome criteria to measure the effectiveness of the program. Its companion bill in the Senate was S. 898, introduced by Senator Kay Bailey Hutchison. The proposed legislation had broad, bipartisan support and passed both houses of Congress. On June 29, 2005, President George W. Bush signed the Patient Navigator, Outreach and Chronic Disease Prevention Act (PL 109-18, Section 340A) into law (GovTrack, 2005). In fiscal year 2008, $2,948,000 was appropriated for competitive grants. HRSA awarded six grants, totaling almost $2.4 million (USDHHS, 2008b).

Studies attest to the importance of patient navigators in minority populations. Researchers at the City University of New York and Mount Sinai School of Medicine in New York City conducted a cohort study of Hispanic patients referred from their primary care clinics for screening colonoscopies between November 2003 and May 2006. Of the 688 patients who were eligible to participate in the study, 532 had a female, bilingual, Hispanic patient navigator assigned to assist them with successfully completing the procedure. Of the navigated patients, 66% completed their screening colonoscopies. The vast majority—95%—had adequate bowel preparation; 16% were found to have adenomas. The "no-show" rate for urban minority patients dropped from a high of 40% before implementation of the navigator program to a low of 9.8%. Most (98%) of the patients reported being satisfied with the navigator program, and 66% indicated that they probably, or definitely, would *not* have completed the procedure if the patient navigator program had not been in effect (Chen et al, 2008).

In 2009, citing the demonstrated effectiveness of patient navigation programs, especially in minority communities, HRSA chose to not allocate any additional funding for ongoing research in this area after 2008 (USDHHS, 2008a). This is a good object lesson about competing demands in an environment of increasingly scarce resources. It is incumbent on APNs to translate their patient advocacy role into political and legislative action. Public laws that are unfunded, such as the Patient Navigator, Outreach and Chronic Disease Prevention Act (PL 109-18, Section 340A), cannot deliver on the legislative intent for which they were enacted.

Even in the best of worlds, with full funding of PL 109-18, Section 340A, successful patient navigator programs present a real conflict to their parent health-care institutions or plans. Implementation of a successful program requires a substantial investment in personnel and training. A successful program will produce measurable improvements in patient outcomes, such as fewer patient visits to EDs for routine care, decreased incidence and severity of complications in patients with chronic disease processes, fewer hospital admissions, and so on. Although all these are highly desirable outcomes for patients, these outcomes translate into significantly less reimbursement to health-care facilities and providers. From a business perspective, it makes no sense to implement a program that will generate less revenue. A similar situation is seen in managed care programs weighing the pros and cons of implementing or expanding health promotional programs. If a few managed care plans take the lead in offering such expanded programs, they run the real risk that the long-term benefits that would accrue to the programs through a reduction in the care costs of their enrollees will not be realized to the investing program if the enrollees subsequently switch to another managed care plan. The managed care plans

that exhibited a commitment to health promotion could end up bearing all the costs for implementing these programs and realize none of the benefits. Indeed, the benefits could flow to other managed care plans that had not made such an investment in the health of their enrollees. Reimbursement needs to be redesigned to incentivize and reward delivery systems that produce positive health outcomes and lower overall health-care costs. Medicare reimbursement has already adopted this approach through provisions in the ACA of 2010— the Hospital Readmissions Reduction Plan (HRRP), effective October 2012 (CMS, 2016a). Hospitals that exceeded the national average for readmission rates within 30 days of discharge for patients treated for myocardial infarctions, congestive heart failure, or pneumonia lost 1% of their Medicare payments in 2013. This increased to 2% in 2014 and 3% in 2015. In addition, patients with chronic obstructive pulmonary disease and total hip and knee replacement were added to the patient conditions being tracked. More than 3,400 hospitals had their condition-specific readmission rates tracked for 2015. Of these, only 799 were not subject to the CMS monetary penalty, and 38 hospitals incurred the maximum 3% penalty (CMS, 2016a; Rice, 2015).

ASSESSMENT

The first step in providing culturally competent care is assessment—of ourselves, of our patients' needs, and of our existing organizational resources. Each of us brings the influence of our own cultural heritage, experiences, biases, beliefs, and expectations about patient-provider relationships to the care that we give. Evaluation of the effect of these influences on our caregiving practices is the first step to achieving cultural competence as a practitioner. The NCCC at the Georgetown University Center for Child and Human Development offers an exceptional array of tools for assessing cultural competence in individuals and organizations, as well as a wealth of instructional materials.

An excellent self-assessment tool is a 37-item checklist, Promoting Cultural and Linguistic Competency Self-Assessment Checklist for Personnel Providing Primary Health Care Services, available from Georgetown University's NCCC. Its content is applicable to all advanced practice nursing roles. The individual responds to specific examples about values, attitudes, communication styles, the practice environment, and patient materials and resources. For example, item 7 asks the practitioner to indicate the frequency with which he or she would do the following:

> For individuals and families who speak languages or dialects other than English, I attempt to learn and use key words so that I am better able to communicate with them during assessment, treatment or other interventions.

The tool may be downloaded by visiting the NCCC Web site at http://nccc.georgetown.edu and clicking on Self-Assessments.

Another newly developed self-assessment tool, the Cultural and Linguistic Competence Health Practitioner Assessment (CLCHPA), was made available on the NCCC Web site in the fall of 2016. It is an extremely valuable self-assessment and educational activity tool that will significantly improve your ability to deliver culturally and linguistically competent care to meet the health and mental health needs of your patients and to take a leadership role in promoting cultural and linguistic competence in your community and in the health-care organizations in which you practice. Upon completion of the assessment, you receive your score relative to the norming sample, analysis of what your score represents (i.e., level of cultural and linguistic competence), and a list of educational resources and professional development activities to facilitate continued growth in your knowledge and skill in the areas of cultural and linguistic competence as well as health and health-care disparities. The assessment tool is unique in that it assesses your ability to communicate effectively with persons from diverse populations, including those with LEP, disabilities, and hearing deficits. The CLCHPA takes approximately 80 minutes to complete. It *does not* need to be completed in a single session; just save your answers and log in again.

Language gives voice to cultural expression. Many cultures have rich oral traditions that transmit the stories, traditions, and beliefs that define their cultural heritage from generation to generation. Language serves as the primary vehicle for most of our interpersonal communication, from patients' descriptions of their health-care needs to interprofessional collaboration. Linguistic competence is essential to the delivery of culturally competent health care. A fundamental tenet of advanced practice nursing is patient empowerment: patients as informed, full partners in decision making about their health care.

Operationalizing this core belief clearly requires effective provider-patient communication, a condition that does not exist when linguistic barriers are present. At the very least, lack of linguistic competence makes patient assessment and intervention difficult; at worst, patient safety may be fundamentally compromised. See **Box 19.7.**

Box 19.7

Buenos Días, Señora

Mrs. W, a 43-year-old married Hispanic woman with three children, came to the neighborhood health center complaining of tightness in her chest and difficulty in coughing up her secretions. Her usual bilingual care provider was unavailable, so she was seen by another practitioner who was not proficient in Spanish. Her records revealed that she had been diagnosed with mild intermittent asthma, for which she had been prescribed albuterol to be used as necessary. Mrs. W reported that she had not filled her last prescription because of the cost.

Mrs. W's physical examination was unremarkable except for a slight increase in respiratory rate and scattered expiratory wheezes. To save her the cost of prescription medication, the provider recommended that she purchase the over-the-counter product Robitussin and take it four times per day. She was advised to return to the clinic if her symptoms did not improve. No written follow-up instructions were available in Spanish.

Four days later, Mrs. W came to the clinic in acute distress. Because of her limited understanding of English, she had purchased Honey Cough by Robitussin. The provider had not thought to explain, or to give her written instructions, about the difference between guaifenesin (the active ingredient in plain Robitussin, which acts to liquefy pulmonary secretions and promote expectoration) and Honey Cough, which contains only dextromethorphan, a potent cough suppressant. Instead of relieving Mrs. W's symptoms, the provider's lack of linguistically appropriate intervention significantly worsened her condition by depressing the very mechanism that would have allowed her to expel her secretions.

The process of self-assessment must be approached with a willingness to confront and modify or discard those inaccurate and uninformed preconceived cultural beliefs and attitudes that detract from providing care. Many of our attitudes and beliefs are so ingrained that we may never scrutinize them in the course of our daily practice until, and if, we become aware of their negative effect on our care. Even then, long-held biases may limit our introspection. Ethnocentrism, or the belief in the relative superiority of one's own cultural group, is a common phenomenon. Often operating at an unconscious level, ethnocentrism can exert a powerful influence on our patient interactions and care practices.

Organizational assessment is likewise essential to providing culturally competent care. The NCCC has produced another excellent tool that details the process for conducting an organizational self-assessment (Goode, Jones, & Mason, 2002). The process, which stresses community involvement and a nonpunitive approach with an emphasis on self-knowledge and growth, is also available at the NCCC Web site listed previously. Knowledge of our individual and institutional strengths and weaknesses in the area of cultural competence is a prerequisite to corrective action (NCCC, 2016b).

Culturally competent patient assessment is indispensable to appropriate diagnosis and treatment and promotes patient participation in decision making about health and treatment regimens. Although an understanding of the beliefs and practices of a patient's cultural group facilitates such assessment, respectful questioning wherein the patient becomes the teacher about his or her culture produces data to support your clinical judgments and helps build trust between patient and provider. See **Box 19.8**. A particularly valuable resource for drawing out a patient's beliefs about health and illness is a work by an early pioneer in culturally competent care, "Understanding, Eliciting and Negotiating Clients' Multicultural Health Beliefs" (Jackson, 1993).

Note that all the questions in Box 19.8 are framed from the perspective of the patient. They acknowledge the patient's ownership of his or her unique illness experience. Framing the questions in this way allows the APN to enter into the patient's lived experience. By exploring the patient's perceptions and expectations, the provider is better able to propose a treatment plan that is compatible with the patient's cultural beliefs and practices.

Box 19.8
Questions to Elicit Beliefs and Treatment Expectations From Patients Seeking Illness Care

- What do you think caused your problem?
- Why do you think it started when it did?
- What do you think your sickness does to you?
- How does it work?
- How severe is your sickness?
- Will it have a short or long course?
- What kind of treatment should you receive?
- What are the results you hope to receive from this treatment?
- What are the problems your sickness has caused you?
- What do you fear most about your sickness?

Adapted from Jackson, 1993, p. 30.

Culturally competent assessment also requires that the clinician apply ethnically appropriate parameters when interpreting physical findings. Body mass index (BMI) is widely used as a tool to assess patients' risk for diabetes and cardiovascular disease. There is a growing body of evidence to suggest that the current, European-derived, "one size fits all" BMI classifications for overweight (25.0 kg/m^2 or greater, but fewer than 30.0 kg/m^2) and obese (equal to or greater than 30 kg/m^2) may not be appropriate across all ethnic groups. A seminal study (Razak et al, 2007) reported in *Circulation* sought to determine if the current cut point for determining obesity that is used in clinical practice is appropriate for use in non-European populations. A random sample of 1,078 subjects was recruited from participants in the Study of Health Assessment and Risk in Ethnic Groups (SHARE) and Risk Evaluation in Aboriginal Peoples (SHARE-AP). The subjects, from four ethnic groups (South Asians [$n = 5,289$], Chinese [$n = 5,281$], Aboriginals [$n = 5,207$], and Europeans [$n = 5,301$]) were evaluated for 14 variables: 2 clinical (systolic and diastolic blood pressure) and 12 biochemical (fasting and 2-hour glucose; fasting and 2-hour insulin; HbA$_{1C}$; Homeostasis Model Assessment-insulin resistance [HOMA-IR]; high-density and low-density lipids and triglycerides [HDL and LDL, respectively]; fasting and

2-hour free fatty acids) cardiometabolic markers. Factor analysis revealed three latent factors that accounted for 56% of the variation in the subjects' cardiometabolic markers and blood pressure. The main effect of ethnicity was highly significant for each factor ($P = 0.001$). Compared with European subjects for a given BMI, South Asian, Chinese, and Aboriginal subjects had elevated glucose and lipid metabolism-related factors. The South Asian subjects had the worst glucose and lipid profiles, the highest 2-hour oral glucose tolerance test levels, the highest LDL levels, and the lowest HDL levels (Razak et al, 2007, p. 2113). Elevated blood-pressure–related factor was found in Chinese subjects at a BMI of 25.3 kg/m^2 compared with a BMI of 30.0 kg/m^2 in Europeans (p. 2114). In discussing their findings, the authors conclude the following (Razak et al, 2007, p. 2114):

> Use of BMI cut points derived among Europeans understates the cardiometabolic risk associated with weight gain in other ethnic groups. The pathway linking obesity to clinical events is mediated partially through its strong association with the development of diabetes, hypertension, and dyslipidemia. This suggests that to minimize the development of cardiometabolic risk factors, lower BMI targets should be used by health-care professionals in some non-European populations.

Major sources of best practices, such as the Joslin Clinic, have already incorporated ethno-specific and gender-specific BMI recommendations in their clinical guidelines. The Joslin Diabetes Center and Joslin Clinic Clinical Nutrition Guideline for Overweight and Obese Adults With Type 2 Diabetes, Those With Prediabetes, or Those at High Risk for Developing Type 2 Diabetes uses BMI or waistline measurements to identify target populations. Persons from Asian populations (South Asian Indians, East Asians, and Malays) with a BMI greater than 23 kg/m^2 and a waistline greater than 35 inches (90 cm) in men, or greater than 31 inches (80 cm) in women, are considered to be target individuals. This is in contrast to the guideline's generic criteria of BMI greater than 25 kg/m^2 or a waistline greater than 40 inches (102 cm) (men) and 35 inches (88 cm) (women) (Joslin Diabetes Center & Joslin Clinic, 2011).

Although the Joslin Clinic took the lead in applying ethnocentric guidelines for the identification of Asian persons at risk for type 2 diabetes, it was not until December 2014 that the American Diabetes Association (ADA) announced that it was adopting the same BMI measures and was incorporating them into their 2015

Standards of Medical Care for Diabetes (ADA, 2014). The BMI cut point for screening overweight or obese Asian Americans for prediabetes and type 2 diabetes was changed to 23 kg/m2 (vs. 25 kg/m2) to reflect the evidence that this population is at an increased risk for diabetes at lower BMI levels relative to the general population (ADA, 2014, 2015).

Many of the national guidelines for clinical assessment of wellness and major health conditions affecting large segments of the U.S. population now reflect a cultural congruence not seen in previous guidelines, as in the Centers for Disease Control and Prevention (CDC) growth charts released in 2000. Before the release of the revised guidelines, clinicians had to rely on growth charts developed in 1977 by the National Center for Health Statistics (NCHS), which were derived from data drawn primarily from 10,000 white, middle-class infants and children living in Ohio between 1929 and 1975. In contrast, the current CDC guidelines are based on survey data of children from diverse ethnic and racial groups and incorporate data on breastfed children in proportion to the rate of breastfeeding in the general population. Fourteen percent of the data from which the current guidelines were developed represent information collected in surveys of African American children. This figure reflects the proportion of African American children living in the United States from 1971 to 1994 ("New Growth Charts a Welcome Improvement," 2002).

Treatment regimens should always strive to incorporate the cultural practices and preferences that are most valued by the patient. For example, Muslim patients may observe strict dietary laws that include a prohibition against eating any pork products. Practicing Muslims may also pray five times a day and may be reluctant to eat or to take medications during daylight hours at certain periods of the year. Tradition also dictates that Muslims fast from dawn to sunset during the observance of Ramadan. Ask your Muslim patients if they plan to observe a strict or a modified fast (Ethnomed, 2016). The scheduling of diagnostic testing and use of treatment plans that are congruent with patients' valued cultural beliefs and practices are more likely to generate positive outcomes. Outcomes data are key determinants of reimbursement, provider recognition by third-party payers, and institutional accreditation. Culturally and linguistically competent patient assessment is the foundation of successful outcomes.

KNOWLEDGE

As an APN, you are well aware of the value of knowledge. Evidence- and research-based practice is the standard to which you are held. Just as you are expected to incorporate the latest clinical guidelines for the management of conditions such as diabetes and lipid disorders into your practice, so, too, must you inform yourself about the beliefs and practices of the cultural groups in your patient population. This can seem to be a daunting task, especially if your patient population is quite diverse. The task becomes even more complex if you have a rapid influx of immigrants from a cultural group new to the setting. Many sources of help are available to assist the individual practitioner and organization to care effectively for diverse populations. Every cultural group has its community leaders. Often they are religious leaders and professionals who are more than willing to assist local health and social agencies in meeting the needs of their community. Many culturally affiliated church and social organizations have developed literature and other materials to help non-community members better understand their cultural beliefs and practices.

All APNs are partners with their patients in providing culturally competent care. Recognizing that individual patients may or may not adhere to cultural norms, key questions to explore about any cultural group for whom you care are in **Box 19.9**. Here is a phrase that may help you to remember these key questions and be a better partner:

Partners **I**n **D**elivering **C**ulturally **C**ompetent, **R**esearch-based **C**are **F**or **D**iverse **P**opulations.

The Internet is an extremely valuable resource for gathering information on various cultural groups. The culture-specific materials developed by the University of Washington Medical Center are invaluable to APNs practicing in culturally diverse settings. Culture Clues are brief, provider-friendly overviews of the dominant beliefs and practices of the major cultural groups cared for by the medical center staff. Examples of the types of information included in the clues are essential information about the cultural group's

---

Box 19.9

Key Questions Used to Explore Cultural Groups: PIDCCRCFDP

Partners In Delivering Culturally Competent, Research-based Care For Diverse Populations

- *Perceptions:* How are health and illness defined?
- *Interpersonal behavior:* Does the cultural group have particular norms for interpersonal behavior regarding beliefs about touch, eye contact, personal space, modesty, sexuality, and so on?
- *Decision making:* Who makes health-care decisions?
- *Communication needs:* Be particularly sensitive to how the patients wish to be addressed and how and by whom health-care information is communicated **(Box 19.10).**
- *Complementary medicine:* What are the group's folk medicine beliefs and practices to maintain wellness and to treat illness or injury? Explore their use of complementary and alternative medicine.
- *Religion/spirituality:* To what extent does spirituality or religious belief affect health-care beliefs and practices (e.g., specific dietary practices, prayer rituals, and such)?

- *Care:* What are the patient's expectations for the outcomes of health and illness care? What cultural preferences and practices does the patient wish to have incorporated into his or her plan of care (e.g., the diet of some patients may include the use of selected foods or herbs to maintain a balance between complementary forces [yin and yang] of hot and cold, light and dark)? Is this the patient's first formal experience with receiving care in a structured health-care setting; the first experience of being cared for by an APN?
- *Family:* What is the primary social unit—the individual, the family, or the community? What are the family and kinship structures and roles in health care?
- *Death and dying:* Explore the meaning of and rituals associated with death and dying.
- *Psychiatric/mental health:* How are mental health issues perceived by the group?

Box 19.10

My Name Is Mr. Roberts

Mr. John Roberts, a widower, was a 68-year-old black man of African American descent. Retired for 10 years, he lived independently in his private home. His civilian and military pensions allowed him to live comfortably and to meet his health-care costs. He was active in several church and community groups and expressed a high degree of satisfaction with his life. A heavy smoker for many years, he had recently agreed to enroll in a smoking cessation program in an effort to better control his hypertension. A chest x-ray examination performed during a comprehensive physical examination revealed a large, previously undetected mass in his right lung. Further testing determined that the mass was malignant and that metastases had occurred. Mr. Roberts declined any treatment, saying that he wanted to live out his remaining life as fully as possible.

When his condition deteriorated to the point at which his comfort and safety were at risk, he agreed to enter a hospice home-care program. The APN coordinating Mr. Roberts's care collaborated with him and his son in ensuring that all aspects of his physical and psychosocial needs were respected and met. Late in the terminal phase of his illness, Mr. Roberts fell and fractured his right hip, necessitating hospitalization. In the hospital, he was frequently addressed by his first name, especially by younger staff members. Despite his repeated admonishment that his name was Mr. Roberts, many of the staff persisted in calling him John.

The small, community hospital to which Mr. Roberts was admitted did not have pain management specialists. The attending hospitalist physician and the nursing staff caring for Mr. Roberts were predominantly Caucasian and found him to be very resistant to switching from the oral analgesic medications that he had taken for pain while at home to intramuscular and/or intravenous administration of

his analgesics. His primary nurse consulted with the clinical nurse specialist for the unit and a meeting was set up with Mr. Roberts's son. His son revealed that Mr. Roberts had always been fearful of being hospitalized or taking anything other than oral medications after he read about the Tuskegee Study of Untreated Syphilis, begun in 1932 and continuing until 1972. The 600 study participants were all black males, 299 of whom had syphilis, none of whom gave informed consent. The men with syphilis were followed for the next 40 years to determine the natural course of untreated syphilis. None of the men received penicillin, even after it became known as the drug of choice for treatment in 1947. Mr. Roberts's son also shared that his father had preferentially sought out an African American as his primary care physician. The hospitalist asked Mr. Roberts's son for help in allaying Mr. Roberts's fears so that his analgesics could be administered by injection. His son helped to bridge the cultural gap and his father experienced significantly better pain relief.

Mr. Roberts died while hospitalized. He had been brought up in a traditional home in which older persons were addressed by their last name by all except family members and close friends. Younger individuals never presumed to call an older person by his or her first name. To do so would have been considered disrespectful and rude.

An accident denied the fulfillment of Mr. Roberts's wish to die at home. However, the indignities that he experienced while hospitalized were totally preventable had his caregivers been more respectful of his communication needs and knowledgeable about the potential for patients to mistrust medical recommendations based on their own personal experiences of racism or knowledge of unethical medical practices in the past. A useful article is Benkert, Hollie, Nordstrom, Wickson, and Bins-Emerick (2009).

(USDHHS, OMH, 2013)

perception of illness, how medical decisions are made, how prognostic information should be handled, and cultural norms about touch and modesty, among others. Culture Clues have been developed for the care of Albanian, Chinese, Korean, Latino, Russian, Somali, and Vietnamese patients, as well as deaf and hard-of-hearing patients. End of Life Culture Clues for the Latino, Russian, and Vietnamese cultures have also been developed. They are available at https://depts.washington.edu/pfes/CultureClues.htm. Each of the Culture Clues provides the reader with additional resources about the cultural group and health care. The University of Washington also maintains a Web site called EthnoMed at www.ethnomed.org that is a treasure trove of information. The culture-specific materials include comprehensive discussion of the barriers to health care. The Web site provides access to an extensive compendium of clinician support resources in the following areas:

- *Cultures:* There are cultural profiles on multiple cultural groups, including Hispanic/Latino, Iraqi, and Chinese cultures. You can also access resources on Refugee Health when you browse the Clinical Topics portion of the Web site.
- *Clinical topics* (including clinical pearls and case studies): The topics range from commonly encountered disease conditions, such as asthma and diabetes, to modesty, sexuality, and breastfeeding in specific cultures, domestic violence, genetics, and end-of-life care.
- *Patient education:* These include extensive patient education materials; browse by topic or language (e.g., literature on cholesterol HDL/LDL, diabetic diet, diabetic foot care, and so on) as materials are available in Spanish and English. Literature on colorectal testing, mammograms, and cervical cancer is available in Chinese and English. Languages supported in the patient education resources portion of the Web site are Amharic, Chinese, Hmong, Karen, Khmer, Oromo, Somali, Spanish, Tigrinya, and Vietnamese. There are also audio resources for blind or low literacy patients. The patient education materials are exceptionally culturally congruent (e.g., the resource entitled *Diabetes During Ramadan* [WellShare International, 2013], which educates the patient about healthy ways to fast during the month of Ramadan).

Finally, honesty is the best policy. If you are unsure whether your approach to a patient is culturally appropriate, acknowledge your unfamiliarity with the patient's cultural norms and ask for guidance in how to best deliver care. Most patients perceive this as being a thoughtful response to their right to respect and will be happy to help inform you. They may become your best teachers. It will enhance their trust in you and allow you to provide care until you research additional information on the patient's cultural group.

COMMUNICATION AND PATIENT TEACHING

Communication is a critical element in the self- and institutional-assessment process. It encompasses provider-patient communication in all its forms, from assessment to patient education, counseling, and documentation. How do you assess a patient or community whose primary language is other than English? What technologies (e.g., Language Line Services) or interpreters are at your disposal to facilitate assessment, intervention, and teaching? What is your own level of proficiency in languages other than English? Linguistic competence is essential to quality patient care. With our multicultural patient populations, most of us are, or soon will be, linguistically challenged. This becomes a practice issue only if we ignore the need and make no attempt to modify our practice environment to meet the comprehensive needs of our patient base. Multiple texts and e-learning programs exist to develop basic foreign language skills.

Patient teaching raises major ethical issues regarding equality of treatment. Whether the patient is an individual, family, or community, many patient education materials are available primarily in English. A substantial number have also been translated into Spanish, with fewer translated into other languages. For most other languages, the practitioner depends on interpreters or English-speaking family members to assist in the education process. The availability of these supports may be limited, and as we know patients need supplemental materials to reinforce direct teaching, especially if the patient is anxious or the encounter is hurried. Cost-containment efforts focus on increased staff productivity, which translates into more patients in less time. This, coupled with a linguistic barrier to teaching, is a recipe for a poor outcome. Collaborative decision making with your patients, a defining characteristic of advanced nursing practice, mandates the ability to communicate effectively. Advocacy begins in your own practice environment with your own patients. You have an ethical and legal obligation to work toward ensuring equality in the treatment of all patients.

Federal agencies such as the CDC, the CMS, the AHRQ, and the HRSA play a critical role in promoting health equity. Their work guides the development of our country's health-related legislation and regulations. They also produce multiple online resources that you can use for your own ongoing education regarding health literacy, to train health-care staff, and to develop culturally and linguistically appropriate patient education materials.

An indispensable resource is the AHRQ's second edition of the Health Literacy Universal Precautions Toolkit (AHRQ, 2015a). Citing statistics showing that 88% of the adults in America have health literacy deficits that limit their ability to manage at least some aspect of their health or health care, and that 36% have documented limited health literacy (Brega et al, 2015, p. 1), the Toolkit provides a wide array of guidance and resources to assess and improve the practice environment, patient provider interactions, and patient education materials in four key areas of primary care practice: spoken communication, written communication, self-management and empowerment, and supportive systems.

The CDC Web site (www.cdc.gov/healthliteracy/index.html) has multiple topical areas, including Learn About Health Literacy, which includes numeracy; Find Training; Plan and Act; Education and Community Support for Health Literacy, Develop Materials, and a Contact Form. You can subscribe for free e-mail updates of Health Literacy and the CDC-sponsored Bridging the Health Literacy Gap Blog. The *Develop Materials* (CDC, 2016) content area is a *must* for anyone developing patient education materials. Click on Guidelines and Standards under the menu header *Develop Materials,* and a document entitled "Communication Guidance" will come up. It provides information on NIH's Health Literacy Initiative; the Federal PLAIN Language Guidelines; a Health Literacy Online Guide that assists in developing online health information that is user friendly; the CLAS Standards; and access to the TOOLKIT that follows.

Toolkit for Making Written Material Clear and Effective (CMS, 2012) is a resource developed by the CMS that contains essential tools for developing patient education materials and for evaluating those currently in use in your practice setting. The Toolkit may be accessed through the CDC Health Literacy Web site by clicking on "Testing Messages and Materials" under the menu header *Develop Materials* or retrieving it directly from https://www.cms.gov/Outreach-and-Education/Outreach/WrittenMaterialsToolkit/index.html?redirect=/WrittenMaterialsToolkit/

One final critical document from the CDC is the resource entitled "Older Adults: Steps to Ensure the Understanding and Use of Health Information" (CDC, 2015) available at www.cdc.gov/healthliteracy/DevelopMaterials/Audiences/OlderAdults/steps.html. It contains information essential to culturally competent care of older patients, including access to such resources as Talking With Your Older Patient: A Clinician's Guide, produced by the National Institute on Aging of the NIH. The Clinician's Guide covers multiple topics (e.g., Working With Diverse Older Patients; Breaking Bad News; Supporting Patients With Chronic Conditions, and so on).

The National Institute of Diabetes and Digestive and Kidney Diseases (NIDDK) Web site at www.niddk.nih.gov provides an extensive listing of patient education materials that are available in Spanish as well as English for urological diseases, kidney diseases, diabetes, digestive diseases, liver disease, weight control, and physical activity. Many may be downloaded and reproduced. The Web site also has clinical practice tools and patient education resources for health-care professionals.

Many additional organizations are actively engaged in addressing health literacy. Two of the most innovative resources now available to APNs are the Asian American Diabetes Initiative (AADI) sponsored by the Joslin Diabetes Center and "The Debilitator." The AADI, directed by Dr. William C. Hsu, author of "Identification of Linguistic Barriers to Diabetes Knowledge and Glycemic Control in Chinese Americans With Diabetes," previously discussed in the health literacy section of this chapter, has developed a wide range of teaching-learning tools for use by patients and health-care professionals. The tools range from clinical guidelines and video clips to a Head Start: Parent Café where parents can learn ways to help their children exercise, maintain a healthy weight, and minimize their risk of developing diabetes. One in five Asian Americans develops diabetes. Materials developed by the AADI, including many free educational resources, may be found on the Internet at https://aadi.joslin.org/en. The information on the Web site is available in English, traditional Chinese, Simplified Chinese, and Japanese. Be sure to click on the Web site's "Drag 'N Cook" (AADI, 2012) to access an app, developed in 2012, that provides digital guidance for the preparation of both delicious and healthy Asian (Chinese, Indian, Japanese, Korean, and Vietnamese) meals. Nutrition facts for ingredients commonly used in Asian cooking, such as soy or oyster sauce, canola oil, brown long grain rice, and carrots, as well as the nutritional breakdown of recipes, are prominently displayed. Drag 'N Cook even sponsors recipe contests with the winners receiving prizes that encourage exercise such as pedometers. Good to eat and good for you—now that's a winning combination!

"The Debilitator," developed by African American independent filmmaker Maurice Madden, is a 30-minute DVD designed to increase awareness of the devastating effects of diabetes in the black community. "The Debilitator" was a film originally produced by Millennium Filmworks. It won a 2006 "Life Making a Difference in Diabetes Award" and was the impetus for the development of the original version of the New Beginnings: A Discussion Guide for Living Well With Diabetes by the National Diabetes Education Program (NDEP). An updated version of the New Beginnings discussion guide (NDEP, 2014) was released by the NDEP in 2014 and may be downloaded in PDF format from http://www.cdc.gov/diabetes/ndep/pdfs/132-new-beginnings.pdf.

RESEARCH AS A CRITICAL DETERMINANT OF PRACTICE

Another thought for consideration is your role as a nurse researcher. Do you or the institutions with which you are affiliated conduct evaluation research to determine whether you are accomplishing desired patient outcomes in your area of specialty practice? Think of how valuable it could be to collect and analyze outcomes data, not only to compare the relative efficacy of the different types of practitioners but also to examine outcomes as a function of patient cultural groupings, primary languages spoken and read, and other factors. Outcomes data from evaluation research are often the catalyst for bringing about organizational change. A recent example of a very powerful piece of retrospective evaluation research is an article entitled "Culturally Tailored Group Medical Appointments for Diabetic Black Americans" by Newby and Gray, which was published in the *Journal for Nurse Practitioners* in May 2016. In the study, half of the 250 adult (mean age 57 years) subjects with type 2 diabetes received standard, 15-minute primary care appointments, whereas the remaining 125 diabetic patients participated in single-session, shared medical appointments (SMAs). The SMAs had 9 to 12 patients/SMA and were held once a month for 120 minutes, led by a collaborative, interdisciplinary team—a nurse practitioner (NP) who was a certified diabetic educator (CDE), a physician, and an additional CDE. The SMA was structured so that each patient received a brief, individual examination and the specific laboratory results to refer to during the 30- to 45-minute educational component that followed the examinations. The participants were then split into two, 30-minute interactive group sessions, led by a CDE, which focused on critical skills for diabetic self-care (e.g., glucose monitoring, reading and interpreting food labels, strategies for healthier food preparation). The small group sessions also provided an opportunity for peer support and self-empowerment. As an added bonus, during the educational component, the SMA members ate a dish that was frequently consumed in their black community (e.g., sweet potato pie) that had been specially prepared to conform to the American Diabetes Association's recommended nutritional standards. The SMA participants had a "lived experience." They got to see that they could still eat the foods that they loved to eat if they prepared them differently, which was a powerful motivator to make the necessary dietary modifications to control their diabetes. The data were collected retrospectively over a 1-year period of time, comparing patients who had received a usual office visit or had participated in a single SMA. Within and between groups, pre- and postclinical measures were assessed over a 3-month period of time. When the researchers compared (paired t-test) the HbA_{1C} pre- and postclinical values of the SMA and usual office visit appointment patients, the SMA patients showed a significant reduction in their HbA_{1C} values (1.26%), whereas the usual office visit patients did not (0.05%) (Newby & Gray, 2016, pp. 317–323). This study is a very powerful example of how clinical research can have a significant impact on how care is delivered.

AMERICAN NURSES ASSOCIATION—ADVOCATE FOR CULTURALLY CONGRUENT PRACTICE

Commitment to the provision of culturally competent care is an integral component of advanced practice nursing, as reflected in the ANA publication *Nursing: Scope and Standards of Practice,* Third Edition (2015b). The document reemphasizes the client's right to self-determination, privacy, confidentiality, full and truthful disclosure, and care that is respectful and inclusive of the client's cultural beliefs and practices. Standard 8 addresses "Culturally Congruent Practice" and Appendix F provides a very valuable list of resources to promote the delivery of culturally congruent professional nursing care. The client advocacy role of the nurse is stressed, as is the importance of empowering the patient for effective clinical decision making and self-care (ANA, 2015b).

NEXT STEPS

I submit that the defining characteristic that has led to widespread use of APNs across multiple care settings and earned them unparalleled patient acceptance is their ability to truly partner with their patients to provide care that the patient perceives as being respectful and inclusive of his or her uniqueness as a human being. A major component of that uniqueness is associated with culture: its values, beliefs, and attitudes toward caring.

The delivery of culturally congruent care is not optional, but mandated by the ethical standards of our profession, as well as by legal and accreditation requirements. The challenge is for us as individual APNs, and collectively as practitioners within a variety of health-care institutions, to consistently practice in a manner that is personally sensitive to our own biases and culturally astute.

20

Conflict Resolution in Advanced Practice Nursing

David M. Price and Patricia A. Murphy

Learning Outcomes

Learning outcomes expected as a result of this chapter:

- Recognize conflict as common and unavoidable in advanced practice nursing.
- Identify conflict management as an essential competency.
- Appreciate that conflict situations are of different types, but have common features, challenges, and recommended responses.
- Relate ineffective responses to conflict.
- Demonstrate effective responses to conflict and describe how they can be learned.
- Set clear, desirable, and achievable *goals* in anticipation of conflict.
- Justify that learning to deal with conflict is a career-long process.
- Describe the vast resources available for learning effective conflict management, including ethical codes, the social science literature, and mentoring by other professionals.
- Appreciate that the basic nature of conflict management is always service to the patient, whether directly or indirectly.

INTRODUCTION

All nurses encounter conflict. *Advanced practice* nurses (APNs) should expect to encounter even more conflict than other nurses do and realize others expect them to be more proficient in the face of it. *All* nurses should develop effective ways to resolve conflict. *APNs* really must commit to a career-long effort to develop these skills. *This is an essential competency of advanced nursing roles.*

In this chapter we will defend the previous assertions, illustrate the varieties of conflict situations common in advanced practice nursing, examine dysfunctional responses to conflict all too common in nursing, and identify ways to deal *effectively* with conflict. We will also recommend resources for continuing development of one's conflict management skills and convey pearls of wisdom about this essential competency that the authors have drawn from long practice and from applicable literature.

DEFENSE OF BASIC ASSERTIONS

Conflict is common in all human endeavors and unavoidable in complex social systems, such as families, voluntary associations, or health-care organizations. In any of these social systems, one should expect differences in personalities, role relationships, assumptions about what decisions belong to whom, and even styles of verbal expression. These differences make conflict not merely likely, but inevitable.

Emotionally charged situations occurring within these social systems bring into the open disagreements, resentments, or mistrust that otherwise might remain under the surface. In the clinical realm, a sudden illness or an exacerbation of symptoms in a chronic illness can trigger open conflict because of heightened emotion. Such developments may alter the social roles of involved parties, even including the role of the APN, creating further confusions of expectation, shifting of responsibility, unfamiliar challenges, and, hence, increased anxiety on the part of some or all the parties. Anxiety arising from changing circumstances or unfamiliar challenges is very common in health care; it is frequently seen in patients and families and occasionally even in experienced professionals (Rushton, Caldwell, & Kurtz, 2016).

APNs, as the very title suggests, have education and professional responsibilities that are more extensive and deeper than is typical of registered nurses. Because we take it to be self-evident that *all* nurses encounter conflict in the ordinary conduct of their work, it follows that APNs will not only encounter more conflict but should be expected to respond to conflict situations with more skill and effectiveness. APN roles often entail role modeling, mentoring, and teaching of nurses and, sometimes, other professionals. Because learning to deal effectively with conflict is a common concern for all health-care professionals to the extent that role modeling and teaching is part of an APRN's responsibility, she or he should regard advanced facility in conflict management as an essential competency (Kritek & Joel, 2013).

ILLUSTRATION OF COMMON CONFLICT SITUATIONS

The following scenarios, all related to a single patient, illustrate potential conflicts that may be encountered by APNs. All three cases are set in a hospital, not because the authors are unaware that APNs also work in long-term care, small clinics, private offices, and elsewhere, but because hospital settings are within the educational, if not workplace, experience of all nurses. The cases will be further discussed later in the chapter.

Case 1

You have arranged to meet with family members of your patient, an elderly woman in the medical ICU. The woman resides in a nursing home and this is her third admission in recent months, all for the same indication: shortness of breath caused by chronic heart failure. She is now resting quietly without apparent distress.

The consensus among her professional caregivers is that the goal of care from this point forward should be comfort, including either return to the nursing home with a care plan, including a "Do Not Hospitalize" order and appropriate medications to treat dyspnea, or to the home of a family member on hospice.

The nursing home staff members have documented that the patient has not completed an advance directive or otherwise expressed preferences about care at the end of life. Based on experience from this and previous admissions, you (and others on the team) expect the principal family members used to making decisions on behalf of the patient will resist the team's recommendations.

Case 2

A pulmonologist consulting on Case 1, but not involved directly in team discussions about the discharge plan, corners you in the hallway. With obvious annoyance, he says that you "have no business" initiating a family meeting about a treatment plan. You reply that you are recommending a treatment proposal representing an interdisciplinary consensus. He counters, "That is a job for a physician!"

Case 3

You have had a subsequent meeting with the physician. In your opinion, this attempt to reach an understanding failed. You decide to alert the director of nursing. She tells you that this physician has made similar complaints before and that she has "had some success in calming him down." You leave her office thinking that you did the right thing by alerting her to the conflict with him.

Later, when reminiscing about your visit to the director's office, you feel disappointed. Thinking more about it, you conclude that the director's response to you was inadequate. You decide that simply "calming him down" is not enough, either for you or for the professional staff as a whole. He is widely viewed as a disruptive presence on the Med-Surg floors. Apparently, the medical staff leadership has long been aware without taking effective action.

You believe that trying to stimulate more effective action by the institution would be professionally responsible. You also remind yourself that doing so would be at least uncomfortable, if not risky, for you.

These three cases illustrate three distinct kinds of conflict situations common in the experience of APNs. Case 1 involves conflict with one's own patients or their families. Case 2 is an instance of conflict with another professional. Case 3 illustrates conflict with administrative leaders and/or institutional procedure. Each of these types of conflict, though distinct, has much in common with the others, especially regarding the attitudes and habits with which parties to the conflict approach it.

We all have noticed that our own family members, neighbors, and coworkers vary from individual to individual in how they tend to respond to conflict. Some of us have realized about ourselves that we tend to respond to conflict differently depending on who else is involved or on the role relationship (i.e., whether we are sister or sister-in-law, social friend or institutional colleague, new friend or old friend).

DYSFUNCTIONAL RESPONSES TO CONFLICT

The Thomas-Kilmann Index (TKI) identifies five distinct kinds of responses to conflict: avoiding, accommodating, compromising, collaborating, and competing. This index has been used to study the relative frequency of preference for each mode of conflict management in various populations. Valentine (2001) analyzed eight studies that applied the TKI to nurses. Nurses in these studies predominantly used two conflict management modes: avoiding and compromising. The third most frequently identified response was accommodation.

The significance of these data lies in the results that typically follow from each of these styles of conflict management. Conflict management experts have found that avoiding and accommodating (going along with or acquiescing) end up in disadvantaging oneself. Compromising leads to all parties to the conflict being *equally* disadvantaged. Collaborating and competing are the only two response modes that lead to a robust gain for one's own position. Because the previously cited data indicate that nurses tend to avoid conflict, go along with the other's idea, or compromise, it appears that nurses generally respond to conflict with ineffective strategies, *if ensuring gain for one's self is the desired end.*

Getting one's own way is not an ethically worthy goal *in and of itself.* Indeed, self-effacement of a certain kind is a professional virtue. Putting the patient's welfare at the center of one's concern is the enduring core of the Hippocratic Oath and all health professional oaths since. In the American Nurses Association *Code of Ethics for Nurses with interpretive statements (2015),* this first principle of professional obligation is most directly expressed in the preface: "The nurse's primary commitment is to the patient. . . ."

However, this ethical promise to always put the patient first does not mean that nurses should simply accept the ideas of their patients. On the contrary, if one believes that his or her own point of view or proposal may lead to a better outcome for the patient or family in question, fidelity to the patient-first principle would *require* the nurse to advocate for her or his own position. Stated differently, rather than being seen as respect for patient autonomy, merely going along with a patient's (or surrogate's) perspective in such instances *should* be interpreted as a failure of the professional obligation to put the patient's welfare first.

Furthermore, when members of a group typically behave in certain ways, others may form unfortunate expectations. To the extent that nurses frequently or characteristically avoid and accommodate, other parties to decision making are conditioned to not look to them for input. Nurses have relevant knowledge, training, and professional perspectives that can lead to better outcomes for those we all are pledged to serve. This systemic lack of expectation of nurse input further disadvantages both nurses and, more importantly, patients and their loved ones.

Finally, nurses can become discouraged and frustrated after habitually practicing avoidance and accommodation. Chronic discouragement and frustration after many experiences of failing to adequately cope with perceived wrong leads to moral distress (Rushton et al, 2016) and to compassion fatigue, sometimes called "professional burnout." Compassion fatigue is a form of spiritual withdrawal that has devastating consequences, both on nurses who succumb and on the human resources of institutions. If we again push the ethical analysis of compassion fatigue to what is *ultimately* at stake, we see that it is of professional concern, not primarily because of its effect on *us,* but because it robs *our patients* of the full measure of our healing presence.

EFFECTIVE WAYS TO DEAL WITH CONFLICT

When encountering any conflict situation, one should pause to identify, review, and clarify one's own goals. What do I want to happen here? Is my preferred outcome really desirable? Is it achievable? Does it accord with professional ideals? What are my motives? How does it affect my relationships with those I am pledged to protect and serve?

Efforts to effectively manage conflict should be in service to goals that are both clear and professionally defensible. Thoughtful clinicians know that much avoidable suffering and waste of resources is caused by medical interventions that have little chance of working, let alone being what furthers the patient's goals. The same is true of conflict strategies. Indeed, much conflict arises in the first place because the parties to it are either unclear about their goals or pursuing goals that are unrealistic or otherwise unworthy.

Let us consider Case 1. You are about to meet with family members of a decisionally incapacitated patient with no advance directive. The patient was admitted to the ICU for shortness of breath but is now stable enough to leave. This is her third admission in recent months. The consensus view of the treatment team is that optimal care is hospice care. The family is expected to resist this recommendation. *What is your goal for this meeting?*

Surely, to answer that the goal is "to find out what the family wants to do" is not acceptable. Such an answer totally ignores the ethical obligation to present the best judgment of the treatment team. That is not primarily an obligation to your team; it is an obligation to your patient and to her surrogates. It is also an obligation that arises out of your professional role as an advance practice nurse.

If your first answer is that your goal is "to get consent for admission to hospice care," you may want to reconsider. That goal may not be achievable and it is ethically suspect. It violates professional principles in that it does not sufficiently respect the patient's right to self-determination as expressed through her surrogates. It may also short-change the meaning of "informed consent." Informed consent is not mere assent to a professional proposal; rather, it is a process of dialog leading to a joint decision.

A better formulation of goals would be "to negotiate a mutually agreeable plan of care." Note the words *mutually agreeable.* This formulation of the goal leaves plenty of room for advocacy of the team's consensus view and for you to push back against unrealistic or otherwise inappropriate ideas, although still acknowledging that the patient and surrogate(s) must agree to the goals of care.

Now that you are clear about your goal for this probably difficult family meeting, you would be well advised to review *how* one might best approach this task. David Weissman, MD, an emeritus professor in the Palliative Care Program at the Medical College of Wisconsin, has trained thousands of health professionals to conduct family meetings focused on treatment decisions for patients at or near the end of life. He calls these meetings "family goal setting conferences" and describes 10 steps that should be taken when conducting these meetings.

The first and longest of Dr. Weissman's 10 steps is headed "Preparation"; the second step is "Establish proper setting" (Weissman, 2016). Thus, he reminds us that, just as we would prepare in advance for a surgical operation, there are very important steps that must happen before starting the intervention itself.

Dr. Weissman proposes that the person conducting such meetings state his or her goal for the meeting and ask others present if they have any other goals. He insists that this happen *immediately after everyone states their names and relationship to the patient.* Again, we are reminded of the primacy of thoughtfully formulated and clearly articulated goals in any enterprise and especially in ones that may involve emotional difficulty or conflict. As part of his "Goals/Relationship" step, Dr. Weissman proposes that the person conducting the meeting ask a "nonmedical" question such as "Can you tell me something about your mother?" The purpose is to build a relationship with the family *before* tackling the hard and potentially contentious main agenda. This advice is entirely in accord with the counsel of conflict management experts (Kritek & Joel, 2013).

Weissman's next step is "Understanding of Condition." The logic of treatment planning requires this step near the outset because instituting interventions without taking account of the patient's condition is a leading cause of avoidable suffering and waste of resources, especially in the elderly and other patients with factors that inhibit recovery. Effective and efficient communication also commends Weissman's suggestion that one ask *all* the family members to respond. Asking, rather than telling, furthers relationships by eliciting what they think, as well as providing additional evidence of what misperceptions are in play, what divisions may exist, and who might be an ally in moving the family toward a plan most consistent with the advice of the staff.

The remaining steps in David Weissman's guide to Family Goal Setting Conferences may be found in the invaluable, comprehensive online resource *Fast Facts,* which is available as a smartphone app and is a useful tool to have instantly accessible (Weissman, 2016). An open-minded and thoughtful reading of Weissman's compact summary of advice for conducting a family meeting, while thinking about the theme of conflict management, should make it readily apparent that, if one masters this set of skills, she or he is probably prepared to deal with all manner of conflict situations likely to arise in clinical settings.

Case 2 shifts attention from conflict with patients or families to conflict involving another professional. The particular instance in Case 2 pits you in conflict with a physician upset upon learning that an APN is convening and conducting a family conference focused on treatment decisions. This physician confronts you in a hospital hallway. With "obvious annoyance," he states that you "have no business" discussing therapeutic plans with a patient's family. He brushes aside your explanation that you will be recommending a treatment proposal that represents the consensus of the interdisciplinary treatment team, declaring, "That is a job for a physician!"

Though this conflict situation may be importantly distinct from Case 1, some recommendations from that discussion are fundamentally applicable. First, preparation is essential for effective conflict management. One should have all

relevant and available information well in hand and be clear about one's goals. One should, in David Weissman's terms, "Check one's own emotions." Second, one should prepare the setting. A hallway is surely not anyone's well-reasoned choice of setting for effectively dealing with this situation. These considerations alone are sufficient reason to postpone further exchange to another time and another place.

One *could* simply turn away and leave the scene. It could be argued that the arrogance and disrespect displayed by the physician "deserves" no more. However, it would be naïve for an APN to be totally unprepared for the possibility of encountering such attitudes and opinions. Furthermore, it seems to the authors of this chapter that returning disrespect for disrespect is both unprofessional and very likely to be totally counterproductive. In sober consideration, an APN's optimal goal in this situation would not be well served by an abrupt withdrawal, with or without an insulting retort.

Accordingly, we recommend that APNs have ready some stock responses for conflict situations of this kind that arise without warning or in circumstances that do not favor effective attempts at resolution. One such response might be, "Dr. X, we clearly need to pursue this matter at a better time and place. I will be in touch." Such a response has several features that commend it:

- It accepts neither the correctness of his position nor that he will have the last word.
- In the terms of previously discussed concepts, it is neither avoidance nor accommodation.
- It is respectful in that you are not outright dismissing his perspective or his right to have one.
- It acknowledges that the issue remains in play and that you expect to engage further.
- By taking responsibility for initiating further discussion, you gain influence over when, where, and how to attempt resolution or, at least, more understanding and respectful disagreement.
- This is consummately professional behavior. Even if he does not perceive it that way, others will.

Assume that you were practiced enough to respond to the Case 2 situation approximately as recommended previously before breaking free of Dr. X's ambush. You are now in a position to plan for your next move. First, your professional stature, as well as optimal management of this conflict, requires that you follow through within a timely period. Second, you need to be clear about your *goal* for the meeting, that is, clear about what you hope to accomplish. Your goals should be both professionally desirable and achievable. Here, it may be helpful to seek some consultation. Consulting peers may be preferable to seeking advice from administrators whose counsel may be geared more to their conception of institutional reference points than to your clinical and collegial objectives. You might decide to do both.

The items that Weissman envisions as appropriate for planning a family meeting are similar to the checklist for preparation of this nonclinical encounter. "Reviewing relevant information" in the context of Case 1 meant making sure that you had a firm grip on prognosis, treatment course, and options for clinical care. In this instance, the relevant information would include the professional, legal, and institutional stipulations about the scope of advanced practice nursing roles. Deciding who you want to be present at the meeting is similarly important and, similarly, might require input from colleagues. Finally, checking your own emotions is especially critical in the Case 2 scenario because your own professional legitimacy is the very subject of the conflict. An adequate plan for the meeting ought to include some provision for a follow-up with other players in case an initial one-on-one with the physician proves inadequate. As much as you prepare for success, you must be realistic.

Finally, even though your efforts to address this conflict in a face-to-face meeting with this particular physician may not meet your goals, it is nonetheless important that you make your very best effort. The professional literature has long addressed the duty to report bad behavior of other professionals (AMA, 2016; Murphy & Price, 1999). Some of this literature is filed under the heading "Whistleblowing," particularly when addressing situations in which first-line superiors do not take effective action. Common advice in this literature is to not report until you have attempted to resolve the situation directly. The fact that a well-executed effort has already been made, without success, is generally thought to be a stronger inducement for action by higher authorities.

Therefore, even if you doubt the efficacy of the meeting you are preparing to have, you should proceed with it. This advice may seem to be at odds with previous discussion about how goals should be achievable. The apparent inconsistency dissolves if one also recalls the suggestion about formulating your goal for this anticipated meeting to include the possibility of a follow-up step. That way, your

goal would not be unachievable, no matter the extent of your pessimism about the sufficiency of the initial meeting.

Case 3 illustrates a distinctly different arena for conflict. Here, the conflict—or—anticipated conflict—is with administrative leaders or institutional procedures. The conflict in Case 1 was "anticipated" in the sense that it emerged unavoidably in the course of ordinary clinical work. The conflict in Case 2, thrust upon you by surprise by an angry coworker, was clearly unanticipated, except in the sense that one should have imagined that such a thing might happen sometime. Differentiated from either of the other cases, Case 3 is a conflict situation that *you* will precipitate . . . *if, indeed, you choose to do so.*

Should you? ("Should" questions are *ethical* questions.) This is not an easy question. On the one hand, the ethical principle is clear enough: *The Code of Ethics for Nurses* devotes a whole section (Provision 6) to the nurse's responsibility to maintain and improve the ethical environment of work settings. "Respect and trust" is a fair characterization of the professional virtue violated by the physician in Case 2. "Respect and Trust" also leads the list of virtues in the Code essential to a flourishing moral milieu that nurses are charged to promote. Lest this language seem too vague, the Code includes a subsection (6.3) stating that the nurse "participate(s) in interprofessional workplace advocacy to address unethical practice." So, yes: an APN has a professional responsibility to protect the hospital from the threat posed by this physician's attitude and behavior.

However, clear statements of professional responsibility do not, *by themselves*, dictate specific answers to concrete actions. Indeed, the immediately preceding section of the Code speaks to an equally important duty to care for one's self, including both one's safety and health and one's professional integrity. So, moral choices are not always easy and citing only *one* obligation is rarely sufficient (and often a feature of craftily misleading arguments).

Facts also count. So does context. Because good ethical choices depend on good information, action without knowledge is reckless and thereby unethical. The Case 3 scenario includes some general information that begs for fact checking and development of further understanding:

- Dr. X is "widely regarded as a disruptive presence." How widely? Only by nurses or by others as well?
- He has complained before. Only to the director of nursing or also to others? What others?

- The medical staff leadership has "apparently" been aware of his disruptive behavior. Is this true? If so, for how long? Has he ever been sanctioned by the medical staff or by any other oversight body? If so, for what?
- How long has he been on the staff? Is he active in staff affairs? Does he, or has he recently, served on important hospital committees? Is he well known to nonphysician hospital administrators?
- Is he an employee of the hospital or in private practice? If in private practice, is it a group practice? Does he have a history of moving around?
- *And about you:* How long have you been at this hospital? How long in your APRN role? Are you well established (i.e., secure in your present position)?
- Who do you regard as your mentors? Who are your champions on the nursing staff? Who are your physician champions?
- Have you initiated complaints or undertaken institutional advocacy before this? Here or elsewhere? How did that go? What did you learn from that experience?

All these are potentially relevant questions. Answers may prompt additional questions. How complete the answers to each should be is unknowable at the outset. Developing the information will remain an open process until you decide that you are sufficiently prepared to proceed.

Note that the previous paragraph ends with a presumption that you *will* proceed. Not doing *anything* seems beyond the range of ethical options, given the citations from the *Code of Ethics for Nurses.* A decision to proceed may also be mandated by a more general understanding of what it means to be a professional in a 21st century health-care institution. However, *how* one ought to proceed, *when* one ought to move decisively, and *with whom* one ought to take action all properly depend on information not yet in evidence.

Again, it is ethically relevant that this conflict situation is one in which the APN has *time* on her or his side. Those who have the luxury of moving deliberately and fail to deliberate may be courageous but are also foolish. Courage is a virtue explicitly cited in the part of the *Code of Ethics for Nurses* that deals with this matter; wisdom and patience are also cited in the very same section (4.2). An APN who excels in only one virtue to the detriment of others should not be regarded as a good role model.

Similarly, an experienced, well-established APN who does exemplary work with patients but always keeps his or her head down in the face of suboptimal workplace conditions is not an exemplar of the profession. Indeed, any nurse, and especially an APRN, who fails to act out of undue concern for his or her personal well-being may be justifiably charged with "unprofessional behavior." In support of such a charge, one could surely cite the *Code of Ethics for Nurses* and, probably, the legislation of most states that describes the roles and obligations of nurse licensees. Indeed, this obligation to act responsibly to prevent the immoral, illegal, or incompetent acts of coworkers is common among all health-care professions in the United States and Canada.

Most of us hesitate to directly confront peers, let alone file formal complaints against them. The reasons we give for our failure to call out bad behavior are many:

- "There but for the grace of God go I."
- "We have to work alongside these people."
- "I doubt that he would listen to me."
- "Why should *I* when her own practice partners don't do anything?"
- "I'm not good at confrontation."
- "Maybe it won't happen again."

We all know at some level that none of these adequately justify a failure to act. Almost none of us could offer such excuses without a measure of shame. Yet letting in that uncomfortable truth rarely changes behavior.

These observations are based on more than two decades of experience leading intensive workshops with health-care professionals of all kinds and from all over the United States and Canada who are sent by licensing boards and other oversight agencies (The ProBE Program). Both role-playing and candid discussion in these sessions convincingly demonstrates just how hard it is for most experienced health professionals to directly confront each other about perceived bad behavior. Despite scores of these seminars, the faculty does not claim that such remedial education has actually helped the approximately 2,000 participants to overcome their avoidance and accommodation. On the other hand, seminar participants do often demonstrate heightened appreciation for the ethical mandate that professionals should protect the public from bad behavior of other health professionals (Caldecott & d'Oronzio, 2014). We cling to the conviction that few of us *want* to act irresponsibly once we are helped to appreciate what our responsibility entails.

Returning to the particulars of Case 3, if you decide to proceed after considering all available information, several general procedural guidelines will help ensure success:

- Remind yourself repeatedly that your goal is not retribution against someone who treated you poorly, but reduction of behavior toxic to the culture of an institution committed to healing.
- Keep it factual. A complaint based on objective facts is far more persuasive than one based on subjective opinion. Describe what happened rather than how you felt about it or how you interpret it.
- Prepare and present a written record of times and places. Include the experience of others, so long as it involves directly observed behavior and not hearsay or opinions based on secondhand information.
- If institutional officials ask you about what other nurses have reported or about the attitudes of nurses generally, be prepared to answer in terms of what you have heard directly. Avoid "impressions" and generalizations. Again, keep it factual.
- If institutional officials explicitly ask you questions about your evaluation of the offending physician's behavior, about why you think such behavior is a threat to the hospital, or about what institutional response would satisfy you, be prepared to answer in terms that are brief, clear, and professional.
- Remember your goal: to reduce the incidence of behavior toxic to the institutional culture.
- If asked (and only if asked), propose solutions that are rehabilitative, rather than punitive. Make it about the integrity and effectiveness of the hospital, not about you (and not about nurses vs. physicians).
- Follow up any meetings with institutional officials with an e-mail or memo summarizing what happened at the meeting and what you understand to be the process going forward. Include the date of the meeting and names of those present. Include relevant target dates and the names and tasks of those who took on roles for next steps. Be sure to include yourself if you were asked to do anything further.
- Prepare this memo and all other written materials with care. Keep a dispassionate, professional tone. Edit out emotionally charged adjectives. Avoid any suggestion that you have any interests beyond those stated in your goal.
- Understand that, even as you felt hesitant to take this on, institutional leaders may be tempted to avoid conflict as well. Although your follow-up memo is a nonthreatening way to remind them of responsibilities that they might rather forget, avoid any suggestion that you expect anything other than an efficient and effective process.

CONCLUSION

In summary of this discussion of Case 3, the observations and recommendations offered here are intended to address a conflict situation that most of us find extremely challenging. Indeed, the level of discomfort entailed is likely the most probable explanation why the ethical duty to report (or otherwise act to curtail) bad behavior of colleagues is a duty so often breached. These observations and rather concrete suggestions should help to reduce the anxiety of APNs to more manageable levels.

Lowered anxiety in the face of this challenge, although in itself a good thing, is not what motivated this effort. The ultimate goal of this chapter . . . and of this book . . . is to help APNs to more fully realize their potential in this high calling.

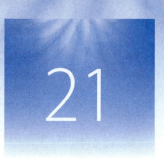

21

Leadership for APNs

If Not Now, When?

Edna Cadmus

Learning Outcomes
Learning outcomes expected as a result of this chapter:

- Understand how health-care reform has created both barriers and opportunities for advanced practice nurses (APNs).
- Distinguish between leadership frameworks and theories and their application to advanced practice nursing.
- Understand what is meant by applying emotional, social, and cognitive intelligence.
- Illustrate the use of power, authority, and influence.
- Demonstrate the creation of change through the lens of complexity science and chaos theory.
- Use disruptive innovation as a means of reforming health care.
- Distinguish between APNs as entrepreneurs or intrapreneurs.
- Explain the use of networking and mentoring to advance one's career.

During the last 15 years an infrastructure for radical change of the health-care system in the United States has been created. Both of the Institute of Medicine (IOM) reports, *To Err Is Human* (IOM, 2000) and *The Future of Nursing: Leading Change, Advancing Health* (IOM, 2011), were prominent in prompting these changes. The latest IOM report has provided nurses, more specifically advanced practice nurses (APNs), with a blueprint to be part of that change. It addresses adjusting their role and functions to ensure access, quality, and value at a reduced cost. The blueprint is further advanced through the Campaign for Action sponsored by the Robert Wood Johnson

Foundation (RWJF) in collaboration with AARP. Their campaign vision is to ensure that "all Americans have access to high-quality, patient-centered care in a health-care system where nurses contribute as essential partners in achieving success" (Center to Champion Nursing in America, 2011). Currently, the Campaign for Action is providing support to Action Coalitions at the state level in every state. These Action Coalitions are charged with implementing the recommendations described in the IOM *Future of Nursing* report. To learn more about these initiatives, visit https://campaignforaction.org/.

Since the initial report was released in 2011, the National Academies of Science, Engineering and Medicine (2015), at the bequest of the RWJF, conducted an assessment of the progress made toward the eight recommendations. In the initial report, recommendation 7 was "to prepare and enable nurses to lead change to advance health." The skills needed to accomplish this recommendation focused on leadership, entrepreneurship, and management. In a follow-up report 5 years later, the findings revealed that although several programs had incorporated courses in leadership, entrepreneurship, and management, the conclusion was that to assess leadership development it would be necessary to track the courses in these areas to determine progress (IOM, 2015).

The Campaign for Action at this point has moved its focus from exclusively building capacity in the nursing workforce toward building a culture of health. Therefore, improving health in the communities is a key priority. This shift underscores the urgency for APNs to lead change and advance health now.

Legislation, including the American Recovery and Reinvestment Act of 2009 (ARRA) and the Patient Protection and Affordable Care Act of 2010 (PPACA), have also contributed to an uncertain health-care environment, but one that holds promise for APNs. These legislative actions provide the technological and financial framework for resource allocation in an evolving health-care delivery system. ARRA defines meaningful use regulations for informational technology. In 2016 the regulations require hospitals, physicians' offices, and critical access hospitals to focus on advancing the use of the EHR to support health information exchanges, interoperability, and advanced quality measures (CMS.gov). The focus of the meaningful use standards are to track a patient's clinical conditions for better coordination across settings and to provide clinical decision support for providers. The anticipated outcomes are to improve quality and safety by providing information in a more efficient and effective manner (Burchill, 2010). Those that do not comply will be fined.

The PPACA has established the Center for Medicare and Medicaid Innovations to ensure coordinated care across the health-care continuum through delivery models that predict improved outcomes for patients. These new care delivery models span the spectrum from preventive to end-of-life care opportunities. This is a unique occasion for APNs to develop and implement evidence-based models of care and to reframe traditional definitions of health and health care. Yet opinion leaders in general do not see nurses as having a great deal of influence in health-care reform. A survey was conducted by Gallup for the RWJF (2010), "Nursing Leadership From Bedside to Boardroom: Opinion Leaders' Perceptions." Telephone interviews with 1,504 opinion leaders throughout the country were conducted from August 19 to October 30, 2009. This study sought to determine the role of nursing in the future and barriers to nurses assuming leadership roles in health care. The key barriers identified were that nurses are not seen as significant decision makers or revenue generators. Several strategies were offered for nurses to overcome barriers and become more influential, including the following: (a) Nurses need to make their voices heard through a unified focus on key issues in health policy; (b) nurses need to demonstrate an interest in health policy; and (c) society and nurses need to have higher expectations for what they can achieve and be held accountable not only for providing high-quality care but also for health-care leadership.

So what does leadership mean for the APN? APNs have a responsibility to lead health-care reform that improves access, quality, and value-based care. Leadership frameworks and theories that have evolved over time will be described and then applied to the APN role. Further, the environments in which APNs practice are described as complex and uncertain; therefore, APNs have a responsibility to make the changes needed for Americans as they traverse this complex health-care system.

EVOLUTION OF LEADERSHIP FRAMEWORKS AND THEORIES

The ongoing changes in the health-care landscape are influenced most by globalization, economic and technological factors, and the aging of the population. The complexity of the health-care environment requires us to examine the leadership theories that are applicable for today and the future. Leadership is often oversimplified into one theory or framework, but the reality is that each situation and how the leader interprets the environment determines the leadership framework that is needed and the process to be employed. To better understand these theories and how they apply to the APN, it is important to appreciate how they have evolved over time.

There have been many definitions of leadership. Leadership has been described as a person or group, a process, or an outcome, depending on the theory utilized. Leadership has moved from leader-centered or focusing on an individual to an orientation of mutual power and influence that results in collaboration and innovation. In the industrial age, leadership was more about control and structure and people were treated as things. It was defined as mechanistic and leadership was considered reductionist. Leadership in the postindustrial age requires a different skill set for both the designated leader and leadership qualities within every follower. Today's leaders must embrace new ways of being and interacting for success.

In the knowledge worker age, Covey (2007) describes the "whole person paradigm" in which the leader taps into each person and maximizes an individual's contributions to create results. Early motivational theories such as McGregor's X and Y theories postulate that employees are motivated by leaders and that the leader can manipulate factors to motivate behaviors within an organization. As leadership theories evolve over time motivation is inspired in the individual through effective communication and a shared vision from the leader. Followers want to meet the challenges and are committed to meeting the goals of the organization. In the whole person paradigm people are engaged in a four-dimensional way, tapping into their mind, body, spirit, and heart. Covey (2007) further describes the four imperatives of great leaders: (1) inspiring trust, (2) clarifying purpose, (3) unleashing talent, and (4) aligning systems. In many situations a lack of any one of these imperatives will not allow the organization to move forward with the speed and efficiency to remain competitive. These imperatives can be applied by the APN in working with patients and other professionals as well. As the frameworks and theories are described, you will see an emphasis on many of these imperatives.

Situational or Contingency Leadership

Situational leadership has been evolving since 1967, starting with the works of Vroom and Yetton (1973) and followed by Fielder (2012) and Hersey, Blanchard, & Johnson(2007). Contingency or situational theories are based on the premise that different styles of leadership are needed in different circumstances. In all these models the most effective style is contingent on the maturity and competence of the subordinates and the situation that is presented to the leader. For example, Hersey, Blanchard, & Johnson's model identifies four combinations that can occur in leadership style based on the situation or level of employee or group that the leader is interacting with. Maturity in this model is focused on competence, which is signified by the knowledge, skills, and commitment of the participants (Blanchard, 2008). The activities of leadership can include (a) "telling" when there is very low maturity, (b) "selling" to those with moderate maturity, (c) "participating" for those with moderately high maturity, and (d) "delegation" for those with very high maturity (Thompson & Vecchio, 2009). Leadership style depends on the difficulty of the task and the maturity of the persons responsible for carrying out the task.

Servant-Leadership

In the early 1970s Robert Greenleaf defined servant-leadership as a leader who wants to serve first versus being the leader first (Greenleaf Center for Servant Leadership, 2010). Servant-leaders focus on meeting the needs of others and accomplishing the work. In this model anyone can be a servant-leader by meeting the needs of others. McCrimmon (2010) describes it as meeting the needs of followers so that they can perform optimally. Spears (2004) defined the characteristics of servant-leadership to include active listening, empathy, healing, awareness, persuasion, stewardship, commitment to the development of others, foresight, and building community. Sipe and Frick (2009) further developed the work of Greenleaf by defining the seven pillars on which servant-leadership will grow and flourish: (1) personal character, (2) an ethic of people first, (3) skilled communicator, (4) compassionate collaborator, (5) possessing foresight, (6) systems thinker, and (7) a leader with moral authority (Sipe & Frick, 2009). These seven pillars translate into specific competencies that define servant-leadership: being visionary, being a good listener, recognizing that there is a higher purpose other than oneself, respecting others, and holding oneself and others accountable for actions that affect the organization as a whole. Although all these competencies are not expected to be fully met by the leader, a large proportion must be part of the persona of the servant-leader.

Some of the advantages of this model are that it introduces the concept of caring and creates a nurturing environment for the followers and ultimately the patient or client. Some of the disadvantages are that it is often confused with transformational leadership and is also seen as a weak form of leadership because of the connotation of the word *servant*. Servant symbolizes the historical religious heritage of nursing where the nurse was called to serve and therefore today seems outmoded. Many of the pillars described in servant-leadership are important characteristics that should be incorporated into a leader's competencies regardless of the model.

Transformational and Transactional Leadership

Transformational leadership has received considerable attention. Burns (1978) defined transactional leadership and transformational leadership. He connected leadership with the need for purpose. Transactional leaders work with their followers to gain some type of exchange for services that are contracted by the leader. Transformational leaders look for the motives of their followers and engage the full person in reaching a mutual purpose. Burns (1978) identified a strong link with morality and ethics in the transformational model, placing emphasis on the wants and needs of the followers as opposed to the leader or the situation at hand. Bass (1985) further defined and challenged transformational leadership, defining the art of transformational leaders as being able to elevate the interests of their followers and their ability to look beyond their own self-interest to that of the group. This type of leadership is most effective in turbulent markets. He further defined transactional leadership as working on the promise of reward or the fear of penalties by the followers. This type of leadership is more effective in a stable marketplace. Bass differs from Burns in that he saw transformational leadership as elevating the performance of followers, yet holding significant cost for them if they were to fail. Burns saw transformational and transactional

leadership as opposites. Therefore, leaders were either transformational or transactional, but not both. Bass, on the other hand, stated that leaders use both transformational and transactional behaviors based on the situation and even within the same situation. Transformational leaders are described as being charismatic and able to bring out the best in their followers. They tend to exude competence and confidence. They are inspirational, individualize the consideration of their followers, and are intellectually stimulating (Bass, 1985; Bass & Riggio, 2008).

Using transformational leadership as a springboard, Kouzes and Posner (2012) developed five practices and 10 commitments of leadership behaviors. They defined leadership not by title, power, or authority but by relationships, credibility, and what we do. The relationship is between the person who aspires to lead and those who choose to follow. Credibility includes being honest, competent, and inspiring and is the foundation of leadership. Credibility is established by doing what you say you will do. Kouzes and Posner's work is different from that of Bass because they put an emphasis on behaviors. Their five principles of leadership are (1) modeling the way, (2) inspiring a shared vision, (3) challenging the process, (4) enabling others to act, and (5) encouraging the heart (Kouzes & Posner, 2012). In each of these principles, there are valuable lessons that the APN can apply in practice.

In practice one, "modeling the way," you need to find your voice and articulate your values. Based on these values, common principles and ideals can be generated with others. Set an example by using actions to speak louder than words. In practice two, "inspiring a shared vision," it is the vision that creates the future state and the enthusiasm helps in getting others engaged. Engaging others through shared dreams is key to successful change. In practice three, "challenging the process," leaders are willing to challenge the status quo and take risks by experimenting with new ways of doing things. Leaders learn from their successes and their failures and continue to adapt to new ways of operating. In practice four, "enabling others to act," the leader recognizes the importance of the team. Building trust and collaboration with others makes them successful. They are considered authentic leaders. In the fifth practice, "encouraging the heart," leaders provide support and encouragement through the change process and recognize the contributions of their team. They celebrate their successes regularly (Kouzes & Posner, 2012).

Relational Leadership

Uhl-Bien (2006) and Rost (1995) describe relational leadership theory as occurring in any direction and reflecting a mutual agenda between follower and leader. It requires an inclusiveness of others and their viewpoints and the ability to persuade others to your way of thinking. This model of leadership focuses on the team as a process, and the team works collectively for the common good of the organization. This is not a single role. In this model teams also evolve their own culture. In the relational leadership model, each individual brings his or her leadership skill set to the table and the collective learning and abilities enable an adaptation to complexity. An example of this type of leadership can be found in the virtual team leadership in which the primary work is conducted using electronic media modalities. This model can be used by APNs as they frequently work in interprofessional teams where they may need to use their expertise in dealing with patient care needs or practice changes.

Clinical Leadership and Congruent Leadership

Theories described in the management literature may not completely translate to clinical practice. Congruent leadership may be a more appropriate theory for the clinician. Stanley (2008) defines congruent leadership theory as "matching the clinical leaders' action and their values and beliefs about care and nursing and is the theoretical foundation on which clinical nurses can build their capacity to be clinical leaders" (p. 519). The concepts that are embedded in transformational leadership—namely, vision and creativity—may not be appropriate to explain clinical leadership; however, the other characteristics remain (Stanley, 2008). Hamric, Hanson, Tracy, and O'Grady (2014) further describe clinical leadership as focusing on the patient first and on building working relationships to problem solve as part of an interprofessional team. Stanley (2006b) further identifies the key characteristics of clinical leaders as being approachable and open; having strong values and beliefs that are displayed in their practice; being effective communicators, role models, and decision makers; and being visible and clinically competent. They do not exhibit the creativity and vision described in transformational leadership (Stanley, 2006). Clinical leaders are not commonly in management positions. This framework may fit more appropriately for the APN.

REFRAMING LEADERSHIP THROUGH MENTAL MODELS

Mental models are needed by leaders to make sense of the VUCA (volatile-uncertain-complex-ambiguous) environment (Bolman & Deal, 2015). Bolman and Deal (2015) use the concept of framing as a mental model and reframing based on the situation. A frame is a composite of beliefs and assumptions used to navigate the world. These frames are filters for problem solving and getting things done in organizations. There are four frames: (1) structural, (2) human resource, (3) political, and (4) symbolic. Leaders of today and the future need to be able to use all four frames based on the situation with which they are presented. Leaders also need to reframe until they understand the situation.

The structural frame focuses on the organization's circumstances, goals, rules, technology, and environment. It addresses how the organizational chart is structured and how work is distributed in the organization. It is the old adage, does form follow function or does function follow form? In times of certainty, relationships are usually hierarchical. Organizations focus on structure in times of uncertainty, looking to reestablish stability (Bolman & Deal, 2013). For example, with health-care reform impending, redesign of the system needs to focus on the needs of the population in the community, building from the bottom up, from the smallest to the largest unit of service. Organizations such as hospitals will shrink over time and other models of care and mental models will substitute, creating newfound relationships.

Structure also applies to teams and requires changes based on the situation. Katzenbach and Smith (1993) identified six characteristics of high-functioning teams: (1) The team shapes purpose in response to a demand or opportunity identified by the leaders in the organization; (2) the team translates purpose into measurable goals; (3) the team itself is a manageable size; (4) the team has the right expertise; (5) the team has a common commitment to the work; and (6) the team members hold themselves collectively accountable. These characteristics should be adapted by APNs as they work in team environments. In comparison, Senge (1994) calls "team" an antiquated concept and claims it takes more effort to maintain the team than to do the team's work. This opinion may be outdated or contingent on the sophistication of team members.

The human resource frame focuses on the alignment between human and organizational needs. The decision that leaders need to make is to either invest in their people or to be lean and mean. Organizations that engage employees and can connect to meaningful work are the organizations that are most successful. How engagement is demonstrated varies based on the organization and the situations. Relationships are key to being flexible and nimble, and are the key to organizational effectiveness (Bolman & Deal, 2013).

The political frame redefines organizations as coalitions in which individuals and groups are competing for scarce resources. Exercising the use of power and influence to negotiate resources as needed is a key skill set for individuals and groups. Being effective politically requires leaders to set an agenda, scan the environment, develop networking skills, and negotiate with those who support their agenda, as well as create relationships with those who do not (Bolman & Deal, 2013).

The symbolic frame focuses on how meaning is perceived by the individual or group. Symbols create that perception and include rituals, values, stories, and myths that are evidenced in our culture. Symbols are created in times of uncertainty and ambiguity to try to make sense of reality and to create a more rational world. Organizations are frequently measured by appearance as well as outcomes (Bolman & Deal, 2013).

Application of Leadership Theories for Advanced Practice Nurses

APNs are leaders both formally and informally in the practice setting. In the clinical setting, they may serve as either the leader or the follower, depending on the situation. There are many common characteristics of leadership regardless of the theory one identifies with. The key characteristics include strong values, clear purpose, bringing out the best in others on the team, strong interprofessional relationships, mutual power and influence, and clinical competence.

The APN uses evidence to support practice, ensures that quality indicators are met, works with the team (having strong collaboration skills), and focuses on the patient and the family. The APN can be the leader as in the primary care model in which he or she manages a practice of patients, or be a member of a team, depending on the environment in which he or she works. In either situation, the APN focuses on the patient and family to ensure that their needs are met and will advocate for them as required to achieve high-quality outcomes. APNs need to be innovators in creating new models of care delivery for the future. Current models under review include accountable care organizations, medical homes, and transitional care delivery models. With the current gap in primary care, APNs need to fill the gap and create new models that are valued by the consumer at a lower cost.

OTHER ASPECTS OF LEADERSHIP

Emotional, Social, and Cognitive Intelligence

Emotional, social, and cognitive intelligence provide the framework for personality. The competencies are clustered as either *personal*, how we manage ourselves; *social intelligence*, how we manage our relationships; or *cognitive*, how we think or analyze information that leads to superior performance (Boyatzis, 2011). The four clusters are self-awareness (emotional self-awareness), self-management (emotional self-control, adaptability, achievement orientation, and positive outlook), social intelligence (social awareness, empathy, organizational awareness), and relationship management (coach and mentor, inspirational leadership, influence, conflict management, and teamwork). The cognitive intelligence competencies include systems thinking and pattern recognition. The emotional, social, and cognitive intelligence competencies are integrated to measure outstanding performance in leaders.

The personal competencies focus on self and include self-awareness and self-management. Self-awareness requires the leader to be honest with himself or herself and with others about his or her strengths and weaknesses. The leader is considered reflective and clear on values and goals and acts with authenticity. Self-management requires us to control our emotions. Leaders who demonstrate self-management are seen as optimistic, enthusiastic, transparent, and adaptable. They are perceived as positive leaders (Goleman et al, 2013).

The social competencies are focused on how we manage relationships and include social awareness and relationship management. Social awareness requires the leader to be empathetic, a good listener, and attuned to the needs of others. Relationship management requires the leader to have a tool set that includes conflict management and collaboration skills. The leader is able to find a common ground in various situations. He or she is considered inspirational, with an ability to influence and develop others on the team. The emotionally intelligent leader is seen as a change catalyst and has the ability to create effective teams (Goleman et al, 2013).

Goleman and Boyatzis (2008) have further developed emotional intelligence based on the breakthroughs in brain science that focus on the emotional centers of the brain. Social intelligence is "a set of interpersonal competencies built on specific neural circuits in the brain and (endocrine system) that inspire others to be effective" (p. 76). They include mirror neurons, which mimic other behaviors; spindle cells, which provide a gut reaction to a situation or person; and oscillators, which coordinate our physical movements with those of others (Goleman & Boyatzis, 2008; Veronesi, 2009). Socially intelligent leaders are tuned in to others so that they can communicate effectively and be effective leaders. The brain can be reprogrammed to learn how to become more socially intelligent through strategies that change behaviors. This requires the individual to be motivated to make the change in behaviors, obtain feedback from others on one's strengths and weaknesses using tools such as a 360-degree assessment, and setting a learning agreement between oneself and a mentor. This calls for intense work on the part of the leader and a socially intelligent mentor. If a leader is mentored by someone who is strong and socially intelligent, who is able to provide immediate feedback on a consistent basis, the neural circuits can be changed (Veronesi, 2009).

Cognitive intelligence provides the leader with the ability to see patterns emerging and the ability to use systems thinking to understand the patterns (Boyatzis, 2011). This is important for leaders in a time of uncertainty and chaos. Leaders need to be able to analyze information and respond to the patterns or changes occurring, specifically in health care. The emotional, social, and cognitive competencies are integrated, can all be learned, and are important for the leader to assess their performance and the performance of others.

Power, Authority, and Influence

Power can occur through persuasion, influence, or control. Bolman and Deal (2013) compare and contrast power from the perspective of structural and human resource theorists. Through the structural theorist's lens, power is focused around authority. The leader makes a decision and then monitors whether the followers carry out the directive. In addition, power is given because of the leader's control of resources. This is an old-world view of power. The human resource theorist changes the concept of power to empowerment. Empowerment fits more appropriately in today's world.

Power is often considered in a negative light. Power can be both negative and positive, depending on how it is used. In the new age, power is needed by leaders in building relationships and getting results. There are various sources of power. These sources can come from one's position, persona, reputation, or expertise, or can come from being coercive or controlling of information or others. Leadership and authority do not necessarily go together. Both are considered voluntary. Leaders cannot lead without legitimacy from their followers. Legitimate authority is a product of influence and acceptance by a group of people. More important than hierarchical authority is the ability to influence others through motivation, persuasion, and negotiation (Jooste, 2004).

Leaders motivate or influence others to follow by creating a shared vision and purpose and providing the environment where change can happen. Alignment of values and purpose is essential to success. This is not an optional step in the leadership sequence; leaders need followers, and vice versa. Both the leader and the follower depend on each other for success, yet each has different talents and skills. Although much has been discussed about leadership, it is just as important to describe key components of being a "good follower." These components include (a) clear role comprehension, (b) service attributes for self and others, (c) integrity, and (d) support for the leader. It is key that the follower be engaged in the organization. The leader needs to create an environment where there is both trust and respect so that the follower can flourish.

ENVIRONMENT

Complexity Science and Chaos Theory

Complexity science and chaos theory create the platform for looking at leadership and organizations collectively in the 21st century. Looking through this lens focuses on leadership as a process and not as an individual. To help explore this basic understanding of complexity science, complex adaptive systems (CAS) and chaos theory are needed.

Complexity science is derived from quantum physics, chaos theory, and systems theory. CAS are a broader context in complexity science and can be applied to health-care systems (Crowell, 2016). Complexity science looks at relationships between and among all things and defines the nature of the relationship by its actions and impact (Malloch & Porter-O'Grady, 2009). Plsek (2003) defines health-care systems as CAS. A CAS is defined as "a collection of individual agents who have the freedom to act in ways that are not always predictable, and whose actions are interconnected such that one agent's actions change the context for other agents" (p. 2). A CAS has the ability to adapt to change. Plsek (2003) defines the following properties of a CAS: (a) relationships as central to understanding the system (i.e., the way in which the system behaves comes from the interactions of the individuals); (b) structures, processes, and patterns; (c) actions based on internalized simple rules and mental models (i.e., the individual's mental model contributes to the patterns in the environment); (d) attractor patterns (i.e., those that help facilitate a change are close to the individual's values); (e) constant adaptation; (f) experimentation and pruning (i.e., support for new ways of doing things and eliminating those that no longer work); (g) inherent nonlinearity (i.e., there is no predictable cause and effect; the shortest distance between two points is not always a straight line); and (h) systems are embedded within other systems and co-evolve (i.e., formal and informal leadership can advance simultaneously and often in different directions). A CAS defines a healthy system as one that is always ready to change because if it is not it cannot survive (Lindberg et al, 2008). Chaos is a key component of change and, in fact, a necessary catalyst for change. Change is constant in the new age; therefore, we need to create spaces for new interactions, structures, and patterns that will be formed (Lindberg et al, 2008).

Wheatley and Frieze (2010) urge us to let go of the traditional paradigm of leadership, which preaches that leaders have the answers and know what to do; people do what they're told and just have to be given good plans and instructions; and high risk requires high control, and as situations grow more complex and challenging, power needs to shift to the top (with the leaders, who know what to do). If we want these complex systems to work better, we need to abandon our reliance on the leader-as-hero and invite in the leader-as-host. We need to support those leaders who know that problems are complex and who know that to understand the full complexity of any issue, all parts of the system need to be invited in to participate and contribute. We, as followers, need to give our leaders time, patience, and forgiveness, and we need to be willing to step up and contribute. These leaders-as-hosts are candid enough to admit that they don't know what to do; they realize that it's foolish to rely only on them for answers. But they also know they can trust in other people's creativity and commitment to get the work done. They know that other people, no matter where they are in the organizational hierarchy, can be as motivated, diligent, and creative as the leader, given the right invitation.

Wheatley (2007) brings together chaos and complexity theories with leadership. She believes that leaders were traditionally focused on transactional functions and that in the new age it is about decentralizing, differentiation of tasks, spanning boundaries, collaboration, flexibility, adaptability of structures and processes, participation, and autonomy. The journey for the leader is from hero to host. Leaders-as-hosts don't just benevolently let go and trust that people will do good work. As hosts, leaders have a great many things to attend to, but these are quite different from the work of heroes. Hosting leaders must do the following (Wheatley & Frieze, 2010):

- Provide conditions and good group processes for people to work together
- Provide resources of time, the scarcest commodity of all
- Insist that people and the system learn from experience
- Offer unequivocal support—people know the leader is there for them
- Keep the bureaucracy at bay, creating oases (or bunkers) where people are less encumbered by senseless administrative trivia
- Play defense with other leaders who want to take back control and are critical that people have been given too much freedom
- Reflect back to people on a regular basis how they're doing, what they're accomplishing, and how far they've journeyed
- Work with people to develop relevant measures of progress to make their achievements visible
- Value conviviality and *esprit de corps*—not false rah-rah activities, but the spirit that arises in any group that accomplishes difficult work together

The Wheatley model is based on four core principles, which drive change for the host-leader (Wheatley, 2007): (1) Participation is not a choice; in other words, "people only support what they create" (p. 89). (2) Life always reacts to directives, it never obeys them; therefore, "people accept partners not bosses" (p. 90). (3) We do not see reality; we each create our own interpretation of what reality is. (4) To create better health in a living system, connect it to more of itself; therefore, leaders need to increase the number and variety of connections. An underpinning of Wheatley's principles is therefore engagement. The leader needs to encourage engagement and create an environment where there is conversation that fleshes out different perspectives and increases the connections by changing or expanding those needing to be involved.

Change in a Complex World

Understanding complexity science and chaos theory can help create the linkage to change. Porter-O'Grady and Malloch (2015) describe change as a dynamic journey that is everywhere and cannot be avoided but needs to be embraced by leaders. The leaders' responsibility is to help translate the change for their followers and role model a comfort level with the ambiguity generated from uncertainty. The leader is the change agent or catalyst for change in an organization and is under constant observation by followers to determine how he or she adapts to the change. If the leader does not adapt to change, the followers will not adapt.

Creating a vision for the change and why it is needed is key to success. The leader needs to work with all the stakeholders in the organization to bring about change. In any change process there are resisters. Resistance occurs if there is a perceived change in vision or values or if the proposed actions cause the stakeholders to be disenfranchised (Raza & Standing, 2011; Trader-Leigh, 2001). Change is not often resisted because of the change itself but because of the role the person or group plays or does not play in the change process. Conflict occurs as an output of resistance. In dealing with conflict the leader needs to create an environment that is supportive so that the conflict can be discussed and ultimately resolved. It is the leader who needs to bring the resisters on board with the change through engagement and facilitated dialogue.

Tools are needed to lead change. One approach to change is to use the traditional approach, which is problem

solving. Hammond (1998) describes the basic assumption in this approach as "an organization IS a problem to be solved" (p. 24; emphasis in original). In today's organizations that are viewed as organic and whole systems, appreciative inquiry (AI) has been found to be more successful. Hammond (1998) describes the assumption of AI as "an organization is a mystery to be embraced" (p. 24). In conducting an AI approach, we look at what is working and through asking guided questions explore where an organization wants to base and create new energy and positivism. A positive deviance approach is used by AI to optimize solutions already seen in the organization. Positive deviance distributes leadership. The leader can serve as the leader, follower, or inquirer (Crowell, 2016). The AI model consists of the "four D's"—Discovery, Dream, Design, and Destiny. In the Discovery phase stories are told about when the qualities of the organization were at their best. The Dream phase explores what it could and should look similar to. In the Design phase the new norms, values, structures, patterns of relationships, and systems emerge. In the Destiny phase transformation occurs through innovation (Ludema et al, 2003; Trajkovski et al, 2012). Using the AI process facilitates engagement, strengthens relationships, and produces results.

Learning Organizations

Creating a learning organization is important in today's environment. The impact of implementing a successful learning organization is that it helps in improving quality, creating a competitive environment, gaining commitment of the workforce, managing change, being proactive, and generating collective thinking opportunities to improve organizational performance.

Senge (1990) defined the five disciplines of a learning organization: personal mastery (members of the organization develop themselves based on goals and purpose), mental models (how we shape actions and decisions), shared vision (building mutually agreeable images of the future), team learning (the sum of individual talents), and systems thinking (interrelationships that shape the system—the whole is greater than the sum of its parts) (Senge, 1990). Fillion, Koffi, and Ekionea (2015) have added two new concepts to the five core disciplines of Senge: (1) knowledge generation and sharing and (2) organizational behavior. Knowledge management requires maturity in organizations. There are two categories of maturity: evolution and revolution. The evolution level is focused on (a) localized exploitation of knowledge and (b) internal integration of knowledge. The revolution level includes (a) reengineering, (b) networks redesign, and (c) redefinition of the business. This requires finding new ways of doing things that does not require more work by individuals in the organization.

The second concept described is organizational behavior. With the complexity and uncertainty in the environment, change in how leaders adapt is important. The leader needs to use innovation to create and define the problems and to generate new ways to resolve them. This includes using emotional intelligence, new ways in motivating others, effective communication strategies, and teamwork (Fillion, Koffi, & Ekionea, 2015).

Many of the five disciplines have been described in the various leadership frameworks and in the complexity theory of previous sections. It is important for the APN to align himself or herself with an environment where he or she can practice in a learning organization. This is an organization where talents will best be utilized and where positive outcomes will be achieved. APNs also need to use leadership skills to generate new and innovative ways of providing care to the clients being served. This requires the APN to become a disruptive innovator.

Innovation

Change and innovation are needed to move our mental model from a mechanistic or industrial age model, which when applied to health care has focused on disease management as the prime strategy, to the current and future model that requires a focus on a culture of health and wellness. This shift requires innovation and a changed mindset by leaders. Leadership in this context requires distributed leadership, understanding of professional power, relationships among and between providers both discussed and acknowledged, and an inclusive use of talents that are valued and used (Briggs, 2016; Dopson, Fitgerald, & Ferlie, 2008). This distributed leadership and opportunity for innovation can lead to intrapreneurship. Intrapreneurship will be discussed further on in this chapter. White, Pillay, and Huang (2016) have identified 19 innovation competencies and developed a survey tool to measure levels of competence in the innovation domain using a five-point Likert scale (not at all important to very important). The researchers had the participants force rank 19 competencies to identify the top competencies by order of importance. The top five competencies were: (1) the ability to convey a compelling vision, (2) resilience, (3) the ability to recognize an opportunity, (4) tenacity and perseverance, and (5) interdisciplinary teamwork and collaboration (White et al, 2016). These findings identified significant gaps in all but one of the innovation competencies in their sample of nurse leaders in academia and practice. These behaviors, skills, and attitudes are important for APNs to possess. As APNs lead they need to look at the opportunities and innovations that can propel them forward in this new mental model. One strategy is to use disruptive innovation.

Disruptive and Catalytic Innovation

Christensen, Baumann, Ruggles, and Sadtler (2006) created the disruptive innovation model, which challenges leaders to offer simpler, more convenient, and less expensive alternatives to underserved customers. There are many examples in industry, such as Southwest Airlines, which offered inexpensive no-frills flights that served an unserved market and had a major impact on the travel industry. Frequently leaders are either resistant to or cannot see the innovation because of their mental model or patterns of thinking. Christensen and colleagues (2006) developed a subset of disruptive innovation called catalytic innovation with a focus on social change at a national level. They described the five qualities of catalytic innovators: (1) creating systemic social change through scaling and replication; (2) meeting the needs of the overserved (people who receive too many services that are not needed) or underserved; (3) offering services that are simpler and less costly, but perceived as appropriate for what is needed; (4) generating resources that are considered unattractive by competitors; and (5) tolerating being disparaged by their competitors, who see their market as unprofitable or unattractive (Christensen et al, 2006). Being a disruptive innovator requires creativity at all levels within the organization or as an individual.

At a national level, the changes predicted to characterize health-care reform could lead to catalytic innovation. Realigning the health-care system to ensure access, improve quality, and add value while slowing the rate of inflation offers attractive opportunities for innovation. Those who are creative and can adapt their mental models will be successful in future health-care delivery. Transforming the system requires several changes, including (a) matching clinician skills to the level of the problem, (b) investing in technology that simplifies complex problems, (c) creating new care delivery systems, and (d) changing regulations that impede progress toward this end (Christensen, Bohmer, & Kenagy, 2000). These changes require collaboration across the spectrum of health care. One prime example of disruptive innovation is the role of the APN. The APN offers services that meet the needs of both the overserved and the underserved. APNs provide services in communities that physicians may view as unprofitable or unattractive for their practice. The services provided are frequently simpler and less costly and meet the needs of the consumers in different ways from those physicians provide.

Rogers's diffusion of innovation theory explicates the process of change in a complex environment. There are five stages of innovation and change: (1) knowledge, (2) persuasion, (3) decision making, (4) implementation, and (5) confirmation. Decision making is the tipping point in this process. When one gets to the decision-making phase of change one can decide to be the innovator or go to the opposite spectrum and be the laggard. Where one falls is distributed in a normal bell curve.

APNs have a unique opportunity to be change agents based on their educational preparation and their ability to champion best practices in organizations. They serve as leaders in organizations where change and innovation focus. One example is the retail clinics such as CVS. They have served as change agents for primary care. APNs have led this initiative and are another example of disruptive innovation. APNs have carved out a market in primary care by making services more available to the majority of consumers. They have focused on the triple aim of access, cost, and quality in designing this market for consumers.

Blue Ocean Strategy

Kim and Mauborgne (2015) describe the differences between blue ocean and red ocean strategies in their book *Blue Ocean Strategy*. Blue ocean is a strategy used to "grow demand and break away from the competition" (p. xiii), whereas red ocean is a strategy used when there is bloody competition for the same market space. The differences in approach surface from how organizations approach the marketplace, competition, demand, value, cost, and differentiation.

The key to blue ocean success is that it focuses on differentiation of services and providers and low cost. It is not an either/or proposition. In providing a framework to create the new value curve, the authors identify four areas where questions should be asked: raise, reduce, create, and eliminate. For example, in looking at an opportunity for an APN in the new health-care reform environment he or she might ask, "What factors should be *created* in the new health-care industry that have never been offered before?" Similarly, one might ask, "What factors should be *eliminated* in the new health-care industry that have previously been taken for granted?" Blue ocean strategy is defined through a "reconstructionist" lens. In the reconstructionist view there are no boundaries and there is demand that is untapped. The focus is on creation of value innovation, which is similar to the disruptive innovation described earlier.

If we look at the current health-care system and the role of the APN, blue ocean strategy is a perfect framework to change health care and to lead change. APNs need to think about creating new models across the system rather than competing from within the system.

An example of blue ocean strategy is the transitional care model defined by Mary Naylor. Naylor and her colleagues (2004) conducted a randomized controlled trial to examine the effectiveness of a transitional care intervention delivered by APNs to elders hospitalized with heart failure. The sample included 239 patients age 65 and older hospitalized with heart failure. A 3-month, APN-directed discharge planning program and home follow-up protocol was implemented. Results demonstrated that there was an increase in the length of time between hospital discharge and readmission or death, as well as reduced health-care costs. If we look at this model in terms of blue ocean strategy, the APNs were not competing with other services but rather served as a liaison between hospital and home care services. They recognized no boundaries and offered a service that was in demand. They differentiated themselves from other markets at a lower cost and improved outcomes.

ENTREPRENEUR VS INTRAPRENUER

Entrepreneurship and intrapreneurship have been in the business literature for many decades, but have not been seen to a great extent in the nursing literature. The

Oxford Dictionary defines an *entrepreneur* as "a person who organizes and operates a business or businesses, taking on greater than normal financial risks in order to do so." Entrepreneurs are risk takers, willing to work in ambiguity and uncertainty; they are ambitious, determined, and self-challenging and have strong leadership characteristics (Gundogdu, 2012). APNs need to be educated on the entrepreneurial skills needed to open up their own practices. Frequently there are disabling factors that deter them from being entrepreneurs. This includes disablers such as lack of business skills or knowledge of education and training on entrepreneurship, as well as peer mentoring (Elango, Hunter, & Wincell, 2007; Shirey, 2007). Elango et al (2007) further identify three groups of barriers for nurses in entrepreneurship: (1) legal and regulatory barriers, (2) ethical and personal conflicts, and (3) knowledge barriers. Legal barriers and issues include regulatory requirements and legal complications around opening a business. Ethical and personal conflicts surround the general belief that nursing is about caring and business is about making money, in addition to the notion of being competitive. The last barrier focused on knowledge barriers, specifically around business and management skills. These barriers can be overcome through formal continuing education programs, as well as through support from professional organizations and peers, and should not preclude the APN from venturing into business. Some states, however, continue to have regulations that prevent them from practicing to the full extent of their license; this needs to be resolved in those states.

In contrast to an entrepreneur, an intrapreneur works within an existing business or company. According to the Oxford Dictionary, an intrapreneur is a manager within a company who promotes innovative product development and marketing. Pinchot (1985) defines the *intrapreneur* as a person who makes a new business into a reality within his or her organization despite barriers and risks. Intrapreneurs need team-building and leadership skills, must be willing to make rapid decisions, must be innovative, and should have a firm grasp of business and the marketplace. They need to create this change without direction from the top leadership (Gundogdu, 2012; Pinchot, 1985). APNs can become intrapreneurs within the organization or practice in which they work, looking for opportunities and then developing that vision into a reality within an organization.

NETWORKING

Networking is defined by Merriam-Webster's Dictionary as "the exchange of information or services, among individuals, groups, or institutions; specifically, the cultivation of productive relationships for employment or business." Professional networks are important for job opportunities, professional identity, or obtaining available resources for the patients being served. Rojas-Guyler, Murnan, and Coltrell (2007) described some of the key ways to develop a network: (a) identifying contacts from current or past experiences; (b) getting involved in voluntary agencies outside of your work; (c) attending professional association meetings; (d) accepting leadership roles within those voluntary agencies or professional associations; (e) publishing your findings in your area of practice; (f) presenting at national, state, or community groups or associations; and (g) simply providing your business card to others.

For new and experienced APNs, the professional organizations at both the state and national levels provide a formal structure for networking. Frequently, there are specific forums that both address professional development opportunities and bring APNs together to deal with political or legislative issues related to practice. As the health-care landscape changes, it is critical that APNs network to determine opportunities for new areas of practice.

Looking for forums that are interprofessional is also important for gaining perspective from outside of the profession. This can be through participation in committees or consortia that are formed at a community, state, or national level.

MENTORING

Dorsey and Baker (2004) describe mentoring as a planned relationship between an experienced person and one with less experience for the purpose of achieving identified outcomes. Joel (1997) describes mentorship as a "patron relationship/system" with varying levels of power, influence, and engagement on a continuum. The continuum goes from the mentor level, which is the most intense, to the level of "peer pals" (peers helping peers), which is the least intense. Mentors may have been role models or preceptors but the opposite may not be true. Mentoring is helping the protégé develop professionally. Mentoring can be either formal or informal in design. Formal mentoring is where a mentor is assigned within an organization. The question of being assigned a mentor is controversial. Mentor–protégé relationships cannot be forced but must be considered mutually acceptable by both parties. Informal mentoring is where the two parties find each other. Barker (2006) identifies key aspects of the mentor–protégé relationship that should be considered from the beginning. They include the following:

1. Select a mentor who communicates with, and does not talk at, the protégé.
2. It is best if there is no line authority between the mentor and protégé where job security is at issue.
3. The mentor and protégé should have a "good fit" (similar styles, communication patterns, availability, and focus on goal attainment).
4. Mentors who derive energy from oppressive relationships should be avoided.
5. The mentor and protégé should both recognize that relationships will change over time.

When considering a mentor, it is not essential that the mentor be within one's own field; however, he or she must meet the professional growth need identified.

The Fellows of the American Academy of Nurse Practitioners (AANP, 2006) conducted a 1-day think tank with new and experienced NPs. They separated their findings based on years of experience in the field. They found that new NPs needed mentoring in several areas, including time management and productivity; managing caseloads of patients; developing clinical skills; overcoming fear and anxiety; and dealing with isolation, business practices, and work-life balance issues (AANP, 2006). This list could help set goals for new APNs in their mentor–protégé relationships (Harrington, 2011).

Mentoring for experienced NPs took on different areas of need. Their needs included networks for communication;

dealing with burnout; development in education, research, and publishing; need for a change; keeping up skills; and the ability to be a mentor themselves (AANP, 2006). Mentors that could be helpful for this group of NPs included peers, educators, researchers, and leaders both inside and outside the profession (AANP, 2006).

Mentorship is even more critical when there are times of uncertainty. As previously discussed, anticipated health-care reform creates both uncertainty and opportunities for APNs. A mentor can help the APN identify new opportunities and provide advice and support for career development, which is vital. Joel (1997) describes how we can help build strength in the nursing ranks by mentoring others. It is the responsibility of those who have the experience and expertise to become mentors to new APNs. It is also the responsibility of the protégé to ensure that his or her objectives and needs are made evident to the mentor and that there is follow-through with the protégé's career plan.

CONCLUSION

This chapter has provided an overview of the various leadership theories and frameworks and applied them to the role of the APN. There is no more critical time than now for APNs to take the lead in changing the health-care system. This requires engagement by the individual APN, as well as courage to lead in this complex world. Business management skills, entrepreneurship or intrapreneurship characteristics, and innovation competencies are needed for the future. Failure to take on a leadership role is not an option. APNs need to be disruptive innovators and seek out the "blue ocean" opportunities to make a difference in U.S. health care. Networking through professional organizations and utilizing mentors can help provide the support needed to move ahead of the curve.

22

Information Technology and the Advanced Practice Nurse

Robert Scoloveno

Learning Outcomes

Learning outcomes expected as a result of this chapter:

- Describe the existing and emerging technologies available to the advanced practice registered nurse (APRN) to enhance clinical practice.
- Develop an understanding of health information technologies (HIT) available to the APRN.
- Demonstrate the ability to evaluate and utilize different electronic patient record software.
- Understand the three types of health information exchanges (HIE) and how they are utilized in clinical practice.
- Understand the utilization of high-fidelity simulation as an educational pedagogy to train the student APRN and also ensure competency of the practicing APRN.

INTRODUCTION

The rapid changes in health-care delivery require a focus on quality and safety for all recipients of health-care services. The National Strategy for Quality Improvement in Health (National Quality Strategy) (U.S. Department of Health & Human Services, 2014) proposes three goals for quality improvement: (1) improve patient-centered quality care,

(2) support proven interventions, and (3) reduce the cost of care. One of the priorities of the National Quality Strategy is the provision of effective prevention and treatment practices. These aims and practices are affected by health information technology (HIT) innovations that are changing the landscape of advanced practice nursing. The Institute of Medicine (IOM) (2011) in their report on nursing's future emphasizes the expanding role of advanced practice registered nurses

(APRNs) and the need for HIT to coordinate quality and safe care across health professionals. There is no question that there is growing emphasis on HIT in health care as is evident by the increasing role of government in HIT innovation and implementation.

The Health Information Technology for Economic Clinical Health Act (HITECH), part of the American Recovery and Reinvestment Act of 2009, established the Office of the National Coordinator for Health Information Technology (ONC) into law. ONC is charged with ensuring private and protected electronic health information. ONC's authorization includes the implementation and meaningful use (MU) of electronic health records (EHRs) to improve quality, safety, and efficiency of health care (ONC, 2014). The adoption of HIT in the United States has been augmented by the MU financial incentive program offered to individual health providers and health-care systems under the Medicare/Medicaid program. The Centers for Medicare and Medicaid have developed objectives and criteria to determine if a provider qualifies to receive incentives. For example, MU in prescribing and dispensing medications may qualify for reimbursement (Jones et al, 2014; ONC, 2014). The Agency for Healthcare Research and Quality (AHRQ) also focuses on strategies to secure EHRs and to use HIT to improve quality and cost effectiveness in the management of the health and health care of individuals and groups. AHRQ disseminates evidence on how HIT improves quality health care (AHRQ, 2015). Further, the Center for Medicare and Medicaid Innovation (Innovation Center), established under the Affordable Care Act (ACA) of 2010, is charged with testing innovative care and payment models, many of which require an HIT infrastructure (Berenson & Cafarella, 2012).

This chapter will present examples of HIT including the EHR, clinical decision support (CDS), the computerized provider order entry (CPOE), and health information exchanges (HIE). Clinical and educational uses of HIT will be discussed as they are related to genetics or genomics and high-fidelity simulation.

ELECTRONIC HEALTH RECORD

The EHR is a systematic compilation and management of patient health information that can be shared with other providers and across health-care settings. The goals of EHRs include improvement in quality, safety, and efficiency of health care (Centers for Medicare and Medicaid Services [CMS], 2012). The EHR is designed for information sharing not only among providers but between providers and patients. With the provider-patient EHR functionality, patients can have access to their health records, including medical information, laboratory results, summaries, and plans. Patients can also designate individuals who may have access to their records (McMullen et al, 2014). The patient's history, immunizations, laboratory data, medications, progress, and problems are included in the EHR. Advanced EHRs have the additional functions of HIE, the CPOE, and CDS (Menachemi & Collum, 2011).

MU of EHRs focuses on quality, safety, and patient-centered outcomes. The MU program provides financial incentives to qualified providers of Medicare and Medicaid patients to use certified electronic records. The MU EHR incentive program has the following central objectives: (a) protection of patient health record information, (b) use of CDS, (c) CPOE, (d) electronic prescribing, (e) HIE, (f) education specific to the patient, (g) medication reconciliation for transitions in care, (h) patient electronic access, (i) secure messaging, and (j) public health reporting (e.g., immunizations) (CMS, 2015). To receive an incentive payment, a MU-certified EHR that meets MU objectives and criteria must be used (Thurston, 2014). APRNs are eligible for incentives under the Medicaid program but are not recognized as eligible providers under the Medicare MU incentive program (McQuade-Jones, Murphy, Novak, & Sarnowski, 2014).

There are benefits and disadvantages of EHRs. Among the clinical benefits, EHRs and their tools have increased provider adherence to evidence-based guidelines and led to a reduction in medication errors. Specific EHR function and process benefits are e-prescribing, built-in alerts, CDS, and patient access to health records. Organizational benefits include cost savings and accuracy in billing and coding. Potential problems of EHR implementation are costs related to adoption, implementation, and maintenance; ongoing training; and disruption in workflow (Menachemi & Collum, 2011). There also have been problems with how EHRs are designed and how they perform, fragmentation in interoperability, lack of training and competence among uses, and fear of privacy and safety of health information (Narcisse, Kippenbrock, Odell, & Buron, 2013).

McMullen et al (2014) discuss the possible threats to privacy and security of EHRs. These threats may emerge because of transparent security measures and poor password management. The Health Insurance Portability and Accountability Act of 1996 (HIPAA) expanded its privacy and security rules to adopt national standards for electronic health-care technology. The Privacy Rule provides standards for protection of individual health information, whereas the Security Rule sets standards for electronic protected health information (e-PHI) (Office for Civil Rights [OCR], n.d.). APRNs can play an important role in the privacy and security of records by using predetermined secure passwords, sending e-mail or texts only if there is certainty that only the recipient has access to the account, following up when there is a belief that there is erroneous information, and participating in professional development on electronic security and privacy (McMullen et al, 2014).

DATABASES FOR CLINICAL DECISION MAKING/EVIDENCE-BASED PRACTICE

Health Information Exchanges

HIEs are computerized systems that allow patient information to follow the patient from practice to practice and during transitions in care. The goal of HIE is to provide coordination of care in an effective, efficient manner. The three types of HIEs are (1) directed exchange, whereby providers receive or send secure, encrypted patient information such as patient summaries and laboratory data; (2) query-based exchange, allowing the provider to discover health information about the patient, usually in unplanned care such as emergency rooms; and (3) consumer-mediated exchange where consumers are given access to their health information and can share that information with health-care providers and make informed decisions (Williams, Mostashari, Mertz, Hogin, & Atwal, 2012). Fontaine, Ross, Zink, and Schilling (2010) discuss research results of the benefits and barriers in implementing HIEs in primary care. One of the benefits is work efficiency, resulting in improved access to laboratory results, improvement in referrals, and better claims processing. A second benefit is cost savings, especially in the cost of laboratories that deliver test results. Other cost savings reported include reduction in staff time and decreased need for support staff. A third benefit is improvement in

quality and safety of care. Although there is limited research in this area, there is some evidence that HIEs promoted better patient outcomes, reduced patient admissions in hospitals, and led to fewer prescribing errors. Barriers to HIEs include costs for connectivity, hardware, software, transaction fees, and maintenance. Additional barriers include concerns about privacy and liability. Patients may be wary about sharing their health information and providers need to trust entities in which they share patient information. Liability concerns are also a barrier to HIT in general and HIE specifically. Providers worry about not acting on patient data or acting when the data is inaccurate (Fontaine et al, 2010).

Computerized Provider Order Entry

The CPOE is a technology system that allows clinicians to enter medication orders into a computer and transmit orders directly to a pharmacy. At the least, the CPOE has the potential to enhance patient safety by ensuring that orders are legible and complete. The CPOE is paired with the CDS system, which provides prescription-related information on drug safety, allergies, and toxic reactions based on patient laboratory results or drug-to-drug interactions (AHRQ, 2015). A review of studies found that CPOE reduced the number of medication errors by 37% to 80%. However, some studies found that CPOE did not have positive effects because of incongruent workflows and clinician "alert fatigue," whereby the clinician ignored critical alerts because of excessive nonspecific alerts (Jones et al, 2014). The CPOE and CDS technologies are complex and require health-care organizations to identify goals and workflow needs (Kuperman et al, 2007). CPOE and CDS systems also need to guard against "alert fatigue" by designing systems that provide more specific, evidence-based alerts.

Clinical Decision Support

CDS provides timely evidence-based information to clinicians, staff, patients, and others to inform decisions as care is being delivered. CDS tools include particular condition order sets, focused patient data sets, health preventive care reminders, computerized alerts, clinical guidelines, and health information databases (AHRQ, 2015). Examples of the use of CDS applications in a variety of clinical areas of care include (a) screening, immunizations, guidelines for secondary prevention; (b) diagnosis-specific treatment guidelines, drug management, dosage, alerts for drug interactions, and drug formulary guidelines; and (c) alerts about duplicative testing (Berner, 2009).

Operational Applications of HIT

Human resources will be affected because of HIT implementation. Changes may include decreases in some areas such as administration and increases in specialty areas such as health-care informatics. There will also be a heightened focus on a geographical shift of health professionals from big cities to rural communities and a shift of health-care delivery from tertiary care facilities to the community and home. Roles of health-care professionals will also change. For example, APRNs may be able to do minor surgical procedures in rural settings with medical assistance through telecommunication and robotics (Anvari, 2007).

The adoption of EHRs, HIEs, and CDS has facilitated health-care management, improved coordination and communication between patient and provider, and reinforced safety. However, as the focus of care management shifts to the community and a population health focus, there is a gap in technology and HIT interoperability (Allen et al, 2014). In a model care management program in communities, Allen et al highlight the efforts and challenges of data standardization, system interoperability, and HIE in community settings. Because no community is the same, work needs to be done on policy and implementation of HITs in these settings.

Staffing decisions in organizations using HIT focus on the organization's priorities in maximizing quality and safety, as well as improved efficiency. These staffing decisions depend more on retraining staff than on staff reduction. A different care management approach is optimizing the roles of the interdisciplinary team because of HIT implementation (Goldsack, Chem, & Robinson, 2014).

CLINICAL AND EDUCATIONAL APPLICATIONS

Genetics and Genomics

Scientific discoveries in the field of genomics are rapidly changing the delivery of care by APRNs and other health-care providers. Genetic or genomic information personalizes care because much of individual disease susceptibility

and response to medications is thought to have a genetic component (Bancroft, 2013). Leading causes of morbidity and mortality such as cardiovascular disease, cancer, and diabetes all have a genetic element that is influenced by lifestyle and environmental factors. Although medications are given in accurate doses and taken correctly, adverse drug effects may occur because of individual genetic markers (Calzone et al, 2010). Pasche and Absher (2011) postulate that the advances in genetics and genomics have the potential to provide personalized genomic treatment to the patient. An example of personalized genomic treatment is found in the field of oncology. Cancer research and treatment has been spearheaded by the sequencing of the person's entire genome and the tumor genome (Pasche & Absher, 2011). Cancer risk assessment, tumor outlining, pharmacogenomics treatment, and targeted therapy are now possible (Monteiro-Santos et al, 2013).

It is evident that genetics and genomics research and technology will provide APRNs and other health-care providers as well as the recipients of health care with important diagnostic and therapeutic information. Screening of individuals across the developmental spectrum can identify and characterize health conditions, spotlight the risk of genetic abnormalities and disease, and inform management (McCormick & Calzone, 2016). Brennan (2015) points out that the pharmacological management of individuals often depends on the APRN's knowledge of genetics and pharmacogenomics testing. Microarray testing can identify individuals who are poor metabolizers, slow metabolizers, or normal metabolizers of specific drugs. APRNs need knowledge from relevant HIT databases to increase their knowledge of pharmacogenomics and to decide which patients to test and how to interpret the results (Brennan, 2015).

APRNs also need to be aware that there is an industry for direct-to-consumer (DTC) personal genetic and personal genomic testing to explain susceptibility to disease. The expectation of the consumer may be for the APRN to interpret the findings and help in their health-care decision making (Loud, 2010). The dilemma is that there are insufficient regulations on DTC genetic tests or the laboratories that perform the tests. Knowledge of the risks and benefits of these tests are relatively unknown (Loud, 2010; Thrush & McCaffrey, 2010). With the advances in genetics and genomics, APRNs need knowledge of genetics and genomics, predictive genetic testing, and DTC testing. They must also be aware of ethical challenges, policies, and standards relative to genetics and genomics and how advances in knowledge in the field will improve interventions.

High-Fidelity Simulation and Advanced Practice Nursing

Simulation is defined as a technology for practice and learning in health care that can be applied to many disciplines (Gaba, 2004). It has been a teaching strategy for educating nurses for many years. It is a recommended strategy to teach safe clinical practice, in part because initial learning for health-care professionals in a real patient setting is hindered by shorter length of patient stays, higher patient acuity, staff shortages, and greater emphasis on medical errors (Medley & Horne, 2005).

Maintaining skills competencies can be challenging for advanced practice nurses (APNs) (Stephenson, Zeynep, & Cullen, 2015). It is important for APRNs to maintain competence in not only high-risk, low-frequency skills but also with emerging HITs such as EHRs. High-fidelity simulation is a strategy that can allow APRNs to maintain competency as well as develop more confidence in the use of HIT in a wide variety of situations and clinical settings, including complex patients, emergent situations, and low-frequency patient encounters; all without risk to actual patients. Utilizing simulated experiences in advanced practice curriculums as well as in competency measurement can ensure successful outcomes for patients. Simulation has also been shown to improve clinical reasoning skills in APN practitioners (Mompoint-Williams et al, 2014).

Individual high-fidelity scenarios can utilize other technologies available to APNs such as noninvasive testing and electronic patient records. The technology of simulation allows for additional training beyond the traditional didactic approach. Because the clinical environment may not lend itself to routine exposure to certain skills, the simulated environment becomes paramount in maintaining competency and positive patient outcomes. Setting up the simulation experience is very important to ensuring learning objectives are met. The participants will be able to perform realistic scenarios only in environments that mirror the real world setting. Also, participants must be able to reflect on their experience during a debriefing period. This important learning tool should immediately follow the simulated experience and allow participants to give honest feedback on what went well and also what they may have done differently.

There is evidence that simulated experiences are beneficial to APNs. In a study by Kowitlawakul et al (2015) APN students in Singapore reported increased confidence in their ability to care for patients in the clinical setting after participating in various simulated experiences. Participants also felt the experiences were useful in helping to develop skills in history taking, communication, and caring for patients with rapidly changing conditions. Simulation is also effective for APNs in maintaining competency. In a study of neonatal nurse practitioners, Stephenson et al (2015) found that nurses who participated in a respiratory distress simulation had better retention of knowledge and were all able to successfully intubate the simulator at 3 and 6 months post-simulation experience.

CONCLUSION

Health care is becoming more and more global and the effective use of technology will be necessary for APNs to provide effective nursing care. Emerging technologies such as telehealth will be available to health-care professionals and patients. Telehealth and any new emerging technological advancement should be integrated with existing HIT systems to increase the quality of care in patients in underserved areas. APNs have used information technologies to document health history and physical findings, evaluate laboratory and procedure findings, order tests and medications, and to bill for patient services (Swenty & Titzer, 2014). It is imperative that with the use of emerging HITs, APRNs have the education to implement and evaluate these technologies in patient care.

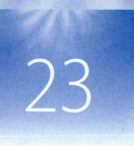

Writing for Publication

Shirley A. Smoyak

Learning Outcomes

Learning outcomes expected as a result of this chapter:

- Design personal strategies for getting into the habit of writing for publication.
- Select from the many types of publications for which to write, including letters to the editor and professional newsletters.
- Understand the differences between writing for refereed journals vs. book chapters and other non-refereed media.
- Determine how to know what is known and what is not about a particular topic.
- Write in an expository style.
- Design literature reviews by selecting key words and search options.
- Understand how the review process is designed and how the reviews affect potential authors.

INTRODUCTION

Nurses have good ideas. These stem from their education and experience, where observation was learned as the bedrock of practice. Nurses observe not only by using their eyes but all their other senses as well, including intuition. Sharing these observations leads to improved clinical practice. Others with whom these observations are shared can create a scholarly dialogue, the outcome of which might be evidence-based practice or hypotheses for study.

Although all RNs are good observers, advanced practice nurses (APNs) include within their domain the need to share by writing for publication. Unfortunately, the skills for such writing are often not within their curricular plans in their academic programs of study. The intent of this chapter is to provide the needed background so that writing becomes not only a goal but an actual achievement.

Before delving into the specific suggestions for writing for publication, I first want to let you know what *not* to do. *Never* attempt to write your first sentence first. This should be the last thing that you do. Concentrate instead on what your final message will be. What is it that your readers should have as a "take home"? What points do you want them to remember? The second thing *not* to do is to write in the second person, because usually that sounds too preachy. However, you will see that I am already doing that. I chose to use the second person because I am trying to have my messages to you delivered as if I were actually facing you in a conversation. It's unfortunate that chapters in books don't allow easy dialogue with authors.

HOW TO GET THE WRITING HABIT

Eons ago, when a guest lecturer at the Rutgers University Alexander Library in New Brunswick, New Jersey, delivered his suggestions to the invited audience of editors and authors, this piece of his advice remained with me: "Writing should be like brushing your teeth or walking your dog." His points were: (a) Habits are automatic; make writing automatic. (b) Select the time of day when you are at your sharpest. Are you a morning or evening person? When do you do your best thinking and working? (c) Assure a space where you will not be interrupted. Choose a place at home where your closed door means to others that you are not to be disturbed. It is probably much more difficult to dedicate such a space and time at work. (d) Limit your writing to 30 minutes; fewer minutes might work, but don't try for an hour.

What you write should be simply what comes to your mind. Develop sentences from the rambling thoughts that go around in your head. Don't worry about punctuation and syntax. Just commit words to your document. These words should come from your own experiences, ideas, issues, or concerns. They might also be observations (any of your senses) that you had never articulated as written descriptions. If you are staring at your blank screen and seem at a loss about what to write, start with what you observed yesterday, or this morning, or what happened as you dreamt.

Making a commitment to yourself to make daily writing automatic will assure that writing will become a part of yourself, a new You. You might find it useful to share this commitment with a relative or close friend. If you have children or teens, they need to know about this new approach of yours and honor your request to be left alone during your writing time. If need be, walk the dog first. Your teeth can probably wait.

APPROACHES TO WRITING

Just as I suggested that you never try to write the first sentence first, another thing not to do first is to attempt to write an article for a professional journal. There are easier, simpler approaches (e.g., the first few items in the text that follows) more likely to have you see your name in print.

Published Minutes

Organizations that publish their minutes, either digitally or in print, need someone to write articulate sentences. If the organization wants others (members and nonmembers) to know what their meetings have addressed, then a fuller account of what happened is necessary. Reprinting the agenda with associated resolutions is not sufficient. This role does not have to fall within the domain of the elected secretary; volunteers may offer to take this on with the approval of the president or board. There needs to be an agreement about whether or not these full minutes will be edited and by whom.

Letters to the Editor

Letters to the editor are welcomed by most professional nursing societies and associations for their newspapers or shorter, published reports. Local and state lay newspapers also welcome such letters. The letter may be about agreeing or disagreeing with a recent news report or article. Be sure to cite the entire source to which you are referring. Your statements may be based on your own experiences or you may use resources from the literature. Your letter should follow the format of those that have already been printed. Timeliness is a factor; waiting too long (more than a week) after the item to which you want to respond is not a good idea. If your letter refers to a journal article, then the prior issue should be the focus. If you are writing about a book, then the most recent printing is needed.

Another format is to write about an issue that you think needs more attention by the press. For instance, for a nursing journal, you might address a new clinical phenomenon that has not been covered in recent months. You might also want the editor to develop a special issue addressing the DNP/PhD approaches to the doctorate or why all specialty associations should be integrated with the American Nurses Association.

Newsletter Articles or Reports

The previous paragraph might also serve as the array of topics about which you might write. New clinical ideas or interventions that are not systematic studies or actual research can be described as innovations. To do this, of course, the management of the unit, agency, or hospital must agree that they want this to be disclosed. If you are writing a short "opinion" piece, unless management or administration is addressed, then it can be offered as yours alone. Minutes sometimes refer to a project having been completed by the association or one that is being planned. Expanded descriptions would lend themselves to reports.

Also, associations sometimes publish reports of proceedings of a convention or conference. These include short synopses of keynote addresses or major presentations. The next section describes how these may become monographs.

Monographs

Societies or associations occasionally publish the proceedings of conventions or conferences in an expanded format. To produce a monograph, the keynote and major presenters must submit an expanded synopsis of their talks or workshops, sometimes including illustrations, tables, or graphs. Your role in such an endeavor might be (a) that you are the presenter who submits your document for the monograph, or (b) that you volunteer to be the editor who prepares the separate pieces for publication.

Book or Video Reviews

Nursing journals and newspapers are publishing book or video reviews much less frequently now that online avenues for dissemination of such reviews have entered our media possibilities. Ten years ago, many journals had a specific column for reviews, and even a column editor. That is no longer the case. On the other hand, if there is a groundbreaking book, such as that by the Institute of Medicine (IOM), *The Future of Nursing* (2011), then not only is there a book review but many more reviewers expressing analyses.

The previous subsections are volunteer efforts; writers rarely are paid for their products. For the next sections, there may be payment of some form such as an honorarium.

Chapters in Books

To be asked to write a chapter for a book, you first have to be an expert in your field and recognized as such. You will have come to the attention of your colleagues by having presented speeches, lectures, workshops, videos, or journal articles with increasing frequency. The focus of these books may be entirely clinical phenomena, or policy issues, or compendia on new teaching/education/administration matters.

Mason and her associates (2002) served as editors for *Policy & Politics in Nursing and Health Care,* one of the first books to have this focus. Although this first issue is more than 10 years old, it is still widely quoted from and is an excellent source for historical issues. Each chapter stands alone and is written by experts in their fields.

An example is a chapter written by Beverly Malone (when she was the CEO of the Royal College of Nursing, London) and me, titled "Managed Care and Mental Health: A Mixture of Optimism and Caution" (Malone & Smoyak, 2002). In retrospect, more should have been said about the "caution" part.

Occasionally announcements about a book being planned are advertised via various professional social media. Topics and required expertise are listed.

If you know the book editor, then a phone call or e-mail would be in order. If the editor is not known, then your response or proposal should be sent the way that the announcement directs. Attaching not only your area of expertise or idea for a chapter but also a one-page, abbreviated curriculum vitae (CV) is a good idea. This short CV should highlight your areas of expertise; note should be made of any recent works of yours that have been published. Be sure to include an e-mail address that you check daily, as well as a cell phone number.

Journal Articles (Refereed and Non-Refereed)

Writing articles for journals requires the greatest skill and expertise or experience.

- Identifying your audience is the first step. To whom are you writing? Are they novices or expert clinicians? Are they associate, baccalaureate, or master's and above prepared?

- Are you writing about what is new to you, alone (you have just discovered this), or is the topic or issue new to others, too? In order to answer this question, a thorough search of the literature must be done.
- The first question that journal editors ask is: "What's new?"
- How will you select the journal for which your article is written? Searching the literature, to answer the point in the second bulleted item in this list, will also lead you to the journals whose domain is yours.
- What does the selected journal require for submissions? Guidelines for authors appear in journal websites and are occasionally printed in hard copy. These guidelines are very detailed; authors would do well to become familiar with all their rules and requirements. More will be said in the text that follows under The Formal Review Process and about the role of editors.

Books

There is a very wide variety of books. Their domains, formats, length, authorship (solo author, edited), and so on, differ considerably. This is not an avenue to which a novice author might aspire. The exception is that the research undertaken for a PhD might lend itself to becoming a book. For instance, years ago Carol Germain studied cancer wards and how patients, families, physicians, and professional staff interacted. Her book, *The Cancer Unit* (1979), was highly acclaimed and is still being used as a resource today.

Editorials

The majority of the nursing journals publish editorials in each issue, whether the journal is published monthly or less frequently. Usually the editorial is written by the editor-in-chief, but sometimes it is delegated to a guest. Editorials also appear in newsletters and lay newspapers.

The following are the most common formats for editorials: (a) They may simply "point" to what is in the current issue, making note of the importance of the topics and articles. (b) They may give a scholarly opinion about issues facing the profession. (c) Similar to (b) is an editorial suggesting questions that should be asked but have not been covered by the press. (d) There may be an interpretation of facts about current findings, reports, and literature. (e) The editor may ask: "What's right and what's wrong?" in the lay press about how health care is addressed.

Recent editorials I have written focus on a few of the previously noted points. In June (Smoyak, 2016a) I asked whether our readers considered themselves to be coddlers or challengers. The impetus for this topic was the unfortunate new expectation that students should be protected against intrusions into their personal comfort. In August (Smoyak, 2016c) I asked: "What's in a name?" The new alphabet soup was the topic, and readers were asked how familiar each of the new designations was to them.

PREPARATION FOR DOING THE WRITING WORK

The previous section listed the types of approaches you might take when considering in what venue to write. This section will provide some preliminary steps to take as you prepare to become an author.

Step One: Get Organized

Gather your data, ideas, vignettes, case examples, notes about opinions, and other material in a filing system that works for you. Younger folks are more committed to digital files and folders into which they put their own documents, as well as PDFs of articles to which they might refer, or news reports of interest, or other graphics that might be used at a future point. Older folks, such as me, prefer the old-fashioned three-cut file folders that can be labeled and then put into large accordion folders. My current folders are titled: Nurse-Physician Debate/Dialogue; Coddling or Challenging; Electronic Files and Health Records; Ethics of Publishing. Flip through the contents of these folders every few weeks to be reminded of your interests and what you have collected.

Step Two: Sort Out the Following Areas or Questions

As previously mentioned, you need to be in touch with what you have just discovered, but is it something that others already know about? If this item is new, how has it been covered in the recent literature?

From the literature, what are the recurring issues that we should be thinking about or studying? Hand-in-hand with these suggestions, of course, is the fact that reading widely is mandatory. Reading should include worldwide news beyond health care. Coverage on TV or various news clips is not sufficient to tell the whole story, nor to get both sides of a story. Often, of course, there are more than two sides, with opposing sides being divided into further, nested subcategories.

Step Three: Use Expository Style

Practice daily, writing marvelous, complete, engaging sentences. Putting words around observations is a good way to begin. In my folders, I collect great sentences that others have written. From an unknown source, there is: "Eschew obfuscatory scrivenry!" (Avoid convoluted writing.) This would be a fine sign to place above your computer.

Aim to be clear and explicit rather than vague and ambiguous. Every controversial statement needs to be documented. Journal editors, including me, frequently query: How do you know that?

Work on transitions between paragraphs. The end of each paragraph should signal what will follow. The entire document should have integrated paragraphs. My best role model for such writing was Gerald Grob, a Rutgers historian known worldwide for his analysis of mental hospitals and institutions and the patterns that patients endured over the years. Select books of his are in the Bibliography. If transitions occur between paragraphs, then the main points, from beginning to end, are not lost.

There should be no surprises. New ideas should not appear in the summary or conclusion.

Step Four: Know Your Resources

Become familiar with manuals of style, handbooks for writers, copyright law, expectations regarding reporting conflicts of interest, and how to assign the order of authors when there are more than one.

A classic handbook is Strunk (2009), *The Elements of Style*. My favorite "how to" is William Zinsser's, *On Writing Well* (1980). Among his marvelous sentences: "Clutter is the disease of American writing. We are a society strangling in unnecessary words, circular constructions, pompous frills and meaningless jargon" (p. 7). There is never a need to use "utilize" or "utilization" when "use" will do.

Step Five and Beyond

Get rid of the belief, if you harbor it, that you can write something and it will be perfect with no revision needed. Abraham Lincoln's famous: "Forgive me, I did not have time to make this brief," illustrates that the way to perfection is to take the time to analyze, re-write, and revise. Think drafts, not final products. Ask colleagues to read your drafts and to make comments. Resist the urge to be defensive; rather, consider their suggestions seriously.

Not a Step: Query Letters

Novice authors sometimes believe that writing a query letter to the editor of a journal to which they wish to submit an article is a good idea. It is not. Any question can be answered by consulting the Guidelines for Authors or reading several issues of the proposed journal. Asking an editor if a proposed topic is of interest is a waste of the editor's time. He or she does not know how well you write, what literature you have searched, or what your plan is. If anything, you will get a standard, boiler-plate response such as, "Without further information, I cannot answer your query."

Query letters have been addressed by editors of nursing journals when we meet annually for conferences for the International Academy of Nursing Editors (INANE). The consensus among these editors is that the perpetrators of the bad advice to write query letters comes mostly from faculty. We know that faculty assign graduate students the task of writing a query letter as part of a course. We have a suspicion that these faculty members are not published authors themselves. Students should be wary about those from whom they receive such advice. My advice is that you ask a faculty member making such an assignment to show you a letter that she or he has written and ask for the response. Then, be sure to examine that faculty member's CV and study the published articles in refereed journals. Unfortunately, this bad advice also appears in books and articles about writing.

REVIEWING THE LITERATURE

A careful and thorough review of the literature will answer two questions: (1) What is it that I should know? and (2) How will I know what's fact or fiction, opinion or science, and how writers derived their sources?

Evidence-based practice is the expectation today not only for clinical matters but also for administration, management, and teaching. Evidence-based practice and science are closely intertwined but are not the same. In a recent presentation to editors of nursing journals, Goldacre (Smoyak, 2016b) challenged us to do better about how we report science. Using his book, *Bad Science* (2008), he provided definitions and illustrations of accurate evidence-based practice and good science, showing how a great many of the supposedly scientific articles about health care are seriously flawed.

Bad science is ignoring the consensus built during decades by researchers about how to conduct a proper study. Goldacre provides gentle reminders about the processes that scientists must execute in order to test theories adequately and publish them fully. He documents the wrongs perpetuated when only positive or significant findings are reported and promotes evidence-based health care built on science, not opinion or hearsay. This reader-friendly book can serve as a reminder about the steps in research and how reports should be written.

Goldacre's second book, *Bad Pharma* (2012), is a more in-depth documentation of problems in medicine, particularly missing trials. When randomized clinical trials (RCT) could have easily been done, he shows that shoddy short-cuts and misrepresentations about the data occur regularly. In the process of documenting poor research designs, he provides very clear short lessons and reminders about what good science is. You would do well to place this book on your "must read" list.

Goldacre's third book (2014), *I Think You'll Find It's a Bit More Complicated Than That,* is a very good illustration about how alternative paths may lead to a book. This is a collection of his columns and papers, published in newspapers and journals, and delivered at conferences and conventions. Beyond being an author, he is a broadcaster and an entertainer, so these pages are filled with stories that have delighted audiences and produced gales of laughter.

Goldacre's nearly 400 pages are arranged as snippets from his columns and lectures. Each can be read individually, selecting from the fascinating titles. These include: "Kids Who Spot Bullshit, and the Adults Who Get Upset by It"; "The Stigma Gene"; "A New and Interesting Form of Wrong"; and "Pornography in Hospitals." My personal favorite is "How Do You Know?" I make this query very often when I write to prospective authors, telling them that their manuscript needs serious revision. I am always amazed at the controversial statements potential authors make as if they were conclusive facts (Smoyak, 2016b).

Revisiting your academic library is also a very good idea. Librarians are excellent sources for how to access databases; they all have their favorite search engines and methods and are quite willing to share them. Many of the larger libraries have an "Ask a librarian" feature whereby you can e-mail your question but also set up face-to-face help appointments. Several times each semester, as a service to new faculty and students, there are refresher courses that include topics such as selecting key words, Boolean logic, and what articles or books can be accessed for free from their cooperating network of academic libraries.

Large hospital systems and other institutions (such as insurance agencies) frequently have arrangements with university libraries, allowing their employees to use the reference materials. Alumni associations also are sources for avenues to using libraries.

Beyond the wealth of data and information about literature sources, many libraries also have their own version of reference management systems, such as End-Note. Depending on the library, a personal reference system that a person may have set up while a student can continue to be accessed after graduation. However, there may be time limits imposed or fees attached.

Databases are described in the text that follows, but university libraries are also grand sources beyond the specific systems mentioned. Exploring their home pages and what exists in the many drop-down menus yields a wealth of opportunities for countless options that can be accessed. Users need to become aware of the access rules. Current full-time faculty have the widest access options but alumni can use these resources also.

Databases

The two databases most frequently used by nurse writers are MEDLINE (Medical Literature, Analysis and Retrieval System Online) and CINAHL (Cumulative Index to

Nursing and Allied Health Literature). MEDLINE was developed originally in 1949 by the National Library of Medicine (NLM) and is continuously updated. The National Center for Biotechnology Information (NCBI) is within NLM. Today, there are more than 20 million journal citations gleaned from more than 5,000 biomedical journals worldwide. Searches can be conducted via PubMed at http://www.ncbi.nlm.nih.gov/pubmed/. MeSH stands for Medical Subject Headings, but you may also use key words, authors, titles of journals, or publication dates. Depending on your access route and what your library has paid for, abstracts only may be available, but full text is also possible.

CINAHL is more recent, beginning in 1961, and is a comprehensive database of nursing and allied health literature, whereas MEDLINE includes all biomedical sources. CINAHL indexes more than 3,000 journals; nearly 100 are full text. Digital access is via EBSCO, http://www.ebscohost.com/cinahl/.

The Cochrane Collection is an international not-for-profit organization of health professionals who also hold academic appointments. Sir Iain Chalmers is its founder. For more than 30 years they have produced systematic summaries of the research literature on health-care studies, many of them RCTs, and many meta-analyses. They also invite people to submit clinical questions that need answers to inform clinical practice. As Goldacre notes (2008), "This careful sifting of information has revealed huge gaps in knowledge . . . revealing that 'best practices' were sometimes murderously flawed, and simply by sifting methodically through pre-existing data, it has saved more lives than you could possibly imagine" (p. 99). Goldacre provides an example. The Cochrane Review examined deaths from any cause (230,000 cases) in all the placebo-controlled randomized trials on antioxidants. Some had very high doses, but were in line with what could be purchased in health-food stores. "This (analysis) showed that overall, antioxidant vitamin pills do not reduce deaths, and in fact they may increase your chance of dying" (p. 107).

Another rich and complete source of clinical data is https://www.guideline.gov maintained by the U.S. Department of Health & Human Services as part of its Agency for Healthcare Research and Quality (AHRQ). This system incorporates the National Guideline Clearing House (NGC), which directs the investigator to clinical practice "statements that include recommendations to optimize care that are informed by a systematic review of evidence and an assessment of the benefits and harms of alternative care options" (NGC, 2016). As previously noted, librarians can lead you to still other databases, depending on the topics and areas you are trying to review.

As you are conducting a thorough review of the literature on your given topic with selected key words, these references need to be committed to a chart, such as Excel, with rows and columns. Each row is for a given reference, and the columns need headers that you develop, such as year, number of subjects, type of article, and chief results. The references may also be grouped as (a) opinions or consensus, (b) qualitative designs, (c) quantitative approaches, (d) summaries of other reviews, or (e) systematic analyses. Color coding or other notes can indicate the potential usefulness for your work.

The references should also be placed in End-Note or another referencing system. Such systems are able to provide points in your citations that you may have missed, such as an author, city of publishing, proper name of publisher, and similar items. You also may select the required design, such as Chicago Manual of Style, American Psychological Association, or others. In whatever form you entered items for the citation, the system will order them correctly (including numeric use and upper/lower cases).

Nurse Author & Editor

Nurse Author & Editor is not a database, but it is a very useful international newsletter published by Wiley-Blackwell on a quarterly basis. This free, online, expanded newsletter features articles about creating quality manuscripts, finding publishing opportunities, reporting new developments, and generating topics for articles. It is available at www .NurseAuthorEditor.com.

The Impact Factor

In order to address the question of how credible or important a given journal is, the Thomson Corporation, using the Institute of Scientific Information (ISI), devised the Impact Factor. Broadly speaking, this factor measures the worth of a journal, using the number of citations that articles within it, in a certain time period, are cited by other authors in refereed journals. "Specifically, the Impact Factor for a given year is defined as the total number of citations received by the journal in that year to articles published over the previous two years, divided by the total number of citable items published by the journal in that two year period" (Webb, 2008, p. 18).

Most nursing journals do not yet have Impact Factors. To gain inclusion into the ISI database, journals must be invited to submit their proposals and then a vetting process begins. An ISI editor assesses the proposal by examining the regularity of publication, profile of the editorial team, whether it is peer-reviewed, and whether its contents are relevant and topical. INANE has been very persuasive in getting ISI to include more nursing journals into their invited group.

There is no consensus today among university nurse faculty about whether or not Impact Factors should be considered when reviewing a faculty member's credentials and determining whether promotion or tenure is warranted.

THE FORMAL REVIEW PROCESS

Evaluative Questions

Both small (readership under 500) and large (thousands of subscribers) journals have reviewers use systematic questions when evaluating manuscripts. Although these have a degree of variability in their style and method of questioning, the following questions are asked by most. These questions would be a good checklist for you to use as you evaluate your drafts.

1. Are there new ideas or a new look at old ideas or information?
2. Is the writing clear and reader-friendly?
3. Are the references relevant and up-to-date? Are important ones missing?
4. Is there evidence for conclusions, clinical interventions, or recommendations?
5. Are the sources for the evidence indicated as the author's own or from the literature?
6. Are clinical implications clear, practical, and useful?
7. If relevant, is the cost indicated? Who pays for what and how?
8. If this is a research report, are the methods clearly and adequately described (sample, instruments, design, analysis)?

9. If tables and charts are included, are they complete and clear?
10. If the manuscript is credible and well-written, would it be more appropriate for another journal?

Some journals use a yes/no format for these questions, whereas others use a Likert scale of some type. There is usually space allocated for the reviewer to suggest additional points, in a narrative format, to the editor-in-chief.

Types of Decisions

Again, there is variability in how reviewers are asked for their "bottom line" or what their final suggested decision is. The most common examples are:

- Accept, revise, reject
- Revise—but—an indication that this might be a reject
- Poor, average, excellent
- A numeric scale, with high and low indicated

Required Disclosures

Authors are required to indicate what role they played in writing the manuscript, to acknowledge that they understand what is meant by copyright, and to state any potential conflicts of interest. Each of these points is covered in the text that follows.

Author's Role

Authors are asked to say (mandatory) what part they played in the writing: (a) conception and design, (b) data collection, or (c) analysis and interpretation. Also, did they (a) actually write the manuscript, or (b) critically revise the manuscript? Although not mandatory, they are also often asked about: (a) statistical expertise, (b) obtaining funding, (c) administrative, technical, or material support, or (d) supervision.

Copyright

A copyright transmittal statement is required. For Slack publications, the language is: "In consideration of Slack, Incorporated taking action in reviewing my (our) manuscript, the author undersigned hereby transfers, assigns, or otherwise conveys copyright ownership of the text and any accompanying images (including video) to Slack, Incorporated in the event that said work is published by Slack, Incorporated" (Slack, 2011).

The statement goes on to define worldwide rights, print, electronic and web formats, and what is meant by collective formats, and asks whether the author is a federal employee. Signatures are required of solo and group authors. Bear in mind that copyright refers to printed words, not the ideas or plans that authors may have that are not yet committed to print. Owners of journals determine the methods by which published articles may be shared.

Copyright has been the traditional means by which publishers assure that their printed material is safe from various kinds of theft. However, some publishers now allow the signing of an Exclusive License Form, the general purpose being that the author retains copyright, but that the publisher is given "Exclusive License" to publish the author's material (Webb, 2008).

Form for Disclosure

Most journals use the International Committee of Medical Journal Editors (ICMJE) form for disclosure. This multi-page form has four parts: (1) identifying information, (2) the work under consideration for publication, (3) relevant financial activities outside the submitted work, and (4) other relationships. For the second section, questions include whether payment or an honorarium was received, whether there was grant support, if writing assistance or administrative support occurred, or whether or not travel was supported. Under the third section, questions include board membership, consultancy, expert testimony, or fees for lectures.

Who's Who?

Larger journals have both a panel for new reviewers and people designated as "reviewer," who are more senior folks. The reviewers sometimes are constituted as a "board of review," which generally means that they are expected to write articles themselves, as well as to solicit manuscripts from others. They may be expected to write editorials, suggest new columns and directions, and attend board meetings. Both panels and reviewers represent specialties, geographic areas, and domains such as academics, administrators, managers, clinicians, and consultants.

Very large journals sometimes have panels with hundreds of reviewers, each with a designated area of expertise. This group is only called upon when the editor needs a content expert or a research or statistics expert. Some may only be called on once a year or less often. Their names are not usually listed on the masthead.

The "inside" editor is an employee of the publisher who has expert editorial credentials. She or he may have a staff of additional copy editors, graphic artists, and so on. The "outside" editor is the editor-in-chief, selected by the publisher to head a journal. Terms of office may be designated or not. How they are paid is proprietary information.

For some journals, editor-in-chief means precisely that: "in chief." For others, there is more of a team approach. My journal, *Journal of Psychosocial Nursing & Mental Health Services* (JPN), and I belong to the latter group.

Panel members and full reviewers are selected similarly. They are expected to be experts in their clinical field or specialty or be acknowledged for their administrative, management, or teaching skills. Journals whose mission is reporting research must have a track record of funded and published studies. They generally come from wide geographic areas in the United States and may come from other countries.

Full reviewers are generally more experienced and have considerably more published articles in refereed journals. They may also have served on other editorial boards or been a reviewer for association publications such as newsletters and monographs. The quality of their review is expected to be stellar, and they are expected to be contributing authors. A large part of their role is to solicit manuscripts for submission and to make suggestions for quality improvement in all areas, such as new columns. Frequently, they are expected to submit at least an editorial from time to time.

Most editors-in-chief keep some type of report card for both panel and full review members. These are shared individually, sometimes in face-to-face sessions at meetings.

The final decision about a submitted manuscript is made by the editor-in-chief. Because reviewers are so diverse in their backgrounds and expertise domains, it is not unusual for three reviewers to have three different evaluations: one accept, one reject, and another revise. It is the editor's role to consider all three very carefully and then make a judgment about the final outcome.

Ideally, the editor then constructs a letter to the potential author relaying the decision, along with the reasons for it. For instance, if the decision is to reject, then the letter must be very clear and exact so that the potential author does not misconstrue what is being said as "revise." If the decision is to revise, very explicit, numbered points must be constructed and the author(s) told to use this numeric system when responding. One author is designated as the one to communicate with the editor. If the decision is to accept, some minor revision points may be needed.

Very occasionally, a potential author might disagree totally or in part with what the editor's letter states. If the objection is that the decision should not have been a reject, the editor may reach out and suggest a telephone call. If the decision is to revise and the author does not want to do what is suggested, constituting major disagreement with the advice, then the decision may shift to reject.

Some editors return revised manuscripts to the original reviewers. This is less likely to be the case when the separate reviews are integrated into one complete, thorough letter. Potential authors need clear communication and messages that cannot be flawed or vague. Editors who send all the comments from the reviewers to the authors are doing them a disservice.

When I encounter authors during exchanges about their submissions and I sense an air of defensiveness, I always point out the following: (a) Editors are your best friends. They want to help you to improve your writing, not just criticize or dismantle. (b) Editors will never become your co-authors. They work only behind the scenes. (c) If you disagree with what the editors are saying, take care to be thorough and explicit about your objections.

OPEN ACCESS

According to the Budapest Open Access Initiative (OA): "By 'open access' to this literature we mean its free availability on the public Internet, permitting any users to read, download, copy, distribute, print, search, or link to the full text of these articles, crawl them for indexing, pass them as data to software, or use them for any other lawful purpose, without financial, legal, or technical barriers other than those inseparable from gaining access to the Internet itself." OA can be accessed at http://www.budapestopenaccessinitiative.org/read.

Types of Open Access

OA may be classified as either gold or green. Gold OA occurs when authors publish in an OA journal that provides immediate free access to all its articles on the publisher's website. Hybrid OA journals provide gold OA only for those individual articles for which their authors (or their author's institution or funder) pay an OA publishing fee.

Green OA, also known as self-archiving, occurs when authors publish in any journal and then self-archive a version of the article for free public use in their institutional repository, in a central repository (such as PubMed Central), or on some other OA website (such as a subject-specific one).

Why Open Access?

Usually authors seek OA to their work for one of two reasons: (1) They personally want the article to be freely available on the open Internet, or (2) their funder has specified that the article must be made freely available on the open Internet. NIH is such an organization. This is not to be confused with copyright restrictions (see the section that follows on plagiarism) or public domain availability, which may occur when a copyright has lapsed or when no restrictions govern the document, such as occurs with many government publications.

PLAGIARISM

Plagiarism is essentially theft of someone else's words, documents, or materials that have been published. It is a crime of theft of intellectual property. Plagiarism occurs whenever an author fails to acknowledge the source of words, phrases, or entire paragraphs, charts, or tables. Adequate and appropriate documentation needs to be provided for any printed material that is not the author's own. Another version of plagiarism occurs when authors use words or statements that they have made in other published work, but do not provide the citation or reference. This is "self-plagiarism."

If exact words or statements are borrowed, these need to be placed within quotation marks and the page number(s) given. If graphs or tables are borrowed, there must be a statement from the publisher of this work that such a copying has been permitted. This permission, of course, must be in writing.

Cross-referencing is the term used when editors hire outside sources to check for plagiarism. One system is CrossRef's Similarity Check, which can be used for all submissions to a journal, or the editor might select only those about which there is a question. Some reviewers have asked journal editors to purchase such systems if they are not in a university setting that has already made a blanket purchase. There is agreement about the importance of being able to identify content similarity issues that may signal plagiarism. CrossRef can upload every manuscript before the author notification of acceptance and have them checked against a growing database of millions of published papers by 800+ publishers. Potential "flagged" papers are sent to the editors with notes. Editors determine potential barriers to publication, recognizing that a certain level of self-plagiarism might be acceptable.

WORKSHOPS FOR WRITING

Buyer beware!! Before registering to be a participant, make sure you know the credentials of the person who is the presenter. You might want to refer to the previously mentioned Who's Who.

If the presenter's plan is to give specific feedback about drafts of manuscripts, then the authors need to know in what form this will happen. Will the manuscript be projected in some way and comments made to statements? Or will the courtesy review be private? Will this happen during the convention or workshop time, or afterwards?

During Q & A periods, a question I am frequently asked is whether I ever do or did ghost-writing. My answer is "Yes." If I am then asked if that doesn't bother me, if what I have written is a grant that a dean submits, or a report to the president, that is forwarded from the dean's council, I say "No." I explain that my background is having written for a squirrel. When I was in elementary school, a teacher asked if I wanted to develop and write a column for the broadcaster at the Samuel E. Shull School. I thought a bit—and then offered, "I want to write as if I were the school's mascot, Squiffer E. Squirrel." The teacher was a bit surprised but gave me free reign. My first column was about what Squiffer saw in the teachers' lounge when he visited there. Teachers were smoking!! Of course, in those days teachers were allowed to do this, but many of the students did not know that the teachers smoked, nor that they ate lots of candy and sweets. A big tribute to my teacher, Miss Drysdale, who did not alter what I wrote. And, after some chagrin, the teachers laughed.

So—if I can write for a squirrel, writing for a dean is no problem.

SHARING WHAT'S IN MY FOLDER

At the top of one of my folders, which is marked "Inspiration," are the following sentences by John Gardner (1959) speaking about "On Excellence."

An excellent plumber is infinitely more admirable than an incompetent philosopher. The society which scorns excellent plumbing because plumbing is a humble activity, and tolerates shoddiness in philosophy because it is an exalted activity, will have neither good plumbing nor good philosophy. Neither its pipes nor its theories will hold water.

UNIT

4

Ethical, Legal, and Business Acumen

24

Measuring Advanced Practice Nurse Performance

Outcome Indicators, Models of Evaluation, and the Issue of Value

Shirley Girouard, Patricia DiFusco, and Joseph Jennas

Learning Outcomes

Learning outcomes expected as a result of this chapter:

- Describe the value, quality, and accountability context surrounding advanced practice registered nurse (APRN) practice.
- Understand APRN performance expectations in general and those specific to specialty practice.
- Develop quality and performance measures for use in practice at the individual, group, systems, and societal levels.
- Demonstrate the ability to design a model for assessing structures, processes, and outcomes within a framework of national standards.
- Plan actions to enhance the APRN impact in patient care, education, research, administration, and advocacy or policy.

INTRODUCTION

Performance measurement in the health-care system is ubiquitous and complex. Whomever the provider, whatever the geographic location, whatever the setting, whatever the organization, whomever the stakeholder, whomever the payer, advanced practice nurses (APNs) can expect to have their performance evaluated. APNs, along with other individuals and organizations, must demonstrate that their performance enhances the triple aims of improving care experiences for patients and families, improving the health of populations, and reducing the per capita costs of health care (Berwick, Nolan, & Whittington, 2008). As Whittington, Nolan, Lewis, and Torres (2015) suggest, the triple aims are an integral part of the United States' strategies to improve health outcomes and health care. These aims provide a framework for state and federal initiatives and the work of credentialing, accrediting, and regulatory agencies at all levels influencing the organization, delivery, and financing of health-care services.

To improve care experiences, individual patients and families are encouraged to become more engaged in care and to participate in planning and assuring they receive quality, safe care. To improve outcomes for population health, providers and communities are expected to transform the organization and delivery of services. To reduce health-care costs, care providers and payers are engaged in payment reforms and developing more cost-effective interventions. Reimbursement structures are also being modified. These aims are influenced by several trends related, in part, to the implementation of the Patient Protection and Affordable Care Act (PPACA; Public Law [PL] 111-148) and subsequent policy and administrative changes. Trends and issues include increased access and, thus, more demand for services; drug pricing; mergers of providers, organizations, and insurers; technologies such as telehealth and mobile apps; and data security (Blumenthal, Abrams, & Nuzum, 2015; Lorenzetti, 2015). Superimposed on all these changes—and influencing them—are political and power issues.

Given the demands facing the health-care system, the voice of nurses and the leadership of APNs are essential to meet our professional and societal obligations to improve health and health care. APNs are uniquely positioned to contribute critical knowledge, skills, and attitudes, as well as their values of civic professionalism and compassion,

to political and decision-making dialogues. The purpose of the health-care system is to continuously reduce the impact and burden of illness, injury, and disability and to improve the health and functioning of the people of the United States. Although providing direct care and influencing the direct care provided by others are necessary work and contribute to meeting this goal, they are not sufficient to meet growing professional and societal quality and accountability demands. By demonstrating their contributions; continuously improving their performance; and being accountable to the profession, employers, and the public for all components of their role, APNs can make a difference.

As the nurse moves from novice to expert, responsibility for and accountability to self and others for the structures, processes, and outcomes of health care increase proportionally. Achieving the status of APN is not a terminal event and the role assumes ongoing and increasing professional and societal obligations. Responsibility for meeting the triple aims means that the APN must serve the profession and society as a primary agent contributing at the level of individual care, in the practice setting, and at the tables where organizational and public policies are made and implemented. In addition, the professional and societal trust afforded to the APN obliges meaningful contributions—beyond individual patient care—to meet the purpose of the health-care system. APNs must not only do good, they must demonstrate their value to society through performance assessment and its documentation and dissemination at every level of care and decision making so their voices are heard. The importance to health outcomes, the profession, and society cannot be underestimated or ignored.

The Case for Accountability

Why should APNs be concerned about these issues? A Web search of the terms *health care AND accountability* resulted in more than 130 million hits. This reflects the importance of this issue in our society. The search revealed that accountability for the quality and costs of health care—its value—are of interest to consumers, purchasers/payers, employers, insurers, the government, and professional provider organizations. Although the demand for accountability for the value of health care is not new, growing complexity and changes in the health-care system raise the issue to a level that cannot be denied or minimized. This demand requires the APN to measure and disseminate information on the value of the role. Nurses in advanced practice, similar to other providers and health-care system components, need knowledge and skills to assess and measure quality and determine the costs of their services if they are to demonstrate value. It is not enough to "do good"; the APN must demonstrate how "doing good" translates into outcomes and costs.

Accountability for practice has been and continues to be embedded in APN standards, education, and position descriptions. As Buerhaus and Norman (2001) suggest, the improvement of health-care quality is an "authentic commitment" (p. 68) for all stakeholders and will shape how health-care services are delivered. Given the definition of advanced practice and its role components, APNs must contribute to and lead broad efforts to improve quality. Their actions in defining, measuring, and reporting on their performance will determine their future and that of the health-care system. The advanced practice framework includes patients, health care, nursing, and individual outcomes. Thus, the APN is accountable for performance in all these domains.

These concepts and obligations are further reflected for the graduate-level student (American Association of Colleges of Nursing [AACN], 2011). Prepared at this level, the nurse is expected to have advanced role skills, possess refined analytical skills, operate from a broad-based perspective, have the ability to articulate views and positions, and connect theory and practice. He or she is expected to engage in quality and safety initiatives and collaborate inter-professionally to improve patient and population health outcomes.

The Quality Context

If the health-care system is to reduce the effect and burden of illnesses, injuries, and disabilities and improve outcomes and functioning, all involved in the system must be responsible for identifying and improving the structures and processes for achieving positive outcomes. Research has shown that consumers and society are not getting what they want or need from the health-care system. Errors continue to occur and patient experiences with care continue to be issues with outcomes becoming part of pay-for-performance determinations. The Institute of Medicine (IOM) (1999, 2001, 2006) identified problems with the quality of care and safety concerns that continue to be reported in the literature. Reports of consumer satisfaction or experience with the health-care system, such as those of the Commonwealth Fund (Commonwealth Fund, 2016b; Davis et al, 2002), found that patients were not satisfied with the quality of care they were receiving and reported continuing concerns on their summaries of assessment data. Hero, Blendon, Zaslavsky, and Campbell (2016) found that concerns about access to preferred care were a major concern. Managed care, cost concerns, and the growing consumer movement in health care have increased the demand for information about the value (quality in relation to cost) of health-care services and the performance of health-care providers in delivering quality, cost-effective services across all components of the health-care system.

Led by advocacy organizations, consumers are demanding greater accountability from health-care providers and the health-care system. They want quality, cost-effective services delivered from a patient-centered perspective. Federal and state government agencies and other purchasers want to know if the services they pay for are achieving the best possible outcomes at the best price. Organizations that accredit health-care organizations are increasingly seeking evidence that the structures and processes of care produce positive health outcomes.

All these demands to demonstrate and be accountable for value- and cost-effective high-quality care require individuals and groups of providers to measure performance and share their assessments with stakeholders. Organizations such as the National Committee for Quality Assurance (NCQA), the National Quality Forum (NQF), The Joint Commission (TJC), and several agencies of the federal government lead efforts to measure and report on the quality of care provided by various health-care system components. Federal and state agencies, independently and in collaboration with private sector organizations, are collecting and disseminating information about the quality of services provided by the health-care system's various providers. Health-care "report cards" are mechanisms widely employed to address the concerns of consumers, payers, employers, and others about the quality of health care being provided. Report cards are done for hospitals, health plans, and provider groups with the intent of informing consumers and improving quality.

Public reports of health-care quality are done by state and federal governments and private sector organizations. Implementation of the PPACA has resulted in greater reporting at the state and federal levels. Although these reports, especially those related to patient satisfaction and experience with care, remain controversial (Rosen & Chen, 2016), they are being widely reported and linked to pay-for-performance initiatives. Quality in service is demanded by anyone seeking that service. This is especially true for health-care services, both by the person receiving services and also for regulating bodies. Nurses must recognize the part they play in quality and safety in an obvious way, measuring, reporting, and articulating their role. The importance of quality and safety is evident in the APN Consensus Document (NCSBN, 2008) that articulates the parameters and standards for licensure, accreditation, certification, and education (LACE). The APN's performance will be measured and reported; thus, he or she must be engaged in determining best practices to meet patient and outcome expectations.

Values and Value in Health Care

To contribute effectively to fulfilling the purpose of the health-care system, the APN needs a clear vision derived from personal and professional values. The APN needs to embrace society's mandate for health-care value and clarify how the quality and cost issues relate to personal and professional goals. Explicit incorporation of quality and cost values and critical thinking about these issues will result in actions and activities consistent with social demand. Therefore, the APN role can be justified and the needs of society will be better served. APNs will be well positioned to provide leadership in affecting quality and costs, the "bottom line" of health-care system performance.

To be effective leaders and advocates for value issues associated with patients and the role, the APN must know and appreciate what other stakeholders want. Thus, it will be easier to understand their behavior and thinking about health and health care and to develop and implement strategies to address value conflicts, thereby resulting in better health-care outcomes. For example, the APN's employer may value reducing costs to ensure organizational survival, whereas the APN's highest value is meeting the diverse needs of patients served by the organization. Negotiation, compromise, and collaboration are necessary to incorporate both values into strategic planning efforts. Awareness of the importance of values, understanding the value equation, and possessing the skills to address value conflicts are critical for APN survival and health-care system improvement.

The purposes of this chapter are to introduce APN students to quality frameworks, performance measurement, and accountability and to suggest approaches to current issues and responses to trends. For the graduate APN, this chapter can enhance knowledge and skills that will promote the quality activities, better demonstrate accountability, and foster actions to justify the role of the APN in meeting societal demands for quality, cost-effective health care. The complexity of the quality movement and the value equation are discussed. As the health-care system becomes increasingly complex, as stakeholders' values and visions clash, and as there is growing dissatisfaction with the health-care system, APN leadership is critical. The challenge to establish value and be accountable at all levels may appear daunting, but it is exciting and potentially rewarding for the APN, the profession, and our society.

THE QUALITY ENVIRONMENT

Beginning with Florence Nightingale, nursing has always given attention to quality issues. Despite our historical roots as leaders in this area, the profession has drifted to a more internal, narrow perspective. Until recently, this mirrored the attention our society gave to the quality of health care. In the United States especially, the values of individualism and self-determination, science and technology, a disease and medical focus, the free-market economy, and nongovernmental interference shaped both the structures and processes of the health-care system, thus influencing its outcomes. Access and cost issues have, until recently, received more attention than quality, particularly at the societal level. As cost concerns increased and new delivery systems—such as managed care—were implemented, greater attention focused on quality and value. In addition, industry and quality theories and practices in business suggested that lessons learned in these arenas could be applied to the health-care sector.

Definitions and Frameworks

With greater attention being given to quality, long-standing terms and processes were dusted off and a new vocabulary evolved. As shown in **Table 24.1,** a plethora of terms are used to describe quality concepts. The APN, to operate effectively in the new health-care quality climate, must be fluent in the new language.

One of the earliest conceptual frameworks to describe quality was developed by Donabedian (1966). It is widely used by the nursing community and others in the health-care system as a way to identify the structural and process factors that affect outcomes. Hamric (1983, 1989) provided a model for APN patient care evaluation using Donabedian's framework. Girouard (2000) identified structural elements that include the APN's education, the time the APN spends in role components, reimbursement levels, and organizational characteristics. Process elements include APN behaviors, referral patterns, prescriptive practice behavior, collaboration, and APN satisfaction. The outcomes related to APN structures and processes include mortality, morbidity, patient knowledge, patient satisfaction, service use, and health status.

Quality of care can be viewed from a micro or macro perspective. At the micro level, quality is conceptualized and assessed for the patient, the provider, or the institution. Clinical and technical care, satisfaction with care, and quality of life represent components of a micro view (Shi & Singh, 2005). Although always an important component of any quality approach, increasing attention is being given to the macro level—looking at outcomes and cost effectiveness for populations and society. Examples include the efforts of private sector organizations such as TJC (formerly the Joint Commission on Accreditation of Healthcare Organizations), NQF, NCQA, and the work supported by private foundations. State and federal legislatures and the agencies implementing public policy decisions are also involved in macro-level quality approaches.

TABLE 24.1	
The Vocabulary of Quality	
Access	Ability to obtain care or health and related services (also defined as use or insurance coverage)
Accountability	The demonstration of value (e.g., quality care, patient satisfaction, resource efficiency, and ethical practice); liability for actions
Cost	To the individual paying for services; to the provider to produce services; for society
Outcome	The end result of structures and processes of care; the goal or objective of health and health care
Performance	Assessment of how individual providers behave; measurement assessment of processes of care; may be compared against standards or benchmarks
Process	Method in which health care is provided; provider behaviors; includes technical and interpersonal elements
Quality	How well services increase chance for desired outcomes; knowledge based and evidence based
Quality assessment	Process of defining and measuring quality Quality assurance Process of measurement and quality improvement; may also be defined as the minimum standards approach
Quality indicator	Trait or characteristic linked with evidence to desirable health outcomes; may serve as proxy for outcome
Report cards	Collection and reporting of performance and other quality-related data to the public or other targeted groups
Structure	Tools and resources for care (e.g., facilities, licensing and regulation, staffing, equipment)
Total quality	Includes an environment for quality, involves continuous measurement and improvement activities (often called total quality management or continuous quality improvement)

One example of such an approach is the Child and Adolescent Health Measurement Initiative (CAHMI), a national initiative based out of the Bloomberg School of Public Health at Johns Hopkins University. In collaboration with consumers, they developed an experience of care framework and measures for children and adults. This framework and the measures developed to date are widely used by such organizations as the NCQA, the NQF, the IOM, and the Robert Wood Johnson Foundation (RWJF) for measuring the quality of care provided to large population groups. In addition, federal government agencies, such as the Agency for Healthcare Research and Quality (AHRQ) and the Centers for Medicare and Medicaid Services (CMS), and state government agencies have adopted the framework and adapted the measures for a macro approach to quality.

Access, Cost, and Quality

The growing demand for quality requires that attention also be given to access because improved health status and other outcomes of care depend on the individual's ability to receive needed services across the continuum of care. Although often discussed as an issue of access to insurance for the uninsured and the underinsured, a payment mechanism is not sufficient to improve outcomes. The providers, services, and goods individuals and groups have access to are major factors in achieving desired outcomes and cost efficiencies. Thus, payment levels, what is paid for, and who gets paid are important access considerations in the quality equation. Well-known deficiencies currently exist in mental health-care services, oral health-care services, and care of persons with chronic conditions. The APN should pay particular attention to and justify the needs and benefits resulting from advanced practice nursing services in all health-care settings and for all levels of care.

Cost issues are the third component (along with access and quality) of the health-care system triangle and are essential to establish the value of health care. Cost can be considered from the perspective of the society at large—the total costs of health care or the percentage of national dollars for health-care expenditures. Global expenditures include provider services, insurance, goods and supplies, pharmaceuticals, research, education, core public health services, and institutional costs for delivering health-care services. Consumers and employers are concerned about the direct costs of care. For employers, their insurance costs, loss of productive work time, and health-care program administration costs are considered as a percentage of expenditures needed to conduct their business. Individual consumers, although most often focused on their out-of-pocket costs, are also concerned about the costs of insurance, the price of services and goods needed, and pharmaceutical costs. A third approach when considering health-care costs is the perspective of the health-care professional or health-care organization in which the focus is on expenditures, such as costs for personnel, administration, physical plants, and supplies and equipment, to produce services for groups of patients.

To adequately assess quality at the individual, societal, or organizational level, the APN must be cognizant of access and cost issues and the role they play in determining outcomes. Access and cost issues reflect structural and process elements, the factors that influence health-care outcomes. In addition, this approach holds opportunities for representing the APN as a solution to access and cost concerns. Thus, the APN can make a strong case for the role's value in the health-care system.

Recent Quality Initiatives

A growing number of national quality initiatives reflect the importance of this issue and support the assertion that quality efforts will remain a significant factor in shaping the future of the health-care system. The identification of standards and expected outcomes for access, costs, and quality; their measurement; and public dissemination and discourse are ongoing and expanding. To ensure quality and cost-effective care, quality must be defined; performance expectations specified; and performance and outcomes measured. These are the bases for the quality efforts of national health-care organizations.

Quality measurement is needed to understand the effects of services on individuals and populations and to make improvements in the organization, delivery, and financing of health care. According to the IOM's National Health Care Quality Roundtable (Donaldson, 1999), still valid today, health-care quality measurement objectives include:

- Gathering and analyzing data to inform quality improvement efforts
- Assessing facilities and individual performance in relation to established standards

- Comparing providers to inform purchaser and consumer choice of providers
- Informing all stakeholders about decisions and choices
- Identifying, rewarding, and sharing best practices
- Monitoring and reporting on quality over time
- Addressing the health-care needs of communities

In response to the demand for quality, performance measurement, and accountability, federal and state governments and the private sector have taken action. Government agencies, with congressional policy direction and as major purchasers of health-care services, need information about the quality of health care to guide policy and program decision making. Two government agencies, the AHRQ and CMS, are worthy of particular attention because quality is a major focus of their activities. The AHRQ, through its internal and external research programs and educational initiatives, is charged to improve the outcomes and quality of health care. In addition, the AHRQ's goals include addressing patient safety and errors, increasing access to effective services, and reducing costs. As a major purchaser (Medicare and Medicaid), CMS must ensure that its program beneficiaries receive quality, cost-effective care. In addition, through its regulatory functions it sets quality standards for the health-care industry.

An example of a recent AHRQ initiative is a synthesis of completed research to answer questions about which prescriptive drugs reduce costs and improve outcomes. AHRQ is also evaluating pilot projects that reward providers for delivering high-quality health-care services. They have disseminated a synthesis of studies so clinicians can make better decisions about treating patients with community-acquired pneumonia. Clinicians will also find AHRQ's "Child Health Tool Box" and other collections of guidelines and measures useful in establishing their own performance measurement and quality programs. AHRQ's more than 10 years of reports on health-care quality and disparities (AHRQ, 2015) provide the APN with important information to guide thinking about the foci of quality initiatives.

Because Medicare and Medicaid beneficiaries use a wide array of health-care services, the CMS's quality efforts are far reaching. Among its initiatives are programs to assess quality and performance in hospitals, home care, and long-term care. The quality improvement system for managed care sets regulatory standards and guidelines for quality assessment and improvement and health services management in managed care organizations (MCOs). To address quality in nursing homes, the CMS is assessing and disseminating information about quality in Medicare- and Medicaid-certified long-term care facilities. Through the collection and analysis of uniform patient level data (outcome and assessment information set [OASIS]), the CMS is fostering outcome-based quality improvement in home health care.

The initiatives described previously reflect only a few of the federal government's quality-related activities. Other Health and Human Services departments, such as the Centers for Disease Control and Prevention (CDC) and the Maternal and Child Health Bureau (MCHB), are actively engaged in similar activities. State governments are also involved in quality measurement and reporting. For example, New York, Florida, and Washington are measuring provider performance in children's health care.

Private sector organizations representing foundations, purchasers, employers, and professional organizations also measure and report on quality. Accrediting organizations, such as TJC, are moving from assessing only structures and processes of care to outcome evaluation. For example, TJC-accredited organizations, through the ORYX initiative, are required to measure specific patient outcomes and provider performance standards. ORYX is TJC's performance measurement and improvement initiative, first implemented in 1997. Safety, medical errors, and infection rates are also being used by TJC as performance indicators. Through annual reports on health-care quality, NCQA looks at plan performance related to quality, access, and consumer satisfaction. NCQA's health plan report cards are shared with employers and purchasing groups and are made available for consumer use in choosing health-care plans. They have played a major role in accrediting medical homes and advanced medical homes.

Three national organizations exemplify the private sector's role and collaboration with government agencies to address quality: the CAHMI, the American Health Quality Association (AHQA), and the NQF. The CAHMI evaluates health system performance for children covered by Medicaid and private insurance and reports on gaps in care to consumers. It is dedicated to helping parents and children make better decisions and choices by informing them about what to expect from the health-care system and by fostering their involvement in holding the health-care system accountable.

The AHQA represents professionals involved in quality and CMS's quality improvement organization (formerly the peer review organizations) by implementing best practices and fostering quality improvement. By supplying providers and the public with regular updates on quality-of-care research, standards, and other related issues, they educate a wide audience of health-care system stakeholders. The NQF, created in response to the President's Commission on Quality in Health Care, states that its role is to develop and implement a national strategy for quality measurement and reporting. It uses its members and other experts to assess research and performance reports and provide guidance for improving health-care quality. For example, it issued a report that identified disparities in health care for minority populations and suggested priority activities to address these disparities.

Employers are also involved in health-care quality through their demand for information about quality and performance. Accountability is achieved through the measurement and reporting of performance measures and though incentives for providers. For example, large employers in Massachusetts are offering bonuses to providers who improve the care of patients with diabetes and who use an electronic database to follow chronically ill patients.

As these initiatives suggest, the APN's performance is already being measured—directly as a primary care provider and indirectly as a contributor to the health-care team's performance. Thus, the APN must be aware of national issues, trends, and approaches in quality measurement and improvement to guide practice and other professional activities. As discussed later in this chapter, there are additional actions to be taken to participate more fully in the quality movement.

ADVANCE PRACTICE NURSE PERFORMANCE EXPECTATIONS

The transition to the role of APN involves a steep learning curve that recognizes the complexity of health care. The APN will be involved in many aspects of health care that were not often thought of as part of direct, day-to-day practice. Quality improvement and evidence-based practice activities are being given much greater attention in all health-care settings. These, along with quality, safety, and performance measurement, have grown exponentially in

recent years and are a priority in the health-care system. Quality in service is demanded by anyone seeking a service—this is especially true for health-care services. The person receiving service, the organization providing the service, those paying for the service, and those regulating the service (and providers) are demanding performance assessment and accountability. The APN, given the components and core competencies required of the role, is expected to be engaged in all aspects of the quality and safety movement including the development, implementation, and evaluation of the performance measurement and reporting process.

As reflected in the LACE discussion in the APRN Consensus Model (2008), quality and safety activities, assessment, and accountability are essential for all APNs. It is not sufficient for the APN to simply be aware of quality improvement initiatives and requirements; the APN must now be an active participant in the process. The National Quality Strategy, part of the current health-care reform initiatives, is the first policy to set national goals to improve the quality of health care. It serves as a guide for all HHS quality improvement programs and regulations and sets standard criteria to measure the quality of health and health care to align national quality and safety efforts. Most of the tasks APNs will be completing in providing care to patients in this new role intersect with some aspect of the National Quality Strategy. The APN is responsible for meeting the demands of patient care while adhering to requirements that have emerged from this strategy.

APNs must also be able to define quality in their own practice. Quality has many definitions, but there is consensus among researchers and policy makers that high-quality care occurs when providers give patients the right care when they need it, such as regularly monitoring chronic conditions to prevent complications. Similarly, quality care is appropriate and cost effective—patients do not receive unnecessary care, such as unnecessary diagnostic tests or treatments. High-quality care is based on the best scientific evidence about what helps people get better and stay well, rather than individual opinions or convenience. High-quality care is tailored to a patient's preferences and values; it is accessible and reliable for all and does not vary because of race, gender, income, or location. High-quality care means that providers are respectful, communicate clearly, and involve patients in decisions about their care (Geisz, 2012). Several

IOM reports are also helpful (as discussed earlier in this chapter) in framing and operationalizing quality definitions. Bunting and Groszkruger (2016), for example, offer an approach to using IOM recommendations to improve diagnostic activities.

The IOM reports and subsequent quality initiatives of federal and state agencies and private sector organizations have identified recommendations—most of which are currently in place—and recognized that a collaborative approach was needed to assure health-care quality and safety. These recommendations included establishing agencies to focus on quality and safety; setting clear standards and expectations; peer review; protection of patient data; and adverse event reporting systems. There are several activities resulting from these reports of interest to APNs. For example, in 2005 AHRQ launched its Patient Safety Network (PSNet), a national Web-based resource that maintains the latest patient safety news and resources. In 2009, the CMS—within the U.S. Department of Health & Human Services—implemented Medicare Part C plan reporting requirements, which mandated the reporting of serious adverse events and hospital-acquired conditions. In 2011, the Institute for Safe Medication Practices (ISMP), the Food and Drug Administration (FDA), TJC, and other organizations began promoting the use of tall man lettering to reduce confusion among look-alike, sound-alike medications such as busPIRone–buPROPion, and PENTobarbital–PHENobarbital.

The IOM identified six aims for quality improvement helpful to the APN developing standards for the practice setting:

- *Safe:* Avoiding injuries to patients from the care that is intended to help them
- *Timely:* Reducing wait times and harmful delays for both those who receive and those who give care
- *Effective:* Providing services based on scientific knowledge to all who could benefit and refraining from providing services to those not likely to benefit
- *Efficient:* Avoiding waste, including waste of equipment, supplies, ideas, and energy
- *Equitable:* Providing care that does not vary in quality because of personal characteristics
- *Patient-centered:* Providing care that is respectful of and responsive to individual patient preferences, needs, and values and ensuring that patient values guide all clinical decisions

Standards for APN master's and doctoral nursing education programs are found in *Health Professions Education: A Bridge to Quality* (IOM, 2003). These widely accepted recommendations called for major restructuring of health professionals' education. All health professionals should be prepared to deliver interprofessional, patient-centered care; practice from an evidence base; engage in quality improvement; and be competent in informatics. Complex practice and delivery system demands create a mandate to expand the clinical education and leadership capacity of APNs. APNs are expected to use advanced communication skills and processes to lead quality improvement and patient safety initiatives in health-care systems (AHRQ, 2015). Similar standards and competencies are found in standards for APNs promulgated by the American Nurses Association and most nurse practitioner (NP) and specialty advanced practice nursing professional associations.

The drive to measure quality is a concern for payers, regulators, and increasingly consumers. As data systems evolve and payers insist on "paying for performance," a level of accountability and transparency will be required regardless of provider type or health-care setting. To address the triple aims of the health-care system to improve the care experience, improve population health, and reduce costs, the National Quality Strategy has key foci for the APN:

- Making care safer by reducing harm caused in the delivery of care
- Ensuring that each person and his or her family is engaged, working as partners in the patient's care
- Promoting effective communication and coordination of care
- Promoting the most effective prevention and treatment practices for the leading causes of mortality, starting with cardiovascular disease
- Working with communities to promote wide use of best practices to enable healthy living
- Making quality care more affordable for individuals, families, employers, governments, and communities by developing and spreading new health-care delivery models

Clearly, professional expectations, such as those discussed previously, embody quality and accountability expectations for the APN in direct clinical care and within the health-care system. The APN is expected to do good for patients, measure performance in relationship to best practices, and be held accountable for practice. But that is not enough; APN expectations include quality-related issues that extend beyond direct clinical care to the health-care system and its quality and accountability issues.

MEASURING QUALITY AND PERFORMANCE

The structures, processes, and outcomes associated with APN practice can be evaluated at the individual's practice level, for groups of providers and organizations, for care systems (such as affordable care organizations), and at the societal level. The APN should be knowledgeable about all these approaches and involved at all levels. He or she will find the literature dealing with research, evidence-based practice, and quality helpful to begin developing a professionally and personally relevant framework to measure quality, evaluate performance, and identify meaningful indicators to justify the role and fulfill the expectations of the role. The intensity of involvement at a given level varies with the position held, employer expectations, level of knowledge, skill in evaluation, and other demands.

Individual Level

APNs can assess their ability to meet the expectations for advanced practice nursing by using core competencies promulgated by the National Organization of Nurse Practitioner Faculties (NONPF) and the Council on Accreditation of Nurse Anesthesia Educational Programs (COA). The competencies are acquired through mentored patient care experiences with emphasis on independent and interprofessional practice; analytic skills for evaluating and providing evidence-based, patient-centered care across settings; advanced knowledge of the health-care delivery system; patient safety; communication; critical thinking; and leadership. Earlier versions of the NPs' core competencies authored in 2002 and 2006 were applicable for master's preparation and for the doctor of nursing practice (DNP) graduate as additive to the core competencies for the master's graduate. As of 2012, there was one set of core competencies for entry into practice on graduation of NPs, regardless of the educational preparation (NONPF, 2012). In June 2016, the COA revised both their master's and DNP program core competencies (COA, 2016).

By 2022 all master's nurse anesthesia programs must be transitioned to DNP.

Most APNs are probably already involved with directly measuring their individual performance. For example, annual performance reviews are a part of most employer–employee relationships. Generally, this type of evaluation focuses on the processes of care, productivity, and position description expectations. When outcomes, such as effectiveness of care, costs, or patient satisfaction with care, are measured by APNs, they generally apply to the individual's work or program-specific goals. Recent quality and performance measurement approaches suggest opportunities for the APN to evaluate performance more broadly and in other domains. For example, some state Medicaid programs are assessing their beneficiaries' experiences with care and providing feedback to individual providers. APNs can use such information to compare their care with other providers and state norms, thus identifying areas for improvement. Although these data are infrequently shared with consumers, it continues to be more widely available.

Group Level

Evaluation of the structures, processes, and outcomes for groups of providers are a growing component of national initiatives to assess quality and performance. APNs may evaluate their practice as a group of APNs or in groups of diverse health-care providers. For example, nurse-midwives can join together to assess the costs, patient satisfaction, and birth outcomes associated with their practice. APNs in a family practice group that includes physicians can determine how their performance compares with that of other group practices. NCQA's performance health plan measurement data can be abstracted to the provider group level and thus can be compared with national or state norms. The hospital-based APN can participate in evaluating patient outcomes for specific populations of patients and in determining performance in relation to issues such as infection rates, antibiotic use, patient safety, and medication errors.

With the advent of setting- and group-specific data collection, analysis, and reporting, opportunities exist for the APN to use findings from these reviews to develop and implement quality improvement in the practice setting. For example, a geriatric NP working with a long-term care facility can use the nursing home-specific reports generated by CMS to design programs to improve structures and processes of care related to specific outcomes. Findings of TJC can guide the hospital-based APN to identify goals for patient care, develop processes for improvement, and assess the effect of changes made.

Systems Level

Health-care plans, ACOs, and Medicaid programs are being evaluated and held accountable to consumers and purchasers of care for the quality they provide. As panel or staff members in these health-care delivery systems, APN care is also being assessed. It is assumed that purchasers of care and consumers will use the information increasingly being made available to make purchasing decisions.

The Consumer Assessment of Healthcare Providers and Systems (CAHPS) Clinician and Group Surveys (CG-CAHPS) ask patients about their recent experiences with clinicians and their staff. These surveys, used by state Medicaid agencies, Medicare, NCQA, and others, ask consumers to report on their care in several domains. Survey questions ask about timeliness of care, appointment, and information; provider communication; attention to mental and emotional health; support in taking care of own health; discussion of medication decisions; and satisfaction with the provider. NCQA uses these tools and the Healthplan Employer Data and Information Set (HEDIS) to evaluate the quality of care in more than 90% of the nation's health plans. HEDIS data are obtained from administrative data sources and chart audits to assess effectiveness of care using indicators derived from research and expert opinion (AHRQ, 2016).

State Medicaid programs use both CAHPS and HEDIS to assess the performance of care provided to beneficiaries. In addition, several states are assessing the quality of children's health-care services using tools such as those developed and tested by CAHMI. For example, one parent survey asks about providers' ability to meet expectations related to promoting healthy development (PHD) in young children.

CAHPS, HEDIS, and PHD measures, as well as other tools used to assess quality at the systems or health-plan level, are evidence based, psychometrically tested, and widely endorsed by providers, consumers, and other stakeholders. Given the current demand for quality information,

these efforts are likely to grow in the future. APNs, as practitioners in most of these settings, should be familiar with the performance assessment measures used in their workplace and regularly review reports to continuously improve quality and meet national performance standards.

Societal Level

At the societal level, there are several existing and evolving approaches to assess the quality of the nation's health-care system and its outcomes. *Healthy People* (ODPHP, 2017) sets health outcome goals, identifies indicators to measure progress in achieving these goals, and lists structures and processes needed to meet the goals. The nation's health quality is also being assessed by several private sector organizations such as advocacy and consumer groups and foundations. Examples include the Commonwealth Fund; high-need, high-cost patients; access to care and patient care experiences; women's health coverage; and local health systems rising to the challenge to improve health care (Commonwealth Fund, 2016b).

Congress mandated that AHRQ produce an annual report to the nation on health-care quality. Also, the AHRQ produces a national report on disparities in health care. The National Healthcare Quality Report (AHRQ, 2016) includes measures of effectiveness, effective treatment, care coordination, patient safety, person-centered care, healthy living, and care affordability. Disparities in quality, access, use, and costs for low-income groups, minority groups, women, children, older adults, and people with special health-care needs are reported in the National Healthcare Disparities Report (AHRQ, 2016).

The Institute for Healthcare Improvement (IHI) focus is to promulgate health-care strategies to reduce errors, waste, delay, and escalating costs (IHI, 2016). It also focuses on improvement capability, person-family centered care, patient safety, quality, cost, and value. The Anesthesia Patient Safety Foundation (APSF) mission is to continually improve "the safety of patients during anesthesia care" (APSF, 2016) through research, education, patient safety programs, and campaigns. APSF provides the platform for exchange of information nationally and internationally about the causes and interventions to prevent anesthetic casualties.

AHRQ has a Patient Safety Organization (PSO) program with 12 participating anesthesia groups. Membership is voluntary and organizations are required to adhere to the criteria set by the AHRQ regarding the Patient Safety Rule. PSOs serve as a repository for which hospitals and all health-care providers can confidentially and voluntarily provide information that will be used for "the aggregation and analysis of patient safety events (AHRQ-PSO, 2016).

The quality and performance measurement approaches discussed previously represent a sample of the increasing number of activities in this area. The models section of this chapter includes more detailed descriptions of these efforts and the recommendations section contains specific actions for the APN's greater involvement at all levels. All are important to the APN to justify the role and to be accountable for meeting the expectations of society for the advanced practice role. All have strengths and weaknesses when considered from the perspective of the APN.

Individual-level performance, especially when evaluated using nonstandardized methodologies, provides information of value to only the APN and the employer. Without comparative data, the APN's performance cannot be assessed in relation to other providers; thus, it is more difficult to justify the role and identify APN contributions to outcomes. Individual-level performance evaluation may be necessary, but it is not sufficient to justify the role or its contributions to quality health care. When performance is assessed at the group, system, or societal level, especially when using standard, tested approaches, the APN is better positioned to justify the role and demonstrate contributions to health-care outcomes. In addition, quality improvement goals derived from these measurement efforts are those that are of greatest social value. However, doing only group-, system-, or societal-level evaluation means that APN-dependent performance may be more difficult to articulate.

APPROACHES AND MODELS FOR PERFORMANCE EVALUATION

As the APN begins or enhances strategies to evaluate performance, quality, and value, a framework is needed to guide decision making and plan for effective and meaningful assessments of the role and its contributions. There are many approaches and models for consideration. The APN should assess the approaches and models in relation to their relevance and adaptability to meet the APN's specific needs, justify the role, and measure APN contributions to health

and health care in choosing an approach to evaluation. The goals of APN quality measurement are the following:

- Develop new and adopt existing data collection methods relevant to the APN role.
- Establish APN competency and practice standards aligned with facility, systems, and societal quality standards.
- Compare APN practice with other providers and groups of providers.
- Improve performance based on evidence.
- Monitor and report quality over time to all stakeholders.
- Address community and societal health-care needs.

Donabedian (1966) provides a basic framework for quality measurement at all levels. Although structures, processes, and outcomes of care can all be examined and used as quality indicators, it is important to provide evidence that measures of specific structures and processes are related to outcomes. In addition, outcomes chosen should be those of importance to health-care stakeholders. Selecting indicators that are of interest only to the APN does not serve to establish the role's value or its contributions to meeting the purpose of health care and the health-care system. Studies of the relationship of nurse staffing or the APN (a structural measure) to patient outcomes demonstrate how this can be done (Aiken, Clarke, Sloane, Sochalski, & Silber, 2001, 2002; Needleman, Buerhaus, Mattke, Stewart, & Zelevinsky, 2002; Needleman & Minnick, 2008; Pine, Holt, & Lou, 2003; Simonson, Ahern, & Hendryx, 2007). The researchers provide evidence for selection of the structural variables (nurse staffing and APNs) and for the relationship between nurse staffing and patient outcomes. The importance of their work to a variety of stakeholders, such as TJC (Joint Commission on the Accreditation of Healthcare Organizations, 2016) and the American Hospital Association (AHA, 2016), is reflected in the media attention given to these studies.

Structure, Process, and Outcome Measures

Structural measures related to quality and specific to the APN role include characteristics of the APN (education, experience, legal aspects, and role expectations), the practice or organizational setting (group resources, organizational structure, and provider relationships), and access to services (referral mechanisms, collaboration, and geographical location). Process measures focus on the nature of the APN's interventions and interactions with patients. In current quality terminology, process and performance measures are synonymous. Process measures include the APN's competence in diagnosis and management of health-care problems, prevention, teaching and counseling, interpersonal aspects of care, and technical care (e.g., errors and medication misuse). Outcomes reflect the results of structures and processes for individual patients, groups of patients, or society. Traditional quality outcome measures are mortality and morbidity. With increasing attention to assessing the quality of health care, patient experience, or satisfaction with care, costs and access are important outcome measures. The framework and evaluation models selected for use by the APN and the purpose and goals of the quality assessment process determine how the APN views patient satisfaction, costs, and access as indicators of quality.

A common model for measuring APN effectiveness encompasses structures, processes, and outcomes. Structural variables include legal issues and funding, organization of care delivery, and use of the APN. Process and performance measures reflect the direct and indirect patient care activities of the APN. The model includes both short- and long-term outcomes. Short-term outcomes include accessibility, satisfaction, patient knowledge and health behaviors, and complications of care. Optimal health status, experience with care, morbidity, mortality, and costs of care are long-term indicators of quality.

Individual Level

Because APNs are involved in evaluating their performance as a component of their organizational responsibilities, approaches to this level of evaluation are important. In addition, individual-level performance processes can be designed to address evaluation needs at the group and organizational, system, or societal levels. The purpose of the individual evaluation is to assess APN achievement of competencies and to measure performance in meeting position or job description expectations. The APN works with peers, physician collaborators, and supervisors to determine the specific factors to be assessed and to identify or design an evaluation methodology. Approaches to individual-level evaluation may include structures, processes, and outcomes. Hansen-Turton, Ware, Bond, Doria, and Cunningham (2013) examined the structural issue of MCO and HMOs credentialing and found that 25% of NPs are not credentialed by HMOs. Other studies focusing on structure have looked at patient characteristics within APN practices, providing valuable information about the types of patients served (Hamric, Worley, Lindeback, & Jaubert, 1999; Paine et al, 1999). Other APN-related structural variables studied include uses of technology (Borchers & Kee, 1999), identification of activities (Knaus, Felten, Burton, Fobes, & Davis, 1997), and the use of hospital data systems (Bozzo, Carlson, & Diers, 1998).

Satisfaction with APN care is a traditional part of APN evaluation. Oermann, Lambert, and Templin (2000) found that having access to nurse-midwives was an important quality of care element for parents. Larrabee, Ferri, and Hartig (1997) found high levels of satisfaction with most aspects of NP care and used those areas with lower ratings to guide quality improvement efforts. Numerous other studies have demonstrated that patients and other providers are satisfied with the care delivered by APNs (Aquilino, Damiano, Willard, Momony, & Levy, 1999; Garvisan, Grimsey, Littlejohns, Lownes, & Stacks, 1998; McMullen, 1999). Instruments have been developed, and their psychometric properties tested, that can be useful to the APN in determining patient satisfaction with NP care (Cole, Mackey, & Lindenberg, 1999).

Assessing the processes of APN care focuses on the nature of the APN's activities and interventions for direct patient care and his or her indirect patient care activities such as staff teaching and planning. Examples of instruments developed for this purpose include those of Ingersoll (1988); Tierney, Grant, and Mazique (1990); Kearnes (1992); Houston and Luquire (1991); and Girouard and Spross (1983). Oermann (1999) studied consumer descriptions of quality of care and found that consumers believed quality nursing care meant having nurses who were competent and skilled, communicated effectively, conducted patient teaching, and demonstrated caring behaviors. These elements of quality are consistent with other reports of consumer expectations and thus should be included in the APN's measurement as indicators of care quality. Evaluation of these processes is important for role justification and the identification of nursing processes that affect quality outcomes. Several studies have demonstrated APN contributions to process indicators of quality (Bozzo et al, 1998; Diers & Bozzo, 1997; Diers, Bozzo, Blatt, & Roussel, 1998; East & Colditz, 1996; Jacavone, Daniels, & Tyner, 1999; Pelletier-Hibbert, 1998).

APNs play a major role in the development, implementation, and evaluation of practice guidelines, clinical protocols, and clinical pathways that guide the processes of care. NPs, for example, develop protocols for their collaborative practices with physicians. APNs in hospitals, home care, long-term care, and other settings have leadership opportunities in this area as well. Examples in the literature include the work of Musclow, Sawhney, and Watt-Watson (2002); Morin and colleagues (1999); Sagehorn, Russell, and Ganong (1999); McDaniel (1999); Jacavone and colleagues (1999); Kee and Borchers (1998); and Card and colleagues (1998). APNs have also described and measured processes of care for a variety of patients (Barnason & Rasmussen, 2002; Beal & Philips, 1999; Brooten & Naylor, 1995; Coward, 1998; Strohschein, Schaffer, & Lia-Hoagberg, 1999).

Outcomes as the result of the APN's clinical activities, given their importance in quality improvement and accountability, are the most meaningful components of the APN's evaluation process. The Bibliography to this text includes several studies that illustrate how APNs evaluated the effectiveness of their practice and outcomes. Additional studies described the costs and demonstrated the cost effectiveness of APN practice (Burl, Bonner, Rao, & Khan, 1998; Dahle, Smith, Ingersoll, & Wilson, 1998; Lombness, 1994; Walker, Baker, & Chiverton, 1998). Studies linking structures, processes, and outcomes of APN care are particularly important to document APN effectiveness and to determine best practices for the organization and delivery of patient care services. For example, Rudy and colleagues (1998) examined relationships between staff type, activities of caregiving, and patient outcomes. Other examples of this type of evidence include the work of Mundinger and Kane (2000) comparing NP and physician outcomes in primary care. (Additional examples, including the work of Aiken, Brooten, and others, are included in the Bibliography.)

Little information is available to describe the APN's contributions to achieving broad community- or societal-level health-care goals such as those in *Healthy People* (USDHHS, 2012). Although the effect of an individual APN or even a group of APNs may be difficult to measure on such outcomes as health promotion and disease prevention, given the number of contributing factors, APNs should begin to identify how to address these most important societal outcomes. As national assessments of quality and outcomes are developed, the APN has an opportunity to begin to examine practice in relation to these evolving

indicators. The models for assessing health-care quality described in the text that follows can be used to shape the APN's quality and performance assessment goals, especially at the systems and societal levels.

Group, System, and Societal Levels

During the past several years, there have been several organized efforts to evaluate the quality of health care in the United States. Some are well established as evaluation models, although they are constantly being refined and updated. Other efforts are in earlier stages of development. There is significant consistency and collaboration among all stakeholders to develop approaches and models that will better determine quality, measure performance, demonstrate value, and allow for health-care providers and systems to be held accountable. Nurses, including APNs, and organizations of nurses are increasingly involved in all phases of these activities. Some of the most promising and widely accepted approaches are described to provide the APN with a broad view of current approaches and models.

Although the individual's performance and the APN's care-related outcomes are important, they take on greater meaning when they can be compared. The APN is encouraged to participate in the development, testing, and use of standardized instruments to measure structures, processes, outcomes, and satisfaction with care to allow for comparisons. In the discussion of group, system, and societal measures that follows, it is clear that group- and system-level assessments will, in the near future, allow for individual provider tracking in relation to performance and outcomes of care. The APN can use these data for individual performance assessments.

One of the most widely used frameworks for quality and performance measurement reflects the way consumers think about their care (Foundation for Accountability, 1999). The categories of the framework are the following:

- *The basics:* Satisfaction with the delivery of care by providers, access to care, and receipt of information and services
- *Staying healthy:* Avoiding illness, health promotion through preventive care, reduction of health risks, early detection of illness, and health education
- *Getting better:* Appropriateness of treatment and follow-up care to help recover from illness or injury

- *Living with illness:* Self-care guidance, symptom control, avoidance of complications, and maintaining daily activities for people with chronic illness
- *Changing needs:* Comprehensiveness of services, caregiver support, and hospice care that helps individuals and families when needs change dramatically because of a severe disability or terminal illness

Evidence-based measures are identified or new measures are developed and field tested for each of the categories and are used as standards for accountability. FACCT's framework is widely used by national accrediting organizations such as NCQA and TJC, federal and state agencies, and others, to measure quality and organize quality reporting. For example, the Commonwealth Fund's score card on health-care quality (2016b) uses the FACCT framework to organize the information contained in the report.

Another framework commonly used for quality and performance measurement is that put forward by the IOM (2001). Experts and a wide variety of health-care system stakeholders, including consumers, developed the framework. It includes six dimensions of quality: safety, effectiveness, equity, patient centeredness, efficacy, and timeliness. It, too, is the conceptual framework that guides other organizations and individuals in quality measurement, improvement, reporting, and research.

The Consumer Assessment of Health Plans (CAHPS) (AHRQ, 2012a) is a national quality measurement initiative conducted by AHRQ through several research organizations. It uses elements of the FACCT framework to organize survey questions designed to assess consumer experience with care. There are general surveys and surveys specific to special populations such as children and people with chronic conditions. CAHPS is used by NCQA and others as a standardized approach to provider and health plan quality and performance measurement.

The Obama administration established *Partnerships for Patients: Better Care, Lower Cost.* This public–private partnership focuses on safety and reducing unnecessary hospital admissions (USDHHS, 2011).

The NCQA assesses and reports on the performance and quality of MCOs and health plans, including those that serve Medicare and Medicaid beneficiaries in managed-care plans. Both the FACCT and IOM conceptual frameworks are used by NCQA. Data are collected on individual providers and aggregated to the health organization (plan)

level. HEDIS and CAHPS serve as the measure sets for assessing quality and performance. HEDIS includes more than 60 evidence-based consensus measures of effectiveness of care. Measures such as immunization levels, breast and cervical cancer screening, chlamydia screening, antidepressant medication management, postcoronary beta-blocker medication use and cholesterol management, comprehensive diabetes care, hypertension control, follow-up after hospitalization for mental illness, prenatal and postnatal care, and appropriate medication treatment for people with asthma are included in the data set (NCQA, 2011). The HEDIS and CAHPS data are analyzed and reported publicly.

Another private sector initiative addressing quality and performance in the health-care system is the NQF (National Forum for Healthcare Quality Measurement and Reporting, 2002). NQF is a membership organization representing a diverse group of public and private sector stakeholders, and its mission is to standardize quality of care performance measurement and reporting mechanisms. NQF has endorsed a list of procedures to promote patient safety; developed a framework for achieving their mission; and identified strategies to reduce health-care disparities. Future plans include developing sets of performance measures for hospitals, nursing homes, cancer care, and diabetes care. The hospital performance measures are created using the IOM's six domains of quality: safety, effectiveness, equity, patient centeredness, efficacy, and timeliness.

Purchasers of care and the business community are adopting existing quality and performance measurement models and assessment methodologies to meet their needs to determine the value of the health care they purchase. For example, a Minnesota coalition of large purchasers, the Buyers Health Care Action Group, assesses quality to increase value, choice, and health-care accountability. The National Business Coalition has strategies to improve patient safety and reduce medical errors by fostering consumer awareness; promoting the use of standardized measurement and reporting; rewarding quality; and supporting and using contract standards for safety. Many business coalitions, employers, and purchasers use data from national organizations such as the NCQA to improve their and their employees' ability to make better health plan choices and to hold health plans accountable.

As the major accrediting organization for hospitals, TJC has a long history of assessing structures and processes of care. During the past several years, and with the introduction of ORYX, TJC has moved toward outcomes assessment. Patient safety, including medication errors and infection rates, are receiving greater attention as quality indicators. Nurses involved in the development and testing of models to improve access quality are also an important consideration. For example, patient satisfaction with hospital care was addressed by Dozier, Kitzman, Ingersoll, Holmberg, and Schultz (2001). They developed and tested a tool, Patient Perception of Hospital Experience With Nursing, to assess whether or not patients' needs were met by nurses. These tools, and others developed by nurses to assess other nurse-dependent outcomes, are an important alternative to traditional patient care satisfaction tools that focus on amenities of care rather than competencies of nursing practice and to evaluate nurse-dependent outcomes.

The federal government's Medicare, Medicaid, and State Child Health Insurance Program all use and drive quality efforts through the evaluation of care to their beneficiaries in health maintenance organizations and MCOs, long-term care, and home care. HEDIS and CAHPS are used to assess plan quality. As a purchaser of care, CMS is able to demand quality and accountability and does so through contracts that specify quality measures and the identification of specific performance improvement goals. For example, CMS and states are involved in a voluntary performance measurement project using HEDIS measures. CMS's OASIS uses patient-level home-health agency data to assess and improve quality in Medicare-certified home-health agencies (Shaughnessy, Crisler, Hittle, & Schenkler, 2002).

In 2016, CMS released the Nursing Home Quality Report for 15,634 nursing homes across the country (CMS, 2015). The report includes information about quality, inspection results, and nurse staffing levels that can be compared with state and national norms. The quality measures include ability to perform activities of daily living, numbers of pressure sores, use of physical restraints, infection rates, cognitive impairments, pain management, and ambulation.

Other federal agencies such as the Bureau of Primary Health Care (BPHC) and the MCHB are implementing quality assessment and quality improvement initiatives. For example, BPHC's quality center coordinates quality initiatives and conducts strategic planning to enhance the quality of primary health care, especially for the community health centers it supports. The MCHB, in part using CAHMI measures, has sponsored national surveys of children with special health-care needs to determine their health status and the quality of care they are receiving.

The federal government's Quality Interagency Coordination Task Force represents another model of collaboration in the quality arena. The task force is to coordinate efforts across all federal agencies involved in health and health-care quality and its improvement. Task force participants are the Departments of Health and Human Services, Labor, Defense, Veterans Administration, and Commerce; the Office of Management and Budget; the Coast Guard; the Federal Bureau of Prisons; the National Highway Traffic Safety Administration; the Federal Trade Commission; and the AHRQ. They are to improve safety, improve patient and consumer information on quality, develop the health-care workforce, and improve information systems. The AHRQ's National Healthcare Quality and National Healthcare Disparities Reports use a framework that includes the IOM's dimensions of care and FACCT's patient need frameworks.

State governments, advocacy organizations, professional organizations, provider organizations, foundations, and others are undertaking other efforts and using the conceptual frameworks offered by the IOM and FACCT to guide the development of measures or the use of existing measures in their quality strategies. For example, the states of Vermont and California are using the CAHMI performance measurement tools to assess quality of health care for children who are Medicaid beneficiaries. Children NOW, a California advocacy organization, issues report cards on child health status using the CAHMI measures. School-based clinics are using HEDIS-like measures to assess and improve the quality of care in these settings. FACCT, using its adult and child health quality measures, had consumer-centered tools for use by individuals, employers, and purchasers of care. For example, "Compare Your Care" was a computer-based program that helped consumers compare their care experience to national and regional benchmarks derived from evidence-based practice guidelines. One module provides a formulary to help inform consumers about 10 health conditions and what prescription medications are best for them.

As the preceding discussion suggests, there is consistency and collaboration across the health-care system in relation to the conceptual frameworks used for measuring health-care quality. The FACCT and IOM frameworks guide most of the assessment, research, and reporting related to quality. Similarly, there is a fast-growing consensus for the use of HEDIS, CAHPS, CAHMI, and similar measures to assess quality in the domains suggested by the conceptual frameworks. Another trend is the significant collaboration and cooperation among a wide variety of stakeholders at all levels. The current climate also strongly suggests that health-care quality models and approaches must include the assessment of care in relation to what consumers want from the system, must be evidence based, and must use standardized and tested measurement approaches. The APN will be well positioned to justify the role and operationalize the APN contribution to health and health care if these and related theoretical frameworks are used. In addition, collaboration, the use of evidence in measure development, rigorous measure testing (or the use of tested measures), and linking structural and process factors to outcomes or quality indicators are vital for APNs to achieve the purposes of their quality and performance assessment activities.

RECOMMENDATIONS FOR ACTION

To meet the expectations of advanced practice nursing, the APN must transform expert knowledge and skill into actions that contribute to meeting societal health-care goals. One of the most important opportunities for influence is to affect changes that improve outcomes for individual patients, groups of patients, health-care organizations, systems, and society. The APN can and should exert influence to make this change a reality. To improve quality, it must be defined from an evidence base, have outcome standards identified against which to measure quality and performance, have identified best structures and processes linked to outcomes, be tested and articulated, be assessed at all levels, and be shared with all stakeholders.

The sixth domain of advanced practice (USDHHS, 2012) is monitoring and ensuring the quality of health-care practice. Competency in this domain is demonstrated when the APN engages in quality monitoring and quality assurance activities. Knowledge and skill for these competencies begin with graduate education, building on the student's undergraduate education and professional experience, and are continuously enhanced through education and practice experiences. In addition, nursing research and

other health-care literature should be regularly scanned and the media closely followed to assess trends and keep knowledge up-to-date. Many of the quality-focused and professional organizations (such as the American Nurses Association, nursing specialty organizations, and nursing research societies) provide electronic and paper newsletters and journals that can help the APN stay informed.

Melynk, Gallagher-Ford, Long, and Fineout-Overholt (2014) identified 13 competencies for RNs and an additional 11 competencies for APNs to improve quality and address costs. The basic evidence-based care competencies for all nurses include identifying questions and problems, seeking evidence, evaluating evidence, and implementing and sustaining change. The APN competencies are at a higher level and include comprehensive searches for and assessment of research and other evidence, integration, collaboration, measurement, mentoring, and leading. Representing the thinking of experts in evidence-based practice, these competencies will help the APN to identify strengths and areas for professional development aimed at enhancing knowledge and skills in this area. Holley (2016) calls for APNs to develop a set of competencies specific to APN performance rather than rely on those used for physicians. The importance of APNs and their performance needs to be fully evaluated and their specific contributions to quality and outcomes made explicit (Naylor & Kurtzman, 2010).

The skills needed to effect change in the quality arena are the core competencies of advanced practice, direct clinical practice, research skills, clinical and professional leadership, ethical decision-making skills, collaboration, consultation, and expert coaching and guidance. Applying these skills beyond the individual patient practice level increases the APN's ability to influence quality. Skills grow over time as the APN gets more involved in addressing quality concerns. As others become aware of the APN's expertise in patient care and quality, and as the APN seeks new opportunities, the sphere of influence will grow.

The APN can take action in relation to the practice, education, research, administration, and advocacy roles of advanced practice nursing at all levels. Each role component is discussed and examples of actions are provided. Although challenging, active engagement in the quality movement ensures recognition of the value of the APN role and better outcomes that will improve the health and reduce the burden of illness for U.S. citizens.

Practice

In direct clinical care, the APN should practice from an evidence base; deliver patient-centered care; be accessible to the patient; be responsive to patient needs, preferences, and concerns; and avoid missed opportunities to deliver preventive and health promotion services. The APN's role modeling and expertise in delivery system operations can guide others to provide quality patient care and engage in quality improvement activities. Operationalizing Brown's (2000) characteristics of the clinical role will also result in quality care and quality improvement. Noll and Girard (1993) provide a typology for quality activities related to APN competencies.

At the practice level, the APN can contribute to the quality movement by collecting accurate and timely data for research and quality assessment purposes. The APN should participate in group practice, organizational efforts, and professional organization quality activities aimed at assessing quality, performance, access, and costs. Partnering with consumers on quality issues is also expected and desirable. For example, quality advisory committees that include consumers can be formed at the practice level to identify patients' quality concerns and approaches to quality improvement.

APNs must also participate in formal quality improvement programs and activities at the practice level. Participation and leadership in accrediting and quality reviews by regulators, including TJC, is another action the APN can take to engage in quality measurement and improvement. Professional organizations such as the American Association of Nurse Anesthetists appoint a member to serve on committees such as the Ambulatory Care Professional and Technical Advisory Committee (PTCA). In this position expert advice is given on standards development, environmental trends, education, and other related issues (AANA, 2016).

Another practice-level set of activities that can be used for quality purposes is use of the position description and annual performance reviews. Position descriptions can be rewritten to reflect the elements of the IOM and FACCT models. Clear articulation of the goals and objectives of the review, and the use of standardized measures derived from these models, will foster more meaningful and relevant APN evaluation. Performance standards should reflect the purposes, goals, and objectives of the practice setting and meet external quality demands. For example, the APN in primary care can use an immunization benchmark from HEDIS to assess preventive care objectives and CAHPS questions about patient centeredness to determine patient experiences with the APN's care. Because standardized measures are used, the APN can compare performance to others or to national benchmarks.

The collection of data and information to justify the APN role, measure performance, demonstrate contributions to quality, and guide quality improvement efforts is critical. Suggested strategies include the regular collection and analysis of data on outcomes expected from the APN's practice; the collection of preintervention and postintervention data to track results over time; and assessment of patient experience and satisfaction with care. Possible data sources include administrative data (the data provided to regulators, accreditors, and insurers), chart audits, and client surveys. HEDIS, CAHPS, and other standardized measure use is encouraged to enhance the ability to compare data across individuals, groups, and settings. Data should be analyzed for trends over time: variations among groups of patients (e.g., age, gender, race, and ethnicity); variance from expected outcomes; differences among providers; and variations when compared with regional, state, or national norms. Performance data should be summarized and shared with consumers, other providers, and organizational leaders and used for accountability purposes.

Education

The APN has responsibility for his or her own, consumers', and other providers' education about quality issues and approaches. Consumers need information to be partners in their care, and other members of the health-care team need to better understand the value of APN practice. Sharing clinical expertise and participating in collaborative efforts to measure and improve quality best accomplish this. Offering information about best, evidence-based practices is one example of this type of activity.

Advanced practice and basic education should include content about and experience with all aspects of the quality process. Buerhaus and Norman (2001) give four reasons for including such information in formal educational programs:

1. Given the current economic climate surrounding health-care delivery, competition will increase and providers will be competing on the basis of quality, using quality indicators to distinguish themselves to purchasers and consumers.

2. The nursing shortage will result in greater use of un-licensed personnel and foreign-educated nurses, but nurses will still be accountable for nursing care and will need to ensure quality and quality improvement.
3. Nursing is responsible for quality and quality improvement to meet health system goals.
4. Nurses can capitalize on emerging evidence about the relationship of staffing to outcomes to advocate for structures and processes that will improve outcomes.

The Council of Accreditation of Nurse Anesthetist Educational Programs (COA) requires the master's and the doctoral nurse anesthesia curriculum to integrate evidence-based practice throughout the curriculum. Resident nurse anesthetists are expected to use critical thinking and provide nurse anesthesia services based on evidence-based principles (COA, 2016). Additionally, the certifying arm, the National Board of Certification and Recertification for Nurse Anesthetists, incorporate evidence-based practice in their recertification program (NBCRNA, 2016).

The APN may be involved in formal classroom or clinical teaching of undergraduate and graduate nursing students and should incorporate quality information and experiences in teaching strategies. The APN is also encouraged to include quality-related content during in-service and continuing education offerings. For example, the pediatric NP giving an in-service on assessing early childhood development should discuss how outcomes will be assessed using the CAHMI PHD measures.

As a professional organization, the AANA provides professional practice resources on evidence-based practice for resident nurse anesthetists, CRNAs, and anyone who is interested in gaining knowledge or greater understanding (AANA, 2016).

Research

APN research-related competencies include critically evaluating and applying research to practice, monitoring and evaluating practice, and participating in research. Research knowledge and skills are directly applicable to quality measurement and the interpretation of data. APNs can contribute by building an evidence base for their practice through collaborative research efforts. Using data collected and analyzed to assess performance, the APN can use research knowledge and skills to promote and improve quality. APNs have contributed to building a knowledge base and the methodologies needed to assess quality. Duffy (2002) described the clinical leadership role of the APN in identifying nurse-sensitive and multidisciplinary-quality indicator sets. The author advocates for using a phased, organization-wide process for incorporating these indicators into data collection efforts. Dunbar-Jacob and Schron (2002) suggest using ancillary studies to clinical trials to study questions relevant to nursing practice. Both of these suggestions provide examples of actions the APN can adopt at the practice level.

Administration

APNs in leadership positions can create a climate that fosters and supports quality and quality improvement. They can also propose structures and processes needed for quality and quality improvement such as available information systems for patient-level data collection. Even if the APN does not have administrative responsibilities, efforts can be made to promote the climate and the structures needed. Cubanski and Kline (2002) suggest several system challenges the APN can help address:

- Redesign care to better serve patient needs.
- Improve the use of information technology for practice and make it available to clinicians.
- Develop systems to coordinate care across conditions, services, and settings.
- Promote team effectiveness.
- Incorporate process and outcome measures into the delivery of health care.

Another administrative opportunity is providing incentives and awards for quality performance or quality improvement. Praise, recognition, promotion, raises, or other monetary contributions can provide incentive to staff. Awards, public acknowledgment, and offering special educational opportunities are other possible actions to foster continuous attention to quality and its improvement. The APN may do these things directly or by promoting their use by leaders in the setting. Rewards and recognition can also be provided through professional nursing organizations.

Advocacy

As another core competency of APN practice, advocacy can be applied to advancing quality measurement performance and improvement. Clearly, patient advocacy has always been a hallmark of professional nursing practice. The APN can further develop this competency by providing consumers with quality-related information, including what to expect from health care and the health-care system. Advocacy and the development of partnerships with patients can be enhanced when patients have their personal health record and information about their condition and treatment options (Davis et al, 2002). Armed with this information, patients can make better informed decisions and participate in all aspects of their care planning. The APN can also advocate for the practice, education, research, and administrative actions described previously.

APNs, especially those in direct practice roles, are not often involved with advocacy at the system or policy level. This is a loss to both the APN and society. With their expertise in practice, who better than the APN knows what is needed for quality care to become a reality? As an exception, CRNAs in academia, clinical practice, and resident nurse anesthetists have continually lobbied at the local, state, and national level for patient safety, access to care, title recognition, and workforce development (AANA, 2016). Additionally, CRNAs have aggressively lobbied to support full practice authority in the Veterans Hospital.

Advocacy is needed at the systems and societal levels to promote more resources for quality measurement and research, improve access for all people, develop better measurement and reporting of quality, support financing of appropriate services, and support government quality efforts. Advocacy with government and private sector organizations means getting involved with the political and policy processes, lobbying, educating consumers and policy makers, and using the media to deliver quality and APN value messages. The APN's expert knowledge and skills should be used to influence legislators, regulators, insurers, and private sector organizations involved (or who should be involved). For example, the APN using the influence of a professional nursing organization should use public comment periods to influence new HEDIS measures, TJC standards, and state Medicaid performance measurement approaches.

The APN should become an insider in the quality movement by participating in local, state, and national committees that are addressing quality concerns. For example, the author serves on the advisory and executive committees of FACCT's CAHMI, thus having influence in the development and adoption of child health performance measures. Nurses are also staff at such organizations as TJC and the AHRQ and review quality-related grants for foundations and government agencies. The APN can also become a leader and advocate for quality in the community, in the state, or in the nursing organization. For example, the APN might chair the town health committee or advisory board and develop community health outcome measures for a report card or promote an annual quality conference by the state nurses association.

CONCLUSION

As the IOM report on the future of the profession (IOM, 2011) recommends, the transformation of the health-care system requires that nurses practice to the full extent of their legal scope and lead change to advance health. The PPACA signals that our society is ready for change in health care. More attention will be directed to primary care, prevention, chronic care, coordination, and other services traditionally provided by nurses. Initiatives to link outcomes to payment will continue. In addition, increasing technology, growing system complexity, and the demands created by an aging population will increase the demands and challenges to ensure the quality and quantity of health-care services. Accountability for performance will be required.

APNs cannot escape their responsibility for clearly articulating their value to the health-care system. Because value equals quality and cost, without evidence of quality the case cannot be made for value. Advanced practice nursing cannot be supported and the purposes of the health-care system are not as well met as when the APN is a major player in the quality movement. Although efforts to define, assess, and improve quality have grown significantly in recent years, APN involvement in this arena has been less obvious. To move the health-care system toward quality, the APN, the health-care team, care organizations, and society must all participate and change. As this chapter has made clear, there are plenty of opportunities for engagement.

This chapter has made the case that the APN must be involved at all levels and in all aspects of the quality movement. The profession and the health-care system are ready for greater nursing and APN leadership. As Stanik-Hutt et al (2013) found in a systematic review of the literature, there is no doubt about the quality of APN care. The health-care system needs to take full advantage of this resource. Recent and ongoing quality initiatives offer clear direction for the APN in evaluating performance, measuring quality, and articulating value to a variety of stakeholders. The competencies expected of the APN are explicit to the quality domain. If the profession's clinical leaders do not get involved, who will fill the gap? The challenges are many, but the potential outcomes for the APN and society are great.

25

Advanced Practice Registered Nurses

Accomplishments, Trends, and Future Development

Jane M. Flanagan, Allyssa Harris, and Dorothy A. Jones

Learning Outcomes

Learning outcomes expected as a result of this chapter:

- Identify diverse practice settings in which advanced practice registered nurses (APRNs) are employed.
- Discuss the role of APRNs in their respective practice settings.
- Describe the impact of education level and experience on APRN reimbursement.
- Demonstrate the impact of health-care quality improvement initiatives and nurse-sensitive indicators on the role of APRNs.
- Describe and discuss the impact of discipline changes (i.e., licensure, accreditation, certification, and education [LACE] model, doctorate of nursing practice [DNP], doctoral education) on professional nursing practice.

INTRODUCTION

The major roles within the framework of the advanced practice registered nurse (APRN) are the clinical nurse specialist (CNS), certified nurse-midwife (CNM), certified registered nurse anesthetist (CRNA), and nurse practitioner (NP) (APRN Consensus Work Group & National Council of State Board of Nurses Advisory Committee, 2008). Historically, the APRN roles developed out of an identified need for improved continuity of care and increased access to health services. APRNs are registered nurses with advanced education. They work with diverse populations in a variety of settings, often where access to health care is limited.

According to the International Council of Nurses (ICN, 2016) the APRN has an expert knowledge base along with the ability to make complex care decisions and clinical competencies for expanded practice. Although acknowledging that the specific attributes of the APRN are informed by the needs of the country and credentialing body within an individual country, the ICN has identified that there are commonalities in terms of educational preparation and key components of the APRN role. Internationally all APRNs are prepared at the advanced level through formal programs that are accredited or otherwise approved and require a formal process for licensure, registration, certification, and credentialing (ICN, 2016).

Key components of the role include the integration of research, education, practice, and management; a high degree of autonomy and independent practice; managing a direct patient case load; acquisition of advanced health assessment decision-making and diagnostic reasoning skills; advanced clinical role and skill competencies; independent consultation with patients and other providers; the aptitude to plan, implement, and evaluate programs of care; and being designated a "first point of contact" to initiate patient care (ICN, 2016). The ICN also recognizes that individual countries and states within countries have regulations restricting practice and the full potential of patient care delivered by APRNs including the right to diagnose, prescribe, consult, and admit to a hospital. However, internationally there are officially recognized and protected titles such as NP or APN for nurses working in advanced practice roles.

Over the years, patients, administrators, family, and physicians have all acknowledged the contributions made by APRNs to enhance patient care (Auerbach, Chen, Friedberg,

Reid, Lau, Buerhaus, & Mehrotra, 2013; Cipriano, 2012; Institute of Medicine [IOM], 2011; Yang & Meiners, 2014). The value and efforts of APRNs have extended well beyond the United States and are gaining increased attention worldwide. The demand for APRNs is even more pronounced in areas where there is pandemic disease and concerns about safe childbirth (World Health Organization, 2016). Despite this acknowledgement of APRN's contributions to health care, there are continued challenges that affect role implementation and utilization.

As APRNs continue to grow in number, numerous studies over a 30-year period have supported their efficacy and impact on health-care outcomes. As these outcomes are now more widely acknowledged, new challenges arise about the blurring of nursing's distinct professional identity. The movement toward the educational preparation of APRNs more aligned with the medical model of cure rather than the advanced practice nursing model of caring and healing stimulates further debate. A nursing-informed model of relationship-based care, intentional presence, mutuality, health patterning, facilitating humanization, and health and healing in living and dying has been described as core to nursing (Newman, Smith, Pharris, & Jones, 2008; Willis, Grace, & Roy, 2008). However, as APRN educational programs expand, nursing theory has been eliminated from the curriculum and instead the focus is on preparing APRNs to be "as good as" medical providers. Some have suggested that this expansion into medical practice is a "natural evolution" of the APRN role, whereas others have argued that the recent changes foster professional abandonment. Unaddressed, this challenge could result in a diminished voice for nursing, decreased collaboration, a loss of professional autonomy, and reduced public legitimacy.

This chapter explores the current realities of APRN roles and the recent trends affecting APRN education and practice. APRNs are discussed within the context of nursing science and a changing clinical practice environment.

THE APRN: ROLES, PRACTICE SETTINGS, AND OUTCOMES

APRNs practice in their expanded roles with increasingly diverse populations in a variety of settings including large medical centers, physicians' offices, community health centers, ambulatory care practices, and emergency departments, as well as the traditional community and rural hospitals and clinics. Nursing and other disciplinary knowledge, along with information about populations and settings, further inform and define each of the APRN roles.

The national Consensus Model for advanced practice nurses regulation (APRN Consensus Work Group & National Council of State Board of Nurses Advisory Committee, 2008) recognizes four roles—CNM, CRNA, CNS, and NP—working with six population foci: adult-gerontology, family, women's, pediatric, neonatal, and psychiatric. APRNs may choose to specialize in areas such as oncology or palliative care, but they cannot be solely licensed as an APRN within a specialty area. The scope of practice for APRNs is not setting specific, but varies according to the needs of the patient or population.

In a changing health-care environment driven by economics and physician residency education, some APRNs (NPs and CNMs) have been used as physician substitutes in disease-based specialty care (Hurlock-Chorostecki, Forchuk, Orchard, Soeren, & Reeves, 2014) within the hospital setting. This phenomenon has resulted in shifts in practice settings for NPs and CNMs who formerly were more home and community based, but now are more acute and hospital based.

Certified Nurse-Midwives

The American College of Nurse-Midwives (ACNM) reports that in 2015 there were 11,194 CNMs. Since 2010 a graduate degree has been required for entry into CNM practice, but early CNM programs did not require baccalaureate preparation, nor did they award a master's degree at the completion of the program. So although most CNMs (82%) now have a master's degree, some report having a diploma or associate's degree in nursing as their highest academic degree. Sipe, Fullerton, and Schuiling (2009) report that 4.8% of CNMs have doctoral degrees, which is proportionally the highest of all APRN groups.

CNMs provide gynecological care to healthy women and low-risk obstetrical care. CNMs care for women in the home and the hospital setting. More than two decades of research consistently supports that CNMs have increased patient satisfaction with care, lowered incidences of cesarean births, decreased use of forceps delivery, resulted in less medication use, decreased length of hospitalization, and, overall, led to fewer complications with the delivery. Further,

mothers cared for by CNMs have a greater tendency to breastfeed their babies, improving both infant immunity and rates of infant mortality (Newhouse et al, 2011).

Collectively these studies suggest that CNMs provide effective prenatal, labor, and delivery care and postbirth assistance, especially in terms of supporting breastfeeding. A body of evidence indicates that CNMs provide obstetrical care that is accessible, safe, and low cost with lower rates of neonatal mortality and cesarean births. CNMs have reinforced the fact that pregnancy is a normal health transition for most women, competently managed by the CNM.

Certified Registered Nurse Anesthetists

There are approximately 40,000 CRNAs practicing in the United States (American Association of Nurse Anesthetists [AANA], 2016a). CRNAs are registered nurses who have completed 2 to 3 years of higher education beyond a bachelor's degree (typically a master's degree) and hold national certification to practice in this role. Most CRNAs have had previous experience in critical care, a criterion often used as part of the admission requirements to a graduate program.

CRNAs work in hospital settings, outpatient surgical centers, and practices where anesthesia is needed and administer more than 65% of the anesthetics given annually to patients (American Associations of Nurse Anesthetists, 2010). From its inception, the role of the CRNA has focused on providing safe, effective anesthesia care to patients in the hospital setting. No particular groups of patients have been identified (i.e., healthier, more stable, poor, ethnically diverse, rural, or inner city) as a specific focus of CRNA care. In response to a critical shortage of anesthesia providers in the 1980s, the American Association of Nurse Anesthetists (AANA) established the National Commission on Nurse Anesthesia Education (NCNAE) to oversee all aspects of CRNA preparation and develop strategies that would enable nurses to respond to this crisis.

Multiple research reports suggest that the care provided by CRNAs is comparable to care provided by physicians who are anesthesiologists (Dulisse & Cromwell, 2010). CRNAs provide cost-effective, safe care and are increasingly in demand as the population ages and more people are enrolled in health-care plans (AANA, 2016b). Despite these positives, physician anesthetists continue to regulate CRNA practice and limit their work as independent providers of anesthesia care; however, the CRNA role has prevailed, especially in underserved and rural settings (AANA, 2016b).

Nurse Practitioners

NPs have traditionally focused on primary care for under-served populations within the inner city, rural areas, and other nonhospital settings. NPs continue to deliver patient care in settings in which traditional physician providers are unavailable. More recently, and in growing numbers, NPs provide care in the hospital setting.

In 2012 there were an estimated 154,000 NPs in the United States. The majority of NPs practiced in ambulatory care settings and nearly one third practiced in hospitals (U.S. Department of Health & Human Services, Health Resources and Services Administration, National Center for Health Workforce Analysis, 2014). More than 94% of these NPs had a graduate degree. Compared with primary care physicians, it has been reported that the majority of primary care NPs practice in urban primary care settings providing care to elderly, poor, and ethnically diverse populations with otherwise limited, or no, access to health care (Buerhaus, DesRoches, Dittus, & Donelan, 2015).

Keough and colleagues (2011) found that among the American Nurses Credentialing Center (ANCC) certified NPs they surveyed, a large number (42%) of acute care NPs were practicing in nontraditional settings; of that group, 90% were practicing in primary care. Other findings of this study suggest that less than 10% of primary care nurse adult–gerontology and family NPs were practicing in acute care settings. This trend of primary care NPs practicing in acute care settings and acute care NPs practicing in primary care settings requires monitoring to assure that NPs are practicing in the role for which they were prepared (Blackwell & Neff, 2015).

Numerous studies over a 40-year period focused on the care provided by NPs when compared with that provided by physicians for a variety of primary care-related conditions. These studies have demonstrated that NPs provide care that is as safe as and as effective as physicians. Additionally, patients often report higher levels of satisfaction with NP practice, particularly related to increased time spent with the patient for information gathering and teaching. Although patients cared for by NPs may have more return visits, they focus heavily on teaching, health promotion,

and self-care, which collectively contribute to a decrease in overall health-care costs. More importantly, NPs practicing within a nursing framework come to know the patient in a holistic way, including exploring meaning associated with sociocultural, financial, and other life situations as they relate to their health. This knowledge may significantly affect the NP's ability to provide care that is responsive to cost, quality, and effectiveness for both the organization and the patient.

NP practice settings have expanded to include NPs in urgent care, emergency department, and acute care settings. Outcome studies are needed to understand and evaluate the effectiveness of the NP role in these care settings.

Clinical Nurse Specialists

There are 59,242 CNSs who are registered nurses with advanced degrees at either the master's level (92.8%) or doctorate level (7.2%). This number represents an 18.4% decline in the CNS (HRSA, 2010). The CNS role developed because of fragmented health-care services and a lack of expert nursing care at the bedside, along with limited continuity in care across settings. With changes that have emerged in health care and cost containment, the CNS role has been affected. More than any other group of APRNs, CNSs report not "functioning in the role" (18.8%). Some CNSs who are dually certified as NPs work in that role (15.8%). Other roles of the CNS include management (17.8%), instruction (21.1%), and staff nurses (16%) (HRSA, 2010).

The CNS is an autonomous nurse clinician who provides specialized care in the community or hospital setting, usually through referral from other providers such as physicians and other nurses. The CNS is recognized as a clinical expert in a specialized area of patient care such as wound care, pain management, or diabetes care. Most CNSs work directly with patients and staff and in conjunction and collaboration with multiple members of the health-care team. With the exception of the psychiatric or mental health CNS, most CNSs do not have prescriptive authority.

According to the National Association of Clinical Nurse Specialists (NACNS) 2014 survey (NACNS, 2016), one in ten CNSs holds a doctorate; the primary area of specialty for CNSs is adult gerontology (71%) followed by psychiatric at 9.3% and pediatric at 8.5%. Most CNSs work in hospitals (59.4%); of that group, 38.84% work in hospitals that have achieved Magnet Recognition by the ANCC.

Although research has provided supportive evidence to link the contributions of the CNS to (a) reduced length of hospital stay, (b) reduced use of emergency rooms for care, (c) decreased hospitalization admissions and recidivism after discharge, and (d) diminished cost and increased satisfaction with care received (Fulton, 2010; Newhouse et al, 2011), the CNS has been challenged in many institutions by budget cuts. It is essential that CNSs conduct outcomes evaluation research that clearly links cost savings, patient care effectiveness, and improved satisfaction to their role (Erickson, Ditomassi, & Jones, 2015; Fulton, 2010).

APRN REIMBURSEMENT

Salaries for APRNs vary by region within the United States and are also influenced by years of experience, practice setting, specialty area, and education. According to the Bureau of Labor Statistics (2016) salaries of CRNAs are the highest of all APRNs, at an average salary in 2015 of $160,250 per year. The average annual salary in 2015 was $72,856 for CNSs, $101,260 for NPs, and $93,610 for CNMs. As in the general public, gender plays a significant role in APRN salaries, with women earning approximately $10,000 less than men (Wolfgang, 2014). It has been suggested that practice settings are the greatest determinant of salaries, with $30,000 separating the most profitable from the least profitable (Rollet, 2010).

Educational level and experience influence compensation. APRNs with approximately 11 to 15 years of experience earn the most (HRSA, 2010). In the United States, more APRNs are obtaining a doctorate, with enrollment in programs up 21.6% from 2012 to 2013; meanwhile, enrollment in PhD programs is up 49% since 2004 (AACN, 2013). Although some have indicated there are no differences in salary for the doctorate in nursing practice (DNP) as opposed to the master's prepared nurse, others report that DNPs earn $4,585 more than their colleagues with a master's degree (Jones, 2013).

To date there are no studies comparing outcomes of master's prepared NPs to the DNP prepared NP. Similar to other APRNs, NPs typically have additional benefits

such as health insurance, paid vacation and sick time, malpractice insurance, credentialing support, continuing education support, and, in some cases, incentives related to outcomes.

The reimbursement rules detailed in the *Federal Register* (1998) that revised Medicare reimbursement for physicians also included other health-care providers. Currently, Medicare payment has allowed CNSs, NPs, and physician assistant (PA) services to be reimbursed in selected situations. The Balanced Budget Act of 1997 facilitated direct Medicare reimbursement for the NP. Expanded Medicare reimbursement for acute-care NPs continues to be reviewed. The American Nurses Association (ANA) is working with a variety of federal agencies to improve direct reimbursement for APRNs, regardless of specialty and geographical location. Challenges associated with reimbursement in today's health-care environment are often linked to care outcomes and reimbursement policy established by insurers, mostly controlled at the state level. It is critical for APRNs to document their contributions to care and patient outcomes. Data that link the work of the APRN to improved patient outcomes, reduction in costs, enhanced patient and family satisfaction, and increased efficiency can be used to examine care and provide compensation recognizing the contributions of APRNs.

FUTURE TRENDS: THE IMPACT OF ADVANCED PRACTICE NURSES

Research comparing the effectiveness of APRN practice suggests that APRNs provide care that is comparable to and in some cases better than care provided by medical doctors (Newhouse et al, 2011). Key components of the APRN role include direct, comprehensive patient care; support and advocacy within the health-care system; monitoring and ensuring quality of and satisfaction with care; and education, research, publication, and leadership (Fulton, 2010; Gordon, Lorilla, & Lehman, 2012; ICN, 2016; Newhouse et al, 2011).

The ANA (1996) identified nurse-sensitive indicators in both the acute-care and community-based settings. They include care outcomes related to activities around pain management, patient satisfaction, cardiovascular disease prevention, pressure ulcer prevention and treatment, identification and prevention of risk for patient falls, nosocomial infection rate, and nurse satisfaction. Such indicators offer all APRNs a focus as well as an opportunity to research and disseminate findings about practice outcomes as suggested by Erickson, Jones, and Ditomassi (2012).

In addition, the Agency for Healthcare Research and Quality (AHRQ) Quality Indictors, Hospital Consumer Assessment of Healthcare Providers and Systems (HCAHPS), and ANCC Magnet Designation initiatives have greatly affected the roles of the CNS and inpatient NP. The AHRQ outlines nurse-sensitive indicators such as falls, skin ulcerations, and hospital-acquired infections (including ventilator-associated pneumonia and catheter-associated urinary tract infections) as conditions responsive to nursing care. These quality indicators are now linked to Medicare reimbursement through the Centers for Medicare and Medicaid Services' (CMS's) program. HCAHPS publicly reports patients' perspectives of hospital care. Magnet Status, a designation developed and rewarded by ANCC, recognizes excellence and innovation in nursing practice as it relates to quality outcomes (ANCC, 2008).

These agendas have spurred studies that aim to link the work of the CNS to improved patient care outcomes. In one study, CNS initiatives resulted in an 86% reduction in the incidence of catheter-associated bloodstream infections, a 47% reduction in catheter-associated urinary tract infections, and a 39% reduction in hospital-acquired pressure ulcer prevalence (Muller, Hujcs, Dubendorf, & Harrington, 2010). This type of compelling evidence provides support for the CNS role and decreases their vulnerability. Other trends such as enhanced safety and risk reduction and the goal of achieving Magnet Status have begun to revive the CNS role.

Although these nurse-sensitive quality indicators do much to support the CNS role, more-specific nurse-sensitive indicators are needed to distinguish the contributions of other APRNs such as the CNM, NP, and CRNA. As such, in January of 2016 Press Ganey (2016) started collecting data for the Outpatient and Ambulatory Surgery Patient Experience of Care Survey (OAS CAHPS), which provides information about patients' experiences of care in hospital outpatient surgery departments (HOPDs) and ambulatory surgery centers (ASCs). After 12 months of data collection, the CMS has announced that findings will be publicly reported in 2018 (Press Ganey, 2016). This is the first such expansion of measuring quality indicators in the outpatient arena and outcomes will shed light on outpatient APRN roles. Further expansion of such quality indicators will provide further evidence to support these roles.

CHANGES AND CHALLENGES IN HEALTH CARE

The past decade has presented many challenges to health-care organizations and the delivery of safe, quality, timely, cost-effective patient care. Currently, reforms include an overhaul of the current health-care system, with increased emphasis on (a) the need for continued cost reduction, (b) the identification of potential risks to existing and new services, and (c) vigilance and monitoring over rare, serious, and reportable medical events by the National Quality Forum.

From a national health policy perspective, implementation of the Affordable Care Act of 2009 has resulted in an increased demand for all APRNs, and NPs in particular. Millions of previously uninsured people are now able to obtain health insurance, resulting in an increased demand for APRNs in primary, long-term, and community-based settings. Care groups made up of physicians and APRNs will be organized to provide care to patients with high-risk problems, such as diabetes and heart disease, and other high-risk chronically ill or dying patients. These care groups will bring both specialists and primary care providers together to provide the best, most cost-effective, high-quality care.

The Institute of Medicine (IOM) 2011 report calls for initiatives that focus on changes that will enhance the potential of nurses to have a positive impact on the future of health care. They include the following:

1. Nurses should practice to the full extent of their education and training.
2. Nurses should achieve higher levels of education and training through an improved education system that promotes seamless academic progression.
3. Nurses should be full partners, with physicians and other health-care professionals, in redesigning health care in the United States.
4. Effective workforce planning and policy making require better data collection and information infrastructure.

Collectively, these agendas will affect care delivery, outcomes, and reimbursements. Additional changes in the health-care landscape have affected and will continue to affect APRNs. Since 1980, emphasis has been given to preparing medical doctors as primary care providers. However, 75% of physicians chose specialty practice over primary care, and this trend toward specialization continues (West & Dupras, 2012). Over the past 30 years, physicians are being prepared at a rate that is greater than the growth of the United States. Population estimates of current shortfalls in primary care physicians range from 33,100 to 65,000 (Iglehart, 2013; West & Dupras, 2012).

In addition, federal regulations, which limit the resident work week to 80 hours, have added a new burden to health-care delivery, creating a void in medical management within the acute-care setting. This trend presents added challenges to NPs, requiring them to fill this gap in care (Blum & Ellis, 2012). The added skills and competencies needed in such roles often focus more on medical specialty knowledge rather than on advanced nursing knowledge, such as being with, listening to, and coming to know the patient as a whole, complex person.

As the number of APRNs increases, competition for reimbursement and questions about the delivery of safe, effective, high-quality care and evidence-based patient or family practice continue to present challenges. Limited time during patients' visits coupled with reduced follow-up visits because of cost constraints may compromise the full impact of APRNs on patient care immediately and over time.

FUTURE DIRECTIONS AND FUTURE CONSIDERATIONS

Emerging changes within professional nursing have affected and will continue to affect APRN practice. The Consensus Model (2008) introduced standards for the licensure, accreditation, certification, and education (LACE) of APRNs. This model seeks to provide consistency and clarity around population-based health and areas of specialization. Further, this model will affect blended education programs that have attempted to merge rather than distinguish roles such as the CNS and NP.

With the American Association of Colleges of Nursing (AACN) recommendation that the DNP be the minimum degree for APRNs to enter practice (AACN, 2011) a growing number of APRNs are being prepared with a clinical doctorate. Since 2010 there has been a 51.2% increase

in the number of nurses pursuing this degree. Although there has been tremendous growth in DNP programs, it is not yet clear what added roles and responsibilities the DNP nurse will assume. The research-focused doctorate (doctorate of philosophy [PhD], doctor of education [EdD], or doctorate of nursing science [DNSc]) continues to be the highest academic degree for nurses, and currently all but seven states have research-focused doctorate programs. Recent statistics suggest that more than 28,369 nurses have a research-focused doctorate in nursing (HRSA, 2010).

Skills Versus Knowledge

APRN preparation includes knowledge, skills, and the resultant competencies for a particular role and populations plus advanced knowledge in the discipline of nursing itself. The graduate curriculum includes content on role preparation, research, and health policy, as well as knowledge that reflects disciplinary theory and concepts (e.g., holism and healing). In addition, specialty content related to populations, diagnoses, procedures and treatments, and disease management enhances an APRN's ability to care for patients.

The ability to blend components of both medicine and nursing makes the APRN unique, but too often the work of nursing becomes invisible as APRNs assume more of the medical role while underutilizing the domains unique to advanced practice nursing. This lack of nursing identity plagues the APRNs responding to the fiscal demands of health care.

Advancing the Discipline

APRNs need to continue to focus on cost-effective, outcomes-based practice and demonstrate patient satisfaction. Along with this work, APRNs must work to lift barriers to practice so they can practice to the fullest extent possible (Dower, Moore, & Langelier, 2013; IOM, 2011). Further, several troublesome issues have emerged in APRN practice: (a) Roles are consistently developed and morphed in a response to fill gaps in medicine, (b) there is a lack of distinction regarding the uniqueness of the role—either in comparison to medicine or to each other, and (c) there remains a lack of nursing-based outcomes to support the contribution of APRNs to individuals' heath, healing, and well-being within the current delivery system.

Despite the need for evidence-based practice, research supporting the APRN role is not a priority in clinical settings. When it does exist, the primary focus is to describe how APRNs are similar to rather than unique and distinct from their physician counterparts. The growth of the APRN role appears to be a response to shortages of physicians, rather than a complement or alternative in care, with clear distinctions about why a consumer would prefer one to the other. It is this lack of evidence that has negatively affected the CNS in the past decade (Fulton, 2010).

Some of the NP roles in acute care have been created in response to cuts in the hours worked by medical residents, and evidence suggests NPs are "as good as" or a welcome complement to physician care teams. However, it is troubling that studies focus on proving that NPs are "equal to" rather than providers of care with a unique focus. Limited use of standardized nursing language that communicates NP care beyond medical concerns is needed to provide evidence linked to outcomes. In articulating the language of nursing, APRNs are able to distinguish their practice and knowledge, as compared with other providers. The care provided by NPs in acute and chronic care settings is comprehensive specialty care that is sought by patients with complex medical and psychosocial problems.

Research, practice, and education are central to the APRN role. Without research that is sensitive to the breadth and depth of APRN practice, the role of the APRN will lack the needed evidence to advance professional nursing practice. Nursing studies that link nurse-sensitive quality indicators to patient care outcomes are essential to advancing the discipline. Doctorally prepared APRNs in clinical settings are critical to achieving this goal (Erickson, Ditomassi, & Jones, 2015).

Often the most critical element in any health-care setting is the nurse–patient relationship. Within this context there is the potential to discover meaning, affect individual choices, and promote health, healing, and personal transformation as suggested by Newman et al (2008) and Willis et al (2008). APRNs attending to this mandate may promote new behaviors that influence health-care outcomes in a cost-effective, efficient, timely, and safe manner.

CONCLUSION

This chapter focused on the role of APRNs and the contributions they have made to improve health care for all. Care provided by APRNs is safe, cost effective, and satisfying to patients and families. Trends in care suggest that both the practice settings and roles of APRNs have changed greatly since their inception. It is important for nurses practicing in these roles to continue to document and research practice outcomes so that when evidence is needed to support a role, it can easily be made available.

As health care evolves, it is important that APRNs reflect a clear image of professional nursing as opposed to changing in response to the call of medicine. Loss of disciplinary focus creates nurses who may be technically skilled and competent but unable to discuss their unique contributions. It is essential that an evaluation of the impact of the APRN take into account accomplishments that are often silent in a medically driven health-care system. These events may require the transition from "fix it" models of care delivery to frameworks guided by nursing knowledge to achieve personal changes and improved life for the patient.

26

Starting a Practice and Practice Management

Judith Barberio

Learning Outcomes

Learning outcomes expected as a result of this chapter:

- Consider the public policies that directly affect practice management such as reimbursement, billing and coding, and collaborative agreements.
- Identify barriers and facilitators of independent practice.
- Describe the growing presence of "pay for performance" models and "shared savings" programs.
- Characterize the development of niche markets.
- Demonstrate the relevance of licensing, taxation, and insurance to practice.
- Justify the hiring of ancillary personnel.
- Distinguish the legal differences between and among varied business structures.
- Create an image for the services offered by the advanced practice nurse (APN).
- Create a business plan for start-up of an independent practice.
- Recommend financial options for business start-up.
- Discuss the technicalities of documentation and the quality assurance process.

Advanced practice nurses (APNs) increasingly strive for greater autonomy in their practice. This desire to have control over their work environment has led to the emergence of independent nurse-managed health-care practices.

However, one must consider: Is an entrepreneurial spirit, a fine-tuned knowledge base and clinical skills, and the desire to provide quality health care enough to succeed? Over the past 25 years, individuals, as well as schools of nursing, have increasingly opened nurse-managed health centers only to see their viability threatened because of a lack of financial self-sufficiency (Brown, 2007; Ely, 2015; King, 2008; Vincent et al, 1999). New areas of concern revolve around shifting reimbursement models, care coordination models, and the implementation of ICD-10 coding. Additionally there is concern over the doctor of nursing practice (DNP) degree and how it affects master's-prepared APNs and their ability to continue to practice, as well as the impact on health-care policy issues such as reimbursement and independent practice without joint protocols.

ADVANTAGES TO INDEPENDENT PRACTICE

With the passage of the Affordable Care Act (ACA) and the resulting increased access to health care for many Americans, there came a need for more primary care providers (PCPs) and more cost-effective services. Nurse-managed practices are positioned to play an important role in access to cost-effective health care; however, for these practices to survive and grow, APNs must acquaint themselves with the emerging realities of the new health-care policy agenda and display the business acumen and financial know-how that is essential to create practices that are efficient and fiscally viable.

Independent nursing practice continues to garner support and become a reality. The ability to maximize care of the client is dependent on having time to provide an educational base for consumers that will enable them to become true partners in the health-care regimen. The ACA, along with the American Recovery and Reinvestment Act (ARRA), has the potential to remove many of the barriers to independent APN practice (Kocher, Emanuel, & DeParle, 2010). See **Box 26.1**. The time to embrace an entrepreneurial spirit may be *now*.

BARRIERS TO INDEPENDENT PRACTICE

With all the advantages to independent practice, why do so few APNs consider this alternative? APNs have long been lauded in the literature with respect to their high quality

---

Box 26.1

Opportunities That Can Come With Independent Practice

1. You have the freedom to focus the practice and your energy on your interests, such as alternative therapy or acupuncture, or specialty populations such as women's health or geriatrics.
2. Time management becomes flexible. You have the ability to structure your workload and allow time to examine, counsel, and educate clients.
3. The quality of your practice becomes your responsibility and is under your control. You are able to include the preventive health care and education needed at each client encounter.
4. Multiple sources for reimbursement can be identified and pursued. Besides third-party reimbursement, contracts for service can be sought out in industry and community groups. Income can be tied to workload.
5. New opportunities and requests for service provide a challenge to expand services and promote the growth of the practice.
6. Staffing becomes your responsibility and provides the opportunity to work with people you respect and who share your philosophy of health care.
7. Enhanced problem-solving skills and self-esteem are positive by-products of independent practice for the entrepreneurial APN. Learning to constructively deal with change, resolve conflicts, and successfully implement strategies creates a profitable practice and enhances self-confidence and self-esteem.

---

of patient care and cost-effectiveness (Carzoli et al, 1994; Newhouse et al, 2011; Office of Technology Assessment, 1986; Spitzer et al, 1974). Their practice has been compared with physicians in primary care practices and findings suggest that APNs provide comparable high-quality care with similar positive health outcomes (Mundinger et al, 2000; Newhouse et al, 2011). What barriers to practice are so prevalent that they dissuade this competent, highly educated, and cost-effective group of health-care providers from establishing independent practices?

In 2007 Pearson identified four major roadblocks to independent APN practice, which still exist today:

1. The need for direct reimbursement from third-party payers
2. Statutory limitations to the APN's scope of practice
3. Inconsistent and restrictive prescriptive authority
4. The inability to obtain hospital privileges

Many factors contribute to the roadblocks that stand in the way of independent APN practice. Throughout the 20th century physicians have controlled health-care practice and health information, partially because they were the first health-care providers to be granted legislative autonomy. This legislative autonomy and recognition enhanced the public's confidence that the actions of physicians were always directed for the good of the public and not for personal gain. Financial security, legislative strength, and a unified medical community also played a role in organized medicine's control of hospital policy and third-party reimbursement (Brassard & Smolenski, 2011; Mirvis, 1999).

Over the past decade the clinical doctorate with a focus on administrative leadership, clinical practice, and clinical education has evolved. Supporters of this terminal clinical degree cite the need for nursing to attain parity with other health-care disciplines. They argue that increased knowledge is needed to provide leadership in health-care system effectiveness and optimal patient outcomes. Advocates maintain that educational credentials are needed to be included in high-level health-care management and policy decisions (Cronenwett et al, 2011; Fain, Asselin, & McCurry, 2008). Some master's-prepared APNs fear being marginalized to second-class status as the DNP becomes the preferred educational degree for APNs. The potential for devaluation of MS-prepared APNs exists, as does the possibility of being replaced by APN providers with a clinical doctorate (Meleis & Dracup, 2005). This fear of becoming obsolete may discourage an entrepreneurial spirit.

In addition to persuasive national barriers, common problems applicable to most new start-up businesses contribute to the demise of independent APN practices. Major obstacles to overcome with the start of most new businesses include the following:

1. Start-up costs for the practice
2. Cash-flow and financing an ongoing practice
3. Accounting practices, billing, and collection of receipts

4. Day-to-day management of the practice
5. Compliance with city, state, and federal regulations
6. General and malpractice insurance for the practice and individual providers
7. Hiring, training, and retaining competent, enthusiastic personnel

The obstacles inherent in starting a business coupled with the unique barriers confronting independent APN practice have provided a challenge to many individuals. This chapter acknowledges their struggles, learns from their mistakes, and provides guidance to the entrepreneurial APN who is about to embark on this journey.

FIRST THINGS FIRST

The decision has been made: You want to be your own boss and deliver health care *your* way. No more time clocks, overbooking clients, or cutting short the patient visit because of time constraints. But where do you go from here? Key considerations and decisions must be made to get your business up and running. The items listed in **Box 26.2** will focus your operation and provide the organizing details

---

Box 26.2

Key Business Decisions

- Develop a clear-cut strategy
- Determine the area's need for the service
- Develop a timeline for business start-up
- Determine licensing, tax, and insurance requirements
- Select your consultants
- Decide on the appropriate business structure
- Create the business name and image
- Select a practice location
- Develop a business plan
- Determine financing options
- Develop fees, reimbursement, and billing procedures
- Purchase equipment and select suppliers
- Hire and manage personnel
- Develop an organized documentation and quality assurance process
- Develop policies and procedures
- Develop marketing strategies

that determine start-up efficiency in the world of shifting reimbursement models and changing patient care models.

KEY QUESTIONS

As you embark on the key start-up decisions to be made, pay attention to the questions that may arise. A major question to consider is the scope of independent APN practice in the state in which you practice. Twenty-nine states currently have statutory or regulatory requirements for physician collaboration, direction, or supervision. Only 21 states and the District of Columbia have independent prescriptive authority that does not require physician involvement or delegation (AANP, 2016). If your practice is not located in one of these enlightened states, carefully read and clarify the policies regarding collaboration or supervision of your practice and the regulation of your prescriptive authority. Developing a collaborative agreement with a physician and creating appropriate protocols, including protocols for controlled dangerous substances (CDSs), are other areas to investigate if this is a state requirement for APN practice.

Reimbursement is another major question to consider. Where will it come from and will it be enough to cover your expenses? Payment for services and procedures have changed to the new ICD-10 diagnosis coding system as of October 2015. This new system requires much more specificity in clinical documentation in the medical record to support the diagnosis code used for billing (Breen et al, 2015; Fleming et al, 2015). Emerging reimbursement models are moving the health-care system away from fee-for-service to rewarding improved health-care quality and patient outcomes. Models to investigate are "pay for performance" models that work well for solo or small practices. These models compensate the care-provider on clinical and cost-saving outcomes rather than payment for services and procedures. Accountable care organizations (ACO) are examples of "shared savings programs" where provider-led organizations or practices are collectively accountable for quality and costs for a patient population across the continuum of care. This can lead to lower costs where savings are shared with the ACO members or higher costs absorbed by the ACO members. Other new models of reimbursement to explore include bundled payments, capitation, and hybrid payments that share the costs and quality of health care with providers and payers (Gosfield, 2013; Navathe et al, 2016; Ritchie et al, 2016; Terry et al, 2014).

Investigate whether managed care is pervasive in your practice location and determine if APNs are admitted to managed care panels and are listed as PCPs. If APNs are accepted in your state as PCPs and practice independently, how do you deal with the patient whose condition exacerbates and needs hospitalization? Investigate the area hospitals to determine if APNs are given hospital privileges. Even if APNs are admitted to hospital panels in your area, you will need a collaborative arrangement or referral agreement with various physicians in the area for management of your patients when they are acutely ill. Evaluate new models of care such as patient-centered medical homes, patient navigators, and care coordinators as a means to improve quality at reduced cost. Payment in revised models of care to improve quality and reduce risk includes care coordination for their members. Care coordination models are especially attractive to payers to mitigate the high cost of care for patients with increased health risks and those with complex and chronic health conditions (Steaban, 2016).

These and other questions will arise as you carry out the myriad tasks needed to launch a new business. Pay attention to detail and carefully consider each question and decision you make. These decisions will structure your practice operations and ultimately enable you to attain your personal and professional goals.

DEVELOP A CLEAR-CUT STRATEGY

Strategy distinguishes your business. It tells the consumer what differentiates your practice from the competition. It is the foundation of your business plan and dictates the day-to-day operations of your practice. How does one develop a strategy? Look around you and consider the market, consumer needs, the competition, your practice's strengths and weaknesses, and your philosophy of health care and personal goals.

Focus the nature of your practice and do not try to be all things to all patients. Competitive personal service businesses, such as a health-care practice, will commonly use the strategy of specialization. Specialization reduces competition and drives reimbursement. Initially, you may want to see any patient who elects to seek your help. As you begin to develop your practice, simultaneously begin to advertise, write articles for the local newspaper, and hold seminars on topics that focus on your expertise. This exposure will promote the area in which you wish to specialize and will allow you to phase out other aspects of your practice.

Specialize by developing a niche market, one that you know extremely well. A niche market is one with a unique service or product that services a particular clientele. You may decide that you want the focus of your practice to be on wellness. You can then tailor your practice to offer individual health risk assessments, counseling on behavior change, work site wellness programs, smoking cessation and weight loss programs, and countless other health promotion activities that may be needed in your location. One word of advice: Know your service. Do not begin a practice marketing alternative therapy without an exhaustive knowledge of these services or competent, knowledgeable staff. Remember that your competition is already established and knows the business aspects of the practice better than you do. You want to present yourself as an expert in the field.

DETERMINE THE AREA'S NEED FOR THE SERVICE

Determine who the potential clients are and then attempt to ascertain their needs. If you decide that your practice will serve the health-care needs of inner-city, low-income residents, you must investigate the most prevalent reasons for health-care use and follow-up care. This information can be gathered from various sources. The state nurses association, state division of health, and county and local health departments may be helpful in providing important data. Topics you may want to explore include health provider demographics for an area, medically underserved areas, and health-care delivery systems in an area such as ambulatory care centers, urgent care centers, and family planning clinics. Local businesses, such as pharmacies and medical device companies, may also provide information about the health-care needs of the local population, as well as advertising and articles in the local newspaper.

DEVELOP A TIMELINE FOR BUSINESS START-UP

Organization is the key ingredient to developing a business plan and moving your practice from the planning stage into action. A minimum of 9 months should be allowed to complete this project. Designate yourself as the project leader and determine other individuals who may assist you with start-up tasks. The key undertaking of business start-up is persistence and attention to detail. A sample timeline for completing major tasks is presented in **Box 26.3.**

Box 26.3

Practice Start-Up Timeline

Nine Months Before Practice Start-Up

1. Select a geographical location.
2. Obtain contracts from third-party payers and hospitals you wish to join.
3. Determine start-up costs of a practice and your net worth.
4. Develop a business plan.
5. Investigate sources of capital investment in your practice.
6. Obtain loan applications, speak to various loan officers, and submit applications.
7. Determine when telephone books are printed and list your practice.

8. Open a business checking account.
9. Obtain state nursing license, advanced practice license, and federal DEA number.

Six Months Before Practice Start-Up

1. Investigate practice locations for rent or purchase.
2. Inquire about zoning laws regarding your type of practice and signage requirements.
3. Determine utility requirements for your practice, sources, and cost.
4. Determine office layout, design, and necessary structural improvements.

Continued

BOX 26.3

Practice Start-Up Timeline *(Continued)*

5. Determine needed office and medical equipment and determine cost of lease versus buy.
6. Explore and select business consultants, specifically a lawyer, accountant, banker, insurance broker, and medical biller.
7. Determine form of the practice, such as solo practice, partnership, or corporation, and have your attorney draw up all legal documents for your signature.
8. Evaluate all contracts with your attorney before signing.
9. Investigate medical practice systems that contain scheduling, billing, and records.
10. Make application for federal Medicare, Medicaid, and NPI numbers and obtain fee schedules.
11. Obtain current procedural terminology book (CPT-4) and *International Classification of Diseases, Ninth Revision, Clinical Manual* (ICD-10-CM) and the HCFA 1500 insurance claim forms.
12. Formalize a collaborative agreement with an area physician if required by law.
13. Apply for an office laboratory license or a CLIA waiver.
14. Apply for provider status to managed care provider panels.
15. Apply for hospital privileges to local health-care institutions.

Three Months Before Practice Start-Up

1. Arrange for professional malpractice insurance for providers and liability insurance for the practice and equipment.
2. Arrange for health and disability insurance for yourself and employees.
3. Arrange for telephone service installation and an answering service for the practice, beeper service, and call forwarding service.
4. Order signage for the practice.
5. Investigate and arrange for the acceptance of credit cards as a payment option.

6. Design and order announcements for the opening of your practice.
7. Apply for your federal and state EIN through your local IRS office and state labor department.
8. Review federal and state tax requirements with your accountant and obtain booklets describing federal, state, and city tax withholding requirements.
9. Develop a policy and procedure manual for the practice.
10. Develop job descriptions for all employees.
11. Begin advertising and interviewing for office personnel.
12. Arrange for needed services such as biomedical waste management, specimen pickup, janitorial services, laundry services, and ground maintenance and snow removal.
13. Order clinical supplies and set up an inventory control system.
14. Order business supplies such as state prescription pads (if mandated), appointment cards, business cards, letterhead stationery and envelopes, stationery supplies, deposit stamp for checks, petty cash vouchers, purchase order forms, telephone message pads, and patient referral forms and disposition forms.
15. Order office equipment and arrange for delivery.
16. Determine office hours.
17. Determine fee schedule.
18. Develop advertising information such as a patient booklet of services, press release, and introduction letters to local health-care providers, pharmacy and medical equipment suppliers, and pharmaceutical representatives in your area.
19. Develop your practice Web site and professional Facebook page, and explore Twitter and YouTube for their advertising potential for your practice.

One Month Before Practice Start-Up

1. Set up your office.
2. Arrange for utility start-up, including telephone, gas, electric, and water.

Box 26.3

Practice Start-Up Timeline (*Continued*)

3. Hire a medical biller and obtain your Medicare, Medicaid, NPI, and MCO provider numbers.
4. Hire office personnel and train them with respect to office policies, telephone procedures, appointment scheduling and collection of fees, and use of the medical office system.
5. Establish the office cash flow procedures and a petty cash fund.
6. Install your office sign.

7. Accept patient appointments.
8. Place announcements, advertisements, and press releases in local newspapers and send to local community groups and area professionals.

Opening Day

Congratulations, you have started an independent APN practice!

DETERMINE LICENSING, TAX, AND INSURANCE REQUIREMENTS

To open an independent APN practice, several licenses must be obtained. After choosing a location for your practice, your next priority should be to apply for all state and federal licenses. Besides state licensure for nursing and advanced practice nursing, you must also obtain state and federal identification numbers and a federal Drug Enforcement Administration (DEA) number, as well as others to open your door and do business. The most commonly required licenses and tax identification numbers have been listed.

State Nursing License and Advanced Practice License or Certification

The state board of nursing will be able to provide information and a list of documents you need to apply for these licenses. Be aware that in some states the board of nursing or the board of medicine oversee the advanced practice nursing license or certification.

State-Controlled Substances License

Check with your state concerning the requirement for a state license to prescribe federally controlled substances. This is not a requirement in all states, but if it is, it must be obtained before application for a federal narcotics license. Your state's board of nursing will be able to inform you

if this license is necessary and the procedure to obtain this license.

Federally Controlled Substances License

APNs do not have legal authority in all states to dispense all categories of controlled substances. You will be able to obtain the necessary information from the board of nursing in your state. DEA numbers are assigned for your lifetime; they will not be reassigned if you move to another location. If you move to another state, you are required to notify the DEA authorities of your new address. If you do not have a DEA number and can legally prescribe controlled substances in your state, you can obtain this license from the DEA, Office of Diversion Control, Registration Unit. Their toll-free number, answered 24 hours a day, is 1-800-882-9539. The DEA also has forms online for registration of APNs. The application form can be found on the Web at the Diversion Control Program Web site at www.deadiversion.usdoj.gov.

Medicaid Provider Number

Medicaid is a jointly funded, federal-state health insurance program for certain low-income people. The people covered include children, the aged, blind, disabled, and people who are eligible to receive federally assisted income maintenance payments.

You can apply for this provider number through the state Medicaid agency. Obtain a provider application for

APNs from the provider relations department of your state health department. The state Medicaid agency is billed using the Centers for Medicare and Medicaid Services (CMS) 1500 form unless the client is enrolled in Medicaid managed care.

The number you receive from your state Medicaid agency will remain with you while you practice in the state. If you move within the state, you only need to notify the carrier of your new address. If you move out of state, you will need to obtain a new number in the new state.

Medicaid Managed Care

Some patients who have health insurance through the state Medicaid program will be covered under a managed care organization (MCO). To obtain a provider number for Medicaid MCOs, you must contact the provider relations for each MCO and apply for admission to the panel of providers. APNs are not admitted to provider panels in all MCOs. In some states, MCOs cannot discriminate among providers on the basis of type of license held. In other states, an MCO can accept or reject any provider. Check your state law concerning managed care and provider panels. If you are initially rejected, request a meeting to present your case. Pursue the MCO to reevaluate your application and go up the chain of command with your request.

Medicare

Medicare is a federal health insurance program for certain groups of people including the elderly over age 65 and the permanently disabled. This program covers hospitalization (Part A); provider services, home care, and outpatient health care (Part B); and medication (Part D).

If you will be providing health-care services to this population, you need to apply for a Medicare number. This number will only be valid in the state in which you currently practice. If you move out of state, you will be assigned a new Medicare number for that state.

An insurer in each state that has contracted with the CMS manages the administration and payment services for Medicare. You can find the Medicare carrier for your state by going to the CMS Web site at www.cms.hhs.gov/ or Medicare at www.medicare.gov/. Once you are aware of the carrier for your state, you can obtain an application and apply for a provider number. Medicare is billed on a form called the CMS 1500. The preferred method of billing for Medicare is electronic funds transfer (EFT), which can be selected when enrolling in Medicare for the first time or when making a change to your existing enrollment information. If a patient is enrolled in Medicare managed care, reimbursement is handled by an MCO and the provider must be admitted to the MCO provider panel.

National Provider Identifier

The national provider identifier (NPI) is a unique identification number given to each health-care provider and used in standard transactions, such as claims for reimbursement for health-care services. This number may be used to identify health-care providers on several documents including prescriptions, patient medical records, and coordination of benefits between health plans. Once assigned, the NPI is expected to remain the same regardless of change of name, change of address, or change of other information provided on the original application. The NPI is the only health-care provider identifier that can be used for identification purposes in standard transactions including electronic billing.

Health-care providers may apply for an NPI number through the national plan and provider enumeration system (NPPES) available at https://nppes.cms.hhs.gov. The phone number for the NPI Enumerator is 800-465-3203 (voice) or 800-692-2326 (TTY/texting). They can be reached online at customerservice@npienumerator.com. There is no fee associated with obtaining an NPI.

If health-care providers do not have a Medicare or Medicaid provider number, they are encouraged to apply for the NPI before enrolling in these programs. Health-care providers who already have enrolled in these programs are encouraged to include their Medicare identification number, Medicaid identification number and state, and any other provider numbers issued by health plans in which they are enrolled when applying for the NPI.

Clinical Laboratory License

CMS regulates all laboratory testing performed on humans in the United States through the Clinical Laboratory Improvement Amendments (CLIA). The objective of the CLIA program is to ensure quality laboratory testing. These amendments require that all health provider office laboratories must be licensed according to the types of tests they perform. Office laboratories are subject to federal and state inspection and approval. The more complex the testing, the more stringent the state and federal laboratory requirements. However, any laboratory testing done on-site will require the facility to have a CLIA number.

Laboratory tests are divided into categories, and there are several waived tests that can be performed in the office setting. A practice that only performs waived tests can apply for an exemption from inspection and the requirement of a medical director to oversee the laboratory. Federal CLIA regulations can be found on the Internet at www.cms.hhs.gov/clia/ and state CLIA regulations can be obtained from the state health department. The state will provide forms for the federal and state application for a CLIA number. Pay particular attention to the state regulations because many times the state regulations are more restrictive than the federal guidelines.

Employer Identification Number

The employer identification number (EIN) is a tax identification number and is needed for all communication with the Internal Revenue Service (IRS). You can apply for an EIN number online at https://www.irs-taxid-number.com or by phone at 888-321-6690. The EIN will be used to report compensation from third-party payers such as private insurance companies, Medicare, or Medicaid.

State Tax Identification Number

Contact your state to confirm if there is an additional need to apply for a state tax identification number. The local phone number can be found in the White Pages listed under United States or the name of your state. Your accountant will be able to inform you of all identifying numbers needed to satisfy federal and state regulations.

Professional Liability Insurance

Many carriers cover APNs, including traditional insurance companies, self-insured companies, and group purchasing programs. Not all companies conduct business in every state. Choose a company that has experienced claim adjusters and a formidable legal network. Inquire about the company's service orientation and its capacity to offer risk management and loss prevention assistance and advice. Consider a company that has been in business for at least 10 years and has a good financial standing. Litigation can take many years to come to fruition, and you want a company with the capability to remain in business to defend you.

Some points to consider when evaluating insurance policies:

1. How comprehensive is the policy? Make sure you read the policy thoroughly and note the inclusions as well as the exclusions. Question anything you do not understand; it may save you a great deal of stress and money if litigation ensues.
2. What type of insurance should you purchase: "claims made" or "occurrence"? A claims made policy will cover the APN only when the insurance policy is active, no matter when the incident occurred. If you were to retire and cancel your insurance policy, you would no longer be covered for any prior incident if litigation ensues at a later date. An occurrence policy will cover the APN for any incident that occurred while the insurance policy was in place.
3. Are the limits of coverage adequate? Many APNs purchase insurance based on the minimal coverage of $1,000,000 per occurrence and $3,000,000 cumulative. We reside in a litigious society, and this amount of coverage can easily be exhausted. Consider purchasing cumulative insurance that is at least double to triple the occurrence amount.
4. Should you purchase "tail coverage"? Frequently, APNs may join a group practice that already has a group policy for professional liability coverage. If you currently have malpractice insurance that you plan on canceling, consider purchasing tail coverage. This policy will cover any prospective legal action from events before joining the group practice.
5. Do you own the practice? If so, you may want to name the practice on your insurance policy. If litigation ensues, usually the practice, as well as an individual, is named.
6. Is business malpractice insurance necessary? Absolutely. Cover the practice. Inquire with the insurance company about the rates for covering an independent APN practice. This coverage will be in addition to your individual plan and can prove quite cost effective in the event of litigation.

Conventional Commercial Insurance Policies

Besides professional and business malpractice insurance, consider purchasing insurance protection for your office, the employees, and the equipment you have purchased. Some types of insurance to consider:

1. *Equipment insurance:* The expenditure for medical and office equipment is costly. A reasonably priced property insurance policy will cover the cost to replace the tangible assets of the practice. This policy should cover all medical equipment and supplies, office equipment and supplies, textbooks, and journals. Insurance premiums typically decrease as deductibles rise.

2. *Equipment malfunction insurance:* Many companies sell product warranties to cover equipment malfunction, repair, and replacement. Investigate commercial insurance companies for a blanket policy that covers all major equipment purchases. Many policies will also cover lost revenue for the time period that the equipment is unproductive.

3. *General liability coverage:* This is comprehensive insurance coverage that protects your practice in the event of litigation by a third party. It does not cover the policy holder or other parties specifically excluded. This policy typically includes lawsuits for personal injury, equipment failure, contractual liability, and advertising liability.

4. *Office disability insurance:* If your office becomes inaccessible because of property loss, your practice could go out of business in a short period of time. This policy should include reimbursement for lost revenue and profit; continuous expenses such as the lease on the copy machine; funding to temporarily relocate your office, purchase supplies, and advertise your new location; and finally the cost to return to your office after it has been restored.

5. *Workers' compensation insurance:* Most states require this insurance for any business that has employees. The owner of the business is usually not covered by this insurance unless the business is a corporation. This policy can be purchased from a commercial insurance company, but the state will regulate the benefits and cost of the policy. Therefore, most policies are comparable.

SELECT YOUR CONSULTANTS

Starting a health-care practice requires knowledge of state and federal laws, as well as general legal and accounting procedures. It is highly advisable to consult with these professionals as you set up your practice. Seek recommendations from other APNs, colleagues, business associates, the state nursing organization, and the board of nursing.

Attorney services will focus on setting up the legal structure of your practice and provide legal advice and contract development and review. When you interview attorneys, pay particular attention to their health-care law experience, especially with respect to independent APN practice.

An *accountant* is another professional whose expertise can be cost effective for the short term as well as the long term. Initially, consult with this professional to develop an accounting system, initiate internal controls, and establish an operating budget. As the practice develops, the accountant may suggest operating procedures that will provide for the best tax advantage and provide tax-planning consultation.

A *medical biller* is an essential component of any health-care practice that intends to receive reimbursement from third-party payers. Medical billers will be involved in all aspects of billing and collecting accounts receivable. They may set up and track a charge account with a major credit card company for patients who self-pay and send billing statements to patients who have been extended credit by the health-care practice. Medical billers frequently make application to insurer provider panels for the health-care providers in the practice. Additionally, they will make applications to NPI, Medicare, and Medicaid for provider numbers for the practice and all professional staff. Once avenues of reimbursement are established, the medical biller will ensure that the patient and medical information requested by the payer is completed and will submit the bill for payment. Tracking accounts receivable and questioning and resubmitting denial of payments is another aspect of the services provided by a medical biller. The scope of services from a medical biller will depend on the expertise and experience of this consultant. Many practices find it more cost effective to hire a full-time medical biller, whereas smaller practices may hire an off-site independent service to handle the billing aspect of the practice. Judiciously assess the qualifications and reputation of the employee or service you are contemplating.

A *practice manager* might be just the person or service you need if you are taking over an established practice or have a large patient following. An experienced practice manager may provide accounting and bookkeeping services, as well as total practice management. Services offered can vary greatly by consultant and fees will increase as services provided increase. Practice managers may perform such services as hiring employees, maintaining bank accounts, paying practice bills, billing and account receivables for services rendered, staffing, payroll, tracking and ordering supplies, and contracting for laboratory, biomedical waste, and janitorial services. Many practice management consultants will develop employee job descriptions, policy and procedure manuals, and fee schedules that are consistent with the local market. Always ask for local references, preferably with other health-care providers, especially other APN practices. Remember to always check references and qualifications to get an idea of the types of services provided by this consultant, his or her experience and expertise, and his or her ability to competently complete the project in a timely manner.

DECIDE ON THE APPROPRIATE BUSINESS STRUCTURE

There are basically four types of business structures for a practice: sole proprietorship, partnership, corporation, or a limited liability corporation (LLC). The legal differences between these forms of business are contained in three issues: liability, the number of owners, and tax ramifications.

Sole Proprietorship

This is the simplest form of business, where the owner of the business and the business are one and the same. All the assets and liabilities of the business are also the personal assets and liabilities of the owner. The owner of an independent APN practice is personally liable for any debt or legal infractions of the practice. There are no explicit prerequisites to establishing a sole proprietorship. A sole proprietorship can have only one owner of the business and is established when you go into business by yourself. This gives the APN the advantage of "running her own show" and establishing a practice according to specific beliefs and preferences. A sole proprietorship is not taxed

per se. Because the business and the owner are one and the same, the owner completes an individual tax return along with a Schedule C, a "profit and loss from business" form, which is used to file the practice earnings and expenses. Year-end profits and losses from the practice will be added to or subtracted from the owner's personal income.

Benefits from this type of business structure include autonomy, flexibility, and the ability to make practice decisions based on your individual philosophy. Any losses suffered by the practice, which is common in the start-up phase of a business, can be deducted from your personal income. Control of the profits is another benefit of this business structure along with a simplified tax return. A major disadvantage of a sole proprietorship is the total liability for all start-up and maintenance costs of the practice, as well as the negligence of any employees.

Partnership

A *partnership* is defined as the association of two or more people to carry on as co-owners of a business to make a profit. Although a partnership agreement is not required by law, most parties will spell out the relationship in a legal agreement. In a partnership there is a differentiation between the partnership and the partners. Partnerships cannot sue or be sued. However, all partners are personally liable for losses, wrongful acts, and omissions or commissions assumed by the partnership. Partners share in the profits, administration, decision making, and workload of the practice as defined in the partnership agreement. In this type of practice, earnings or losses pass through to the individual partners and appear on each partner's personal tax return.

A major benefit of this type of business structure is the shared financial and professional risks and responsibilities. Decision making remains fairly flexible and it is generally easier to attract venture capital for financing the practice. The disadvantages of a partnership include the unlimited personal liability of each partner and the responsibility of each partner to pay taxes on business income.

Corporation

A corporation is an individual legal entity without ties to the individual business owner and is generally formed as a C corporation. It has the legal status to buy and sell assets and enter into contracts. It has its own tax identification number as well as tax return. A professional corporation enjoys limited liability in that only the corporate assets can be used to satisfy judgments; therefore, it reduces the personal and financial risk of the APN owner and shareholder. In a professional practice, the APN is paid a salary, and as an owner or shareholder receives the profits of the corporation as dividends throughout the year. The downside of this arrangement is that the corporation is taxed on its profits and then the individual is taxed on the dividends. The owner of a small corporation can elect to be an S corporation that offers special tax advantages. All profits of an S corporation are taxable only as they are distributed as dividends to shareholders. Because of the intricacies of the law and the ever-changing tax laws, it is essential that the APN consult a tax professional.

Advantages of a corporate structure are the limited liability of the shareholders, centralized management, tax advantages for pension and profit-sharing plans, and a larger talent pool for decision making. Disadvantages of a corporation include the costs involved to establish and operate the corporation. There are also time-consuming federal, state, and local government requirements and filings to deal with, as well as the possibility of double taxation on corporate profits and shareholder dividends.

Limited Liability Corporation

A LLC is another form of corporate structure that provides the best aspects of a partnership and a corporation. Income and losses pass through to the shareholders or owners as in a partnership and there is no limit on the number of owners or shareholders. Legal liability is also limited and members are not liable for the overall obligations of the LLC, although an individual would still be liable for professional malpractice. This type of corporate structure is also easier to set up and is subject to less government regulation. Be aware that LLCs are not recognized in all states, so be sure to check with your accountant or attorney.

Benefits of this type of corporate structure include limited liability and taxation only on the member's share of the LLC's income. An unlimited number of shareholders are allowed and the shareholders or an appointed manager can manage the LLC. Disadvantages include limited recognition of this corporation by individual states and limited legal precedent addressing this form of corporate structure.

CREATE THE BUSINESS NAME AND IMAGE

Image plays an important role in how your practice is perceived in the marketplace. Your image is reflected in the office environment, advertising materials, your personal presentation and that of your staff, and written communication. Determine what image you want to present to your patients and convey this in your business name and practice style.

Ascertain what image would generate a positive response from prospective patients. Would a warm, homey atmosphere or a high-tech, professional office create more appeal for your target population? Are you trying to convey the notion of alternative therapy or new concepts in health-care delivery? Investigate what the potential consumer expects in his or her health-care provider. Above all, project high quality in every aspect of your practice, from the service you provide to the image you present.

Carefully evaluate the image you project in every patient encounter. Pay attention to every detail of the practice even if you delegate responsibilities to staff or consultants. Make sure the staff conveys their commitment to patient care and service during each interaction with patients. Consider the advantages of consulting with experts for certain aspects of the practice. A graphic artist may be better able to create a logo or brochure for the practice. Perhaps a marketing expert can develop a more effective advertising strategy. Keep in mind that image considerations play a part in all your practice decisions and should be used as a guide for future decision making.

A business name should convey the image you want to present to the public and will basically take on one of two forms: your name or a name you have created for the practice. By selecting your name as the legal name of the practice, you are conveying a professional image and making the patient aware of the health-care provider in this practice. If you have been part of another practice in the area or are well known in this location, your name recognition may draw in several patients. The addition of "and Associates" to your name will convey the appearance of a larger practice with additional resources.

Professional practices do not always convey the names of the health-care providers. Many APNs prefer to project the name of what they do to reflect their business focus. Lois Brenneman of NPCEU decided to market her product versus her name. NPCEU offers continuing education programs to APNs nationally. An individual was purposely not identified with this practice to project the image of large numbers of programs with a variety of speakers. *Elder Choices* is a health-care counseling practice that was developed by a group of APNs with expertise in gerontology and counseling. The name of this practice conveys the target population and the focus of the practice. Ultimately the choice is yours. Consider the image you want to project and use this as a guide in choosing a name.

SELECT A PRACTICE LOCATION

Location, location, location. This will be one of your most important business decisions. Think about your ideal geographical location, knowledge of the marketplace, professional relationships, and professional climate. Remember, health care is local, not global. The highs and lows of the local economy will have an effect on the success of your practice. Several factors will play into your ultimate choice of practice location.

Geographical Location

When you consider your practice location, think about convenience for your patients and the niche market you want to attract. A pediatric practice located in a downtown business location will not be as appealing as a practice location in a growing suburb. Ascertain parking availability in your practice location and determine if it is adequate to meet the needs of your clients. If on-site parking is limited or unavailable, investigate the proximity of public transportation to your practice location. If you hope to attract walk-in patients, determine if your practice is located in a heavily used pedestrian area. Remember that your services must not only be high quality, be cost effective, and have public appeal, but they must also be convenient.

Demographics

The demographic makeup of your location will provide a snapshot of your market. The U.S. Census Bureau; local, county, and state governments; and private demographic services can provide the data necessary to evaluate a location. Pay particular attention to a few key factors.

1. *Male versus female population in a given area.* Women are the primary purchasers of health care and typically direct the health care of their families.
2. *The age distribution of the local population.* Age dictates the type of services chosen. New-age therapies might not be as eagerly accepted by a rural aging clientele as they would by upwardly mobile city dwellers. Age also influences the types of care used. Pediatric and midwifery services are sought after in a childbearing, child-rearing population, whereas wellness programs, health education, and chronic illness management may have a higher use among an older population.
3. *The income distribution in the local population.* Income influences the probability of and type of health insurance coverage, as well as disposable dollars for noncovered therapies and preventive programs. A stable or growing population is frequently associated with higher incomes and employment security.
4. *Cultural and language influences on the local population.* Cultural background, values, and practices of particular groups of people will influence their use of health care and wellness programs. Language barriers can be a significant factor to patient use of your services. Consider hiring personnel from the neighborhood who are familiar with the culture and speak the language of the local population.

Professional Relationships

Do not discount the professional relationships you have made along your professional career path. Prior employment, educational training, preceptorships, and professional associates are all sources of reference and referrals for your practice. These people already know you, your competence, and your skill. They can provide references or testimonials to your practice, as well as opportunities to expand the services provided by your practice.

Professional Climate

Consider the professional climate in the area where you are considering opening an independent APN practice. What are the legal restrictions to practice in your state? How will the local medical and nursing community respond to your practice? Will collaborative protocols with an area physician and hospital privileges be difficult to obtain? Will physician consultation and referrals pose a problem? Do not abandon a location because of these obstacles, but know if they exist. When you are aware of potential barriers, you can address them and seek solutions.

DEVELOP A BUSINESS PLAN

A business plan is a written document that encapsulates the practice strategy for the future direction of the business and an action plan to achieve the practice objectives. Formulating a business plan is an effective way to plan for the practice and anticipate business decisions. Business plans may be developed for several reasons such as a new business start-up, business expansion, financing of the business, or as an ongoing plan to manage the business. An effective business plan will describe the elements needed to run the business. Items should include a summary, business concept, market analysis, competition, competitive analysis, marketing plan, management team and personnel, operations, financial plan, and repayment projections. A business plan should give a clear picture of what is really required to start the business.

Summary

This should be a short and concise explanation of the major features of the practice. In one to two pages you should describe your practice strategy, practice development, financial objectives, and business organization. It is important to describe your service and why it has promise. Describe the status of the practice with respect to a start-up timeline and marketing research. Include information about the business structure and the location of the practice, as well as financial projections, financing needs, and the projected return on investment. Be sure to focus on the key elements of the plan. Give the reader an overview of the practice, not a reiteration of the business plan.

Business Concept

This section should contain a clear explanation of the practice strategy. What sets your practice apart from other health-care practices in the area? Focus on the individuality of the practice and how this compares with the competition. Include areas that might have a significant impact on your strategy such as unique services, marketing ploys, or management team.

Market Analysis

This is where you document the need for your practice in a specific location. Has your location been designated as a health professional shortage area (HPSA)? If so, include citations of the documentation that supports this statement. Describe the marketplace and your potential competition. Discuss the size of the potential market and where patients are currently obtaining health care. Assess your competitors with respect to the size of their health-care practice, the clientele, the types of insurance accepted, and their fee structure. Determine if the population of the area is generally growing or shrinking and if there is a segment of the population that is medically underserved. Learn all you can about the population of your targeted location and consider this information when developing your marketing plan.

Where do you obtain this information? Seek out reports from various area trade associations and the chamber of commerce, as well as city, county, and state government reports. Research published material distributed by your competitors and reports published by area nursing organizations, hospitals, medical associations, and health departments. Conduct focus groups of area residents to determine what residents identify as a priority and the extent of these types of services in the specific location.

Competition

Know your competition and exactly what threat they are to your practice. Do they have a better location or a more convenient public transportation network than your practice? How do the services they offer and the quality of care compare with those of your practice? What are their practice fees and insurance reimbursement arrangements? Explore the reputation and image of your competition and the appearance they present to the public. Research the stability of the other health-care practices in your area, paying particular attention to staff turnover, reorganizations, and the announcements and cancellations of new initiatives. Pay attention to the advertising and marketing efforts of your competition and new health-care practices that may open in your area within the near future.

Competitive Analysis

This section of the business plan deals with an analysis of the strengths and risks associated with your practice. Be sure to include in your business plan a strategy to address these risks. An example of a business risk might be two established family medical practices within a 10-mile radius of your practice, thereby contributing to the risk of an inadequate patient caseload to financially sustain your practice. You can address this risk by renting highly visible space in a heavily trafficked area and target your services to a segment of the health-care market. A suburban storefront operation with convenient hours and walk-in appointments located in a strip mall next to the grocery store and cleaners may appeal to a large segment of the busy, well-woman population.

Marketing Plan

Develop and describe your overall promotional plan. What strategies will you use to reach your target population? Explain the reasoning behind your choice of advertising media, use of publicity, and other promotional plans and how they will enable you to get your message across to the target audience. Be realistic in your determination of a marketing budget and advertising timeline. Remember that effective marketing relies on repetition of your message. If your marketing budget is limited, concentrate your efforts on a smaller geographical area and the target population.

Management Team and Personnel

Focus your attention on key personnel. Describe the skills and competencies your staff and consultants bring to the practice. This is the section to highlight the relevant experience of your consultants, management team, and personnel. Stress the training and experience of your team and correlate their abilities to their role in your practice. Résumés of each team member should be included in the appendices. Include an organizational chart and job description for each member of your practice staff and any incentives for significant performance such as bonuses or potential ownership privileges.

Operations

Discuss the major business functions of your office and describe how the work will get done. Note any services that are "special" for a practice that deals with your target population. For instance, your specialty area may be women's health care and your practice provides the services that are typically expected for this type of practice. However, you may also provide a special service such as bone density scanning, which is not typically offered in the area. This specialty service should be highlighted in the business plan. This could be the reason why your practice may be more effective in soliciting and retaining patients than the competition.

Financial Plan

This section of the business plan should discuss projected income, balance sheets, the income or profit-and-loss statements, cash flow projections, and the break-even analysis. You should plan to show financial projections for 3 to 5 years.

Projected income statements should describe the amounts and types of costs associated with the practice and the receipts and profits on both a monthly and annual basis for each year of the plan. Balance sheets should summarize the assets and liabilities of the practice and should be prepared for the practice start-up interval, then semiannually during the first year of operation, and annually for the remainder of your financial plan. The profit-and-loss statement will discuss the costs to run the practice and income projections. The projected income minus the practice costs will enable you to infer proposed profits. Cash-flow projections describe the management of the practice funds. These projections should be made annually for the time period discussed in the financial plan and monthly for the first year of the plan. The break-even analysis identifies the amount of cash that will cover all practice costs. In the financial plan describe how you would reduce the break-even point if practice receipts fall short.

The financial plan should include all information that will assist potential lenders in understanding your revenue calculations. These projections will be as important as the assumptions on which they are based.

Repayment Projections

When preparing your financial plan, be sure to specifically discuss how and when any borrowed funds will be repaid (see next section). Discuss the sources that will provide the funds for repayment, as well as any collateral you propose to use to guarantee the loan. Most individual investors typically prefer short to intermediate loans with repayment of the loan within a 5-year period. Commercial lending institutions frequently consider longer term loans and lines of credit.

DETERMINE FINANCING OPTIONS

Setting up a health-care practice involves many anticipated and established costs regardless of the target population or practice use. The most common source of start-up capital is personal funds or an investment in the business by family or friends. Personal loans are another alternative for attaining funds to use in setting up a practice. Equity in a residence is frequently used as collateral to attain personal bank loans or establish lines of credit with a financial institution. Personal loans are generally easier to obtain through a bank than a business loan unless the business has a history of being profitable. Bankers may look at the hard assets of the practice, such as equipment, as collateral for a business loan. Criteria for securing a business loan vary among lenders, as does the emphasis they place on particular factors such as hard asset collateral, profitability, or years in business.

The Small Business Administration (SBA) offers many financial programs for the small business owner. The SBA frequently funds federally specified projects and objectives. Frequently the SBA will guarantee up to 90% of a bank loan for a small business rather than make a direct loan to the business. The amount of the loan that the SBA will guarantee depends on the business equity. This guaranteed loan protects the lender in case of default by the business owner and is made available to small businesses unable to secure funding from conventional lenders. Information about SBA programs and requirements for participation can be obtained on their Web site at www.sba.gov/financing.

State and local government agencies are other sources of assistance for the small business owner. These agencies have a vested interest in enhancing the economic well-being of the community and many offer various services to the entrepreneur. Information about programs offered by government agencies can be obtained by contacting the local chamber of commerce or state and city government offices.

Foundations frequently provide grants to businesses that focus on a specific area or related project and are another good source of funding. Geographical limitations are not often imposed on foundation funding.

DEVELOP FEES, REIMBURSEMENT, AND BILLING PROCEDURES

Establishing Fees

In the managed care world in which we practice, fees for health-care services are usually set by MCOs. The usual, customary, and reasonable fees of indemnity insurers are largely being replaced by a contracted fee schedule of the MCO. The APN can charge anything he or she wants; however, the MCO will reimburse only up to the maximum contractual allowance determined by its fee schedule. Is it worth the time and effort to develop a fee schedule?

Definitely develop reasonable fees for your services. In developing these fees, you will have to consider a multitude of factors, including the work performed, clinical skills required, time spent with a patient, practice expenses (e.g., rent, staff salaries and benefits, supplies, utilities, insurance, etc.), and risk involved in treating the patient, as well as indirect care such as making referrals to other health-care professionals and reviewing and evaluating laboratory and x-ray results. Ultimately, your fees should reflect what you feel your services are worth. They should not vary according to the type of insurance plan a patient carries or an MCO's maximal allowable fees.

Another yardstick for measurement of your fee schedule is the MCO allowance for the service. If your fee is less than that approved by the MCO, your fee is unreasonably low. Finally, consider your comfort in charging this fee to the self-pay patient. If you feel it is a reasonable cost for your services and you are not consistently writing off a percentage of the fee, it most likely is a reasonable fee.

Reimbursement

The National Center for Health Statistics (NCHS) updates contain estimates for 15 selected health measures based on data from the 2015 National Health Interview Survey

(NHIS) with one such measure being the lack of health insurance coverage. This report shows that 28.6 million people were without health insurance coverage in 2015. Although this is a decrease of 7.4 million people from 2014, it is still a staggering number of people without health care (Ward et al, 2016). Many of these consumers will seek out services on a self-pay basis and become part of your patient caseload or go out of plan because of the service you provide or the convenience of your service. Many patients will pay the fee for service in a walk-in, fast-track, health-care center, for example, because of the convenient location or extended hours. The best opportunity you have to collect a fee for service is while the patient is still in your office. Set up and publicize your policy that payment is expected at the time of service. Initial paperwork given to the patient on the first visit should include a financial policy that explains your payment expectations, any financial arrangements available, and your policy on filing insurance claims. Consider the acceptance of credit cards for payment of your fee for service. This provides a convenient method for your patient to pay your bill in full and transfers the risk of nonpayment to the credit card company. Most banks will process credit card transactions for a fee, and many credit card companies will electronically transfer funds to your bank for immediate access to the money.

Reimbursement from third-party payers can usually be done electronically using Electronic Data Interchange to submit the claim file to the payer directly or via a clearinghouse. Historically, claims were submitted using a paper form, usually the CMS 1500, and submitted to the CMS, indemnity insurers, or MCOs for payment. The coding required on the claim forms refers to nationally accepted, standard billing and coding systems. As of October 1, 2015, the American Medical Association's CPT codes, the *International Classification of Disease 10th Revision* (ICD-10), and CMS's Healthcare Common Procedure Coding System (HCPCS) for durable medical equipment, medical supplies, and drugs are required by CMS and other health-care payers.

Indemnity insurers are the traditional insurance companies who usually have no relationship with the health-care provider other than paying the bill for service for a covered patient. These insurers typically require an annual deductible paid by the patient and then they pay 80% of the health-care provider's bill with the remaining 20% being the responsibility of the patient. Be aware that these insurers pay "usual and customary reimbursement" (UCR), which is rarely equal to the fee you charge for your service. The patient is responsible for any charges not covered by their insurance in addition to their 20% copay.

MCOs contract with health-care providers for patient services. Contracts may set specified fees for services provided to the patient or may be based on a monthly capitated fee, regardless of patient use. In either case, the health-care provider cannot bill the patient for the difference between the contracted or capitated fee and the provider's regular fee for service. The exception is patient copayment requirements for each MCO plan. Copayments may be different for each plan and are based on many factors, including the family's annual income level, the frequency of multiple encounters with the practitioner, or the nature of the health-care problem. To contract with MCOs, the APN must apply and be accepted to each individual MCO provider panel.

The ACA payment models, with a focus on value versus volume, is driving health-care providers to deliver high-quality care at decreased cost. Shifting reimbursement models include pay-for-performance models, shared savings, bundled payments, and capitation payment models. These value-based programs share risk with the provider and payer and usually include a fixed payment for a group of services. A hybrid approach that combines a fee-for-service payment with a pay-for-performance bonus based on patient outcomes and satisfaction may be an effective way to achieve cost containment and value-based care (Navathe et al, 2016; Ritchie et al, 2016).

Billing

There is a variety of medical management software that will automatically submit insurance claim forms. However, monitoring the claims submitted and tracking the date and amount of payments received requires an organized system. Controlling reimbursement will ensure the success and continuation of your practice. A billing protocol such as that shown in **Box 26.4** will allow you to track the timeliness of insurance payments and the number of insurance reductions and denials.

Box 26.4

Billing Protocol

- File claims daily or at least twice per week.
- Check all claims for accuracy and completeness before submission.
- Develop a "claims pending" report and revise and print it daily. Most insurers guarantee payment within 30 days of filing an accurate and complete claim.
- After 30 days, call all insurance companies about unpaid claims and make a notation.
- Refile the claim if it has not been received by the insurer.
- Develop and print an "aged accounts" analysis for each insurance company to track payment patterns longer than 30 days.
- Contact the plan administrator of habitually poor payers and request an explanation. This could be a sign of a financially troubled insurance plan.
- Periodically review the explanation of benefits (EOB) sent by the insurers that explains reductions or denials of claims.
- Contact the insurer to discuss reductions or denials of claims, and revise and refile the claim if appropriate.

PURCHASE EQUIPMENT AND SELECT SUPPLIERS

Weigh the pros and cons of leasing versus buying equipment. Keep in mind that although leasing does not require the large up-front outlay, it does entail monthly payments with interest. Vendors typically have varied leasing options with opportunities to purchase the equipment at a lower price at the end of the lease. Look at the total cash investment requirements for practice start-up, the capital you have available, current equipment costs, and interest rates on loans versus equipment leasing.

A phone system is the communication system of your practice. Choose a system that will meet your needs and one that has expansion capabilities for the future. Besides front office phone lines, consider phone lines for the examination rooms and your office, as well as dedicated lines for the computer modem and the facsimile machine. Typically, six lines are the minimum needed in a health-care practice, with costs for a basic system in the $3,000 range. Other phone costs you might incur include a Yellow Pages listing and an after-hours answering service.

A computer system is another essential need for your office. Consider the number of computers needed for the medical biller and front office staff and the need for laptops for the providers to access patient files, document clinical encounters, formulate treatment plans, and prepare referral and consultation reports. Many health-care offices have multiple computers attached together to form a local area network (LAN). This allows multiple staff members to access and share patient files, printers, hard disk drives, and CD-ROMs. A computer consultant will be able to recommend and install a system that will meet your practice needs.

Practice management software focuses on two basic areas for health-care practices. The medical care areas have a patient-driven management focus. They typically include copies of all front office forms, have the ability to generate insurance claims, assist in patient scheduling, bill insurance companies, and have a complete electronic charting and clinical documentation system. The management focus is profit based and provides managerial and cost accounting information to maximize time and profits. Items contained in this section include the general ledger, accounts payable and receivable, monthly and annual financial reports and ratios, capitation disbursements and utilization rates, and the detection and tracking of trends for each patient encounter.

CTS (Computer Training Services) *Guide to Medical Practice Management Software* is a software evaluation program that reviews and analyzes the strengths and weaknesses of the leading medical management systems available in the marketplace. CTS has been publishing managed care software selection tools since 1983 and enables the practitioner to make an educated choice of a management system that best fits his or her individual needs. Information about this software can be obtained at www.ctsguides.com. Before purchasing any medical management system, contact several vendors and request a demonstration of their product. It is also wise to obtain references and contact local practices that use a particular system and ask about ease of use and satisfaction with the system.

Durable equipment, such as office furniture, examination tables, electrocardiogram machines, and so on, can be obtained from vendors such as durable equipment companies and medical supply companies. Investigate the purchase of secondhand medical equipment through brokers or through advertising in nursing and medical journals. Occasionally you may find office and medical equipment for sale because of the retirement or death of a practitioner or the downsizing of a health-care facility. If you purchase equipment through a vendor, be sure to compare costs by obtaining quotations on equipment, warranties, and services offered. Be sure to include "hidden" costs, such as termination fees, if leasing; federal, state, and local taxes, if applicable; shipping and installation charges; postwarranty maintenance charges; and interest costs for installment purchases.

The purchase of disposable medical supplies and periodic reordering of supplies is another financial consideration. Establish an organized purchasing system by centralizing the ordering process. Consider assigning one person in the practice to be responsible for tracking and ordering supplies. The designated person will talk to sales representatives and will become familiar with suppliers and prices to comparison shop for the best-quality supplies at the cheapest price. Centralized ordering will enable the purchaser to ascertain the quantity of supplies used per month, which will assist in the development of an inventory process. This will decrease unnecessary inventory, prevent running out of needed supplies, and avert higher prices because of "emergency" ordering.

HIRE AND MANAGE PERSONNEL

APNs who open an independent practice and hire employees must have a working knowledge of the laws and statutes regulating a health-care practice, as well as a working knowledge of how to develop internal personnel guidelines for hiring and managing personnel. Human resource management incorporates all the federal, state, and local laws and regulations that must be complied with by the health-care practice. These laws govern how employees must be treated and paid and they protect the rights of the employees in the workplace. The components of human resource management include the following:

1. *Administration:* Activities include developing and updating employee handbooks, guides and regulations, and posters; developing procedures for recruiting, hiring, review, discipline, and termination; and having labor law expertise or a consultant.

2. *Labor and liability issues:* Knowledge of and compliance with a multitude of government regulations such as the Civil Rights Act of 1964 and the Equal Employment Opportunity Commission (EEOC), Federal Age Discrimination in Employment Act (ADEA), Americans With Disabilities Act (ADA), and the Fair Labor Standards Act (FLSA). These laws deal with wrongful termination, unemployment, discrimination, sexual harassment, and employee rights. The practitioner additionally must deal with immigration regulations and other government rules such as personnel record-keeping (W4, I-9, etc.).

3. *Payroll information and processing:* Knowledge and management of activities that include employer tax administration, record keeping, reporting, payroll calculations and deductions, paycheck imprinting and distribution, W2 and W4 and quarterly reports, unemployment administration, management reports, and time-off use and accruals.

4. *Workers' compensation:* Knowledge of state law requirements and purchase of insurance from a qualified carrier, state insurance fund, or becoming self-insured according to state law regulations. Activities include claims filings, management and administration, fraud investigation and defense, audits and loss control, communication with injured employees, and return-to-work procedures.

5. *Safety:* The Occupational Safety and Health Administration (OSHA) regulations require that employees have a workplace safe from recognized hazards. Employer activities include the establishment and implementation of an illness and injury prevention program that includes general and specific safety training and required protective equipment.

6. *Benefits:* Knowledge and compliance of mandatory benefits that include overtime pay, unemployment insurance, and work breaks. Development and management of optional benefits such as health insurance, pension plans, vacation time, sick time, personal time off, continuing or advanced education credits, travel, bonuses, and so on.

There are many government regulations and time-consuming human resource responsibilities that must be dealt with before you open up your practice. Some practitioners hire an experienced office manager and rely on outside service providers such as a payroll service, insurance agent, and bookkeeper, as well as the expertise of an accountant and lawyer on retainer. This still leaves the responsibility of developing the employee handbook and job descriptions and advertising, interviewing, hiring, training, and evaluating personnel to the APN or a designee.

An innovative alternative to in-house human resource management is to outsource this responsibility to a professional employer organization (PEO). The PEO specializes in labor management and cost control and handles all the human resource issues whereas the APN maintains functional control of the employees. The PEO becomes the "employer of record" for your workplace employees; by combining your employees with the employees of many other practices, the PEO is able to offer the employees better benefits such as health insurance, retirement plans, credit unions, and so on. As the owner, the APN benefits because the PEO has relieved the APN of the liability of compliance and administration of mandated government regulations and payroll administration and management. The PEO has no financial interest or ownership in the practice and only deals with employee issues. An example of a PEO is Medical Management Consultants, Inc., which can be accessed at www.mmchr.com.

DEVELOP AN ORGANIZED DOCUMENTATION AND QUALITY ASSURANCE PROCESS

Documentation

Organizing documentation for a health-care practice will facilitate the smooth flow of business activity. In addition to the front office forms such as patient intake forms, patient rights forms, and release of information forms, the APN must develop and organize the medical record, patient educational materials, and patient authorization forms such as the "informed consent to treat" forms. One of the most important documents of an APN practice is the medical record. A well-documented, legible, and structured medical record will facilitate claims processing and may serve as a legal document to substantiate patient care. The medical record is confidential and can be released to third parties only with patient consent. Frequently the consent to treatment includes a "release of records"

statement allowing records to be sent to third-party payers, if requested. Key elements of an effective medical record are as follows:

1. *Organizing format:* All medical records should be uniform with separate sections for patient information, annual screening list, problem list, medication list, test results, consultations, daily encounter or progress notes, and other forms necessary for your particular practice. Information contained in these sections must be adequately secured and in chronological order. All coding on the charts, such as allergies or chronic health problems, must be uniform and the interpretation of the coding must be well known to all personnel.

2. *Timeliness:* Medical notations must be written at the time of the patient encounter. Always include the date and time of the patient contact in the progress notes. If notes are dictated, this should be at the time of the patient encounter. The notes must be proofread and signed by the health-care provider, preferably before they are entered into the medical record.

3. *Accurate records:* Record all information using a concise and accurate format. Many APNs use a SOAP format to concisely record the patient's **s**ubjective statements and the provider's **o**bjective findings, **a**ssessment, and **p**lan of care. Handwritten progress notes must be legible to prevent misinterpretations and clinical errors.

4. *Corrections:* Alteration of a medical record is unlawful. If an error has been made, draw a single line through the entry and add the correct information. Be sure to include the date, time, and your signature next to the correction or in the margin of the record. An addendum is also acceptable and can be added at the end of the record with a cross-reference to the original note. The date and time of the addendum are noted and signed by the author.

5. *Telephone conversations:* Document all patient calls in the record with time, date, nature of the conversation, actions taken, and signature of the provider. Calls or conversations with family should also be included in the progress notes with the date, time, nature of the conversation, and provider signature. If calls were placed for consultations, appointments, or equipment rentals for the patient, this should also be recorded in the progress notes, dated, and signed.

6. *Treatment plan and instructions:* Record your plan of treatment for your patient including important instructions, educational information given verbally or in writing, and warnings about interactions or complications that may occur. A well-written and organized medical record will be your first line of defense against a malpractice claim and will facilitate accurate and timely claims processing.

Quality Assurance

MCOs, insurers, and the public are increasingly asking health-care providers to demonstrate the value and improve the quality of their services. If outcomes management (OM) and performance improvement (PI) processes are put into place when the practice opens, then data collection about the quantity, quality, and cost effectiveness of the practice will be built into the foundation of the practice. OM is the process by which you measure, track, modify, and achieve the best clinical outcomes (quality) while incurring the fewest overall costs such as economic, intellectual, technical, and time spent (cost effectiveness). PI involves the measurement, evaluation, and improvement in the quality of the services of the practice and the patient care received through a systematic and collaborative examination of the practice's entire operation (quality and quantity).

The initial step of OM is to determine what outcomes are to be measured (e.g., up-to-date immunization status of children under age 6) or what change in functional status will be noted (e.g., maintain fasting blood sugar lower than 130 for the diabetic patient). Outcome measurements vary between what is valued by the patient and what provides information to the health-care provider to improve care and reduce cost. The diabetic patient values a good quality of life free from complications of diabetes mellitus, such as decreased vision, peripheral neuropathy, fatigue, and polyuria. The health-care provider values 100% immunization coverage of the pediatric patients to prevent unnecessary illness and complications that could lead to serious injury and costly health care. Both of these examples represent appropriate areas to monitor outcomes of patient care.

In addition to monitoring clinical outcomes measuring the effects of treatment and the functional status of patients receiving treatment, other areas to monitor include patient satisfaction and financial and economic factors. Patient satisfaction evaluates the patient's satisfaction with the services provided by the practice staff and the health-care provider. Although not an indicator of the clinical quality of the provider, it does measure the provider quality. A review of the literature suggests that patient satisfaction highly correlates to clinical outcomes. A patient who feels respected by the staff and informed, educated, and considerately treated by the health-care provider is more apt to follow a treatment regimen and return for follow-up care.

To maintain cost effectiveness while offering quality services, financial and economic factors must be evaluated. Measuring the cost of resources consumed to produce a clinical outcome will evaluate these factors. Patients diagnosed with diabetes mellitus frequently require large amounts of time to educate them about the disease and possible complications, treatment plan, and medications. Measuring the time the health provider spends to maintain the health of these patients and the costs involved might justify the purchase of additional patient education materials or hiring a registered nurse (RN) who is also a diabetic educator.

PI integrates the concepts of OM by evaluating the data received from the patient and the provider and using the findings to improve patient care and practice services. The benefits of PI include continuous monitoring of health-care delivery, effective use and cost containment, and the development of practice guidelines for your health-care practice. PI processes should permeate all facets of the practice to ensure high-quality health care at the lowest cost.

Primary accrediting bodies in health care and third-party payers are increasingly using and requiring OM data from providers to accredit or evaluate their performance. Insurance companies use this information to evaluate the retention of practitioners on their provider panels, as well as to sell services to employers. Health-care providers are increasingly subject to clinical and economic profiling by MCO plans, insurance companies, and consumer groups.

The National Committee for Quality Assurance (NCQA) has included in its health plan employer data and information set (HEDIS) the monitoring of additional quality criteria such as access to and availability of care, health plan stability, use of selected services, patient orientation, and translation services, to name a few. The NCQA is the primary accrediting body of MCOs and health maintenance organizations and is a major organization looking after consumer interests and rating health plans and providers. Annually, the NCQA requests that all managed care plans submit information about themselves and publishes a report card titled "Quality Compass" that rates the health plans. This document is sold to medical plans, employers, and various other health-care consultants. For information about this report or to obtain a copy of this document, visit the NCQA Web site at www.ncqa.org.

Performance standards will become increasingly more important in the years to come as health-care providers are asked to document the value and improve the quality of their services. Strategies for complying with performance criteria must be a top priority for health-care practices. Delegating responsibility for continuous quality improvement monitoring and implementing tracking systems for compliance will greatly improve the use of performance standards for the practice. Revising practice services based on data from the performance standards and rewarding staff and providers for compliance and high scores will improve the practice's entire operation and increase the value and reputation of the practice.

DEVELOP POLICIES AND PROCEDURES

Practice policies, procedures, and protocols should be written in great detail and should be part of every employee's orientation. Employees are expected to know these guidelines to ensure the smooth functioning of the practice. Additionally, important procedures and protocols such as a protocol for handling a medical emergency, a policy on confidentiality or annual equipment maintenance, and a procedure for handling patient complaints or termination of the professional relationship should also be outlined in this manual. Because this manual is essential to providing organized, high-quality services, each employee should sign a written acknowledgement that the practice manual has been read and this form should become part of the employee's personnel record.

Specific office policies, procedures, and protocols that should be developed are listed in **Box 26.5**. Responsibility for the initial development of the practice policy manual should be the APN's. However, updates and maintenance of this manual can be delegated to the office manager or another employee after the manual is established.

Box 26.5
Necessary Policies, Procedures, and Protocols

- Communicating practice fees
- Office collection procedures
- Billing policies and follow-up
- Release of records procedure
- Registering a patient
- Source of patient referral log
- Setting up the patient record
- Completing the superbill
- Scheduling patient appointments
- Closing and reconciling daily cash collections and disbursements
- Cleaning laboratory equipment
- Performing an electrocardiogram
- Scheduling a laboratory test
- Handling test results and consultation reports
- Referring patients for consultation
- Arranging services for patient care
- Protocols for purchasing equipment and supplies
- Equipment maintenance policy
- Handling a medical emergency protocol
- Confidentiality policy
- Protocol for handling patient complaints
- Procedure for termination of patient care

DEVELOP MARKETING STRATEGIES

Marketing can take many forms from word of mouth to high-priced television appearances. These external marketing strategies are tangible ways of reaching your target population to advertise the location of your practice and the services you provide. There are also internal strategies that you can employ to retain your patient base and increase your patient loyalty. For example, the internal strategies of competence and concern can be expressed through efficiency and friendliness of the staff and health-care provider.

A marketing budget should be an essential part of your start-up operational budget. Marketing is your practice's form of communication to the target population. This is how you inform patients about your location and what you can do to help them maintain their health or resolve a health problem. Marketing is not an optional expense.

A marketing plan helps you to organize your activities and prevents "lost opportunities" to showcase your practice, or high-cost "emergency" printing of practice brochures or appointment cards. Opportunities to showcase your practice can be found in many areas. Contact your local chamber of commerce to see if there is a "Welcome Wagon" service for new residents in your town and inquire about including your practice brochure for distribution to these consumers. Join community organizations to become known in your area and volunteer to offer free seminars on health-care topics. Inquire about membership in local speakers bureaus in your community or through professional organizations such as the state nurses association or the state board of nursing. Offer to participate in community and organizational health fairs and screenings that are being planned in your area. Repetition is the name of the game. Your name, location, and services need to be repeated many times before they are remembered. Before opening your practice, be sure to order stationery, appointment cards, brochures, and announcement cards with your practice name, address, and telephone number engraved. Also order an inscribed stamp to imprint the name, address, and phone number of your practice on educational materials or any other forms of information that may be distributed to patients in your office or potential patients at speaking engagements and health fairs. Develop and submit articles that highlight health topics to local newspapers and community bulletins, being sure to briefly describe who you are, where you are located, and what services you offer. Before opening your doors, submit practice announcements to local media services such as cable television bulletin boards, community radio programs, local newspapers, and community bulletins, brochures, and calendars.

Don't underestimate the power of the Internet and social media networking. Patients search for health-care providers on the Internet using Google, and with more than 88 billion Google searches per month, search engine optimization is a necessity (Jackson, Schneider, & Baum, 2011).

Developing a Web site to advertise key information about your practice is essential. Getting that Web site seen by consumers requires a strategy to reach the top of a search engine list. Two such strategies are repetition of key words in the title and beginning of any article and the frequency and repetition of these key words throughout the Web site, article, or advertisement (Maley & Baum, 2010). Additional social media networking includes advertising via YouTube, a professional page on Facebook for your business, and even having a following on your blog on Twitter. With 35- to 55-year-olds being the fastest growing segment on Facebook with an average daily use of 20 minutes, you will quickly build up an online community for your professional page. Twitter helps you build a community of people interested in what you have to say. Twitter reaches 800 million search queries each day and searches have increased by 33% in the last year (Schneider, Jackson, & Baum, 2010). These 21st century marketing tools will become a mainstay of your marketing plan.

Lastly, be sure to educate your staff about your credentials and what services you offer. Your staff is marketing your practice every time they answer questions or speak to a potential patient. Be sure they know about your education, experience, and specialty training, as well as what services you offer.

27

The Advanced Practice Nurse as Employee or Independent Contractor

Legal and Contractual Considerations

Kathleen M. Gialanella

Learning Outcomes

Learning outcomes expected as a result of this chapter:

- Describe the differences between an employee and an independent contractor.
- Discuss liability concerns for an independent contractor if a negligence case arises.
- List two sources of whistleblower protection.
- Categorize the types of terms contained in employment and independent contractor agreements.
- Explain a covenant not to compete.
- Assess possible exposure to charges of fraud and abuse.

INTRODUCTION

Advanced practice nurses (APNs) need to be clear about whether they are practicing as employees or as independent contractors. The difference between an employee and an independent contractor is a legal one based on common law or statutory definitions (Internal Revenue Service [IRS], 2016a). In general, if the individual or entity for whom the APN performs services controls what the APN does and when and how he or she does it, the APN is an employee. If, however, the individual or entity oversees only the result of the APN's work and not the manner or method in which the work is done, the APN may be considered an independent contractor (IRS, 2016b). The distinction between the two has significant legal, tax, and financial implications. This chapter explores these implications and includes a discussion of the various contractual issues that apply to employment and independent contractor agreements. Pertinent case law is discussed as well.

EMPLOYEE OR INDEPENDENT CONTRACTOR: WHAT DIFFERENCE DOES IT MAKE?

An APN's status as an employee or independent contractor is a significant factor when considering issues pertaining to professional liability and other legal, tax, financial, and contractual situations.

Professional Liability Considerations

With regard to liability exposure, employees alleged to have engaged in negligence or malpractice will likely find a safe harbor in the doctrine of *respondeat superior*. This doctrine holds that an employer is responsible for the acts of its employee. Thus, if an employee is acting within the scope of his or her employment and is sued for negligent treatment of a patient, the employer is vicariously liable for the damages sustained by the patient. Although this doctrine will not prevent an employed APN from being individually named as a defendant in a lawsuit, it does give the employee a level of protection that is unavailable to APNs who function as independent contractors. An in-depth discussion of these considerations and the liability insurance implications can be found in Chapter 29.

Financial and Tax Implications

APNs who practice as employees receive paychecks that have monies withheld by the employer. The monies that are withheld include state and federal income tax payments, payments to Social Security and Medicare, as well as unemployment and disability taxes. In addition, the employer is responsible for paying its share of any Social Security, Medicare, and unemployment and disability

taxes due on that employee's wages. The employer is responsible for forwarding any amounts withheld from the employee's paycheck, as well as its share of such payments, to the government. The employer must also issue a Form W-2 statement to each of its employees showing the total amount of taxes that were withheld from the employee's pay during the previous year.

Employees may deduct unreimbursed business expenses (e.g., dues for professional organizations, subscriptions to professional journals, qualifying work-related education, and premiums for professional liability insurance) on their tax returns, but only if the deductions are itemized and only for unreimbursed expenses that exceed 2% of the employee's adjusted gross income (AGI) (IRS, 2015). For example, an employed APN with an AGI of $100,000 in 2016 could deduct unreimbursed employee expenses that exceeded $2,000 (2% of AGI). If the APN spent $3,500 that year on professional dues, subscriptions, continuing education, and liability insurance, the APN can deduct only $1,500—the amount that exceeds 2% of the APN's AGI.

If the APN practices as an independent contractor, the organizations to whom he or she provides services must issue a Form 1099-MISC showing the total amount of money it paid to the APN during the previous year. Unlike the employee, the independent contractor is responsible for paying his or her income and self-employment taxes, and will be required to pay quarterly estimated taxes to avoid penalties (IRS, 2016c). The organization is not required to withhold any taxes or make any Social Security or Medicare payments that an employer of an APN would be required to make. The savings in time and money that independent contractor arrangements present to the organization make it an attractive alternative.

If the APN is an independent contractor, his or her business expenses are reported annually on the income tax return. Unlike the unreimbursed business expense threshold of 2% of AGI that an employee must meet before being allowed to take a deduction, business expenses incurred by an independent contractor do not have to amount to any specific percentage of AGI to be deducted (IRS, 2016c). Thus, in the example previously given, the APN would be able to deduct the full expenses incurred of $3,500.

The APN must keep other trade-offs in mind when contemplating employment versus an independent contractor arrangement. Employers often provide certain benefits to their employees (e.g., health insurance, pension plans, and paid personal time off for holidays, vacations, illnesses). These benefits are not made available to independent contractors. Some organizations prefer to offer an independent contractor arrangement to an APN to avoid the cost of providing such benefits. If an APN wants or needs these kinds of benefits, an independent contractor arrangement is not advisable.

Factors Used to Determine Status

Because the liability, financial, and tax implications of one's work status can be significant, it is important for APNs to understand the factors that are considered to determine whether an APN is an employee or an independent contractor. A determination is based on the facts. The IRS (2016b) considers common law and looks at the degree of control asserted by the organization versus the degree of independence maintained by the worker. To determine whether an APN is an employee or an independent contractor from a federal tax perspective, the IRS would evaluate behavioral and financial controls and the type of relationship that exists between the APN and the organization for which the APN provides services.

Questions the IRS would pose to evaluate the status of the arrangement include the following:

- What instructions does the organization give to the APN? If the organization instructs the APN about when and where to work, the equipment and supplies to be used, who will assist the APN, and what work must be performed (or even how the results are to be achieved by the APN), these are factors that indicate the APN is employed by the organization.
- Does the organization educate and train the APN to perform services in accordance with certain policies and procedures, or does the APN have his or her own protocols for providing services? The former arrangement points to an employer–employee relationship. The latter would indicate the APN is an independent contractor.
- Does the APN have significant fixed unreimbursed business expenses (e.g., office rent, telephone and computer services, professional dues, and support staff to pay) in connection with providing services to the organization? If so, this generally indicates that the APN is an independent contractor.

- Does the APN advertise and are his or her services available to more than one organization or to various individuals? If so, the APN is likely to be considered an independent contractor.
- How is the APN paid? Does the APN receive a set amount of pay over a certain period of time and receive benefits from the organization or is the APN's compensation based on a flat fee without the provision of benefits? The former arrangement indicates an employment situation, whereas the latter arrangement would suggest the APN is an independent contractor.
- Does the APN realize a profit or take a loss? If so, it indicates the APN is an independent contractor.
- What type of relationship exists between the organization and the APN? Is it for an indefinite period or will it end on completion of a particular project? Is there a written contract that describes the type of relationship that exists? (For example, if the contract is called an "employment agreement," the employer–employee relationship is obvious because it is specifically stated within the agreement.) Does the APN receive benefits such as health insurance, a retirement plan, and paid time off? If so, it indicates the APN is an employee.

State taxing authorities make similar inquiries for state tax purposes. The factors relied on by these taxing authorities can differ from the IRS and vary from state to state. Some states are more stringent than the IRS and other states when classifying workers as employees versus independent contractors. Thus, it is important for an APN to be familiar with the federal bases used to distinguish between employee and independent contractor arrangements, as well as the bases used by the states in which the APN practices. APNs should seek out sound legal and accounting advice to address these issues.

Failure to properly classify the work status of an APN can be costly to the APN if he or she is treated as an independent contractor but is, in fact, an employee. A case filed years ago by individuals who had been classified as independent contractors rather than employees at Microsoft illustrates this and is still relevant today. *Vizcaino v. Microsoft Corporation* (1997) arose out of a tax audit of Microsoft conducted by the IRS. The audit concluded that several of the individuals classified as independent contractors needed to be reclassified as employees and the requisite taxes paid. The IRS concluded that the individuals were employees because Microsoft controlled the manner and way in which the individuals performed their services for the company. Microsoft ended up paying the required taxes and overtime that resulted from the reclassification and it reclassified some of the individuals as permanent employees. Eight of these reclassified individuals demanded that they receive all the employment benefits they did not receive during the time they were considered independent contractors, including participation in Microsoft's 401(k) plan and employee stock purchase plan. Microsoft refused to issue these benefits, so the individuals sued the company. The Ninth Circuit Court of Appeals in *Vizcaino* ordered Microsoft to provide employment benefits to its employees for the periods of time that those individuals had been erroneously classified as independent contractors.

A similar decision was reached by the Ninth Circuit Court of Appeals in *Alexander v. FedEx Ground* (2014), in which the court examined the many factors that California considers in determining whether a worker is an independent contractor or an employee as a matter of law. The court found that although the written agreements between FedEx and its drivers designated the workers as independent contractors, FedEx had a broad right to control the way the drivers performed their duties. The drivers were reclassified as employees.

The financial impact that the decisions in *Vizcaino* and *Alexander* had on the companies involved in these lawsuits was significant, as were the financial gains realized by the reclassified workers. Although the workers in these cases were not health-care providers, the findings and results would apply equally in the health-care industry.

The Advanced Practice Nurse as Employee

Employees working without a contract guaranteeing a specific position for a definite time at a designated pay rate are referred to as employees "at will." In the past, this kind of employment arrangement allowed employers to terminate any at-will employee for any reason or for no reason. Although the general rule that an employee can be hired or fired for any reason or no reason continues to exist, there now are many exceptions in place. These exceptions include public policy concerns, antidiscrimination laws, and whistleblower statutes. Thus, employers no longer enjoy the unbridled latitude the general rule of law previously afforded them.

Although the absence of job security continues to be an issue for at-will employees, federal and state statutes have been enacted and judicial decisions have been made to ensure that employers treat employees more fairly, regardless of the employee's status as a contract or at-will employee.

One of the key limitations on an employer's ability to terminate an employee at will is called the "public policy" exception. It is a judicially mandated exception that permits a terminated at-will employee to pursue a wrongful termination claim against the employer in cases where the employee has a reasonable basis to believe he or she was terminated in violation of a clear mandate of public policy. *Landin v. Healthsource Saginaw, Inc.* (2014) is an example of such a case. Mr. Landin worked as a licensed professional nurse (LPN) at the hospital until he was terminated. He was an at-will employee who reported a coworker's negligence that he believed caused the death of a patient. Mr. Landin alleged the hospital retaliated against him and ultimately terminated him for reporting his concern. He filed a lawsuit claiming wrongful termination by the hospital. The case was tried and the jury awarded substantial damages to Mr. Landin. The hospital appealed. The Michigan Court of Appeals upheld the jury award and agreed that Mr. Landin's actions warranted protection under the public policy exception.

Another whistleblower case that gained national attention involved two Texas nurses employed by Winkler County Memorial Hospital. The nurses were concerned about the incompetent practice of a physician who was treating patients at the hospital. They reported their concerns to hospital administration, and when the hospital failed to act they reported the physician to the Texas Medical Board. The hospital fired the nurses, who were also criminally prosecuted. They were charged with improperly releasing official hospital information to the medical board. The charges against one nurse were dropped and the other nurse was acquitted of wrongdoing at trial (Murray, 2011). The nurses then sued the hospital, the physician, and others based on several claims, including wrongful termination, and recovered $750,000.

APNs practicing as employees have the opportunity, similar to Landin and the two Texas nurses, to pursue wrongful termination causes of action if they believe that adverse employment action was taken against them in violation of the common law public policy exception. In addition, many states and the federal government have adopted strong whistleblower statutes that enhance the common law protections available to employees. (The protections afforded to employees under some of these laws also have been extended to independent contractors, but on a very limited basis.) Some of these laws have specific protections for health-care professionals. An example of such a statute is the New Jersey Conscientious Employee Protection Act (1986, as amended). It specifically prohibits employers from taking retaliatory action against health-care professionals, such as APNs, who disclose information about employers who provide improper patient care.

Whistleblower claims alleging improper patient care are not always successful. *Hitesman v. Bridgeway, Inc.* (2014) is an example. Mr. Hitesman was employed as a registered nurse (RN) in a nursing home that also had a subacute unit. He claimed there was a significant increase in the number of patients at the facility with respiratory or gastrointestinal symptoms and was concerned about inadequate infection control. He brought his concerns to the attention of the medical and nursing directors, but was dissatisfied with the facility's response. He next reported his concerns anonymously to municipal, county, and state agencies as well as the media. He released information to the media that the employer deemed a violation of its confidentiality policies and the Health Insurance Portability and Accountability Act of 1996 (HIPAA). Mr. Hitesman was terminated. He then sued the employer alleging violations of the Conscientious Employee Protection Act (CEPA). He relied on the American Nurses Association (ANA) Code of Ethics, the employee handbook, and a statement of resident rights to support his case. The trial court ruled in Mr. Hitesman's favor but the decision was reversed on appeal. The appellate court found Mr. Hitesman's reliance on the previously noted resources insufficient to establish that the employer had provided improper patient care. The New Jersey Supreme Court affirmed the appellate court's decision. APNs who find themselves in situations that seem to require whistleblowing pursuant to law or the ANA Code of Ethics (2015a) should consider consulting an attorney familiar with this area of the law before acting.

Other statutory protections include a variety of antidiscrimination laws. There are several federal laws that protect workers from discrimination based on age, race/ethnicity, sex/sexual orientation/gender identity, religion, marital or family status, genetic information, and disability. Many states have their own laws as well. These laws

continue to evolve and are the subject of much interpretation by the courts. Employees are afforded additional protections under federal and state laws that provide for unemployment benefits, payment for injuries on the job (workers' compensation), the need for family and medical leave, and continuation of health-care benefits. APNs who work as employees should be aware of their many rights under these laws.

Some APNs may have written employment contracts that provide them with additional rights. Contractual issues are discussed in greater detail later in this chapter.

The Advanced Practice Nurse as Independent Contractor

An APN who is an independent contractor has a contract, which may be verbal, written, or implied, with another party to provide specific services. The contract does not stipulate a level of behavioral and financial controls over the APN that would be associated with an employer–employee relationship. If an APN is working as an independent contractor, he or she is not entitled to benefits that the organization provides to its employees. The APN also would not be able to obtain unemployment compensation, workers' compensation, or family and medical leave protections through that organization if the need arose. This is because the legal relationship is not an employment relationship. Of equal concern is the impact that potential professional liability claims would have on the APN who is an independent contractor. For example, an APN who is not employed by the hospital but has privileges there would be individually responsible for his or her negligent acts that occur in the hospital.

The case of *Hansen v. Caring Professionals, Inc.* (1997) is illustrative. Although it does not involve an APN, it does involve a nurse; the issues presented in the case also would apply to APNs who work as independent contractors. The case examines whether the nurse, who was retained by Caring Professionals to provide temporary nursing services to a local hospital, was an employee or independent contractor of that agency. The distinction was fundamental in determining whether or not the agency could be held liable for the alleged negligent acts of the nurse. Mr. Hansen, the plaintiff in the case, claimed that a malpractice occurred when a central venous catheter that had been inserted into his wife's jugular vein became dislodged. It was alleged that air entered the intravenous line and created an embolus that caused Mr. Hansen's wife to sustain severe brain damage and total disability.

Eileen Fajardo-Furlin, RN, was named as a defendant in the case because she cared for Mrs. Hansen while she was in the hospital. Ms. Furlin was working at the hospital on temporary assignment through Caring Professionals. Caring Professionals also was named as a defendant. The patient's husband sought to hold Caring Professionals responsible for the alleged negligence of Ms. Furlin. Caring Professionals sought to be removed from the case, asserting that there was no employee–employer relationship, but rather an independent contractor relationship, thereby absolving Caring Professionals from any liability for Ms. Furlin's actions. The trial court agreed and dismissed Caring Professionals from the case. An appeal followed, but the appellate court agreed with the trial court. Caring Professionals succeeded in getting removed from the case because Ms. Furlin was an independent contractor. The nurse remained in the lawsuit as an individual defendant. This case illustrates how the type of working relationship an APN has with an organization could have a significant impact on the outcome of a negligence or malpractice case. This case also illustrates the importance of having individual professional liability insurance. Nurse Furlin, as the only remaining defendant in the case, would be responsible for the cost of her legal fees and any judgment or settlement unless she had carried her own malpractice policy.

CONTRACT ISSUES FOR APN EMPLOYEES AND INDEPENDENT CONTRACTORS

APNs should have a basic understanding of contract law. It is often advisable and sometimes a requirement for APNs to have written agreements in place to address certain work and practice issues. The remainder of this chapter introduces the APN to these types of considerations.

Types of Contracts

Contracts are promises or sets of promises that outline the rights and responsibilities of the parties. They are legally binding, and if valid they can be enforced. When one or more parties fails to perform in accordance with articulated rights and responsibilities, that failure is termed a *breach*. When a breach occurs, remedies outlined in the agreement or contract are available to the nonbreaching party. In addition, when an agreement-related dispute is tried in the civil justice system or is the subject of binding arbitration, the nonbreaching party can obtain damages if a breach is found to have occurred.

Contracts are usually categorized by the way in which they are formed. They can be express contracts, implied contracts, or quasi-contracts. Express contracts are promises or sets of promises to which the parties agree either verbally or in writing. Implied contracts are promises or sets of promises that are derived from the conduct of the parties to the contract. Quasi-contracts are not considered contracts *per se,* but they are used by courts in some jurisdictions to allow one or more parties to the quasi-contract to avoid unjust enrichment at the expense of the other party or parties. This is known as *equitable relief.*

Some contracts, whether express or implied, are considered invalid for various reasons. An invalid contract will not be enforced by the courts. An example of an invalid contract is one that is illegal because fulfilling its terms would be considered a crime. For instance, if an APN enters into a contract that provides he or she would receive financial incentives for referring patients to a health-care facility, this would be an anti-kickback violation. Taking kickbacks for patient referrals is a crime; thus, a court would not enforce such a contract. The contract is considered to have been void at its inception. Some contracts can be considered voidable. For example, if one of the parties to the contract is a minor or has a level of mental illness or dementia that prevented him or her from understanding the terms of the contract, the contract is considered voidable by that party. Unenforceable contracts are those that may be valid but not enforced because of some defense that may be asserted by one or more parties to the contract. An example would be if a party were tricked into signing the contract or entered into the contract by mistake.

For any contract to be enforced, the parties must have reached a "meeting of the minds" about its terms. When the parties have reached a meeting of the minds, the result is called *mutual assent.* Mutual assent is achieved when one party makes an offer and the other party unequivocally accepts the offer. In addition to offer and acceptance, there must be an exchange of consideration for the contract to be valid. For example, an APN can enter into an employment contract with a physician practice. The consideration received by the APN is monetary compensation. The consideration received by the physician practice is the services that the APN provides to the practice.

Contracts can be unilateral or bilateral. A unilateral contract is one in which there is no opportunity for negotiation. An example of such a contract is a professional liability insurance policy. The insurance company promises to defend an APN in a malpractice case pursuant to the terms of the insurance policy in exchange for the payment of premiums by the APN. The terms of the policy (contract) are not negotiated. Once the APN pays the premium, the policy becomes effective. A bilateral contract is one in which the parties negotiate the terms. APNs often negotiate the terms of their agreements and should not be reluctant to do so, whether it is an employment contract to obtain compensation and benefits that are acceptable or an independent contractor agreement to obtain satisfactory limitations on restrictive covenants.

Common Contractual Terms Included in Written Agreements

Agreements can be struck with a handshake or with the stroke of a pen. Agreements struck with a handshake, although honorable, may prove to be frustrating, unworkable, and largely unenforceable because many of the issues that normally are addressed in written agreements are not addressed in verbal agreements. In addition, it is much easier to prove the terms of an agreement that has been reduced to writing. Written agreements can help the parties avoid the misunderstandings that may arise with implied or verbal contracts. Thus, it is recommended that APNs who enter into employment and independent contractor agreements do so in writing whenever possible.

Written agreements can be brief, limited to just a few pages, or they can be lengthy, detailed documents. The length and terms of the agreement depend on the specific arrangements contemplated by the parties, as well as their needs and preferences. Larger providers, such as extensive health-care systems, hospitals, and large medical practices, tend to enter into very lengthy, detailed agreements with the APN. Extensive negotiations may not be possible. Smaller providers tend to have shorter, more generalized agreements and are more flexible when the APN requests changes before agreeing to accept a contract.

Regardless of the length of an agreement, employment and independent contractor agreements for APNs routinely include certain terms. Among them are the scope of the contract; its effective date; the relationship and responsibilities of the parties; confidentiality; conflict of interest; compensation; indemnification and subrogation; dispute resolution; term, renewal, and termination; remedies for breach; notices; modification and assignment of the agreement; severability; conflict of laws; legal authority; *force majeure;* covenant not to compete; and signatures. Each of these provisions will be discussed.

Scope

The section of a written agreement addressing scope recites the activities governed by the agreement. In this section the services provided by the APN are identified. The services may be stated broadly or they may be listed individually. A broadly written scope statement for an APN might state that he or she agrees to render services that are consistent with the scope of practice (SOP) articulated in his or her state's nurse practice act (NPA) and in accordance with all applicable national practice standards, such as the ANA's *Nursing: Scope and Standards of Practice* (2015b). A more specific scope statement might delineate the APN's job responsibilities and list the individual services to be provided. In either event, it is important to verify that the services contemplated by the agreement fit within the APN's SOP as defined by the state.

Effective Date

The section of a contract addressing the effective date will specify the date on which the agreement begins. It is also the date against which time frames identified in the agreement may be measured. For example, if the effective date of the agreement is July 1, 2016, and the APN is required to provide a certain report to the other party every 90 days, the first report is due on October 1, 2016.

Relationship of the Parties

In the relationship of the parties section of the contract, the APN is identified as either an independent contractor or an employee. If the APN is going to be considered an independent contractor, it is important to keep that status in mind as other contractual provisions are written. Classifying an individual as an independent contractor but prescribing when, where, and how services will be performed may subject an organization to having that independent contractor reclassified as an employee. As previously discussed, this could expose an organization to liability for unpaid taxes and employment benefits, as well as governmental penalties.

In situations in which an APN is going to function in an independent contractor role, the contract should specifically state that the APN is not eligible for paid sick leave or vacation time, health insurance, retirement plans, and other benefits extended to the organization's employees. An employee contract, on the other hand, should specifically include all the benefits to which the APN is entitled.

Responsibilities of the Parties

Once the relationship of the parties has been established, the responsibilities of each party can be more easily identified. Similar to other provisions, this section may be brief or quite lengthy, comprehensively listing what the expectations are of each party. If an APN is going to work as an independent contractor, it is imperative that the APN maintain the decision-making ability with regard to the manner and means by which services will be provided to patients. In addition, the APN should contemplate adding a provision that he or she be consulted about any existing and future clinical practice guidelines the organization may have or consider and be permitted to provide appropriate changes, if necessary, before implementation.

If an APN is identified as an independent contractor in the agreement and then is required to operate in a controlled manner proscribed by the other party, it is likely that the APN will be considered an employee, not an independent contractor. If, on the other hand, the agreement being executed is an employment contract, it is reasonable to identify when, where, and how the APN is to function.

Typically, APNs practicing as independent contractors have the responsibility to ensure that they are and remain properly credentialed, that they have adequate liability insurance, and that they perform contractual services in a manner that complies with professional practice and ethical standards, as well as all applicable local, state, and federal regulations, statutes, and case law. However, APNs might consider including a contractual requirement that the organization with whom they are contracting assist with the credentialing and recredentialing process for area

hospitals, managed care organizations (MCOs), third-party payers, and regulatory agencies. In addition, APNs, whether practicing as employees or independent contractors, may be asked to promptly disclose any disciplinary actions taken against them. If a contract contains this type of provision it is imperative that the APN understand his or her obligation to report and act promptly when the need arises. Otherwise, the failure to report may be an event identified in the agreement that would permit immediate termination of the APN.

The organization with whom the APN is contracting usually requires the APN's assistance and cooperation with the collection of data to confirm the APN's competency and proper credentialing. Required data may include confirmation of educational preparation, specialty certifications, licensure, prior employment, status of existing and past practice privileges, liability insurance, malpractice claims, criminal background information, membership in professional associations, and compliance with the Drug Enforcement Administration (DEA) and any state drug control agencies. In addition, APNs practicing as independent contractors may be asked to provide information regarding the types of client populations previously served, charges per encounter, visits per hour, visit frequency, incidence of diagnostic procedure use, admission and readmission rates, complication and mortality rates, outcomes, accessibility and availability history, appointment waiting times, and after-hours coverage history.

The responsibilities of APNs are delineated in written agreements; organizations with whom they contract should have their responsibilities delineated in the agreement as well. In that regard, it is the organization's responsibility to execute contracts that are consistent with the organizational bylaws. The APN may explicitly require that the organizational bylaws be incorporated into the agreement by reference and that he or she be provided the most current edition of the bylaws. The APN may be obligated to review the bylaws and written policies of the organization periodically or whenever they are amended. The APN may also negotiate involvement on the bylaws committees or other organizational committees or panels.

It is also the organization's responsibility to have sound corporate compliance programs in place and to provide the APN with the information he or she needs to provide the agreed-to services. These and other organizational responsibilities can be stated broadly or can be delineated specifically and in detail with set deadlines and penalties for failure to meet those deadlines.

Confidentiality

The confidentiality section of a contract usually deals with information and documents that the parties wish to protect as confidential. The responsibilities of the parties with regard to this information and these documents is also outlined. Some confidentiality provisions address an organization's exclusive property right to medical, financial, and other records; specifically define what is protected; and contain strict prohibitions on accessing, reproducing, or removing certain information. Other confidentiality provisions simply state that confidential, proprietary, and trade secret information shall not be disclosed to third parties without describing what information is considered to be confidential, proprietary, or a trade secret. If there are questions about what specific information is protected, it is prudent to clarify this so that potential breaches of confidentiality are minimized.

With regard to the privacy and confidentiality of protected health information, many contracts now address the requirements of the Privacy Rule and Security Rule adopted by the federal government in 2003 and 2005, respectively. These rules are commonly referred to by health-care providers as "HIPAA." The protections under HIPAA were expanded with the passage of the Health Information Technology for Economic and Clinical Health (HITECH) Act of 2009 and the subsequent adoption of additional federal rules. These laws enhance the privacy and security protections of the electronic health records (EHRs) that have become prevalent in today's health-care delivery systems. APNs must be fully familiar with the requirements that apply to them under these laws, as well as the HIPAA and HITECH Act policies and procedures of the organizations with whom they contract.

Conflict of Interest

Conflict of interest provisions are contained in written agreements in an effort to ensure that both parties are acting in the best interests of each other and promoting the mutual success of the relationship. Potentially conflicting loyalties can be problematic and should be avoided. Typically, conflict of interest provisions require the party who becomes aware of a potential conflict to promptly disclose it to the other party. When these provisions are included in an APN's written agreement, it is important for the APN to act in a manner that avoids potential conflicts and is not contrary to the contractual requirements, such as always acting in the best interest of the patients and not in the best interest of any other third party. Health-care entities often have written conflict of interest policies and the APN should be fully familiar with the policy. For instance, an APN may be required to disclose an ownership interest in a medical device company or an investment in the pharmaceutical industry.

Compensation

Compensation provisions in written agreements delineate the payment that will be rendered once agreed-to services are provided. The sum may be listed as a total amount of money that will be paid over the course of the contract, or it may be listed as an incremental amount, paid according to established benchmarks. Caps may be identified that limit the total amount of money that will be paid, as well as any bonus payments. With regard to bonus payments, it is important to decide whether bonus payments will be based on profit that is generated from the services provided by the APN, the productivity of the APN, the quality of care given by the APN, or some combination thereof. Not only does the APN need to decide whether or not bonus payments are going to be incorporated into the written agreement, a great deal of attention needs to be paid to the formula used to calculate bonus payments. It is important to be sure the formulas used are reasonable, are regularly audited, and do not benefit one party more than the other. Care should be taken to avoid financial incentives that may be viewed as kickbacks or otherwise illegal.

In addition, health-care organizations, plans, and practice groups will likely include a statement conveying that it is the responsibility of the APN practicing as an independent contractor to pay all taxes associated with contracted services.

APNs executing written agreements need to consider adding specific dates on which payments will be made. When those payments are not forthcoming, a late fee can be imposed so long as it is included in the agreement. Additionally, when the compensation for the APN is based on billing receipts, the APN should be provided with ongoing documentation tracking the billing process and reimbursement levels from each payer, including secondary sources and previously denied claims. Time frames within which claims will be processed should be set and penalties for failure to meet those time frames should be negotiated.

Indemnification and Subrogation

Indemnification and subrogation issues are typically addressed in written agreements. Indemnification is a promise between the parties to hold each party harmless for the wrongdoing of the other party. For example, an APN may enter into a contract with a physician practice as an independent contractor. The contract will contain language that says the APN is responsible for his or her own wrongdoings. If a malpractice claim occurs for which the APN is solely responsible, it is the APN who must bear the loss associated with that claim. The APN must indemnify the physician practice. The contract will also contain language that requires the APN to carry his or her own insurance coverage and provide proof of it. It is important to ensure that an indemnification provision is reciprocal so that both parties are extended the same level of protection. The APN should be indemnified by the physician practice if someone other than the APN is responsible for a malpractice or other type of claim.

Subrogation, on the other hand, permits the substitution of one party for another. In health-care matters, the doctrine of subrogation has been used by health-care facilities to recover from the APN the monetary losses sustained after the health-care organization is found liable for the negligence or malpractice of the APN or other individual to whom the APN delegated any aspect of care or treatment. Similar to indemnification, a subrogation provision will likely be included in certain contracts. If it is, the APN should be sure the provision is reciprocal so that both parties to the contract have a right to subrogation.

Dispute Resolution

Dispute resolution provisions describe the process to be used when the parties disagree about any aspect of the contract. Usually, this provision states that both parties will use their best efforts to promptly resolve all disagreements. In situations in which the disagreement cannot be resolved, there may be a requirement for the parties to submit the dispute to mediation or arbitration as alternative dispute resolution mechanisms. The parties to the contract may negotiate terms that require either binding or nonbinding dispute resolution. If there is binding arbitration, for example, the parties to the contract are waiving their rights to file a lawsuit in the event one of the parties is dissatisfied with the arbitrator's decision. If the parties agree to a nonbinding dispute resolution process, it is important to state that the process must be concluded before filing a cause of action in court.

Term, Renewal, and Termination

Term, renewal, and termination provisions in written agreements specify the length of the contract, usually in months or years, as well as the process for renewing and terminating the agreement. Renewal clauses typically require one or both parties to notify the other party within a certain period of time of their intention to renew the contract. Some written agreements approach the issue differently by providing for automatic renewal for a specific period if one party does not notify the other of its intent to *not* renew the agreement.

Termination provisions in written agreements usually require the terminating party to notify the other party within a specific period, usually 60 or 90 days, of that party's intent to terminate the agreement. Agreements may be terminated with or without cause, and severance payment may or may not be incorporated into the agreement. "Termination without cause" provisions permit the APN to be terminated for any reason or no reason, so long as the termination is not unlawful. Sometimes courts consider "termination without cause" provisions in written agreements to be insufficient or unenforceable, thereby permitting the terminated party to pursue a wrongful termination in violation of public policy. This is especially true if the terminated party is characterized as a whistleblower who reported an allegedly illegal practice and was subsequently notified of the termination of the agreement.

If a "termination without cause" provision is going to be included in the written agreement, it must be reciprocal, permitting the APN to terminate the agreement for any reason or no reason within a comparable period. APNs, similar to other parties to written agreements, need to be sure that their decision to terminate an agreement is lawful.

Not only may agreements be terminated without cause, they may be terminated with cause. An event giving rise to termination with cause usually results in the immediate dissolution of the contract. Terminations for cause are typically limited to instances in which the APN commits a crime, breaches his or her fiduciary duty to the organization, is disciplined by his or her professional board, or acts in a manner that potentially compromises the standing of the organization in the community. These provisions may also be stated more broadly by permitting "for cause" termination with any illegal occurrence. Similar to termination without cause provisions, termination of the agreement "for cause" may be exercised by an APN, so long as an identifiable "for cause" event has occurred and the agreement permits termination. It is, therefore, important to ensure that termination clauses are reciprocal and that the APN articulates the occurrence of those events that would permit the APN to terminate the agreement, as well as the financial consequences for each party if the agreement is terminated.

Remedies for Breach

Written agreements usually identify the remedy or consequence of breaching or failing to perform under the terms of the agreement. In an attempt to limit the circumstances that can give rise to a breach and to establish the amount of money to be paid because of a breach (known as liquidated damages), one party may attempt to define the specific circumstances that would create a breach of contract. An example would be one party's failure to provide the other party with proof of insurance. In situations in which a specific definition of breach is acceptable to the APN, it is important to ensure that the limited definition is reciprocal and that each party be given a reasonable opportunity to "cure" the breach. The APN should pay particular attention to any liquidated damages clause in the contract. The financial consequences of such a clause can be devastating if a breach cannot be cured and the liquidated damages clause is triggered.

Notices

The notices clause in written agreements identifies the individuals who are to receive notice from the other party. The clause contains specific contact information for each of the individuals listed. The provision also outlines the process, such as certified mail, to be used when notifying the other party of any occurrence requiring notification, such as a decision to renew the contract for an additional term. It is important that the notification information be current so that the proper individuals are apprised of any communication between the parties to the agreement.

Modification

Modification provisions in written agreements permit the parties to modify the terms of the agreement without having to execute a new contract. For multiyear contracts, modification clauses are important because they permit an APN to renegotiate the compensation package or any other aspect of the agreement on an annual or other agreed-to basis. Any specific term of the contract may be modified so long as the modification provision states that the contract may be modified at any time and as long as both parties agree to the modification. Modifications invariably must be in writing and signed by all parties to the contract. Sometimes modification provisions will specify only certain components of the agreement that can be modified. Before executing an agreement, it is important for the APN to understand which terms of the agreement are subject to modification and, if necessary, negotiate for the right to modify additional terms before signing. Typically, modifications that occur during the term of the contract accompany the agreement in written form and are attached to the agreement as addendums.

Assignment

Assignment provisions in written agreements either permit or prohibit the assignment of the contract from one of the parties to another individual or entity. When assignment is permitted, one party may pass a contract on to a third party. That third party then assumes the responsibility for performing in accordance with the terms of the contract. On the other hand, when assignment is prohibited, the agreement cannot be transferred to another party. Often, if an APN is contracting with an entity, the entity will want the ability to assign the contract to another entity or subcontractor (such as a hospital or group practice) but will be unwilling to allow an APN to assign the contract to another APN.

Severability

Severability clauses help to keep uncontested and enforceable provisions of the written agreement in effect. Sometimes one specific provision of an agreement is disputed and deemed unenforceable. For example, a provision in the contract that requires the APN to refer his or her patients to a clinical laboratory, imaging center, or durable medical equipment (DME) company owned by one of the physicians in the group practice where the APN works may violate federal or state self-referral laws. Such a provision could be severed from the agreement without voiding the entire contract. The severability clause permits the rest of the contract to remain in full force.

Conflict of Laws

The conflict of laws clause in a written agreement identifies the jurisdiction within which the agreement was executed and the jurisdiction that governs contractual disputes that may arise. It is important for APNs to know which jurisdictions apply. For example, if an APN is contracting with a health-care facility that is owned by a company located in another state, the APN may be subject to that other state's laws if a dispute arises. Sometimes this clause will require the APN to seek relief in the other state's court system rather than the court system of the state where the APN is located. These types of provisions are becoming more prevalent as health-care systems, facilities, and group practices continue to consolidate with other systems, facilities, and practices—sometimes on a national scale. This trend can make it quite difficult for the APN to obtain remedies if there is a breach of the contract.

Legal Authority

The legal authority section of a written agreement states that the parties to the agreement have the authority to enter into the arrangement. This provision ensures that only the individuals with the authority to bind the parties are participating in the negotiation and execution of the written agreement.

Force Majeure

The *force majeure* clause of a written agreement ensures that the contract will not be considered to be breached in situations in which an "act of God" prohibits one party from performing in accordance with the terms of the agreement. "Acts of God" include natural disasters such as floods, earthquakes, tornados, and hurricanes, as well as human disasters such as wars, terrorist acts, and riots. A *force majeure* clause has the effect of putting the

performance requirements of the contract on hold until performance can be reasonably resumed.

Covenant Not to Compete

Covenants not to compete limit an APN's ability to enter into other ventures that would compete with the "interests" of the organization, plan, or practice group with whom he or she is contracting. Typically, covenants not to compete are time limited and may contain geographical limitations. That is, an APN may be prohibited from entering into other ventures that directly or indirectly compete with the other party for a certain period of time, such as 2 years after the contract terminates. The prohibition also may be limited to a certain geographical radius, such as a 10-mile radius from the location of the other party. This type of limitation is meant to protect the organization or practice group from direct competition by the APN, who could otherwise open a practice in the same general location and take business from the other party.

When a covenant not to compete is included in an independent contractor or employment agreement, it is important for the APN to know what organizations or entities the other party considers to be within the scope of the covenant not to compete. It is also important to clarify what the other party means by the use of the word *interests,* to limit the applicable period to as narrow a time frame as possible, to limit the geographical restraints, and, if possible, to include a specific sum of money that will be received by the APN for agreeing not to compete. Often the agreement will include a requirement to pay liquidated damages if the APN violates a covenant not to compete. Each state has laws that govern whether a restrictive covenant is enforceable or not. A few states prohibit restrictive covenants altogether as a matter of law or strictly limit their use. The APN should keep in mind that these laws vary from state to state.

Also, in exchange for retaining this covenant in an agreement, an APN should give serious consideration to requiring the other party to execute an exclusive agreement that would not allow the other party to contract with other APNs. Alternatively, the APN might ask for the right of first refusal on all projects and referrals for which the APN is qualified. An example might be the closure of a pain management clinic because of lack of funding and termination of the APN who functioned as staff, with subsequent reopening of the same service on receiving new grant monies. On reopening, the pain management clinic would give the APN the right of first refusal for rehiring.

Signatures

The signatures section of a written agreement is the place where the parties sign and date the document. After the parties sign the agreement, it is considered to be executed. An agreement that is executed signifies that the parties have reached a meeting of the minds and that both parties intend to interact with each other in accordance with the terms of the contract.

Other Provisions to Consider Including in Written Agreements

Although most written agreements contain some combination of the provisions previously identified, there are contemporary issues that may need to be addressed by APNs as well. Those issues include the proprietary rights of the parties and incentives, as well as the frequency with which clinical practice guidelines and collaborative practice agreements will be negotiated.

Proprietary rights of the parties should be discussed by the parties considering entering into a contractual business relationship. It is important to clarify who owns all tangible and intangible property at the beginning of the business relationship so that issues regarding ownership interests can be explored and restrictions on use, if any, can be articulated. Tangible personal property might include equipment, supplies, or furnishings. Intangible property, on the other hand, includes things such as intellectual property and goodwill. In situations in which these issues have been addressed during the negotiation period, the parties are clear about what property they each own and the expectations regarding the use of that property during the term of the contract and once the agreement expires or is terminated.

With regard to incentives, it is important for APNs to avoid agreeing to participate in any incentive arrangement that is based on schemes to acquire new patients in which the APN knowingly receives inducements. Incentive arrangements that fit into this category include any agreement to pay the APN for referring patients to specific providers. Engaging in these kinds of activities exposes health-care

professionals to fraud and abuse allegations and to breach of fiduciary duty causes of action.

Health-care providers are experiencing the consequences associated with these problems. The Office of Inspector General–U.S. Department of Health & Human Services (OIG-HHS) reported that the federal government obtained $1.9 billion in health-care fraud judgments and settlements in 2015 for alleged kickbacks and false claims—a figure that does not include recovered state Medicaid funds (OIG-HHS, 2016). APNs should be careful to avoid contracts and activities that the government might view as fraudulent. Investigations are on the rise as the federal government actively seeks to recoup significant amounts of money to help fund national health-care reform under the Affordable Care Act (ACA) of 2010. In one case a Texas nurse was sentenced to prison for participating in a kickback scheme with a DME company. The DME company paid the nurse 10% of the Medicare payments it received for each patient the nurse referred to it (OIG-HHS, 2011). The outcome would be the same if the nurse was an APN who had an employment or independent contractor agreement that included a provision for the APN to receive a certain percentage for each patient referred to the entity where he or she worked or elsewhere. APNs need to be vigilant and avoid these and other types of arrangements that may be characterized as kickbacks.

It may be appropriate, however, for APNs to consider including legal incentives that are based on the achievement of quality outcomes. Quality outcomes that might be used as incentives include, but are not limited to, patient satisfaction, length of stay, reduced mortality and readmission rates, and adherence to recommended clinical regimens.

Avoiding Legal Pitfalls Associated With Written Agreements

Written agreements are executed in an effort to establish the ground rules the parties agree to follow. Sometimes, however, these agreements are the subject of litigation. Usually, in litigation arising out of a written agreement executed between two parties, one party alleges that the other has breached the contract and should pay damages to the nonbreaching party. In other instances, one party may attempt to argue that the contract should be deemed illegal or that certain provisions of the contract should be disregarded.

The case that follows is illustrative of some of the contractual terms previously discussed in this chapter, as well as some problems APNs may encounter in situations involving written agreements. *Washington County Memorial Hospital v. Sidebottom* (1999) involved a nurse practitioner (NP) who entered into an employment agreement with a rural Missouri hospital in 1993. The employment agreement contained a covenant not to compete during the term of the agreement and for 1 year following the termination of the agreement. The covenant applied to the geographical area within a 50-mile radius of the hospital. The NP could not "directly or indirectly engage in the practice of nursing [elsewhere] without the express direction or consent" of the hospital. In February 1994, the NP was still employed at the hospital and asked for permission to provide prenatal care for the county health department. The hospital was not providing prenatal care for its patients at the time and allowed the NP to provide the care for the county. However, the hospital reserved the right to rescind its permission if it offered prenatal services in the future.

The employment agreement terminated in 1996 and the NP and the hospital entered into a new employment agreement that had a term of 2 years. The second agreement contained the same covenant not to compete. It also provided for an additional 2-year term unless either party provided written notice of termination at least 90 days before its expiration in 1998. The agreement also gave the parties the right to review the NP's compensation at set intervals.

During the course of the second employment agreement there were some discussions between the parties about increasing the NP's compensation. In January 1998, the hospital unilaterally gave the NP a 3% salary increase, which the NP considered to be unfair, although she did sign a modification to the agreement concerning the increase. The NP resigned a few months later and immediately began employment with a physician practice that was located within the 50-mile radius of the hospital. The hospital went to court and obtained a temporary restraining order. The NP immediately had to stop working for the physician practice. Thereafter, the court issued a permanent restraining order prohibiting the NP from practicing within the 50-mile radius for 1 year from the effective date of her resignation.

The NP appealed and argued the court should not enforce the covenant "because there was no threat of significant patient loss" to the hospital. However, the appellate court found the geographical limitations and time frame of the covenant to be reasonable and protective of the hospital's patient base, which was the source of its revenue. The court noted that the hospital had helped the NP get established in the community by setting up two clinics, advertising her services, and providing her with the support necessary to maintain her practice.

The NP also argued that the hospital materially breached the employment agreement by unilaterally amending the contract with a salary increase without the NP's review or any negotiations. The appellate court rejected this argument as well and found the hospital had acted in good faith by giving the NP an increase equal to a cap it had imposed on salary increases for all employees at the time. The court required the NP to pay for the hospital's costs of the appeal. Had the hospital offered proof of other financial damages from loss of patients because of the NP's violation of the covenant, the court would have awarded those damages as well.

Had the court agreed that the hospital breached the employment contract by unilaterally amending it before the NP violated the covenant, the NP would *not* have been subject to the covenant not to compete. The covenant would have been unenforceable and the court would have allowed the NP to continue to practice within the geographical area excluded by the contract. Likewise, if this case arose in a state where restrictive covenants are prohibited by law, the noncompete language would have been stricken by the court and the NP would have remained employed with the physician practice.

CONCLUSION

Traditionally, nurses have practiced as employees and not independent contractors. However, more and more APNs are embarking on private practice careers and pursuing entrepreneurial opportunities that require the protections of a written agreement. In addition, more and more APNs and their employers are entering into written contracts to define their rights and responsibilities. Because executing written agreements governing the working relationship between the APN and another party is now commonplace, it is important to understand the basic, foundational issues that need to be addressed in written agreements. This chapter has identified several of those issues.

Although written agreements can provide APNs with great flexibility and autonomy, they can also result in the APN rather than the health-care organization being held liable for alleged acts of negligence. In addition, the terms included in written agreements may be the focus of litigation themselves. Cases discussed in this chapter demonstrate how some courts have addressed these issues. In light of the principles discussed in this chapter, it is important for APNs to ensure that agreements regarding their status as employee or independent contractor be memorialized in writing. In addition, these written agreements need to be carefully reviewed for compliance with federal and state laws and regulations and to ensure that the written agreement accurately reflects the mutual assent of the parties. APNs should seriously consider obtaining legal advice to protect their interests.

28

The Law, the Courts, and the Advanced Practice Registered Nurse

David M. Keepnews*

Learning Outcomes

Learning outcomes expected as a result of this chapter:

- Understand the various sources of law.
- Describe the relationship between the law, legislation, and regulation.
- Distinguish between federal and state responsibility for health-care laws.
- Summarize the rulemaking process.
- Justify the functions of the courts.
- Describe the structure of the U.S. court system.
- Explain the role of precedent in the U.S. legal system.
- Illustrate legal scope of practice (SOP) issues.
- Explain fraud and abuse.
- Clarify antitrust law and its relevance to health professional practice.

*Acknowledgment: The author wishes to express his deep appreciation to Kammie Monarch, JD, RN, whose significant contributions to prior versions of this chapter are reflected in this version.

INTRODUCTION

The focus of this chapter is to highlight several areas of the law that directly affect the role and practice of advanced practice registered nurses (APRNs). It gives an overview of the sources of law in the United States; explains how the judicial branch of government works; and discusses some specific areas of law that guide all APRNs in their daily practices. This chapter does not directly address issues related to negligence and malpractice because they are addressed separately in another chapter.

SOURCES OF LAW

The legal environment for nursing practice is derived from several sources, including *legislation* that governs and otherwise affects practice; *regulations* that implement legislation; and the *decisions* of courts that interpret and enforce laws, including both legislation and regulation.

Legislation

Much of the legal context for advanced nursing practice originates in statutes—that is, in legislation passed in Congress and in state legislatures. Legislation defines the legal authority for practice, legal responsibilities of practitioners, many of the penalties for failing to live up to those legal responsibilities, and other critical aspects of practice, including reimbursement.

Different responsibilities fall to the state legislatures and to Congress. Congress votes on legislation that involves the use of federal funds, relates to issues that span across state boundaries, or affects commerce between states.

A large number of health-care issues are the responsibilities of the states. State legislatures define licensure requirements for health-care professionals, hospitals, and other health-care organizations. States also determine issues related to the scope of practice (SOP) of APRNs and other health professionals—these include major issues such as the scope of APRN prescriptive authority and whether APRNs must practice in collaboration with physicians.

In theory, Congress passes laws that deal with national or federal issues, whereas most health-care issues are reserved for the states to address. In practice, this line has become harder to draw. For example, the Medicare program was created by federal legislation in 1965, and Medicare funding, financing, eligibility, coverage, and payment are all governed by federal law. But to qualify for reimbursement, services must be within a practitioner's SOP, which is determined by each state. Although states are responsible for regulating hospitals and other health-care organizations, such organizations must be in compliance with Medicare requirements, including Medicare conditions of participation (COPs), in order to participate in the Medicare and Medicaid programs—that is, to be eligible for payment by those programs. The states have traditionally been responsible for regulating health insurance, but Congress has determined that many insurance issues are areas of national concern. Accordingly, the Affordable Care Act (ACA) (Public Laws 111-148 and 111-152)—the health reform law enacted in 2010—sets out a framework for state health insurance exchanges and requires most large employers to provide health insurance or pay a penalty. It also requires that individuals not covered by their employer or a government health-care program purchase insurance or pay a penalty.

Opponents of the ACA argued that this latter requirement exceeded the authority of Congress—that only the states had the authority to mandate individuals to purchase health insurance. In *National Federation of Independent Business v. Sebelius* (2012), the Supreme Court upheld the so-called individual mandate, finding that Congress's power to levy taxes gave it the authority to require that individuals failing to purchase health insurance pay a penalty.

Generally speaking, when Congress acts in a given area it overrides states' actions in the same area—a doctrine known as *preemption*. For instance, the federal Employee Retirement Income Security Act of 1974 preempts some state laws regulating employee benefit plans, including employer-provided health insurance. This has had the effect of exempting self-insured plans (in which employers bear their own insurance risk directly) from state regulation. It also has had the effect of preempting state courts' ability to try many damage suits based on damages allegedly caused by the actions of an employer-provided health plan.

In some instances, however, both Congress and the states may act—either because Congress explicitly allows the states to act or because Congress and the states address different aspects of the same issue. For example, the federal Occupational Safety and Health Act addresses health and safety issues of employees, but it allows states to pass more stringent laws and regulatory mechanisms to protect employees within the state. Both Congress and many state legislatures have enacted antitrust laws that address anticompetitive marketplace activity. Although Congress has strengthened and broadened federal laws on health-care fraud and abuse, including fraudulent and abusive activities directed against private health insurers, states also have laws that address health-care fraud and abuse.

Government Agency Rulemaking

The actions of federal and state government agencies have a critical role to play in health care, including the practice of APRNs. The rules and regulations they issue have the force of law.

In the United States, government is divided into three branches: legislative, executive, and judicial. Under this framework, the legislature passes laws, the executive branch implements them, and the judicial branch interprets them when controversies arise.

The executive branch is headed by a chief executive—the president at the federal level and the governor at the state level. It includes several different agencies that administer the day-to-day workings of the government. They are headed by officials who report to the president or governor and who (generally) are appointed by him or her. These agencies cover all areas of government. In health care, relevant federal agencies include the U.S. Department of Health & Human Services (DHHS) and agencies within it, such as the Centers for Medicare and Medicaid Services (CMS), the Food and Drug Administration (FDA), the Centers for Disease Control and Prevention (CDC), and the National Institutes of Health (NIH). But many other agencies have an impact on health care and health professionals in one way or another—the U.S. Department of Labor, the Department of Defense, the Department of Veterans Affairs, and others.

These agencies act based on the authority given to them through Congress (for federal agencies) or the state legislatures. A common explanation of these agencies' responsibilities is that they implement legislation. This description is accurate, but it may be deceptively simple. "Implementation" may involve a range of activities, from simply operationalizing a clear legislative mandate to filling

in complex details in a legislatively developed program to acting on its own initiative based on a long-standing, broad grant of legislative authority.

The following examples may help illustrate the differences between each of these types of executive agency action.

In one hypothetical state, following lobbying efforts by nursing organizations, the state legislature passes legislation authorizing APRNs to prescribe drugs without physician supervision or mandatory collaboration. The relevant part of this legislation reads as follows:

1. An APRN shall be authorized to write prescriptions for drugs, regardless of class of drug, provided that the APRN:
   a. Is certified by a national accrediting body recognized by the National Commission on Certifying Agencies or the American Boards of Nursing Specialties; and
   b. Has successfully completed 100 hours of coursework in pharmacology offered by an accredited school of nursing, either as part of an educational program leading to preparation as an APRN or subsequent to completing such program.
2. The board of nursing (BON) shall establish and maintain a mechanism for ensuring that APRNs meet the previous requirements before prescribing drugs.
3. The BON shall maintain a list of APRNs who are qualified to prescribe drugs and shall make this list available to the board of pharmacy.
4. A licensed pharmacist, upon being presented with a valid prescription written by an APRN who is qualified to prescribe drugs, shall fill such prescription in the same manner as a prescription written by any other qualified prescriber.
5. Nothing in this section shall be construed as requiring physician supervision of APRN prescriptions or prescribing practices.

To implement this change in the law, the state BON and state board of pharmacy might propose amendments to their regulations. The BON's regulations would include a process for tracking and verifying completion of required pharmacology coursework and for maintaining a list of APRNs who are authorized to prescribe. The board of pharmacy might amend its regulations to reflect the fact that the law authorizes pharmacists to fill prescriptions written by APRNs.

This is the simplest form of implementation—providing a mechanism to operationalize a clear legislative mandate. Imagine that the law was written a little differently and instead reads as follows:

> An advanced practice nurse shall be authorized to prescribe drugs, provided that she or he has completed coursework in pharmacology, and in accordance with standards and mechanisms determined by the board of nursing.

This law is much less precise. How much coursework do APRNs need in order to prescribe? Where can they obtain this coursework—must it be from a school of nursing or can it be provided by another continuing education provider? Can the coursework be completed online? What other standards should be included—should there be restrictions based on the APRN's area of expertise or certification? Are pharmacists required to fill prescriptions written by APRNs? What role (if any) will physicians have related to APRN prescribing? These are all issues that would be left to the BON to address when it proposes and issues regulations.

Why would a state legislature adopt a law that is so sparse on details? Perhaps it was the result of a compromise following a failure to reach consensus on the details among interest groups and legislators and an agreement to let those details be worked out in regulation. Or, as is often the case, perhaps legislators preferred to leave it to the relevant government agency to set appropriate standards, based on the belief that legislators lack the expertise (or time) to debate whether 75, 100, or 200 hours of pharmacology coursework is appropriate, but that the government agency charged with regulating nursing practice is in a better position to make such a determination.

This type of scenario—the legislature enacting legislation that leaves it to a government agency to determine major details—is fairly common. When Congress passed the Health Insurance Portability and Accountability Act (HIPAA) in 1996, it included requirements for safeguarding the privacy of health information. It was left to DHHS to develop and promulgate rules that spell out the mechanisms for implementing and enforcing standards for doing so. When Congress expanded the scope of Medicare reimbursement for APRNs as part of the Balanced Budget Act (BBA) of 1997, it was up to DHHS (and, specifically, to the Health Care Financing Administration, now the CMS) to address important questions such as who would qualify for reimbursement and how statutory requirements that APRNs work in collaboration with a physician would be implemented.

The ACA introduced several important new measures to expand access to health-care coverage, curb abusive practices by some insurers, and expand primary care and preventive services, among many others. Many of the provisions of the ACA required DHHS and in some cases other agencies, including the Department of Labor and the Internal Revenue Service, to issue implementing rules. These include rules addressing basic issues such as determining what is included in "essential health benefits" and what constitutes "preventive services."

Sometimes government agencies act under a broad scope of authority that has been granted to them in a specific area by Congress or a state legislature, rather than in response to a recent legislative mandate. A state health department may be granted the authority to establish licensing standards for hospitals, for instance. After initially establishing regulations containing standards for licensure, the agency may subsequently decide to revise those standards as part of its broad mandate to protect the public's health.

The Court System

What Courts Do

Courts administer justice by applying laws to controversies. Facts are determined, the law is applied to those facts, and a decision is rendered. Civil courts adjudicate controversies between individual parties and address the rights of the parties. Parties in these matters are referred to as *plaintiffs* and *defendants*. Plaintiffs are the suing party and defendants are the party defending the action filed against them. Criminal courts, in contrast, are charged with administering criminal laws and determining penalties for wrongs against society. In a criminal action, the government prosecutes a defendant (or multiple defendants).

Structure of the U.S. Court System: Federal and State

In the United States, there is a federal court system and each state has its own court system. Types of cases heard in state-based civil proceedings typically include breach of contract, negligence, and malpractice causes of action, as well as domestic relations, real estate, probate, and other state-specific matters. These cases may or may not be heard by a jury, but they are always overseen by judges.

In most states, the party losing the case at the trial court level has the opportunity to appeal the matter to an appellate court. States use different names for this level of court, but they all are considered intermediate appellate courts. Generally, these courts are referred to as *courts of appeals*. In these courts, the appealing party is referred to as the *appellant* and the other party is the *appellee*. Cases coming before a court of appeals are not retried. Generally, appellate judges determine whether or not the trial was properly conducted and/or whether the right law was correctly applied. After reviewing the trial court record, the court of appeals may affirm, modify, reverse, or remand the judgment made at the trial court level. Affirming the trial court decision upholds the original determination made in the matter. Modifying the trial court decision changes the decision in some way. Reversing the decision of the trial court results in nullifying it. Remanding the decision results in the case being sent back to the trial court.

The losing party at the appellate court level may have the opportunity to appeal the matter to the state's high court. (That course is known as the state Supreme Court in most states, but may go by different names in other states. For example, the high court in New York State is the Court of Appeals.) Cases that raise federal constitutional issues may be appealed to the U.S. Supreme Court.

Unlike the varied nature of the state court systems, the federal court system is uniform. Entry-level trial courts are federal district courts. There are 94 federal districts located in each U.S. state and territory. Larger states are divided into two, three, or four federal districts. These district courts are presided over by appointed federal district judges. Federal district courts hear both civil and criminal matters. Cases tried in federal district courts include those in which the United States is a party; disputes between states, between a state and a citizen of another state, between citizens of different states, and between a state or its citizens and a government abroad; disputes affecting foreign ambassadors; cases arising under federal law and the U.S. Constitution; and admiralty and maritime cases.

After a judge in a federal district court has rendered his or her decision, the losing party may appeal that decision to a federal court of appeal (also referred to as circuit courts). There are 13 such courts in the United States. The losing party at this level may request to appeal the decision to the U.S. Supreme Court.

The U.S. Supreme Court is located in Washington, DC, and is composed of nine justices, one of whom serves as Chief Justice. Supreme Court justices—similar to all federal judges—are nominated by the president of the United States and confirmed by the U.S. Senate.

The Role of Precedent

In making their decisions, courts look at how prior cases raising similar issues have been decided. Previously decided cases with similar facts or legal issues are called *precedents*. Courts will look to these prior decisions as guides to deciding current cases by either following them or distinguishing a current case to explain why previous decisions do not apply.

SELECTED LEGAL ISSUES

Legal Scope of Practice Issues

State laws define the boundaries within which members of each health-care profession may practice. This is referred to as that profession's *SOP*. The SOP of APRNs is generally found in each state's nurse practice act (NPA). Typically, scopes of practice for nurses, including APRNs, are written broadly and do not delineate specific tasks.

State laws governing APRN SOP vary considerably. Eighteen states and the District of Columbia currently allow APRNs to practice without any legal requirements for physician supervision or collaboration. Other states require varying degrees of involvement by physicians. State laws also vary in APRN authority to prescribe medications—some require collaboration with a physician, some allow only some categories of APRNs to prescribe, and some impose restrictions in terms of types of medications that can be prescribed. New York State permits nurse practitioners (NPs) to prescribe only within their specialty area.

These varying restrictions on APRN practice have been cited as a barrier to expanding access to health-care services. The Institute of Medicine (IOM) report on *The Future of Nursing* (Committee on the Robert Wood Johnson Foundation Initiative on the Future of Nursing at the Institute of Medicine, 2011) included a recommendation to remove SOP barriers, declaring that "advanced practice registered nurses should be able to practice to the full extent of their education and training" (p. 278).

In 2008, the APRN Consensus Group and the National Council of State Boards of Nursing issued a *Consensus Model for APRN Regulation: Licensure, Accreditation, Certification and Education.* This document sets out a uniform model of APRN regulation with the intent that it be adopted by all U.S. states. The model has been endorsed by a wide range of nursing professional and specialty organizations.

Advanced Practice Registered Nurses in the Courts

In 1936, for the first time, SOP issues between nurses and physicians were addressed in a published opinion. That case, *Chalmers-Francis v. Nelson* (1936), involved a nurse's administration of anesthesia over the objection of a physician and one of his associates. The physician asserted that administration of anesthesia by a nurse was a violation of the California Medical Practice Act and should be immediately stopped. The case was eventually heard by the California Supreme Court. In reviewing the matter, the Court concluded that anesthesia administration by nurses did not constitute diagnosing or prescribing within the state medical practice act.

In *Fein v. Permanente Medical Group* (1981), an NP was alleged to have been negligent when she assessed a patient with chest pain as having a muscle spasm rather than a myocardial infarction. At trial the patient was awarded almost $1 million in damages. The case, which presented several issues, was eventually appealed to the California Supreme Court. One of the issues raised was whether an NP's professional conduct should be judged according to a physician standard of care. The court found that an NP—not physician—standard of care should apply because the NP's SOP includes examining and diagnosing a patient and that the activity engaged in by the NP was within her SOP even though that activity overlapped with activities engaged in by physicians.

In *Sermchief v. Gonzales* (1983), the Missouri Board of Registration for the Healing Arts threatened to charge two nurses with the unauthorized practice of medicine and to charge five physicians with aiding and abetting the unauthorized practice of medicine. These health professionals all practiced at a clinic in which the nurses performed family planning, obstetrics, and gynecology services using standing orders and protocols that were approved by physicians. In an attempt to resolve the issue, the health professionals asked for an injunction prohibiting the board from taking action and to declare that their actions were lawful. The case eventually went to the Missouri Supreme Court, which ruled in favor of the nurses and physicians, affirming the ability of the nurses to practice as APRNs. In reaching its decision, the court reviewed the state's definition of professional nursing; it noted that the SOP for nurses had been expanded and that the nurses in this case were practicing in accordance with applicable laws. Because these nurses' conduct was consistent with the state NPA, they were not engaging in the unauthorized practice of medicine.

Planned Parenthood v. Vines (1989) was decided by a court of appeals in Indiana. In this case, a patient sued Planned Parenthood, alleging that an NP had inserted an intrauterine device (IUD). One of the issues addressed by the court was the standard of care required of the NP. After considering the matter, the court concluded that the NP was a specialist and should be held to the standard of care for a person with superior knowledge and skill, and thus must practice consistent with others with superior knowledge and skill. At trial, expert testimony asserted that the standard of care for inserting IUDs was the same for nurses and physicians. Therefore, the NP was required to insert the IUD using the care and skill of others, including physicians, performing that same task.

Berdyck v. Shinde and HR Magruder Memorial Hospital (1993) was decided by the Ohio Supreme Court in 1993. In this case, the court ruled that the standard of care applicable to any health professional was the same, regardless of the particular professional performing that skill. Here, a nurse and physician were both accused of negligence with regard to recognizing the signs and symptoms of preeclampsia. One of the issues the justices dealt with on appeal was the duty of care owed to the patient. In rendering its decision to affirm the lower court's denial of the hospital's motion for summary judgment, the justices noted that the fact that a physician owes a particular duty of care to a patient does not mean that the nurse is exempt from owing that same duty of care. The court observed that the same act may be within the practice standards for both nurses and physicians, and that both groups of health professionals must embark on the completion of that act in a way that is consistent with their respective duties of care to their clients.

The Ohio Supreme Court's determination in the *Berdyck* case was reiterated in *Ali v. Community Health Care Plan, Inc.* (2002). The plaintiff sued a health maintenance organization (HMO) that employed a certified nurse-midwife (CNM). The plaintiff alleged that she was treated negligently during her pregnancy, thereby causing her to lose the baby. She had reported the development of a vaginal discharge to the HMO's CNM during a telephone conversation approximately 2 weeks after having an amniocentesis. She claimed the CNM failed to direct her to see a physician. The CNM countered that the character of the vaginal discharge reported by the patient was not indicative of a loss of amniotic fluid. The CNM's documentation supported her position. The case was tried and the judge instructed the jury to apply a certain standard of care: what a reasonable and prudent CNM practicing obstetrics and gynecology would have done under the same circumstances. The jury rendered a verdict in favor of the HMO. The plaintiff appealed and argued the trial judge should have directed the jury to apply a different standard: what a reasonable and prudent *professional* practicing obstetrics and gynecology would have done under the same circumstances. The plaintiff contended the CNM standard was a lower standard. The appellate court disagreed and determined that any professional practicing obstetrics and gynecology would be required to direct a patient to be seen if the patient reported signs and symptoms consistent with loss of amniotic fluid. The verdict rendered by the trial court was affirmed.

Spine Diagnostics Center of Baton Rouge Inc. v. Louisiana State Board of Nursing (2008) concerned a Louisiana State Board of Nursing Advisory Opinion, which concluded that interventional pain management falls within the SOP of certified registered nurse anesthetists (CRNAs). A trial court ruled that the Advisory Opinion constituted a regulation expanding the CRNA SOP into a new area. An appellate court affirmed, finding that interventional pain management is "solely the practice of medicine" and agreeing that the Advisory Opinion was a regulation that the BON had issued without providing notice and an opportunity to comment as required by the state administrative procedures act (APA) and finding it invalid. The state supreme court declined to hear the case, allowing the appellate court ruling to stand.

In 2011, an Iowa court invalidated rules issued by the state BON and department of public health authorizing NPs to supervise fluoroscopy. Iowa physician groups argued that the rules were invalid because state law prohibits the expansion of nursing into medicine without official recognition by physicians. The court found that state law also required that the agencies first establish a curriculum, safety standards, and an examination before authorizing NPs to supervise fluoroscopy. Nursing organizations unsuccessfully argued that the law should be upheld (*Iowa Medical Society and Iowa Society of Anesthesiologists v. Iowa Board of Nursing and Iowa Department of Public Health*, 2011).

Professional Discipline

BONs govern the practice of nursing in every state. It is the responsibility of the BON to protect the public from conduct that poses a threat to the public health, safety, and welfare. Each state's NPA or regulations set out specific grounds for professional discipline, but generally they include acts of unprofessional conduct, gross negligence, endangering patient safety, unethical conduct, and acting outside of one's SOP (Monarch, 2002).

In 1980 an APRN was disciplined because he was found to have violated the NPA in Florida. The case was *Hernicz v. State of Florida, Department of Professional Regulation.* Hernicz's license was suspended because he was alleged to have treated two patients without physician supervision. Disciplinary action was taken in this case because the state of Florida required APRNs to work with a sponsoring physician. In this case the Florida Court of Appeals concluded that the disciplinary action taken was proper because the Florida Department of Professional Regulation presented credible and substantial evidence that the NP did not have a supervising physician when he treated two patients.

When an APRN is accused of violating the state NPA, he or she must be notified in the complaint of the specific alleged violations. A disciplinary action process will be held in accordance with the state's APA. It is the provisions of the APA that ensure that individual disciplinary action proceedings occur in a manner that respects the constitutional rights of the nurse. Of particular concern is the nurse's right to due process. This requires that the nurse have a meaningful opportunity to respond to the complaint and to be meaningfully heard.

Following disciplinary proceedings, a BON will issue final agency orders. This document describes any disciplinary action that was taken, outlines the finding of facts, and outlines the conclusions of law that were relied on in rendering the decision. Disciplinary action may include issuing a reprimand, suspending the APRN's license, or revoking it. Once a final agency order is issued by a BON, the matter is concluded, unless one of the parties elects to appeal the decision in court.

Courts will generally not substitute their own judgment for that of the BON. However, there are instances in which a court reversed a BON action. Typically, reversals occur when a court determines that the nurse's due process or other constitutional rights were violated or the board acted beyond its statutory authority, failed to follow required procedures, committed an error of law, or made an arbitrary and capricious decision.

Hogan v. Mississippi Board of Nursing (1984) is an example of a case in which a BON decision involving an APRN—in this case, a nurse anesthetist—was overturned by a court. Hogan was investigated by the Mississippi Board of Nursing for allegedly misappropriating narcotics from the hospital where she worked. The BON conducted a hearing, found her guilty, and her license was revoked. She appealed. The Mississippi Supreme Court found that the BON had applied the wrong standard of proof in determining that Hogan had misappropriated narcotics. Whereas charges of misconduct generally require the BON to prove the charge by a *preponderance of the evidence* (showing that it is more likely than not that the accused party committed the alleged acts), in this case the court ruled that charges leading to license revocation must meet a higher standard—*clear and convincing evidence*—but the BON failed to apply this standard in Hogan's case. The court thus directed the BON to restore Hogan's license.

FRAUD AND ABUSE

Responsibility and accountability are not new concepts for APRNs or for any professional nurse. As APRNs have broadened their roles in health care, areas of potential legal risk have grown. Many of the issues that were formerly of primary concern to other health professionals are now much more clearly relevant to APRNs as well.

As Medicare providers, APRNs are able to receive Medicare provider numbers (known as National Provider Identification, or NPI) and to bill Medicare directly for covered services. APRNs are recognized as providers by increasing numbers of group and private health plans as well. Recognition as providers has also brought an increased responsibility (and need) for APRNs to understand the requirements for sound, legal billing practices.

Federal and state governments have sharpened their focus on fraudulent and abusive practices by all health-care providers. Government agencies have concentrated increasing resources on investigating and prosecuting fraud and abuse. As independently accountable professionals, it is in APRNs' interests to understand what is expected of them as providers under Medicare, Medicaid, and other health-care programs and plans. As in most other areas of law, ignorance of the law in this case does not excuse violations. The fact that a practice may use billing staff or an outside billing specialist does not mean that providers are not expected to know, and to be responsible for, claims and documentation submitted under their names and NPI.

APRNs need to have some familiarity with reimbursement laws and what they are expected to do to avoid violations. Some common examples of conduct that may be considered to violate fraud and abuse laws include billing for services that were not actually furnished to the patient, misrepresenting the patient's diagnosis (providing a false or more severe diagnosis to justify payment or increase the amount of payment), misrepresenting the services provided (billing for more complex or intense services than those that were actually furnished to the patient), misrepresenting the medical necessity of services provided, and billing for services under circumstances in which requirements for payment have not been met.

The federal government and many state governments have been stepping up investigation and enforcement activities related to fraud and abuse for several years. The ACA increases federal sentencing guidelines for health-care fraud that involves more than $1 million in losses; increases coordination between CMS, the HHS Office of Inspector General (OIG), and the Department of Justice (DOJ); and adds greater oversight of private insurance abuse. It expands resources devoted to fraud and abuse enforcement and sets the stage for possible further expansion of fraud and abuse laws.

Assessing Risk and Avoiding Fraud and Abuse

Whether in their own practices, in physician-based practices, or in hospital-based practices, APRNs should be aware of programs in place to ensure compliance with applicable laws on billing for services. APRNs should not assume that billing practices that have been in place for some time must be okay because "we have always done it this way." Enforcement agencies are generally concerned more with *patterns* of inappropriate, illegal billing practices over time than with isolated, accidental events.

The Health Care Fraud Prevention and Enforcement Action Team (HEAT), a joint initiative of DHHS and the U.S. DOJ, includes a Provider Compliance Training Initiative to encourage compliance and to advise providers on how to avoid fraud and abuse. Several resources have been developed as part of this initiative, including instructional videos and podcasts. These can be accessed at http://oig .hhs.gov/compliance/provider-compliance-training/index .asp. In addition, the DHHS OIG Web site (http://www .oig.hhs.gov) includes advisory opinions and compliance guidance resources that can be readily accessed.

Billing, coding, and payment policy are complex. Most APRNs are not experts in this area, but all should have a general understanding of coding, billing, and payment. In most instances, working with a billing specialist—either one employed by the practice or an external consultant—is highly advisable. However, each APRN must have sufficient knowledge to work with these specialists to ensure their accuracy.

One specific area in which APRNs (and the practices in which they work) must be careful is the area of "incident-to" billing. Since its inception, Medicare Part B has paid not only for "physician services," but also for services and supplies furnished incident-to the services of a physician (CMS, 2011). Among other things, this has allowed physician practices to bill for services provided by other staff—not just APRNs, but also staff nurses, medical assistants, and other office personnel. For many years, this was the only way that services provided by APRNs were covered under Medicare. As APRNs won Medicare reimbursement for eligible services, more and more APRNs have been billing Medicare directly for their services. However, many practices have chosen to continue billing APRN services as incident-to services. When an NP or a clinical nurse specialist (CNS) bills

Medicare directly for services (under their own names and NPI), Medicare pays for those services at 85% of what it would pay a physician. (CNMs' services are paid at 100% of the physician rate as of January 1, 2011.) Incident-to services are billed under the physician's name and number and are paid at 100% of the physician rate—in essence, they are treated as if the physician performed the service. Thus, many physician practices that employ APRNs see a financial incentive in using incident-to billing.

Incident-to billing, however, comes with several requirements (CMS, 2011). The physician must initiate the patient's course of treatment and must provide subsequent services frequently enough to reflect the physician's continuing active participation in and management of the course of treatment. The services must be provided under direct physician supervision—the physician must be present in the office suite and immediately available to provide assistance and direction throughout the time the APRN is providing services to the patient. The APRN must be an employee, leased employee, or independent contractor of the physician or of the entity that employs or contracts with the physician. (So, for example, the APRN and physician may both be employees of the same clinic or health system.)

These requirements reflect the fact that incident-to payment was not designed as a mechanism for paying independent providers of care, but rather as a way to reimburse physicians for services provided by office staff. Incident-to billing long predates recognition of APRNs as Medicare providers. Also, keep in mind that these conditions do not apply to APRN services billed under the APRN's name and NPI.

The potential for incorrectly billing for services is increased when practices depend on incident-to billing for services provided by APRNs. Is there a physician on the premises and available at all times or do APRNs cover for physicians during hospital rounds or at other times when no physician is in the office? Are there times when a new patient is seen by an APRN? Are there times when an established patient is seen by an APRN for a new health problem? If the practice complies with all the conditions for incident-to billing, are the details of such compliance adequately documented?

Notably, in addition to the restrictions and risks inherent in incident-to billing for APRN services, it also renders those services invisible—they are reflected in Medicare data as having been provided by the physician, not the APRN.

ANTITRUST LAW

Antitrust is another area of the law that can have an important bearing on health professionals' practices. The first federal antitrust statute, the Sherman Act, was enacted in 1890, followed by the Clayton Act and the Federal Trade Commission Act, both in 1914. Congress's goals in enacting these statutes was to ensure free competition by countering business practices and transactions "which tended to restrict production, raise prices or otherwise control the market to the detriment of purchasers or consumers of goods and services" (*Apex Hosiery Co. v. Leader,* 1940). When competitors work together to restrain competition by others, they deprive consumers of the purported benefits of a free economic market—it removes incentives to lower prices and improve quality. Some activities that had been undertaken by large industries at the end of the 19th century—dividing up economic markets, agreeing on minimum prices, boycotting other competitors—were seen as inherently injurious to consumers. As part of a populist reaction to the "robber barons" in industries such as steel and oil, the antitrust laws were an effort to reclaim the free enterprise system as the United States had previously known it. For instance, in describing the Sherman Act, the U.S. Supreme Court noted that this statute was "designed to be a comprehensive charter of economic liberty aimed at preserving free and unfettered competition as the rule of trade. It rests on the premise that the unrestrained interaction of competitive forces will yield the best allocation of our economic resources, the lowest prices, the highest quality, and the greatest material progress, while at the same time providing an environment conducive to the preservation of our democratic, political, and social institutions" (*Northern Pacific Railway Co. v. United States,* 1958).

The U.S. DOJ and the Federal Trade Commission (FTC) share federal enforcement responsibilities for these antitrust statutes; in addition, state attorneys general and private parties may also bring suit under these laws. Most states also have their own antitrust laws, generally with provisions parallel to the federal laws.

The antitrust laws are written broadly. The application of these laws has been shaped by decades of judicial interpretation. Some activities—price fixing, group boycotts, and market allocation (dividing up markets among competitors)—are considered *per se* violations. This means that once it has been established that a competitor has engaged in one of these activities, the courts do not inquire as to its anticompetitive effects, such as whether and how it has harmed competition or injured consumers. Other activities are analyzed under a *rule of reason* approach. Under this approach, the court analyzes an alleged restraint on competition, weighing the procompetitive effects of an agreement against its anticompetitive effects (Marsh, 2010). This means that the court carefully examines the industry involved, the history and purpose of the restraint, the relevant market, and any special circumstances that exist in that market (*United States v. Topco Associates,* 1972). Meeting this standard is clearly a much more involved, costly, and time-consuming analysis than that required for activities that are considered *per se* violations.

For many years the antitrust laws were considered by the courts to be inapplicable to the activities of most professionals. "Learned professions" such as law and medicine generally were considered sufficiently different from other businesses for concerns about anticompetitive conduct to be relevant. However, in 1975, in *Goldfarb v. Virginia State Bar,* the U.S. Supreme Court found setting minimum attorneys' fees to be a Sherman Act violation, rejecting the defendant bar association's argument that they were exempt because the law is a learned profession. Subsequently, the U.S. Supreme Court made the application of the antitrust laws to medicine explicit in *Arizona v. Maricopa County Medical Society* (1982). In that case, local physicians had agreed on maximum fees that could be charged. This decision indicated that such acts were price fixing and effectively eliminated any belief that health care was outside the reach of antitrust laws.

In *Wilk v. American Medical Association* (1990), the American Medical Association (AMA) was found to have engaged in a boycott of chiropractors. The AMA's Code of Ethics had declared it unethical for physicians to associate with unscientific practitioners and later determined that chiropractic practice lacked a scientific basis. The effect of these determinations was a pronouncement that any physicians who referred patients to chiropractors, accepted referrals from chiropractors, or taught at a chiropractic school would be committing an ethical violation. A group of chiropractors sued the AMA, alleging that it was attempting to eliminate chiropractic care through an illegal boycott. The U.S. Court of Appeals for the Seventh Circuit eventually determined that this AMA policy (which had subsequently been changed) was, in fact, a *per se* violation of the Sherman Act.

In 2010 the FTC issued an administrative complaint against the North Carolina Board of Dental Examiners, which had acted to stop dental hygienists from independently offering tooth-whitening services in mall kiosks and salons. The board, charging that the hygienists were engaging in the unauthorized practice of dentistry, issued cease-and-desist letters to the hygienists and mall operators. The hygienists stopped offering teeth-whitening services. The FTC charged that the board—the majority of whose members were practicing dentists elected by the state's dentists—had engaged in anticompetitive activity in violation of the Federal Trade Commission Act; their activities, the FTC argued, were designed to drive their competitors from the market. The board argued that, as a state agency, they were immune from antitrust laws. Challenges to the FTC's findings eventually reached the Supreme Court, which ruled in favor of the FTC, finding that the board could only be immune if its activities were actively supervised by the state. In this case, the court found, board members had acted to stifle competition (*North Carolina State Board of Dental Examiners v. Federal Trade Commission*, No. 15-534, 547 U.S. ___, 2015). Several nursing organizations hailed the ruling, arguing that it "could strengthen the position of APRNs in their efforts to practice to the full extent of their education and training" (Robert Wood Johnson Foundation, 2015).

In one of the few antitrust cases involving APRNs, a group of CNMs brought suit against hospitals, a physician-owned insurance company, and several physicians. The CNMs charged that the defendants had engaged in concerted actions to prevent them from gaining hospital privileges, required physician supervision, and hampered their ability for their collaborating physician to secure liability insurance. Their thriving practice was eventually forced to close. Eventually, the CNMs won settlements against some of the defendants, and the U.S. Court of Appeals for the Sixth Circuit ruled against the remainder of the defendants (*Nurse Midwifery Associates v. Hibbett*, 1990).

In *Oltz v. St. Peter's Community Hospital* (1994), the Ninth Circuit Court of Appeals examined a case brought by a nurse anesthetist whose contract with a hospital was cancelled after a competing group of anesthesiologists obtained an exclusive contract with the same hospital. The hospital, located in a rural community in Montana, provided 84% of the surgical services rendered in the area. The anesthesiologists did not want to compete with Oltz, who charged a lower rate for anesthesia and enjoyed a good relationship with local surgeons. After the hospital cancelled Oltz's contract, he was effectively put out of business and had to relocate to find suitable employment. Oltz sued the anesthesiologists and the hospital and claimed their actions constituted a violation of the Sherman Act. On appeal from a trial court verdict awarding him no damages, the Ninth Circuit Court of Appeals ruled in his favor, finding that Oltz had presented ample evidence to support his claim that the hospital and physicians had conspired to eliminate him as a competitor.

Promoting Competition

Not all conduct that hinders competition constitutes antitrust violations. The FTC often provides analysis and advice on the potential impact on competition of proposed legislation and regulations. For example, in 2010 the staffs of the FTC's Office of Policy Planning, Bureau of Economics, and Bureau of Competition issued a letter advising that proposed Kentucky rules governing "limited service clinics" (such as retail clinics) would unjustifiably restrict the activities of health professionals practicing there, potentially hindering the ability of these clinics to compete with other types of clinics (DeSanti, Farrell, & Feinstein, 2010). The FTC may also initiate an administrative complaint when it believes that a practice is anticompetitive, as it did after investigating the North Carolina Board of Dental Examiners activities described previously.

In its 2011 report, the IOM Committee on the Future of Nursing took note of these and other opinions and actions by the FTC. As part of its recommendation to remove SOP barriers in order to allow APRNs to practice to the full extent of their education and training, the committee suggested that the FTC and the Antitrust Division of the DOJ "review existing and proposed state regulations concerning advanced practice registered nurses to identify those that have anticompetitive effects without contributing to the health and safety of the public. States with unduly restrictive regulations should be urged to amend them to allow advanced practice registered nurses to provide care to patients in all circumstances in which they are qualified to do so" (Committee on the Robert Wood Johnson Foundation Initiative on the Future of Nursing at the Institute of Medicine, 2010, p. 279).

CONCLUSION

Laws, regulations, court decisions, and other arenas of public policy continue to affect health care and nursing. As important as it is for APRNs to be aware of how the law affects them, it is also critical for them to play a role in shaping laws today and tomorrow. Organizations representing nursing and APRNs have an important role to play in advocating for policies that can expand access to health care, including advanced practice nursing services. Nursing is key to achieving the goals of health reform—something that is recognized not just by nursing groups but also by broader groups of health-care leaders, as demonstrated by the IOM report's recommendation that APRNs should be able to practice to the full extent of their education and training. The opportunity is ripe for APRNs—through increased advocacy and collaboration with a broad array of partners and allies—to shape the legal and regulatory environments to maximize their role in health care and expand consumers' access to their vitally needed services.

29

Malpractice and the Advanced Practice Nurse

Carolyn T. Torre*

Carolyn T. Torre*

Learning Outcomes

Learning outcomes expected as a result of this chapter:

- Describe the legal risks associated with advanced practice.
- Understand the impact of health-care reform and full practice authority on patient access to care and workforce supply and demand.
- Compare malpractice risks and adverse actions for advanced practice nurses (APNs) and physicians by state.
- Demonstrate trends in malpractice claims as reflected in actuarial data.
- Understand the practice characteristics of who gets sued and why.
- Evaluate communications and resolutions programs as an alternative to tort reform.
- Contrast malpractice risks of independent and collaborative practice.
- Weigh the merits of a malpractice insurance policy.
- Propose actions to take when a lawsuit is filed.
- Demonstrate actions to take if going to trial and the possible consequences.
- Illustrate risk reduction strategies (clinical competency, communication, documentation, state or federal law, current malpractice insurance).

*Earlier versions of this chapter were authored by Sharon Muran, Amy Muran Felton, and Marie Infante.

INTRODUCTION

Professional liability insurance is essential for advanced practice nurses (APNs) who, because of their autonomy, exercise of independence in clinical decision making, provision of complex care, and prescription of medications, assume an increased risk of being sued for malpractice. The purpose of this chapter is to provide some basic information about the legal accountability of APNs, an overview of the current health-care practice climate and the process of litigation, the risks that affect being sued for malpractice, and those risks that affect liability insurance availability and cost. Finally, the chapter discusses steps APNs can take to minimize the risk of being sued for malpractice, including (a) maintaining current clinical skills and knowledge; (b) communicating clearly with patients regarding treatment options and ensuring informed consent; (c) documenting clear, supportable reasons for taking or not taking diagnostic and therapeutic actions, as well as recording the patient's response to interventions; (d) recognizing the timely need for consultation and referral; (e) nurturing the optimal professional and business relationships that are a part of advanced practice nursing; and (f) knowing and abiding by state and federal laws governing APN practice.

All nurses, including APNs, should purchase their own individual malpractice insurance. Individual policies cover nurses not only for care they provide in the workplace, but additionally for care they may provide for others, such as neighbors or friends. Finally, they offer protection in the face of licensure actions by state boards of nursing (BONs), which is critical for nurses who cannot work without an active license (Pohlman, 2015). Many nurses persist in their own interests and may choose not to vigorously defend particular nurses. If these nurses do not also have their own individual liability insurance, they can be at risk of financial insolvency, particularly if they decide to settle or are ultimately found guilty. Additionally, employer's and facility's policies may not cover nurses against license protection actions involving reports to BONs. Malpractice insurance, optimally, is a hedge against both risks.

THE PARADIGM SHIFT: ADVANCED PRACTICE NURSES IN AN EVOLVING HEALTH-CARE CLIMATE

A study by researchers at the Rand Corporation of health-care coverage transitions associated with the implementation of the Patient Protection and Affordable Care Act (ACA) between 2013 and 2015 found a net gain of 16.9 million Americans covered by insurance. The number of Americans without health insurance fell from 42.7 million to 25.8 million. The largest gain in insurance was through employer-based plans, though gains were also made by coverage through Medicaid, federal and state marketplaces, nonmarketplace individual plans, and other plans such as Medicare and military policies (Carman, Eibner, & Paddock, 2015). Poor minorities, particularly Hispanics, but additionally blacks, Native Americans, and legal immigrants, have experienced a dramatic rise in health-care coverage (Tavernise & Gebeloff, 2016). The largest number of Americans who remain uninsured, despite health-care reform, reside in states across the south and southwest where Medicaid expansion has been rejected and where many fall into the Medicaid gap: not poor enough for Medicaid but too poor to receive tax credits for plans in the insurance marketplace (Bui & Sanger-Katz, 2015; Garfield & Damico, 2016).

The rise in the number of insured Americans, along with ACA provisions that now reimburse providers for preventive care, a growing population, and a surge in those older than age 65, have increased the demands for primary care providers. These demands are especially acute in underserved, rural, and poor, urban neighborhoods. Primary care physicians, including family practice physicians, internists, and pediatricians, have traditionally been the largest provider source for primary care but this pattern has been steadily changing related to a shrinking pool of U.S. medical school graduates seeking to specialize in primary care (Bodenheimer & Pham, 2010). In 2015 only 11.6% of U.S. residency matches were for primary care, down from 12% in 2014 (Pohl, Barksdale, & Werner, 2015). The Health Resources and Services Administration (HRSA) released a report on the supply and demand of primary care practitioners in 2013, their first since 2008, predicting a shortfall of 20,400 primary care physicians by 2020. However, when nurse practitioners (NPs) and physician assistants (PAs) were included in models among primary care providers, the projected shortfall of primary care providers was reduced to 6,400 (HRSA, 2013). Studies underscoring the value of employing APNs with *full practice authority* (that is, without legally mandated physician supervision, collaboration, or oversight) to bolster the nation's workforce continue to proliferate (Traczynski & Udalova, 2013; Weinberg & Kallerman, 2014): Weinberg and Kallerman found that "allowing nurse practitioners to practice and prescribe drugs without physician supervision or oversight increases medical care for underserved populations and reduces emergency room use for conditions responsive to primary care" (p. 32). Also, a recent survey comparing the practice patterns of primary care NPs and primary care physicians determined that NPs were more likely than their physician counterparts to be employed in urban and rural settings, to accept Medicaid patients, and to work with vulnerable populations (Buerhaus et al, 2015).

The APN title in most states includes NPs, clinical nurse specialists (CNSs), nurse anesthetists (NAs), and certified nurse-midwives (CNMs). Determining which APNs are included when examining data related to malpractice rates is important because some advanced practice specialties such as obstetrics, anesthesia, and pediatrics are riskier than others. Advanced practice nursing programs educate registered nurses (RNs) at the master's and doctoral level in specialties designed to cover primary, specialty, and acute-care needs across the entire age spectrum. APNs work in a variety of practice settings including federally qualified health-care centers, private physicians' offices, nursing homes, correctional facilities, schools, college health centers, hospitals, and patients' homes; as teachers in schools of nursing; and as policy makers at the state and federal level in both governmental departments and nonprofit organizations. Donelan and colleagues (2013), describing a survey comparing perceptions of practice of NPs and physicians in primary care, wrote that although 80.9% of NPs reported working with a physician, only 41.4% of physicians reported working with a NP.

By June 2016 APNs in 21 states and the District of Columbia had achieved full practice authority by legislatively eliminating requirements for supervisory agreements, collaborative agreements, or joint protocols with physicians from their APN statutes (AANP, 2016). White papers published by the New Jersey State Nurses Association describe the need to eliminate legislative, regulatory, and practice barriers for APNs in that state to make them maximally accessible as primary and specialty care providers (Torre & Drake, 2014; Torre, Joel, & Aughenbaugh, 2009). A seminal, comprehensive 2011 report on the future of nursing released by the Institute of Medicine (IOM) emphasizes the cost effectiveness and high quality of care offered by APNs and argues that legislative, regulatory, and insurance barriers must fall for them to be able to practice to their full scope and educational preparation (IOM, 2011). A related article by the primary authors of the IOM report contends that APNs are integral to meeting the nation's primary care provider shortage and concluded that there are "no data to suggest that nurse practitioners in states that impose greater restrictions on their practice provide safer and better care than those in less restrictive states or that the role of physicians in less restrictive states has changed or deteriorated" (Fairman et al, 2011, p. 194). APNs are directly reimbursed by insurers at both the federal and state levels such as Medicare and Medicaid; by private insurance companies such as Blue Cross/Blue Shield, United Healthcare, and Oxford; and by many health maintenance organizations (HMOs) and managed care organizations (MCOs), but outdated Medicare laws and company policies can and do impose significant restrictions on if, how, and at what level this reimbursement occurs. In states without full practice authority, whether or not an APN is credentialed and reimbursed by private insurance companies is frequently dependent upon whether a collaborating or supervising physician is credentialed by that same plan. If the physician leaves the state, loses a license to practice, or dies, the APN and the APN's patients cannot provide or receive care (Torre & Drake, 2014). Limiting APNs' full practice authority and denying them independent reimbursement are both associated with decreased consumer access to care and increased health-care costs (Weinberg & Kallerman, 2014).

With more APNs acting as the primary and specialty care providers of a growing number of insured, APNs can anticipate being subject to an increased risk of professional liability. Because the best defense is a good offense, APNs must actively and continuously engage in effective risk management strategies including ensuring that they have the consistent protection of malpractice insurance.

THE RISKS OF ADVANCED PRACTICE NURSING

There are at least three types of exposure that APNs should seek to avoid: (1) financial exposure in terms of judgments or settlements from a civil lawsuit, (2) licensure or certification actions by the relevant state agencies or private associations, and (3) civil or criminal sanctions and exclusion from participation in the federal health-care programs for fraud or abuse.

Civil Lawsuits

The first type of exposure is liability for professional malpractice. Malpractice is "failure of professional skill that results in injury, loss or damage. A claim of malpractice requires that the patient/plaintiff prove the following: (1) The existence of a client-professional relationship—a duty of care. (2) Behavior below the appropriate standard of care for professionals dealing in like circumstances. (3) A causal link between the practitioner's failure to conform to treatment standards and harm to the patient. 4. Actual injury to the patient" (Buppert, 2015, p. 286).

Negligence includes failure to follow up, failure to refer when necessary, failure to disclose essential information, and failure to give necessary care (Buppert, 2015). When the appropriate standard of care is not followed and results in harm to the patient, financial exposure to compensate the patient or the patient's family occurs. This exposure is the typical risk covered by most malpractice insurance policies.

Licensure or State Certification Exposures

There are other types of direct or indirect financial exposures that arise from breaking state statutes or regulations that control advanced practice. Substance abuse, fraud, unprofessional conduct, failure to fulfill requirements for continuing education, and failure to renew state licenses by deadlines or to have a written collaborative agreement or joint protocol with a physician where one is required are other examples of charges that can result in licensure sanctions or loss of APN certification by a state BON. These types of risks may or may not be covered by a professional liability insurance policy; wise APNs check to make sure they do.

Federal Health Program Exclusion

Another type of legal risk is noncompliance with laws and regulations of the federal health-care programs that provide direct reimbursement for the services of APNs (Buppert, 2015). The penalties can be both criminal and civil. A conviction for fraud is referred by the courts to the state BON for appropriate action with respect to the license of the guilty nurse (Bureau of National Affairs, 2004). The most severe civil penalty for breaking these laws is exclusion from federal health-care programs based on the authority of

the secretary of the U.S. Department of Health & Human Services (DHHS) to ban practitioners from receiving payments from any federal health-care program when they have violated certain laws. These risks are generally not covered in a typical professional liability insurance policy. In addition, all providers (e.g., hospitals, HMOs, home health agencies, nursing homes, and others) and all other practitioners (e.g., physician, group practices, and others) who themselves participate in federal health-care programs are banned from hiring the excluded APN at risk of losing his or her own federal reimbursement. Therefore, program exclusion is a career-ending event for most individuals.

Although a thorough discussion of statutory and regulatory risks is beyond the scope of this chapter, APNs must know the laws that control their practice and their reimbursement, develop behaviors to ensure compliance with these laws, recognize the risks associated with noncompliance with these laws and regulations, and use risk prevention strategies to manage their professional practices and minimize those risks (Buppert, 2015; Infante, 2000). A sensible APN keeps a copy of a current reference book on state statutes and regulations related to APNs at the ready (Torre & Ridge, 2014) and a link to the Centers for Medicare and Medicaid Services Web site (www.cms.gov) handy.

Increasing use of telemedicine will, for example, require knowledge of state laws not only in the state where the APN practices but also where the patient resides. In some states, such as New Jersey, the BON requires that a RN or APN be licensed there to provide clinical care to a New Jersey resident, even when provided remotely. One of the most important ways to keep up with current state and federal laws and regulations and other practice- and policy-related issues is to be an active member of your state nurses association, an affiliated APN group, and at least one national organization representing APNs. Doing so means you can participate in initiating policy changes that control APN practice, stay abreast of changes in state and federal laws affecting APN practice, and develop and sustain supportive relationships and communication networks with other APNs.

MALPRACTICE AND THE ADVANCED PRACTICE NURSE

How frequently are APNs sued for malpractice? There is no reliable way to gather information on the number of lawsuits filed on a national basis. There is also little to stop a patient from bringing a malpractice lawsuit regardless of the ultimate merits of the allegations against the practitioner. The most comprehensive source of reports on verdicts and settlements resulting from malpractice claims against health-care professionals is the National Practitioner Data Bank (NPDB) of the DHHS, HRSA. APNs are being sued more frequently and the cost of both malpractice payouts and average expenses related to defending claims have risen (CNA/NSO, 2012; NPDB, 2015, Table 1). Interestingly, data on physicians shows just the opposite—that in the past decade, reports of malpractice have decreased and payment costs are flat or have declined (Mello, Studdert, & Kachalia, 2014; NPDB, 2015, Table 4). Although reports of malpractice suits and settlements as well as reports of adverse events have risen for the inclusive APN category (encompassing NAs, CNMs, NPs, and CNSs) since 1990, they remain low in number compared with reports against physicians (NPDB, 2015; Tables 1, 2, 3, and 4).

The National Practitioner Data Bank and Healthcare Integrity and Protection Data Bank

The NPDB was established by Congress in 1986 (NPDB, 2015). DHHS is responsible for its implementation and maintenance. The NPDB is intended to improve the quality of care by restricting the ability of incompetent practitioners to move from state to state without disclosure of previous malpractice payments or adverse actions.

In 1996, Congress created a second data repository, the Healthcare Integrity and Protection Data Bank (HIPDB), to combat fraud and abuse in health insurance and health-care delivery. The HIPDB collects, reports, and discloses information regarding licensure and certification actions, program exclusions, criminal convictions, and other adjudicated actions and decisions against both individual practitioners and institutional providers. State licensure boards, hospitals, and other eligible entities access these databanks to assess an individual practitioner's (including APNs') responsibility for errors and professional misconduct when considering applications for state license, employment, staff privileges, or other affiliations. Although there is some overlap between the NPDB and the HIPDB, only the NPDB reports malpractice judgments and settlements (NPDB, 2015).

The NPDB collects information on all malpractice payments made by insurance companies on behalf of individual health-care practitioners. Payments must be reported to the NPDB no matter how small the amount, whether or not the case is settled before filing suit, and whether or not the payment was the result of a confidential settlement. Reporting of malpractice payments is mandatory for all types of licensed health-care practitioners. The NPDB also collects information about adverse licensure or professional sanctions imposed on health-care practitioners. Reporting of adverse licensure actions, clinical privilege actions, and professional society actions is mandatory for all physicians and dentists in the United States. Adverse actions against APNs and other health-care practitioners may be voluntarily reported to the NPDB.

Trends in Malpractice Claims

The NPDB began collecting and analyzing data on malpractice claims in 1990 and issues cumulative reports of its findings. The most recent data are from 2014. Using a data analysis tool available on the NPDB Web site, consumers can create summaries of both malpractice reports and adverse event reports between 1990 and 2014 on classes of licensed health-care practitioners by year and by state (NPDB, 2015). Comparing and contrasting both the number and rates for each of the APN categories, as well as comparing and contrasting them to the reports and rates for two other similar health-care professionals (physicians and PAs), provided the following picture in 2011, the last date for which this kind of comparative data has been available (NPBD, 2011a):

- NAs had the highest number of reports over this 21-year period (1,461 reports out of an estimated 44,000 providers), but CNMs had the highest rate of reports (830 out of an estimated 6,700 providers). This was calculated as 3% (NAs) and 12% (CNMs), respectively.
- NPs had a total number of reports approaching that of NAs (1,150) but a very low rate (0.6%) because of the total number of these providers (167,857) at that time was significantly larger.
- CNSs had an extremely low number of reports: only 13 over 21 years, out of a total of 69,017 providers (0.01%), perhaps reflecting that the CNS category was not separately reported before 2002 and, in addition,

that the role, except for psychiatric CNSs, has been less likely to involve diagnostic decision making and medication management requiring prescription writing than other APN categories.

Summary reports contrasting the rates of NPDB reports of malpractice suits and settlements on APNs to those of physicians (medical doctors [MDs] and doctors of osteopathy [Dos]) over a 24-year period between 1990 and 2014 are in **Tables 29.1** through **29.4.** In 2014, Zthere were estimated to have been 348,430 APNs in the United States, including CNSs, NAs, CNMs, and NPs.* Between 1990 and 2014 there were 4,616 reports of malpractice suits and settlements to the NPDB, *a rate of 1%.* During that same period, they experienced 1,994 reports of adverse events to the NPDB, *a rate of lower than 1%.* In comparison, over the same period an estimated 916,264 physicians had 317,643 reports of malpractice suits and settlements to the NPDB, *a rate of 35%,* and 113,297 reports of adverse events, *a rate of 12%.*** Nurse Midwives: Bureau of Labor Statistics: www.bls.gov/oes/current/oes2911bl.htm

An assessment by Hooker, Nicolson, and Le (2009) of whether or not the utilization of PAs and APNs increases professional liability determined that the probability of making a malpractice payment during the period they examined was 12 times lower than that of physicians for PAs and 24 times lower than that of physicians for APNs. This same study described higher average malpractice payouts for APNs compared with PAs, even slightly higher than those for physicians. The reason for these variations may be found in an explanation provided by the NPDB (2011b, p. 30): Because fewer claims are made against nurses than physicians, one large payment for an APN negatively affects the mean. Hooker and colleagues (2009) also found that female clinicians of all clinical types paid

higher malpractice payments than male clinicians and that, with regard to APNs, female patients were involved in bringing significantly more suits than male patients.

What Are APNs Sued For?

As would be expected, the highest number of claims made for NAs are related to the anesthesia care, and claims are made for CNMs in relation to obstetrics (NPDB, 2011b, p. 29). A 2012 analysis of malpractice claims data for NPs covered by the Nursing Service Organization over the period 2007 to 2011 determined that the "predominant allegations" for open and closed claims were related to diagnosis, treatment, and medication, in that order (CNA/NSO, 2012). Failure to diagnose Down syndrome (where a NP did not order prenatal testing as required by facility policy) resulted in a finding of wrongful life and the highest claim payment of $975,000; a case involving failure to diagnose pulmonary embolism resulted in the second highest payment of $925,000 (CNA/NS0, 2012, p. 18).

Adult and family practice NP specialties had the highest number of claims (75.5%), but the highest average claim paid was related to the pediatric specialty, followed by women's health. In the case of the pediatric NP, a child in intensive care was given the wrong medication, which caused vomiting with aspiration and resulted in permanent brain damage. A women's health NP inserted an intrauterine device into the uterus of a woman (not known to be pregnant), resulting in the premature delivery of a neurologically impaired child. Also in women's health, a student NP failed to notify the physician that a patient was experiencing premature dilation; the woman experienced the premature delivery of a neurologically impaired infant (CNA/NSO, 2012, p. 12). The fact is that pediatric patients have a longer time to sue and are awarded higher damage awards when suits are successful because they have a longer predicted time to live with the pain, suffering, and expense of care related to injury.

NPs in the CNA/NSO (2012) study with claims made against them most often worked in physicians' offices, followed by community-based outpatient clinics and skilled nursing facilities. Descriptive data regarding NPs' practices revealed that most NPs with claims made against them had master's degrees in nursing; higher levels of education were associated with higher-than-average payouts. In general, more time spent with patients was associated

---

*Data used to estimate the numbers of individual APNs in the United States are from:
    Nurse practitioners: American Association of Nurse Practitioners: www.aanp.org
    Clinical Nurse Specialists: explorehealthcareers.org
    Nurse Anesthetists: American Association of Nurse Anesthetists: www.aana.org
**Data used to estimate the numbers of physicians in the United States are from: Young, A., Chaudhry, H., Pei, X., Halbesleben, K., Polk, D., & Dugan, M. (2014). A census of actively licensed physicians in the U.S. Federation of State Medical Boards. *Journal of Medical Regulation, 101*(2), 8–23.

TABLE 29.1

Medical Malpractice Payments: Advanced Practice Nurses: Reports of Suits and Settlements to the National Practitioner Data Bank by State and Year: 1990 to 2014 APNs Include CNSs, NAs, CNMs, and NPs

Location	1990	1991	1992	1993	1994	1995	1996	1997	1998	1999	2000	2001	2002	2003	2004	2005	2006	2007	2008	2009	2010	2011	2012	2013	2014	Row Total
Alabama	0	1	3	3	2	0	5	2	0	1	1	3	3	1	2	5	2	1	1	1	1	3	2	1	5	48
Alaska	0	2	1	0	0	0	0	1	0	0	0	1	3	0	1	0	1	0	3	1	0	0	0	0	3	18
Arizona	1	3	0	0	4	1	3	6	4	5	5	2	4	5	2	5	7	11	4	4	2	5	9	11	3	103
Arkansas	0	1	0	1	0	2	1	1	2	2	1	3	0	3	1	1	2	1	3	2	2	5	3	5	5	47
Armed Forces	0	0	0	1	0	0	0	0	0	0	0	0	0	0	0	0	0	0	0	0	0	0	0	1	0	2
California	1	8	3	7	1	4	3	7	9	6	7	8	12	6	9	14	6	13	15	14	14	9	16	21	12	225
Colorado	1	3	3	1	2	1	3	3	2	7	4	3	2	6	4	6	4	5	5	7	6	3	7	5	2	93
Connecticut	0	0	3	0	1	0	2	0	0	0	1	3	2	1	0	2	3	3	4	1	1	3	0	0	1	32
Delaware	0	1	0	0	2	0	0	0	0	0	0	0	0	1	1	0	0	0	1	1	2	1	0	0	0	10
District of Columbia	0	1	0	0	0	2	0	0	0	0	1	0	0	1	1	3	0	0	0	3	1	1	0	0	0	14
Florida	1	12	14	6	8	13	11	7	13	20	20	25	30	25	29	39	31	33	28	57	28	27	31	39	27	571
Georgia	0	3	4	2	4	3	2	4	4	5	5	6	7	6	7	12	2	7	4	4	8	8	5	11	9	129
Hawaii	0	0	0	0	0	0	1	0	1	0	1	0	0	0	0	0	0	0	3	0	1	0	0	0	0	7
Idaho	4	2	1	0	1	0	1	1	2	1	1	1	1	0	2	3	1	1	0	0	3	0	2	3	3	34
Illinois	1	2	3	1	3	1	0	4	1	3	3	3	4	4	4	2	3	4	10	8	0	11	6	8	10	100
Indiana	0	0	0	1	0	0	2	1	0	0	0	0	0	1	0	0	3	2	1	4	3	4	2	7	3	36
Iowa	1	0	1	2	2	3	3	3	0	0	0	0	0	1	2	2	3	1	1	3	2	3	0	3	4	39
Kansas	1	2	2	1	5	1	4	4	3	3	1	8	1	1	10	7	0	3	4	4	1	3	3	4	5	81
Kentucky	0	2	0	3	1	3	0	3	3	3	2	4	4	2	4	0	4	2	4	3	4	9	3	5	10	76
Louisiana	5	3	7	8	2	1	5	6	2	6	6	5	4	4	8	6	6	7	5	11	5	16	15	14	8	165
Maine	1	0	0	0	0	0	0	2	0	0	1	1	1	1	1	0	1	1	3	1	1	3	0	3	1	22

Continued

TABLE 29.1

Medical Malpractice Payments: Advanced Practice Nurses: Reports of Suits and Settlements to the National Practitioner Data Bank by State and Year: 1990 to 2014 APNs Include CNSs, NAs, CNMs, and NPs (Continued)

Location	1990	1991	1992	1993	1994	1995	1996	1997	1998	1999	2000	2001	2002	2003	2004	2005	2006	2007	2008	2009	2010	2011	2012	2013	2014	Row Total
Maryland	2	0	2	5	9	3	1	2	3	4	1	4	6	4	1	6	12	5	2	5	9	5	9	6	8	114
Massachusetts	1	3	4	0	4	0	2	2	2	7	5	7	7	5	5	8	7	12	17	12	16	10	16	8	7	167
Michigan	1	6	5	3	6	7	1	6	1	5	3	6	6	5	4	8	10	4	7	3	5	9	9	5	2	127
Minnesota	0	0	0	0	2	0	0	0	3	1	1	3	0	2	3	4	3	2	2	3	1	1	4	1	2	38
Mississippi	0	3	0	0	1	2	0	2	0	1	1	1	5	2	3	1	5	2	6	7	1	5	4	8	2	62
Missouri	2	2	7	2	1	2	4	0	2	1	2	5	3	3	8	1	2	5	5	3	5	4	9	6	4	88
Montana	1	0	0	1	0	0	0	1	1	1	1	1	0	0	2	3	0	0	0	3	2	4	1	0	1	23
Nebraska	0	0	0	1	3	1	1	1	0	2	2	2	3	1	0	3	5	2	0	1	1	2	1	1	1	34
Nevada	0	0	0	1	1	1	1	0	1	0	1	6	3	1	1	0	2	2	1	1	4	4	0	0	1	32
New Hampshire	1	1	2	0	1	1	1	1	5	1	1	2	5	0	2	1	3	3	0	1	1	1	3	0	4	41
New Jersey	0	0	2	0	0	2	0	1	5	0	2	5	5	3	8	7	10	8	8	15	13	18	10	15	10	147
New Mexico	0	3	1	0	6	0	1	0	3	1	0	3	6	1	5	2	7	7	6	4	5	2	8	8	4	83
New York	0	7	8	10	2	6	8	3	9	13	11	14	12	16	18	17	30	16	29	21	19	18	30	27	28	372
North Carolina	0	5	2	3	2	0	0	2	1	2	0	4	3	2	1	7	0	4	7	6	2	4	7	2	3	69
North Dakota	0	1	0	1	1	0	0	0	0	0	0	0	0	0	1	1	0	1	1	0	0	1	1	1	0	10
Ohio	3	7	9	5	9	4	1	8	2	4	4	3	5	3	5	3	3	2	3	7	6	7	6	7	4	120
Oklahoma	0	1	3	3	1	2	0	2	5	3	2	3	3	4	3	1	4	5	3	4	3	2	3	3	3	66
Oregon	2	2	0	0	0	0	1	2	0	2	3	3	5	1	5	5	2	1	6	5	5	6	12	1	12	81
Other Territories	0	0	0	0	0	0	0	0	0	0	0	0	0	0	0	0	0	0	1	1	0	0	0	0	0	2

Location	1990	1991	1992	1993	1994	1995	1996	1997	1998	1999	2000	2001	2002	2003	2004	2005	2006	2007	2008	2009	2010	2011	2012	2013	2014	Total
Pennsylvania	2	6	6	2	5	4	1	15	3	5	7	11	7	12	8	12	10	13	15	13	15	12	24	21	15	244
Puerto Rico	0	0	0	0	0	0	0	0	1	0	0	0	0	0	0	0	0	0	0	0	1	0	0	0	0	2
Rhode Island	0	0	0	1	0	1	0	0	0	0	0	2	5	0	1	1	3	2	1	2	1	2	0	0	0	21
South Carolina	0	0	0	0	2	0	3	0	0	0	3	3	3	3	3	5	1	5	3	3	2	3	5	3	6	55
South Dakota	0	1	0	0	0	0	0	0	0	0	2	0	0	2	0	0	0	1	1	1	0	1	1	1	0	9
Tennessee	1	3	2	4	0	3	7	3	3	3	3	8	3	3	7	6	9	6	12	12	10	9	8	9	6	140
Texas	8	8	10	13	15	9	10	9	12	13	13	11	13	13	14	23	19	20	11	18	17	16	12	9	15	331
Utah	0	0	0	1	1	3	1	0	2	1	1	0	1	1	1	1	3	3	2	2	1	3	3	0	2	33
Vermont	0	0	0	0	0	1	0	0	0	0	0	0	0	0	0	1	0	0	0	1	0	0	0	0	0	3
Virginia	0	4	1	2	0	2	3	0	2	4	1	0	4	4	7	4	4	4	5	5	4	2	7	4	3	76
Washington	0	3	1	1	5	0	5	0	7	3	2	0	3	3	4	6	6	9	3	5	4	3	18	6	4	101
West Virginia	0	0	2	0	0	0	0	1	1	0	1	0	2	2	3	0	1	1	2	1	2	2	0	3	4	28
Wisconsin	0	6	0	0	1	0	1	0	2	0	1	4	0	1	0	1	1	0	2	2	3	1	3	1	1	31
Wyoming	0	2	0	0	1	0	0	0	0	0	0	0	1	0	0	1	0	1	2	2	1	0	1	1	1	14
Column Total	41	120	115	89	113	89	94	130	118	134	120	187	202	172	209	247	242	242	263	294	242	272	319	298	264	4,616

Source: Singh, H. (2016, July 14). National Practitioner Data Bank. Location by data year, generated using the data analysis tool. Retrieved from https://www.npdb.hrsa.gov/analysistool.
Data source: National Practitioner Data Bank. (2014). *Adverse action and medical malpractice reports (1990–2014)*.

TABLE 29.2

Adverse Actions Against Advanced Practice Nurses Reported to the National Practitioner Data Bank by State and Year: 1990 to 2014

Adverse Actions Include Loss of Clinical Privileges, Panel Membership, Professional Society Membership, Drug Enforcement Administration Actions, or Participation in Medicare and Medicaid

Location	1990	1991	1992	1993	1994	1995	1996	1997	1998	1999	2000	2001	2002	2003	2004	2005	2006	2007	2008	2009	2010	2011	2012	2013	2014	Row Total
Alabama	0	0	0	0	0	0	0	0	0	0	12	7	9	27	23	57	22	32	7	21	12	7	19	21	8	284
Alaska	0	0	0	0	0	0	0	0	0	0	0	0	0	3	1	3	1	0	2	3	3	4	3	2	10	35
Arizona	0	0	0	0	0	0	0	0	1	0	0	1	3	1	3	1	0	3	0	0	0	0	3	2	3	21
Arkansas	0	0	0	0	0	0	0	0	0	0	1	0	0	0	0	1	0	1	1	2	3	1	2	2	5	19
Armed Forces	0	0	0	0	0	0	0	0	0	0	0	0	0	0	0	0	0	1	0	0	0	0	0	1	0	2
California	0	0	0	0	1	0	0	0	1	0	1	2	1	1	2	0	1	0	11	1	3	0	2	2	6	35
Colorado	0	0	0	0	0	1	0	0	1	0	0	0	0	0	0	0	0	0	1	0	0	0	0	0	1	4
Connecticut	0	0	0	0	0	0	1	0	0	0	1	1	1	4	4	6	3	4	4	3	3	8	7	3	7	60
Delaware	0	0	0	0	0	0	0	0	0	0	0	0	0	0	0	0	0	0	0	0	0	1	0	3	3	7
District of Columbia	0	0	0	0	0	0	0	0	0	0	0	0	0	0	0	0	0	0	0	0	0	0	0	0	0	0
Florida	0	0	0	0	0	0	2	0	0	2	0	0	4	7	13	3	7	9	11	2	1	4	0	4	8	77
Georgia	0	0	0	0	0	0	0	0	0	3	0	2	0	0	0	1	0	0	1	5	1	3	5	3	0	24
Hawaii	0	0	0	0	0	0	0	0	0	0	0	0	0	0	0	0	0	0	0	0	2	1	1	0	0	4
Idaho	0	0	0	0	0	0	0	0	0	0	1	2	2	0	2	0	0	1	0	1	1	0	1	0	0	11
Illinois	0	0	0	0	0	0	0	0	0	0	0	0	2	0	2	1	2	0	3	3	4	2	1	1	5	23
Indiana	0	0	0	0	0	0	0	0	0	0	0	0	0	0	0	0	0	1	0	0	0	1	1	2	9	14
Iowa	0	0	0	0	0	0	0	0	0	0	0	0	0	0	0	0	0	0	1	0	1	1	2	0	0	5
Kansas	0	0	0	0	0	0	0	1	0	0	0	0	0	0	1	1	1	0	2	1	2	0	0	0	0	10

State	Total																		
Kentucky	29	1	2	1	2	3	2	0	2	0	3	3	5	3	0	1	0	0	1
Louisiana	54	1	2	4	6	9	2	6	1	2	4	9	2	4	2	6	0	0	0
Maine	17	4	6	2	0	1	2	0	0	0	0	0	0	0	2	0	1	0	0
Maryland	6	1	0	1	1	0	0	0	1	0	1	0	0	0	1	0	0	0	0
Massachusetts	33	1	0	2	1	1	2	2	0	0	2	0	1	0	5	6	0	0	0
Michigan	87	21	4	0	2	1	1	2	2	2	1	0	4	4	8	9	2	1	3
Minnesota	9	1	0	2	1	0	1	0	0	1	0	1	0	0	0	0	0	0	0
Mississippi	26	4	0	3	4	0	1	1	1	1	1	1	3	0	2	0	1	5	0
Missouri	4	0	1	0	0	0	0	0	0	0	0	0	1	0	0	0	0	0	0
Montana	2	0	0	0	0	0	0	0	0	0	0	0	0	1	0	0	0	0	0
Nebraska	11	3	2	0	2	2	0	0	0	0	0	0	2	2	0	0	0	0	0
Nevada	5	1	0	0	0	0	0	0	1	0	0	1	0	0	0	0	0	0	0
New Hampshire	9	2	1	1	0	0	0	0	0	0	0	0	0	2	0	1	0	0	0
New Jersey	11	1	1	0	1	2	0	0	3	1	1	0	0	1	0	0	0	0	0
New Mexico	10	2	3	0	0	0	0	0	0	0	1	2	2	0	0	1	1	0	0
New York	67	3	3	7	5	7	6	4	7	3	6	7	3	1	4	2	1	2	4
North Carolina	50	6	0	9	4	10	3	2	3	1	2	4	1	2	3	0	0	0	0
North Dakota	9	0	2	1	1	2	1	1	1	1	0	0	0	0	0	0	0	0	0
Ohio	35	6	6	2	3	2	3	0	3	1	0	1	2	0	2	0	1	2	0
Oklahoma	156	24	24	18	22	20	8	14	8	9	8	2	8	0	14	1	0	2	0
Oregon	49	6	4	8	6	9	5	2	5	1	2	4	6	4	2	1	1	1	0

Continued

TABLE 29.2

Adverse Actions Against Advanced Practice Nurses Reported to the National Practitioner Data Bank by State and Year: 1990 to 2014 (Continued)

Adverse Actions Include Loss of Clinical Privileges, Panel Membership, Professional Society Membership, Drug Enforcement Administration Actions, or Participation in Medicare and Medicaid

Location	1990	1991	1992	1993	1994	1995	1996	1997	1998	1999	2000	2001	2002	2003	2004	2005	2006	2007	2008	2009	2010	2011	2012	2013	2014	Row Total
Other Territories	0	0	0	0	0	0	0	0	0	0	0	0	0	0	0	0	0	0	0	0	0	0	1	1	0	2
Pennsylvania	1	0	0	0	0	0	0	1	1	0	0	0	1	3	3	5	10	6	6	4	10	9	4	2	5	71
Puerto Rico	0	0	0	0	0	0	0	0	0	0	0	0	0	0	3	6	1	2	2	0	8	8	3	5	10	48
Rhode Island	0	0	0	0	0	0	0	0	0	0	0	1	2	1	0	0	0	0	1	0	2	0	4	3	0	15
South Carolina	0	0	0	0	0	0	0	0	0	0	0	0	0	0	0	1	5	1	9	11	12	4	3	3	1	50
South Dakota	0	0	0	0	0	0	0	0	0	0	1	0	0	0	0	0	1	0	1	0	2	2	1	1	1	10
Tennessee	0	0	0	0	0	0	0	0	0	0	0	1	0	4	4	2	4	1	7	8	19	17	21	20	41	149
Texas	0	0	2	0	0	0	0	0	1	0	1	2	1	3	1	0	2	1	1	1	1	0	5	4	10	36
Utah	0	0	0	0	1	0	0	0	0	1	0	0	0	0	1	0	1	1	4	0	1	3	10	6	6	35
Vermont	0	0	0	0	0	0	0	0	0	0	0	0	0	0	0	0	0	0	0	0	0	1	1	3	0	5
Virginia	0	0	0	1	0	0	0	2	2	2	3	1	5	2	6	3	5	2	7	7	9	6	7	12	6	88
Washington	0	0	0	0	0	0	0	4	1	3	6	8	6	7	9	6	10	8	8	12	8	9	6	20	25	157
West Virginia	0	0	0	0	0	0	0	0	0	0	0	0	0	0	0	0	1	0	0	0	0	0	0	0	0	1
Wisconsin	0	0	1	0	0	1	0	1	0	0	0	0	1	0	0	1	0	0	0	0	1	1	2	2	1	11
Wyoming	0	0	0	0	0	0	0	0	0	0	0	0	0	0	0	0	0	0	0	0	0	1	0	1	0	2
Column Total	1	6	5	3	5	13	24	20	31	40	46	62	100	110	118	101	104	122	123	180	155	177	190	258		1,994

Source: Singh, H. (2016, July 14). National Practitioner Data Bank. Location by data year, generated using the data analysis tool. Retrieved from https://www.npdb.hrsa.gov/analysistool. Data source: National Practitioner Data Bank. (2014). *Adverse action and medical malpractice reports (1990–2014)*.

TABLE 29.3

Medical Malpractice Payments: Physicians: Reports of Suits and Settlements to the National Practitioner Data Bank. Physicians Include Medical Doctors (MDs) and Doctors of Osteopathic Medicine (DOs)

Location	1990	1991	1992	1993	1994	1995	1996	1997	1998	1999	2000	2001	2002	2003	2004	2005	2006	2007	2008	2009	2010	2011	2012	2013	2014	Row Total
Alabama	24	60	47	54	45	52	63	67	70	54	66	78	80	53	67	45	40	57	50	38	47	48	53	39	40	1,337
Alaska	1	13	30	14	16	31	16	20	16	22	21	24	15	19	15	18	21	10	10	12	19	8	15	11	11	408
Arizona	68	186	196	212	181	191	234	256	240	221	267	293	276	307	209	264	234	210	170	174	171	154	160	167	153	5,194
Arkansas	37	62	70	74	66	57	49	51	82	71	73	89	84	68	78	77	57	57	59	56	52	58	48	47	49	1,571
Armed Forces	1	4	5	1	0	4	3	0	0	2	5	2	2	3	2	2	4	5	2	1	0	2	1	0	1	52
California	447	1,527	1,670	1,800	1,707	1,628	1,519	1,857	1,462	1,467	1,340	1,437	1,394	1,350	1,265	1,180	1,004	987	986	982	914	882	925	954	861	31,545
Colorado	72	148	161	176	174	170	144	146	160	152	150	136	175	170	156	116	146	121	139	128	101	98	69	97	77	3,382
Connecticut	40	140	150	143	117	166	118	138	155	158	168	183	183	220	157	154	157	142	131	117	111	123	84	101	98	3,454
Delaware	10	34	38	31	35	42	40	26	26	29	30	56	48	70	28	34	33	20	28	33	17	21	20	20	21	790
District of Columbia	18	54	53	39	55	52	87	68	57	58	65	76	48	47	54	69	48	26	25	30	25	34	18	9	7	1,122
Florida	274	747	776	750	786	889	1,109	1,076	1,090	1,090	1,174	1,276	1,283	1,323	1,242	1,070	842	851	964	924	810	737	721	732	755	23,291
Georgia	83	194	197	225	216	261	250	262	286	263	271	267	277	326	321	293	267	265	238	211	197	195	177	205	206	5,953
Hawaii	6	27	31	27	41	37	38	23	40	36	37	44	37	47	29	18	20	30	23	28	25	13	13	19	20	709
Idaho	7	29	32	29	31	28	29	31	31	27	35	37	26	37	30	44	29	28	20	29	16	31	22	17	24	699
Illinois	214	778	765	788	656	603	604	584	558	540	575	534	498	499	483	461	404	421	365	352	317	322	298	324	254	12,197
Indiana	83	342	308	230	324	330	260	273	268	286	282	325	287	309	246	191	229	219	210	272	219	218	228	210	245	6,394
Iowa	46	113	108	127	106	114	129	136	108	90	121	134	118	127	102	110	71	67	94	76	74	56	68	60	54	2,409
Kansas	47	139	149	173	183	168	174	163	155	175	184	167	158	155	167	181	149	146	137	122	158	129	133	117	116	3,745

Continued

TABLE 29.3

Medical Malpractice Payments: Physicians: Reports of Suits and Settlements to the National Practitioner Data Bank. Physicians Include Medical Doctors (MDs) and Doctors of Osteopathic Medicine (DOs). *(Continued)*

Location	1990	1991	1992	1993	1994	1995	1996	1997	1998	1999	2000	2001	2002	2003	2004	2005	2006	2007	2008	2009	2010	2011	2012	2013	2014	Row Total
Kentucky	33	133	133	138	145	151	138	151	137	144	186	194	288	195	167	165	141	133	126	132	99	111	118	97	119	3,574
Louisiana	113	237	237	269	224	202	243	245	305	287	285	297	307	288	309	279	355	317	345	298	305	281	258	255	246	6,787
Maine	15	39	36	44	29	37	27	38	32	51	63	42	34	45	34	44	35	50	41	41	38	33	40	45	44	977
Maryland	64	199	194	189	210	230	231	230	280	245	277	249	276	297	268	247	200	222	211	207	216	258	224	342	163	5,729
Massachusetts	82	322	303	297	228	234	235	228	225	269	338	328	261	288	307	274	259	293	254	260	232	224	203	199	220	6,363
Michigan	332	909	870	807	930	1,029	643	656	737	764	721	760	729	625	505	510	436	416	401	375	301	306	315	321	290	14,688
Minnesota	54	155	140	130	134	122	115	98	83	94	91	104	95	94	98	76	69	88	78	67	56	45	50	42	39	2,217
Mississippi	27	70	105	92	119	114	114	119	124	109	124	136	158	102	113	88	98	88	94	77	73	78	106	60	75	2,463
Missouri	105	327	268	280	272	309	282	248	225	253	221	290	271	227	267	221	192	226	154	189	135	163	157	143	145	5,570
Montana	20	67	56	57	53	58	61	65	55	85	70	69	65	58	46	40	55	65	57	41	49	42	39	39	30	1,342
Nebraska	33	46	57	55	63	53	68	58	61	72	72	92	90	89	112	171	66	62	54	53	42	47	40	33	42	1,631
Nevada	19	61	63	68	80	77	70	69	86	89	100	98	118	109	113	108	77	98	80	82	57	67	68	56	41	1,954
New Hampshire	12	47	48	77	68	54	60	52	50	49	62	55	51	46	53	48	49	41	52	52	43	44	36	41	44	1,234
New Jersey	211	553	573	570	539	476	565	500	639	584	687	677	649	584	596	765	525	508	482	587	447	429	425	485	414	13,470
New Mexico	14	90	91	70	87	107	123	119	115	126	101	115	86	102	101	104	109	94	73	89	97	88	146	72	74	2,393
New York	592	1,749	1,993	1,959	1,808	1,698	1,757	1,832	1,975	2,007	1,992	2,040	1,796	1,879	2,000	1,880	1,791	1,595	1,494	1,417	1,389	1,379	1,398	1,307	1,324	42,051
North Carolina	59	230	219	243	216	216	213	239	231	201	205	232	265	209	259	195	164	151	155	133	131	143	137	115	102	4,663
North Dakota	11	21	28	24	33	22	25	23	24	18	21	30	25	28	25	26	15	22	11	21	15	11	5	7	5	496

Location	1990	1991	1992	1993	1994	1995	1996	1997	1998	1999	2000	2001	2002	2003	2004	2005	2006	2007	2008	2009	2010	2011	2012	2013	2014	Column Total
Ohio	215	680	623	576	546	684	603	616	425	911	810	657	552	581	506	416	277	237	246	281	233	216	175	183	175	11,424
Oklahoma	37	115	107	118	95	91	101	65	90	76	100	135	127	153	167	168	148	161	146	159	124	130	102	142	115	2,972
Oregon	32	102	120	111	95	98	68	89	66	88	78	94	103	127	111	83	87	101	108	87	94	82	103	59	79	2,265
Other Territories	1	7	4	7	6	1	0	3	1	1	3	2	4	1	2	4	1	1	1	1	0	1	0	2	0	58
Pennsylvania	564	1,150	1,097	1,125	1,171	1,403	1,401	1,352	1,235	1,508	1,392	1,504	1,262	1,290	1,251	1,060	899	828	845	853	782	806	772	795	638	26,983
Puerto Rico	27	121	80	47	137	155	119	168	144	167	192	230	171	180	225	245	190	229	277	257	291	261	258	277	323	4,771
Rhode Island	18	76	63	64	43	67	51	94	59	70	63	65	44	77	46	44	57	52	49	47	34	48	34	56	40	1,361
South Carolina	31	77	59	63	40	85	87	129	136	145	182	169	151	180	164	185	210	202	155	126	121	121	126	125	112	3,181
South Dakota	6	22	12	27	25	21	23	31	27	23	19	21	29	32	21	32	26	20	37	20	11	16	14	11	26	552
Tennessee	59	161	155	186	146	168	174	167	153	189	178	192	201	181	197	173	165	180	147	161	109	161	117	87	112	3,919
Texas	387	979	1,044	1,011	993	1,010	1,058	915	1,001	1,026	1,093	1,142	1,049	1,115	1,105	974	628	576	498	506	509	420	457	433	407	20,336
Utah	27	76	106	98	109	123	125	91	98	102	105	106	118	100	88	104	91	80	82	97	89	102	78	56	66	2,317
Vermont	11	24	27	28	31	28	28	35	51	30	22	26	25	20	23	16	18	11	20	20	19	16	6	8	8	551
Virginia	66	192	226	205	212	197	206	193	242	229	215	197	216	204	194	174	158	134	116	154	132	157	184	131	110	4,444
Washington	126	175	223	233	211	248	223	258	277	302	205	264	231	223	202	186	200	169	150	138	118	136	144	147	121	4,910
West Virginia	58	158	145	121	128	146	114	183	90	141	156	207	167	110	84	82	74	84	86	86	160	162	78	90	83	2,993
Wisconsin	62	199	174	131	109	113	132	90	73	73	74	114	99	122	86	85	71	63	71	73	40	58	41	43	37	2,233
Wyoming	2	22	20	31	36	15	34	22	31	27	27	25	35	24	20	24	18	11	15	11	21	9	16	14	14	519
Column Total	5,003	14,188	14,444	14,485	14,110	14,665	14,383	14,648	14,387	15,296	15,394	16,116	15,137	15,115	14,516	13,613	11,737	11,256	10,862	10,783	9,885	9,780	9,518	9,447	8,875	317,643

Source: Singh, H. (2016, July 14). National Practitioner Data Bank. Location by data year, generated using the data analysis tool. Retrieved from https://www.npdb.hrsa.gov/analysistool. Data source: National Practitioner Data Bank. (2014). *Adverse action and medical malpractice reports (1990–2014)*.

TABLE 29.4

Adverse Actions Against Physicians Reported to the National Practitioner Data Bank by State and Year: 1990 to 2014

Adverse Actions Include Loss of Clinical Privileges, Panel Membership, Professional Society Membership, Drug Enforcement Administration Actions, or Exclusion From Participation in Medicare and Medicaid.

Location	1990	1991	1992	1993	1994	1995	1996	1997	1998	1999	2000	2001	2002	2003	2004	2005	2006	2007	2008	2009	2010	2011	2012	2013	2014	Row Total
Alabama	14	35	37	39	37	30	36	60	71	73	66	84	84	79	56	70	56	53	49	78	63	75	112	73	82	1,512
Alaska	1	16	7	9	10	10	6	1	25	24	21	19	23	18	19	31	18	46	30	29	22	18	14	16	27	460
Arizona	26	72	69	85	89	90	149	119	92	121	140	210	165	174	142	149	203	194	172	174	172	163	131	111	125	3,337
Arkansas	14	20	28	19	21	23	27	35	49	45	35	31	33	21	9	22	41	27	29	27	40	32	43	46	40	757
Armed Forces	0	0	2	1	3	3	4	4	5	1	0	0	0	2	4	3	1	1	3	3	3	1	2	1	0	45
California	127	321	298	328	361	567	506	587	634	636	520	484	508	517	547	553	554	549	506	577	570	628	598	609	673	12,758
Colorado	29	100	113	117	120	127	126	117	95	74	64	81	110	93	127	125	128	132	114	174	146	131	128	125	123	2,819
Connecticut	24	43	41	49	51	65	63	67	67	58	73	61	64	75	64	67	60	53	57	59	60	107	84	68	60	1,540
Delaware	2	14	3	5	5	2	15	9	3	2	3	4	4	8	9	8	21	15	11	9	27	33	32	42	45	331
District of Columbia	6	15	15	6	4	8	36	32	44	8	4	13	18	18	24	21	33	36	34	30	17	15	29	49	40	555
Florida	82	251	197	220	194	252	246	230	174	232	215	236	181	169	230	266	233	288	199	211	218	307	311	295	332	5,769
Georgia	29	113	104	94	106	135	92	97	124	115	148	196	178	148	138	134	119	85	88	115	100	106	85	84	73	2,806
Hawaii	3	9	10	15	13	8	20	16	18	15	11	9	7	9	7	14	22	20	29	28	27	18	19	15	26	388
Idaho	1	6	9	9	14	12	16	11	18	16	10	18	22	13	14	16	12	14	27	12	15	18	20	10	18	351
Illinois	43	135	99	108	123	97	122	188	146	153	120	133	180	155	213	219	234	221	202	213	245	276	271	504	381	4,781
Indiana	16	61	54	69	62	87	82	25	31	22	39	38	31	23	76	79	89	64	73	84	63	95	121	87	85	1,556
Iowa	25	80	62	38	56	53	59	72	55	57	62	61	55	42	58	54	65	60	49	48	54	45	63	65	57	1,395
Kansas	8	35	39	32	43	36	58	27	42	33	42	48	40	29	42	31	40	32	56	57	41	34	27	43	43	958

Kentucky	27	76	72	102	77	57	66	64	79	68	113	66	78	106	87	88	86	111	96	109	68	97	142	170	160	2,265
Louisiana	33	59	70	59	58	62	59	47	59	60	57	58	61	60	65	66	81	53	64	83	118	66	92	77	76	1,643
Maine	4	12	8	19	14	17	26	24	40	17	17	23	27	24	21	23	42	37	46	35	34	31	36	33	22	632
Maryland	32	65	125	138	156	132	141	124	110	93	78	84	66	61	72	89	93	76	91	124	147	131	203	239	234	2,904
Massachusetts	28	48	67	77	103	99	95	90	92	95	133	164	150	132	173	154	129	106	98	72	92	74	86	88	105	2,550
Michigan	56	88	101	140	141	211	192	227	246	220	210	150	125	112	159	133	117	128	116	135	169	150	162	190	204	3,882
Minnesota	10	49	66	71	54	76	76	50	70	50	52	61	60	40	43	37	24	36	27	52	49	54	41	43	44	1,235
Mississippi	15	56	50	41	47	59	72	63	62	67	41	50	33	18	15	21	12	16	26	27	31	43	42	27	23	957
Missouri	38	77	62	108	99	83	97	89	73	79	101	84	69	90	181	90	92	64	76	107	112	104	101	96	103	2,275
Montana	5	10	11	17	28	15	11	7	12	16	9	15	20	33	21	15	12	17	11	7	13	19	16	12	9	361
Nebraska	4	21	9	19	20	25	20	12	17	11	14	11	17	25	27	26	23	27	18	24	34	34	33	34	30	535
Nevada	5	20	21	17	21	29	18	26	28	45	26	26	34	35	27	41	25	35	38	72	53	65	59	43	56	865
New Hampshire	2	11	12	9	13	9	11	17	18	25	19	27	25	19	30	32	25	17	9	19	35	25	41	31	33	514
New Jersey	62	150	175	172	161	148	154	136	136	145	135	143	151	128	143	85	108	121	109	146	115	122	99	100	125	3,269
New Mexico	2	10	19	13	12	9	28	8	22	12	15	18	28	20	36	28	39	26	31	66	48	55	53	55	55	708
New York	83	213	235	283	344	390	399	460	465	412	485	424	389	427	373	376	359	318	328	364	396	485	487	569	477	9,541
North Carolina	22	51	68	45	59	64	58	83	58	76	72	74	51	70	85	133	179	155	138	162	153	147	171	126	125	2,425
North Dakota	5	12	27	17	17	14	21	18	17	18	23	17	15	24	13	11	10	11	18	19	21	11	12	22	17	410
Ohio	52	141	193	197	212	270	282	246	292	290	134	174	245	239	273	236	269	235	233	270	278	423	406	411	349	6,350
Oklahoma	34	59	80	77	72	64	87	65	85	70	59	74	56	68	37	57	68	47	69	62	58	77	60	62	52	1,599

Continued

TABLE 29.4

Adverse Actions Against Physicians Reported to the National Practitioner Data Bank by State and Year: 1990 to 2014 *(Continued)*

Adverse Actions Include Loss of Clinical Privileges, Panel Membership, Professional Society Membership, Drug Enforcement Administration Actions, or Exclusion From Participation in Medicare and Medicaid.

State																									Column Total
Oregon	21	59	33	45	54	60	47	53	57	66	55	73	61	42	67	60	59	64	67	73	80	63	77	76	1,465
Other Territories	0	1	1	2	0	0	0	0	2	3	2	0	1	0	3	1	2	3	2	0	0	0	1	0	23
Pennsylvania	51	86	96	92	140	163	222	237	156	194	233	183	242	154	185	200	51	170	196	253	230	249	259	228	4,571
Puerto Rico	0	4	2	0	3	1	0	4	13	6	6	13	14	13	11	11	51	46	14	27	22	50	27	10	350
Rhode Island	4	6	15	15	30	20	29	25	27	8	3	14	16	19	17	20	30	21	17	19	28	30	40	30	499
South Carolina	15	46	41	48	52	47	57	56	70	57	39	43	68	50	40	54	43	73	55	69	57	62	56	64	1,321
South Dakota	2	2	4	9	13	7	6	2	6	2	8	6	15	7	5	8	10	10	13	20	24	20	12	24	239
Tennessee	21	45	50	63	62	62	67	52	30	68	63	53	65	80	104	92	81	80	113	122	102	98	87	94	1,792
Texas	62	221	201	214	292	287	278	293	335	187	192	177	229	203	188	178	151	186	189	246	260	281	440	446	6,007
Utah	4	16	13	26	18	11	27	24	33	47	37	41	28	31	34	23	36	17	39	39	39	67	41	47	772
Vermont	2	12	9	11	14	20	14	16	16	15	14	10	25	5	18	25	16	8	13	15	14	11	12	13	349
Virginia	52	152	140	153	174	132	141	139	141	133	117	127	123	143	154	104	141	211	222	166	174	180	158	150	3,695
Washington	32	74	65	92	79	83	57	106	111	77	59	50	75	83	87	115	104	110	143	122	130	125	104	124	2,331
West Virginia	15	51	50	51	65	70	57	49	57	31	42	46	58	35	50	48	33	36	63	57	61	39	47	40	1,196
Wisconsin	17	53	42	48	52	56	67	45	41	43	15	23	37	48	51	59	54	48	64	64	125	119	105	82	1,387
Wyoming	0	3	8	6	7	4	1	9	13	11	15	18	24	5	6	10	9	13	11	16	17	19	11	21	262
Column Total	1,267	3,385	3,428	3,739	4,075	4,461	4,646	4,663	4,780	4,608	4,290	4,373	4,280	4,668	4,591	4,715	4,546	4,462	5,106	5,215	5,678	5,845	5,978	6,148	113,297

Source: Singh, H. (2016, July 14). National Practitioner Data Bank. Location by data year, generated using the data analysis tool. Retrieved from https://www.npdb.hrsa.gov/analysistool.
Data source: National Practitioner Data Bank. (2014). *Adverse action and medical malpractice reports (1990–2014)*.

with lower payouts, as were higher levels of clinical hours and continuing education, the use of electronic medical records, and the use of error disclosure policies (CNA/NSO, 2012, p. 62). Slightly more than half of the survey participants who experienced claims said that a physician was on site during the incident, leading the surveyors to conclude that ". . . the presence of a supervising physician had little impact on the extent of liability (CNA/NSO, 2012, p. 70).

Of the 1,880 closed claims subjected to analysis in the CNA/NSO 2012 study, 504 of them involved incidents involving NPs' licenses; that is, reports to BONs, most commonly with regard to improper treatment and care, unprofessional conduct (most often drug diversion), and medication errors; only 26.4% of these claims resulted in payment, which averaged $4,441.00. These license protection claims most often emanated from office settings, followed by hospitals, patients' homes, and schools, in that order. Board actions in response to license protection claims usually resulted in positive outcomes for NPs; 61.7% of license protection of these cases were closed with no action taken (CNA/NSO, 2012, pp. 52–57).

When the NPDB (2014) data are examined based on reports of payments by state, it is apparent that the number of reports for APNs varies; the highest number of reports for malpractice between 1990 to 2014 was in Florida, followed respectively by New York, Texas, and Pennsylvania. For physicians, the same states were associated with the highest number of reports but in a different order: New York had the highest number of malpractice claims reports, followed respectively by Pennsylvania, Florida, and Texas (NPDB, 2014).

There continues to be little in the scant claims experience or research to explain why APNs are sued so much less frequently than physicians. Although substantial evidence exists that many more medical errors are made than lawsuits filed, little is known about why malpractice claims are filed in some circumstances but not in others, regardless of the type of health-care provider (Buppert, 2015). A 2011 study of physician malpractice risk according to specialty estimates that whereas 99% of physicians in the highest-risk specialties (neurosurgery, thoracic-cardiovascular surgery, and general surgery) and 75% of physicians in low-risk categories (psychiatry, pediatrics, and family practice) are likely to face a claim by age 65, 78% of all claims annually did not result in payments to claimants (Jena,

Seabury, Lakdawalla, & Chandra, 2011). A comparative analysis of lawsuits against APNs, physicians, and PAs in 2006 estimated that the probability of being sued was 1 in 62 for physicians, 1 in 563 for PAs, and 1 in 1,016 for APNs (Hooker et al, 2009).

Physicians see large numbers of patients on a daily basis in an effort to maximize the income stream for a practice; as a consequence, less time is spent with individual patients, which carries increased liability risk. Levinson and colleagues (1997) found that physicians with no claims made against them spent a longer time in an encounter. As noted, in the CNA/NSO (2012) study, generally, the longer the time spent in an encounter, the fewer claims were made against NPs. Logically, spending less time means communicating less with patients about their concerns and about their treatment, which is especially problematic when patients have complicated histories and complaints. A systematic review of 11 randomized clinical trials and 23 observational studies evaluating data on patient satisfaction, health status, cost, and the process of care by Horrocks, Anderson, and Salisbury (2002) determined that NP and physician outcomes were comparable but that patient satisfaction was highest among patients of NPs. This review also found that NPs offered more advice or information to patients, documented findings in greater detail, and had better communication skills than their physician colleagues. No differences were determined between NPs and physicians in the health status of their patients, in the number of prescriptions written, in return visits requested, or in referrals to other providers; these results were confirmed by a more recent examination of primary health-care practice between 1996 and 2011 by Traczynski and Udalova (2013). A meta-analysis of the Cochrane database by Laurant and colleagues (2006) involving 16 studies evaluating primary care provided by nurses and APNs, in contrast to that of physicians, found that resource utilization and costs were equivalent for comparable care but that patients were more satisfied with the care of nurses. It has been suggested that a clinician is less likely to be sued when patients perceive genuine interest in them, when they believe their care to have been competent, and when careful documentation has been made of services provided (Lefevre, Water, & Budetti, 2002; Wright, 2008). Buppert (2015, p. 281) emphasizes that good communication is essential because it leads to satisfied patients and "satisfied patients generally don't sue."

Malpractice Lawsuits and State Laws

Malpractice lawsuits, with rare exceptions, are filed in state court under state law rather than under federal law. State laws pertaining to filing a malpractice claim vary widely and may make it easier or more difficult for patients to sue for malpractice and obtain a judgment or settlement. For example, differences in statute of limitations (the time from discovery of an injury to filing of a lawsuit), burdens of proof, caps on noneconomic damages (e.g., pain and suffering), attorneys' fees, and use of mandatory medical review panels or arbitration to resolve issues make a great difference in the frequency of malpractice lawsuits in a given state and the amount of a judgment or settlement.

Advanced Practice Nurses and Tort Reform

Often health-care professional stakeholders seek state or federal legislation to solve the problems of too many lawsuits and too little access to affordable insurance. Commonly referred to as *tort reform,* these proposed laws seek to make it more difficult or less profitable to file claims against health-care professionals. The intended results are (a) to create a more favorable market for malpractice insurance carriers to continue to provide coverage and (b) for health-care practitioners to continue to provide services. In every session of Congress there are legislative proposals and political calls for tort reform at the federal level (Underwood, 2009). Although there are strong policy arguments to support Congress taking such action, malpractice litigation is a matter of state law and state legal practice. Federal tort reform, although repeatedly proposed, remains unlikely in the foreseeable future. Meaningful state tort reform laws have been passed in several states, and to keep up with the fluid nature of these changes it is prudent to check state-by-state specifics regarding the current nature of medical liability legislation, which can be found at the National Conference of State Legislatures (NCSL) Web site (NCSL, 2014).

An extensive analysis by Mello (2006) of multiple studies examining the impact of state tort reforms on the malpractice crisis concludes that caps on noneconomic damages reduce the average size of malpractice awards by 20% to 30% and have a modest impact on malpractice insurance premium growth but that these caps have "disproportionately" negative effects on the

most severely injured. Mello contends that state reforms such as changes to joint and several liability, statutes of limitations, or attorney contingency fees have not had the expected intent of changing the underlying elements of the malpractice crisis by reducing premiums, making malpractice insurance more readily available, or improving the financial health of insurance companies; that research fails to support the perception that overall physician supply has significantly decreased; or that there is a relationship between malpractice cost and physician supply. Mello agrees that the evidence indicates physicians do practice defensive medicine—ordering referrals, medications, and tests to protect themselves from liability—but says that the impact of these strategies is hard to measure.

More recently, Mello, Boothman, and colleagues (2014) and Avraham and Schanzenbach (2015) described the use of Communication and Resolution Programs (CRPs) as alternatives to current medical malpractice processes. These programs involve recognition of unanticipated adverse events, open communication with patients about the events, and compensation where appropriate. Early adopters of these programs report significant reductions in liability costs and improved patient safety.

Notwithstanding their historically low incidence of claims, some APNs can expect to find themselves increasingly affected by situations that arise in a "hard" malpractice insurance market. The effects are escalating insurance premiums, coverage limitations, insurance company insolvencies, or decisions by carriers to stop covering medical malpractice altogether, limiting access to whatever liability insurance is available (American Association of Nurse Anesthetists [AANA], 2002a; Silverman, 2004). Because of prohibitive insurance costs or complete lack of insurance, some practitioners have taken drastic actions, including early retirement, closure of high-risk practices such as obstetrics, or relocation to a state where the claims experience is more reasonable and insurance is available (Silverman, 2004). Because of the malpractice burden, Xiao and colleagues (2008) found that many Michigan CNMs moved from private practice to salaried employment (where the employer pays the medical malpractice premium); those who were independently covered or who were "going bare" were significantly less likely to provide obstetrical care. In another response, associations such as the American College of Nurse-Midwives (ACNM), the American

Association of Nurse Anesthetists, and other professionals, including several physician groups, have formed their own insurance companies to ensure insurance access to their members in the periodic downturns of the insurance business.

Although the aggregate claims history for APNs may seem modest, a hard market for malpractice insurance affects APNs as well as physicians and all licensed health-care practitioners. The best advice is for APNs to engage in a form of risk management called *risk prevention* and make every effort to reduce errors.

PRACTICE SETTINGS AND SPECIALTY PRACTICE RISKS

As an initial legal principle, each person is always individually accountable for his or her own torts (wrongs). As demonstrated by the NPDB statistics, APNs can and do get sued in their own right. Liability in all cases turns on whether the APN exercised due care under the circumstances. This conclusion is determined by examining the duty owed to the patient, the professional standards that apply to a reasonable APN practicing under similar circumstances, and the causal effect of any act or omission of the APN to the injury suffered by the patient. Whether anyone else, such as collaborating physicians, are accountable and can be sued for the harm caused by substandard acts or omissions of the APN depends on the relationship between the parties and on the facts and circumstances of the incident.

EMPLOYED ADVANCED PRACTICE NURSES

APNs such as NPs and CNSs are employed by health-care systems, as well as by acute-care, extended care, and home care facilities, MCOs, and private physician practices. CNMs and NAs may be employed either by acute-care institutions or by physician groups of obstetrician-gynecologists and anesthesiologists, respectively. As employees, APNs are presumed to be covered by the employer's malpractice program because under the concept of "vicarious liability" the employer is held responsible financially for harm caused to a patient by its employee. The Latin term

for this principle of imputed responsibility is *respondeat superior*. It applies only in an employment situation because the employer effectively controls the manner in which the care is rendered (i.e., the employer has legal control over the actions taken by the employee that are within the scope of the employee's job description). When hospitals or health-care systems are sued, it is typically a result of errors or omissions committed by employees such as physicians, technicians, nurses, and APNs. From an economic perspective, employers have more assets to pay a settlement or a judgment and therefore are better able to bear the risk.

When an APN is in a true employment relationship, liability for negligence continues to flow through to the employer as a consequence of this traditional principle of tort law. The insurance rates charged to the employer reflect the risks associated with the entire pool of employees. However, this allocation of risk also provides the employer with the best opportunity to manage the risk through direct payment of claims. Many health-care employers are self-insured, meaning they personally "retain" risk or fund the settlement of claims to a given dollar ceiling. In effect, they are settling with their own money, thus avoiding the higher insurance premium costs. Self-insured employers are thus strongly motivated to keep claim settlements below their self-insured limit. To achieve this objective, it is common to agree to a settlement without disputing which of the named health-care employees were actually liable.

The danger to the employed APN is twofold. First, if named individually in a lawsuit, the APN can be found jointly and severally liable or liable for contributory negligence as an individual, not just an employee. If, under these circumstances, the APN relies only on the employer's malpractice insurance to cover the claim, the hospital defense counsel could decide to settle the case and leave the remaining liability to the APN individually. Second, an APN without individual malpractice insurance coverage is subject to the decisions of the one hospital lawyer, which may not be in the APN's best interest. Moreover, if the APN is at the mercy of the hospital insurer, a settlement of a suit on behalf of any named health-care practitioner must be reported to the NPDB as required by law. Such a settlement could be negotiated without knowledge or consent of the APN. With the APN's professional reputation and financial well-being at stake, the APN cannot afford to abdicate responsibility to an employer. It is advisable to carry sufficient amounts of individual malpractice insurance to maintain control and to avoid these types of conflicts (Buppert, 2008, 2011, 2015; CMF Group, 2002; Philipsen, 2009). With individual malpractice insurance coverage, the APN has separate counsel who is not conflicted by the interests of the hospital and can zealously represent the interests of the APN.

INDEPENDENT VS. COLLABORATIVE PRACTICE RISKS

The APN, subject to state nurse practice acts (NPAs), is increasingly likely to become an independent practitioner who controls his or her own professional judgments and actions. With greater autonomy comes greater individual accountability for actions. In this type of practice arrangement the APN may deliver health-care services in any one or more of several settings, including traditional employer settings. Independent practice is usually accomplished through solo practice, group practice with other APNs, or business arrangements in which the APN and the health-care system, HMO, physician, or group practice structure their relationship as one of "independent contractor" or as a credentialed member of a hospital's medical staff with defined privileges.

As an independent contractor, the general rule is that no vicarious liability flows from the APN to the institution, physician, or other third party (Ingram, 1993). In real life, however, even when the APN is not the employee of the institution or physician, a lawyer may still argue that the institution or physician is responsible because ostensibly the APN and the hospital or practice encourages patients to believe the nurse is employed by the institution. This type of ostensible agency theory is frequently argued in emergency room and anesthesia cases or whenever the lawyer wants to get to the (presumably) "deep pocket" of the hospital or the physician as a source of money for the patient. A plaintiff's lawyer will argue that responsibility is shared by all who were involved in the events leading to the claim of injury, including the institutional provider and any physician (or APN) involved in the care of the patient at the time under legal theories of joint and several or contributory liability (Buppert, 2015; Philipsen, 2009; Silverman, 2004).

Whether vicarious liability is imputed to the hospital, group practice, HMO, physician, or other party turns on the specific relationships and the degree of control exercised by one professional or party over the APN. A hospital, for example, is not held liable for the professional negligence of non-employed medical staff members regardless of whether they are physicians or APNs. Although courts take many factors into account, the final decision in any case depends on the facts and circumstances particular to that situation (Feld & Moses, 2009; Silverman, 2004). If physicians are, by law or policy, required to supervise APNs, then the degree to which they are held accountable for APN practice is greater than if they are in a collaborative relationship; in the latter case, "some neglect by the physician must be proven" (Buppert, 2008, p. 262). Buppert (2016) reported on her review of 6 out of 12 cases in which a collaborating physician was found to have some liability for care provided by a NP; in these cases either the physician had actually been involved in the patient's care or the judge imputed from the existence of the collaborating agreement that the physician *should* have been involved. From a litigation perspective, this makes the ongoing effort of anesthesiologists to continue to supervise the practice of NAs in states such as New Jersey puzzling. NAs provide 65% of all anesthesia care in the United States annually, are the sole providers in two-thirds of rural hospitals in the United States, and are the primary anesthesia providers for the military. A large study comparing the care of NAs in 14 states (two more, Colorado and California, have now joined them) that had opted out of the Medicare rule requiring anesthesiologist supervision to those of NAs in states that have not opted out found no increase in risk to patient safety in the opt-out states (Dulisse & Cromwell, 2010); congruent results were obtained by Negrusa and colleagues (2016). Multiple court decisions have concluded that surgeons, dentists, and health-care centers working with CRNAs do not accrue increased liability because they are *not in control of the CRNA* (AANA, 2002b).

Because APNs are significantly less likely than physicians to have claims payments made against them (Hooker et al, 2009; NPDB, 2011a; Pearson, 2014), it can be reasonably concluded that physicians should be more concerned about the litigation risk posed by their physician colleagues than their APN colleagues. Still, anecdotal reports of an increasing number of claims made, for example, against obstetricians and gynecologists in New York and New Jersey who work with CNMs and NPs (Silverman, 2004) create anxiety for physicians about APN liability risk and result in some physicians refusing to sign collaborative agreements or joint protocols or demanding large payments because they fear automatic surcharges to or rises in their insurance rates (Torre & Drake, 2014; Torre, Joel, & Aughenbaugh, 2009). When, as happened to CNMs in New York and New Jersey in 2004, insurance rates doubled, physicians or hospitals may be less enthusiastic about hiring these providers, considering them too costly (Silverman, 2004).

Although many APNs work in what they would describe as collaborative practices with physician colleagues, legal parameters set by the Board of Medical Examiners' Corporate Practice Rules in some states (for example, New Jersey) preclude physicians from being a corporate partner with (or an employee of) professionals of "lesser licensure," such as APNs, so most APNs are employees. Where APNs work in practice together and are required to have a joint protocol or collaborative agreement with a physician, they may contract with physicians as consultants. The most prudent business relationship for all parties exists when the APN (and the physician) is an independent practitioner and not an employee because in this circumstance accountability rests with the individual provider. No one practitioner controls or is liable for the activities of another. This risk control strategy does not ensure that an APN or a physician will not be sued, but it does appreciably diminish the chances of unprotected and unwarranted vicarious liability for all parties. Although it is true that the physician who employs an APN can be liable, similar to any employer, for the negligence of his or her employees under the theory of *respondeat superior,* if an independent business relationship exists between the physician and the nurse, there is no legal basis on which to automatically impute liability to the physician.

Removing the statutory and regulatory requirements for supervisory or collaborative agreements and joint protocols from all state statutes will make it clear that the responsibility for the totality of APN care resides solely with them and that should reduce real or perceived physician anxiety about increasing liability risk when sharing care with their APN colleagues (Buppert, 2016; Torre & Drake, 2014).

MALPRACTICE INSURANCE AS A RISK MANAGEMENT TOOL

Liability for individual acts or judgments as a professional cannot be transferred, but financial responsibility for damage awards (indemnity) and legal (defense) fees incurred in arriving at damages may be transferred. The objective is to limit the financial effect should you cause or be accused of causing injury to another (Buppert, 2015; Shinn, 1998). Purchasing professional liability coverage involves thorough investigation and selection of insurance with a regular review of coverage to be sure it continues to meet practice risks. A suggested process includes the following steps:

- *Identify a carrier:* Professional liability carriers differ from one specialty to another. APN professional associations and their Web sites are a reliable source of information about insurers who can be expected to understand and have experience in representing APNs. Practicing colleagues with coverage are another source of information. Choose a company with a sound financial reputation, preferably one with an A to A++ rating (A. M. Best & Co., 2015).
- *Select the type of coverage:* Although it seems to be increasingly difficult to find (and may be completely unavailable for CNMs and NAs), Buppert (2015) encourages practitioners to try to purchase occurrence rather than a claims-made coverage because occurrence policies will cover the APN regardless of when the incident occurred and whether or not the policy is currently active; claims-made policies cover the APN only when the contract is currently active. Additional tail-funding can (and should) be purchased to extend the period of coverage with a claims-made policy, but this will add to the cost of the insurance.
- *Select level of coverage:* Because so many cases occur where damage awards exceed $1 million, Buppert (2011, p. 17) counsels that NPs should purchase "as much insurance as you can get, and afford."
- *Understand the coverage limits:* For example, $1,000,000 each occurrence/$5,000,000 annual aggregate means the most paid for any one claim is $1,000,000 and the number of claims at that amount that can be paid in 1 year is five. Find out if legal costs are included in the

policy. Are they included within the limits of liability or are they in addition to the limits? If they are not included, the APN would be responsible for these costs (CMF Group, 2002).

- *Determine policy settlement provisions:* Look only for an insurer who agrees to consult, will permit choice of counsel, and will not settle without written consent.
- *Understand costs of malpractice insurance:* Rates differ considerably for APN specialties and the cost burden of malpractice insurance therefore also varies by specialty. In 2015, the average annual wage of a CNM in New Jersey was $111,800 (Bureau of Labor Statistics, 2015). The minimum annual cost of an insurance policy for a CNM offered by General Star Insurance, for example, is $5,000. In contrast, the mean total income for NPs in 2015 was $103,000 (Bureau of Labor Statistics, 2015) whereas the maximum cost of malpractice insurance for a family NP in New Jersey in 2016 through Mercer Insurance was $1,467.
- In comparison, costs of malpractice insurance for NPs in those states that have achieved full scope of practice (SOP) independence to those in states that have not demonstrates no significant increases in rates for NPs in the independent states.
- *Know contractual obligations:* In addition to the duties the insurer has to you, there are limitations of which the APN needs to be aware. All policies have specific exclusions under which the insurance does not apply. All policies exclude criminal acts or events that are "against public policy." In general, the broader the coverage, the higher the premiums. Maintaining professional liability protection is a partnership. The insured also has obligations to the insurer that must be honored if professional risks are to be successfully managed. Truthfulness when applying for insurance, timely premium payments, and complying with the conditions of coverage as stated in the policy are essential. Key among all policy conditions is notification of the insurer as soon as possible if an adverse event occurs (Buppert, 2015; CNA/NSO, 2012; Coakley, 2010).

What Happens When a Lawsuit Is Filed?

APNs justifiably dread the prospect of a lawsuit, which will impugn professional competency, create personal and family anxiety, and incur financial hardship. Education about an issue can reduce stress and promote informed decision making. The same approach applies here. Know what to do if a lawsuit occurs. As a practical matter, the lawyer for the patient or the patient's family makes a case assessment before filing the lawsuit to determine whether the case has merit. For a malpractice lawyer who takes cases on a contingency basis (i.e., the lawyer is paid a percentage of any award, but only if the patient wins), the golden rule is to go after only the "live fish." In other words, malpractice lawyers only sue professionals, including doctors or nurses, who have the money or insurance to pay any judgment or settlement. To ensure there will be someone at the end of the lawsuit to pay an award, lawyers for patients frequently name any and all entities or individuals who could possibly have something to do with the claim of injury. Whether or not a NP has malpractice insurance is "usually (revealed) during the discovery process in preparation for trial" (Buppert, 2015).

When a suit is filed, an APN should anticipate the following:

- The APN is served with a copy of the suit that includes the summons and complaint filed by the plaintiff (patient).
- The professional liability coverage must be activated by immediately notifying the insurance agent or the insurance company verbally.
- The specifics of the claim and the date of notification are recorded. Any conversations must be thoroughly documented, including the next steps each party is to take.
- One copy of the summons is retained; one copy is sent to the insurance agent and one to the employer, if applicable.
- Anecdotal documentation is prepared (i.e., all that can be recalled about the incident: who, what, when, where, how, and why). If possible, the patient record should be consulted. Dates, times, and people involved should be noted.
- If employed, the APN is to notify the risk manager verbally and in writing, again documenting the interaction with risk management.
- The temptation to discuss the suit with others should be avoided. Discussions should be limited to the insurance agent, claims representative, attorney, and, if applicable, the employer's risk manager. Do not discuss the case

with anyone related to the plaintiff, anyone who might be a witness for the plaintiff, or the news media.

- Do *not* assume any financial obligation or pay any money without the insurance company's consent. If this occurs, the APN cannot expect the costs to be covered by the liability policy (CNA/NSO, 2012; Shinn, 1998).

Insurer's Response

- Within 24 to 48 hours from the time of notification of the filing of a claim, the APN should be contacted by the insurer's claim representative whose skills have been matched with claim specifics to ensure the best-qualified person manages the claim.
- The insurer will have determined whether other providers covered by the insurer are being sued or have been sued by the same patient. If so, the insurer will determine whether there is any conflict in having one person manage the lawsuit for all the insured providers. The assignment of a single claims representative occurs when all the insured agreed with the carrier that no one is at fault or fault lies with someone not insured by the liability carrier.
- The claim representative interviews the APN by phone and explains what the insurance policy covers. In addition, the claim representative contacts any other carriers (e.g., the employer) that should or might be providing coverage for the APN (Shinn, 1998; Shinn & Curtin, 2001).

Legal Counsel

- Once coverage is confirmed, the APN is advised by the claim representative what law firm will be providing counsel. Attorneys are usually from local or regional firms who have negotiated fee arrangements to handle the insurer's claims and have medical malpractice experience related to the specific claim.
- The assigned lawyer interviews the APN. The objectives are for the lawyer to become more familiar with the case while the APN becomes comfortable with the lawyer. To facilitate this process the APN should ask for (a) the lawyer's credentials, (b) the number of cases of this type previously litigated, (c) the number of cases that have gone to trial, and (d) the outcomes.
- The APN should contact the claim representative immediately if he or she is dissatisfied with the assigned attorney and request that a change be made. Walker (2011) emphasizes that the APN's lawyer should be an expert in APN statutes and regulatory requirements, and fully understand APN SOP and the professional standards of APNs.
- Once the lawyer is agreed upon, the APN should receive a written outline from the insurer's claim representative stating what law firm will provide defense, as well as any investigative firm that will be used, and an explanation of how the claim will be handled. Coverage issues should be described along with current status and detailed resolutions.
- The APN's counsel and the plaintiff's lawyer then engage in discovery (i.e., investigation of the facts of the claim). Written questions called *interrogatories* are served by both sides, followed by written responses and the appearance of the plaintiff, defendant, and witnesses at depositions where a court reporter will take their testimony under oath. In the end all information gathered is used to settle or ready the case for trial (Coakley, 2010; Shinn & Curtin, 2001).

Settlement

- Although each case should be evaluated on its merits, it is possible for settlements to be reached regardless of whether the APN has some fault or not. In the first instance, variables include some degree of fault, social climate, plaintiff socioeconomic factors, local statutes, previous jury verdicts for similar claims, the APN's ability to pay the claim, and the potential for a verdict in excess of the liability limits. Reasons for settlement even when the APN is not at fault include economics, medical records that do not support APN actions, impracticality of having the APN testify in his or her own defense, or the desire to avoid the unpredictability of a jury trial (Coakley, 2010; Shinn & Curtin, 2001).
- In the end the best rule for the APN is never to agree on a settlement until having had the opportunity to express personal opinions about the case, have them seriously considered, and conclude personally that a settlement is the best resolution of the matter (Coakley, 2010; Shinn & Curtin, 2001). Remember that a settlement will be reported to the NPDB. This means it will be part of an APN's permanent professional record.

TRIAL

Risks Inherent in Witness Testimony

In a trial, the patient has the burden of proof. To be successful, evidence must be sufficient to meet the four elements of negligence: duty, breach of duty, causal connection, and damage. The plaintiff's attorney typically presents the case with as many types of witnesses as possible. Witnesses may include the patient, aggrieved family members, APN experts, medical experts, hospital employees, or economic experts. Each of these witnesses plays a different role in the plaintiff's case.

The patient allegedly injured by the APN is often the most powerful witness. If possible, the injured party describes firsthand what he or she thinks occurred, as well as the bad effect caused by the APN's actions or omissions. Family members are effective witnesses because they serve to personalize the patient, demonize the APN, evoke jury sympathies, and inflame jury passions.

The testimony of nursing and medical experts is crucial to a plaintiff's case because it provides a clinical perspective on the problems described by the patient and the patient's family members. The plaintiff's APN experts explain how the APN breached the standard of nursing care owed to the patient. They do so by pointing out problems found in the APN's own clinical records and other ways in which the care was allegedly substandard. They also challenge the adequacy of the APN's continuing education.

Medical experts testify about the nature and extent of the patient's injuries and describe the pain and suffering, disability, or additional health risks resulting from these injuries. In addition, the experts opine on the manner in which the APN's breach of the standard of care directly caused these injuries and point out any ways in which the APN and, often, the collaborating physician failed to comply with the applicable standard of care. Finally, they explain why the patient's injuries were *not* a natural and unavoidable result of the individual's medical condition, known risks associated with the procedure or treatment, the aging process, or a preexisting health problem.

It is not unusual to see experts attack the qualifications, training, and continuing education of the APN. Perhaps of greatest importance are their attempts to increase the opportunity to have the judge or jury assess punitive damages by linking a lack of qualifications to a wanton or reckless disregard for the welfare of the patient. Finding evidence in memos and e-mail files of shortcuts, failure to respond to telephone calls, or undue financial controls is usually not difficult. "Putting profits or self-interest before patients" is a common mantra of the plaintiff's argument.

Testimony of current and former colleagues and employees of a hospital on behalf of the plaintiff presents a danger to the APN because they will claim that the APN treated them badly, was unprofessional and unreliable, and consistently put his or her own self-interests ahead of patient care by consciously not responding when needed or simply not knowing the appropriate thing to do. Employee testimony is orchestrated to increase the APN's punitive damages exposure by showing a pattern of callous behavior toward both patients and employees.

In the trial process, the plaintiff's witnesses are questioned by the plaintiff's attorney and cross-examined by the APN's counsel. Once the plaintiff concludes, the APN's counsel has the opportunity to present witnesses to rebut the plaintiff's allegations. The APN may or may not testify, depending on the specifics of the suit; the APN is held to the testimony presented in the deposition (NSO, 2014).

Trials may end with the successful defense move for a directed verdict against the plaintiff. This means the APN's lawyer asserts and succeeds in arguing the plaintiff failed to meet the burden of proof or has not made a valid case for malpractice. If the trial is a bench trial, the judge rather than a jury decides on the verdict (Aiken, 2004). Most plaintiffs demand a jury trial. If the verdict is against the APN, the APN, counsel, and insurer determine the next steps (Shinn & Curtin, 2001). One option following an unacceptable verdict is to file an appeal to the next higher court (Buppert, 2015).

Risk Reduction Strategies

To avoid malpractice, Buppert (2011, 2015) recommends that APNs be wary of developing a patient-provider relationship (implicitly a duty to the patient) with colleagues, neighbors, family, and friends outside of a formal practice relationship; practice within established standards of care; be sensitive to the limits of education, expertise, and SOP;

consult with and refer to other providers as early and often as necessary, especially if "the history and examinations suggest a deadly condition and it hasn't been ruled out or treated" (Buppert, 2011, p. 17); carefully document so that clinical choices are clear and justifiable; find another work setting if the current one is not permitting safe practice; and purchase an individual occurrence malpractice insurance policy.

Strategies for limiting exposure to a significant malpractice case must focus on neutralizing the factors that are favorable to the plaintiff's case or on turning them to the APN's advantage. In the best of all circumstances, these interventions and practices are put into action to prevent a lawsuit from being filed in the first place and they are thoroughly documented to provide evidence of the APN's good faith in the event of litigation. Broadly, these actions are described as caring, communication, competence, and charting (Giessel & Palentino, 2006).

Caring and Communication: Fostering Positive Relationships With Patient and Family

APNs must manage expectations by providing the patient and family with a realistic depiction of care and treatment needed, as well as expected outcomes. This message should be reinforced consistently in clinical records and written materials, including educational materials and all one-on-one communications. If a significant gap exists between what is promised and the actual capacity to deliver care and services, there is a high risk that the patient and the family will be disappointed.

In addition, when discussing any aspect of care and services, particularly any aspect of informed consent, the APN should present the information in easy-to-understand lay person's terms that take into account the patient's condition and the limitations of treatment. Finally, the APN should explain issues typical to all patients in similar circumstances and encourage the patient and family to work with the APN to identify and prevent problems.

In the event of a poor outcome or adverse reaction, every effort must be made to disclose the events to the patient and family, respond to their concerns, ameliorate the patient's condition, and address either the professional conduct or system's failure that led to this outcome. Making apologies to patients and families for bad health-care

outcomes is an emerging strategy; ethicists and liability experts increasingly argue that providers have a moral responsibility to admit medical error and that disclosure linked with offers of compensation may reduce total liability costs, notwithstanding the complexity of appropriately providing such an apology and the emotional impact of an apology on both the patients and provider (Avraham & Schanzenbach, 2015; Gallagher, Studdert, & Levinson, 2007; Kachalia, 2009; Mello, Boothman, et al, 2014). The good faith effort of this practice standard should be noted by APNs as it is now recognized and protected in many states (NCSL, 2014).

In these days of instant communication, maintaining an appropriate level of accessibility to both patients and institutions is a must. It is far better for patients to contact the APN directly at any time than for them to feel they must call an attorney or a government agency to report substandard care or medical errors. Work hard to avoid making a diagnosis and providing treatment by phone or e-mail.

Office and hospital staff members should be encouraged to get to know the patients. Staff members who know their patients' names and individualized care needs and preferences make better caregivers and poorer litigation targets than staff members who do not take the time to develop such relationships. Emphasize this point to staff whenever possible. It seems too obvious to state, but everyone wants to be treated with dignity and recognition of their individuality. Positive relationships may be one of the primary reasons why people decide *not* to sue a health-care professional.

APNs must pay particular attention to the patient's medical history and understand the patient's underlying medical conditions and concurrent treatment and drug therapies to meet his or her medical needs. In a lawsuit it may be necessary for the APN to address medical progress by explaining how that patient's underlying medical conditions affected any negative outcome experienced by the patient. At the beginning of evaluation and treatment it is prudent, if not always practical, for the APN to obtain from the patient or a legal representative an authorization to release medical information from all other facilities where the patient has been treated and to obtain these materials and review them. This activity not only helps the APN to appreciate and understand the patient's full medical and behavioral picture, but also provides a wealth of information in the event of a subsequent lawsuit.

In turn, the patient's medical history is essential for determining the patient's prognosis, rehabilitation prospects, and medical risks; for developing and carrying out an effective care plan; for providing a context in which to evaluate the patient's progress; and for providing possible medical explanations for negative outcomes experienced by the patient while under the APN's care. Buppert (2015) urges APNs to be alert to high-risk patients characterized by multisystem failure, substance abuse, and cognitive and emotional challenges. She suggests that APNs refer early; carefully document care and failures to follow up; review medications at each visit and provide easily understood and clearly legible dosing instructions; where possible, involve guardians or family members when counseling or teaching patients with cognitive challenges to ensure patients understand their circumstances and have truly consented to treatment; and be aware that if a patient has sued another provider, the patient may seek to sue his or her current one as well.

Fostering Positive Staff Relationships

To cultivate office and hospital staff, the APN should acknowledge and respect them. To the extent possible, APNs should ensure that their own office staff are paid and treated as well as their counterparts at other offices. Acknowledging caring behavior early and often is important. Employees appreciate the opportunity to participate in decisions that affect their work environment. Feedback should always be encouraged on issues of importance to staff. Staff training not only is the key to improving the delivery of care but also may be presented as a benefit, particularly to employees of the hospitals and nursing home where the APN practices. It helps to have employees and staff members improve their business, administrative, and clinical skills. In many ways the APN depends on them for carrying out orders. In addition, staff who are not health-care professionals but filling positions such as receptionist, appointment secretary, or business administrator may be the first and most frequent individuals with whom a patient interacts; it is essential that patients perceive these key people to be accessible and interested in addressing their needs speedily, competently, and courteously. In support of positive conduct, all training efforts by the staff should be encouraged and rewarded.

Fostering Positive Relationships With Professional Colleagues

Maintaining open lines of communication with collaborating and attending physicians, with other health-care providers in the community, and with facility nursing and medical staff is also essential to minimizing the risks of future lawsuits. As for the legal relationship with the collaborating physician, the APN must be informed about the requirements, if any, under the state NPAs for advanced practice nursing and follow them.

APNs must also manage the business relationships between themselves and their physician colleagues and institutions. It is essential to review all written agreements and institutional credentialing procedures and bylaws to be sure they do not create the impression of an employee relationship or impute vicarious liability on the physician or the institution unless that is what both parties intend. Requirements for unnecessary controls, such as supervision or practice restrictions, should be addressed because, as described previously, they could actually increase rather than decrease exposure to legal liability for both the physician and the institution.

APNs should keep collaborating physicians informed of developments in the practice or the care of a specific patient that might create the risk of a lawsuit. The physician-APN team should confer and decide whether changes in care are indicated and whether both need to more closely monitor care delivery systems and identify potential areas of concern. APNs should seek the collaborating physician's help in resolving any concerns about a patient's course of treatment.

Maintaining Competence

APNs are required by both state law and national certification requirements to complete a specified number of continuing nursing education contact hours in their specialty for recertification and it is essential that they keep files readily available to document this education should they be audited by either state BONs or national certification bodies. To provide evidence-based care, APNs must reach out to seek the clinical, procedural, and legal information that will guide "best practice" for their patients. Ready accessibility to online learning options make keeping up easier, and utilization of handheld electronic tools means information can be uploaded, viewed, and used nearly immediately.

Documenting Care

Keeping detailed records of care provided is time consuming and often onerous, but it is imperative for liability risk reduction. Electronic medical records systems, although complicated and often expensive to implement, help accurately share patient information between providers, increase legibility, and may make the process of record-keeping less labor intensive; however, they are only as accurate and complete as the information entered into them. When quotations from patients (who have declined care or been noncompliant with treatment, for example) will help make clear actions the provider has taken, be sure they are included in the record and keep them objective. Include summaries of phone conversations and e-mail messages that contribute to understanding patients' concerns and providers' suggested next steps. If a patient misses an appointment, record that. Document informed consent. Never alter a record, as written, once a lawsuit is filed (Buppert, 2015; CNA/NSO, 2012; Giessel & Palentino, 2006; Miller, 2009).

CONCLUSION

Although APNs are sued for malpractice relatively infrequently, it is an experience to be strenuously avoided. Thoughtfully reviewing liability risk reduction strategies before beginning practice and repeatedly reminding oneself of them thereafter can help achieve this goal: know and follow state and federal laws governing APN practice; know institutional policies and abide by them; maintain clinical competency and expertise through ongoing continuing education; warmly engage patients and families in their own care using clear communication; document care carefully, preferably using an electronic medical record; follow evidence-based practice guidelines; understand the limits of your knowledge and expertise; consult often and refer in a timely and appropriate manner; foster positive relationships with staff and professional colleagues; and purchase, and keep current, the most comprehensive malpractice insurance policy that is available for your specialty and within your budget.

30

Ethics and the Advanced Practice Nurse

Gladys L. Husted, James H. Husted, and Carrie Scotto

Learning Outcomes

Learning outcomes expected as a result of this chapter:

- Identify the essence of practice-based ethics in advanced nursing practice.
- Examine the application of contemporary ethical theories in practice.
- Consider the relevance of a rational bioethical decision-making process.
- Apply the elements of a rational bioethical decision-making process in the current advanced practice arena.

Experience and knowledge alone do not ensure the development of ethical practice. Rubin (2009) described the structure of a type of nursing practice that restricts the development of clinical knowledge and ethical judgment even in experienced nurses. Elements of this restrictive practice include stereotyping patients; failure to recognize qualitative distinctions in physical, mental, or contextual circumstances; failure to accept responsibility for professional decisions; and lack of a sense of agency. This type of practice impedes the progression of nursing practice beyond the novice level.

Benner's (2001) novice-to-expert theory of nursing practice development allows for the newly practicing registered nurse (RN) to begin at the novice level. However, models for advanced practice require expert nursing practice and do not allow for novice practice (Walsh & Bernhard, 2011). Based on *The Essentials of Doctoral Education for Advanced Practice Nursing* (American Association of Colleges of Nursing, 2006), advanced nursing practice education must move the nurse beyond the novice level. Advanced nursing practice education should provide opportunities to achieve essential and specialty competencies of advanced practice. In addition, opportunities for feedback and reflection necessary for synthesis and broader learning must be included to bring the advanced practice nurse (APN) beyond the level of knowledge and practice acquired in baccalaureate education. Therefore, the theoretical foundation of advanced practice education must be based on models that include self-reflection and intellectual dialogue in addition to knowledge and skill acquisition (Fawcett, Newman, & McAllister, 2004).

The symphonological model, as will be demonstrated, ensures that practitioners begin with patient-centered, holistic assessment including the contexts of knowledge, situation, and awareness. The consideration of the bio-ethical standards to direct practice within the patient's circumstances will facilitate the type of reflection that will preserve a nursing model for practice rather than a medical model, thereby enhancing the lives of their patients and of themselves, albeit in different respects.

THE VALUE OF COMMUNICATION

> One day two nurses in a jungle village passed under a coconut tree. As they passed, a coconut fell from the tree to the ground. An argument arose between them as to who had a right to possession of the coconut. Finally, they decided to do what seemed the only fair and ethical thing to do. They would split the coconut in half and each nurse would take one half of the coconut. They shook hands and each prepared to go on her* way.
>
> —(Husted & Husted, 2015, p. 39)

Nurses (and everyone else) sometimes make unfortunate decisions without ever realizing it and without learning anything from it (Tuckett, 1999). This is especially likely to occur when we do not engage ourselves in a process of discursive thought.

> Fortunately, before the nurses parted, a colleague passed them. She was an APN whose years of well-examined experience had developed in her the habit of seeking out reasons and relevance. When she asked them what they were going to do with the coconut, each was surprised by the answer of the other. One wanted the shells to use as cups for holding water and was not interested in the meat of the coconut. The

other only wanted the meat and had no interest in the shells. Because of the APN's intervention, one nurse now has twice as much coconut meat as she would have had otherwise and the other nurse has two cups instead of one.

Responsible ethical decision making and action in health care is somewhat similar to the division of coconuts. It requires awareness and understanding of the context in which the decision is to be made. All health-care professionals should assume the responsibility of seeking out what should be done and *why* it should be done. None of the contemporary ethical systems, as we will discuss, consistently recommends attention to these distinctions. "APNs are frequently at the forefront of advocating for patients seeking primary and/or specialty care and must be knowledgeable about the nature of ethical dilemmas and skilled in making ethical decisions" (Kalb & O'Conner, 2007, p. 197).

Nursing is not only concerned with patients in crisis; it is about patients in temporarily unpleasant conditions. Ethics is not only about difficult dilemmas; it is also about everyday occurrences. "Although ethical issues in health care receive much publicity, attention is rarely given to the non-dramatic, everyday ethics of health care" (Smith, 2005, p. 32). If an APN faces a choice between following present convenience and protecting the welfare of her patient, she should recognize that an ethical responsibility is at play here. And, hopefully, she will choose her patient's welfare.

A practice-based ethical system, understandably, attends to practice. The welfare of her patient is the focus of a nurse whose ethical practice is mature and advanced.

PRACTICE-BASED BIOETHICS

> For bioethics, one disability defines and sets apart every patient regardless of the nature of his affliction. This is the loss of agency—the power of an individual person to initiate and sustain action, the power to act on his purposes. . . . To achieve this purpose [returning agency to the patient], symphonology interweaves professional (therapeutic) practice and ethical interaction.
>
> —(Husted & Husted, 2008a, p. 104)

The purpose of symphonology is to return the patient to a state of agency where he can be his own agent to the extent possible in the context. A practice-based, symphonological (*symphonology* from *symphonia,* a Greek word meaning

---

*We use the pronoun "she" for the nurse or any health-care professional and "he" for the patient. This convention is for the reader's ease of understanding and to keep understanding in context. The singular is preferred to the plural or indeterminate because professionals and patients are individuals, and a practice-based ethic is, and ought to be, an individualistic ethic.

agreement) approach to ethical interaction is an approach from professional responsibility. Symphonology defines ethics as a system of standards to motivate, determine, and justify actions directed to the pursuit of vital and fundamental goals.† Ethics is not convenience, it is not etiquette, and it is not that which brings on a state of self-satisfaction. Symphonology is a *practice-based bioethic* derived from, and appropriate to, the self-determination of a patient, the purposes of a health-care setting, and the role of a health-care professional.

Practice-based bioethics aims to relate professionals and patients internally (to bring them into the same ethical context), to make human values its focus, and to make the health-care setting maximally purposeful. Practice-based bioethics is based on interactions between a professional and a patient who relate to each other through agreement and understanding. When a nurse strengthens a patient's confidence in his recovery or supports him in dealing with a morbid prognosis, she is nursing within a practice-based ethical system.

The measure of success for a practice-based bioethic is a patient's vital objective that he shall regain or retain his power to initiate and sustain actions. An ethic that is not skillfully exercised and harmoniously interwoven with practice cannot justifiably be the ethic of a health-care professional. It is the "ethic" of a nurse who is merely "going through the motions."

The nurses who passed the coconut tree made a valuable discovery. The best action to take depends on the nature of the context, the motivations of the persons involved, and what it is possible to do in this context. The best professional actions depend precisely on the same realities—and on respect for individual rights. These produce relevant, appropriate, and justifiable ethical actions.

RIGHTS

Rights (a singular term denoting a single, noncomplex agreement) is the product of an implicit agreement among rational beings made and held by virtue of their rationality not to obtain actions or the product or conditions of action from one another, except through voluntary consent, objectively gained. It is freedom from aggression—an agreement not to aggress (Husted & Husted, 2015, p. 20). See **Table 30.1.**

In any society, to the extent people recognize and are faithful to this agreement, its members respect and enjoy human rights. When this is lacking, they do not. "When ethical agents live and interact together, the benefit of the

TABLE 30.1	
Individual Rights	
Individual Rights	**The State of Nonaggression That Results From This Implicit Agreement**
Among rational beings	Beings who can think, a capacity of all humans
Made and held by virtue of their rationality	Made because of their rationality and the fact that, being rational, they can see the advantage to it
Not to obtain actions	For example, by coercion
Nor the product of actions	By taking over a person's life
Or conditions of actions	By changing the circumstances of the person's life for the worse
Except through voluntary consent	One is not coerced—the agreement establishes the terms of interaction.
Objectively gained	One is not deluded or deceived, but is fully informed.

Adapted from the digital supplement for educators accompanying G. L. Husted & J. H. Husted. (2015). *Ethical decision making in nursing* (45th ed.). New York, NY: Springer.

---

†All definitions, unless otherwise stipulated, are taken from the text by Husted and Husted, 2015.

rights agreement is so great and so obvious, the detriment of not having this agreement is so manifestly ruinous, that the agreement literally 'goes without saying'" (Husted & Husted, 2015, p. 22).

Ethical practice does not allow a professional to violate the rights of a patient. A dedication to human values is internal to the ethical nature of the health-care setting. This presupposes respect for the rights of patients.

The practice of nursing, ideally, goes beyond respect for rights. However, a professional, practice-based ethic must *begin* with the recognition of a patient's rights. Through this recognition, a nurse provides a bridge between a patient's present condition and situation and the realization of the values her profession promises.

The reality of individual rights is not complex. It is present whenever two or more people are together. Each has a right not to be aggressed against by the other. Rights surround every human interaction, however insignificant. Rights are a reality so familiar and all-encompassing that, in normal circumstances, it is the last thing with which one has to be concerned.

The rights agreement is the ethical foundation for all explicit agreements. It is the already preestablished implicit agreement that explicit agreements will be made without deception and will be honored.

The rights agreement structures and defines *human* interaction and the pursuit of human values. The recognition of rights produces interaction according to the standard of reciprocity—a voluntary process of give and take, without force or deception, and without interference with the other person's pursuit of values.

ADVANCED PRACTICE AND A PRACTICE-BASED BIOETHIC

> Rapid advances in technology make many demands on the character, education, and abilities of the advanced practice nurse. The emphasis on scientific developments throughout the past several centuries has caused ethics to take a quantitative rather than a qualitative approach. Science has sought to separate itself from concerns about human values and values systems.
> —(Callahan & Mannino, 1998, p. 282)

Whenever the need for an ethical decision arises in the health-care setting (and this is daily), it is confined within a specific, radically limited, yet complex context. The more complex the context, the more valuable are the ethical attitudes of a nurse who makes decisions that are based on this context—a nurse who makes practice-based decisions.

All of a nurse's experience that is relevant to her ethical competence is, ultimately, experience with individuals. The health-care setting is defined by the nature and purposes of human beings. A practice-based ethic is defined by the same realities. Each follows and enhances the other.

There is no such thing as skillful nursing without skillful ethical analysis. Ethical reasoning and clinical judgment share a common process and both serve to teach and inform the other. The importance, therefore, of attention to clinical practice, regardless of how far removed an APN is from the clinical setting, cannot be overemphasized (Solomon et al, 1994). A person does not graduate from nursing school or enter a nursing graduate program already skilled in bioethical decision making. Just as clinical expertise requires experience and attention, so does ethical expertise.

THE CONTEMPORARY ETHICAL THEORIES

If professional nursing practice is to be shaped by bioethical concerns, the ethic of nursing, of necessity, must be derived from, and relevant to, the profession and its practice. Attention to the context and careful thought and analysis are the essence of any competence, including advanced practice competence. Contemporary ethical theories do not lend themselves to the health-care professions or to ethically defensible decisions in health-care practice. None of the dominant ethical theories could be discovered in, or derived from, the profession of nursing. None can be made relevant to nursing practice.

> Skillful ethical comportment will deteriorate to a merely competent level if we apply norms and principles to complex practical situations where we have the potential for skillful recognition of patterns. . . . Strategies of adjudication and the search for certitude through the application of norms and principles, though comforting, do not produce skillful ethical comportment.
> —(Benner, Tanner, & Chesla, 1996, pp. 276–277)

TABLE 30.2		
Contemporary Ethical Systems		
Systems	**Defining Characteristic**	**View on Consequences**
Deontology	Following the rule	Not important
Utilitarianism	Doing the greatest good for the greatest number	Consequences to the greatest number
Social or cultural relativism	Beliefs of a particular society, culture, or religion are paramount.	Social mores do not relate to individual consequences.
Emotivism	If I feel it is right, it is right.	The individual determines consequences for self; consequences to others are irrelevant.

Yet, this is exactly what the contemporary ethical theories demand. See **Table 30.2.**

> Things are seldom what they seem. Skim milk masquerades as cream; Highlowes pass as patent leather; Jackdows strut in peacock's feathers.
> —(*H.M.S. Pinafore,* Gilbert & Sullivan, 1885)

A young woman or man entering the profession has every reason to believe that the purposes of nursing are shaped by the deepest and most vital human concerns—those concerns that are related to the life, health, and well-being of those who are sick and disabled. Unfortunately for nursing students, the contemporary ethical theories being taught are not *relevantly* related to these purposes.

The dominant ethical theories of today being taught to nurses are deontology, utilitarianism, and cultural or social relativism. The result always involves an element of emotivism.

Deontology is the theory that actions in conformance with formal rules of conduct are obligatory regardless of their results (Angeles, 1992). Deontology requires a nurse to attend to out-of-context duties. Intention is the overriding ethical concern whereas *consequences* are viewed as irrelevant. The individual motivations and character structures of a patient are secondary, or more often *unrelated,* to the ethics of nursing practice.

There is nothing inherent in the practice of nursing that implies that in a dispute between the requirements of a patient's welfare and the demands of deontology, a nurse ought to choose deontology. Van Hooft (1990)

states, "The idea that we are following rules when we act morally is a tired hangover from the days when the lives of people were controlled by religious and secular absolute rulers who accorded no respect or independence to ordinary people" (p. 211). "Deontology is entirely concerned with an agent's actions. It is unconcerned with consequences. It is also indifferent to the agent's intentions, except his intention to do his duty" (Husted & Husted, 2015, p. 95).

Utilitarianism is the theory that one should act so as to promote the greatest happiness (pleasure) of the greatest number of people (Angeles, 1992). Utilitarianism requires a nurse to pay attention to consequences, but consequences to more than just one patient. It is impossible for a nurse to give her concern to the largest number possible and at the same time provide optimum care for her individual patients. Only optimum care—the best care a professional is capable of—is ethical care. There is no such thing as indifferent ethical care.

There is nothing in nursing as a profession to justify the idea that, once a nurse has accepted a patient, she should never abandon concern for that patient in favor of pursuing the greatest good for the greatest number. The profession of nursing is incompatible with such a demand. Utilitarianism is a theory in which the end is said to justify the means (Gibson, 1993). It would, all too often, make the patient a means and the desires of the patient's family or the nurse's outlook on life, for example, an end. The purposes of individual patients, and not the whims of a greater number, are the reason for being of professional nursing. Nothing in the principle of utility (i.e., the greatest good for the greatest number) establishes the principle of individual justice (Sarikonda-Woitas & Robinson, 2002).

Social or cultural relativism is the theory that what is ethical and what is unethical is determined by the customs, beliefs, and practices of a society or a culture (Angeles, 1992). There is nothing in the purposes or traditions of nursing to suggest that, in a clash between the requirements of a patient's welfare and the demands of one's society or culture, a nurse should choose the sentiments of the society or culture. This would turn a nurse's attention onto the views of a society or culture and away from her patient. Relativism undermines professional practice and the well-being of patients. A patient's culture may be important, but it can be of no greater importance than the importance given to it by a patient. "Culture provides a set of perspectives about how the group interprets its life and what happens to it, including sickness and death. However, culture is not a discrete trait descriptive of all individuals in it. Rather, culture should be understood as having a dynamic nature" (Kim, 2005, p. 164).

Barnes and Boyle (1995) observe that: "Unfortunately, the emphasis on shared patterns has rather rigidly defined nursing's perceptions of people from specific cultures and has not allowed for personal variations [of individual persons] within a given culture" (p. 414). Communication between patients and cultures is, at best, a figure of speech. Cultures, as such, have no tongues, no ears, and no ability to evaluate an individual's values and circumstances. Only individuals have this (Kikuchi, 1996).

> Although cultural factors are a valuable blueprint to caring for a patient, there can be no justification for failing to allow for the patient's personal evaluation of the beliefs of her culture to serve as the standards of culturally congruent care. Otherwise one is caring for the culture and not the patient, and the concept of "care" will have been subjected to a radical change in meaning.
>
> —(Zoucha & Husted, 2000, p. 326)

A flawed definition of a human being is more virulent than a plague.

Emotivism is the doctrine that holds that feelings or emotions are forms of ethical knowledge. The doctrine states that every ethical judgment and decision is simply a disguised description of a person's feelings (Angeles,

1992). The irrelevance of the contemporary ethical systems inevitably leads ethical agents to depend on emotions rather than objective awareness.

There is nothing in the nature of nursing to suggest that, in a clash between the requirements of her patient's welfare and the demands of her present emotional state, a nurse should guide her actions by her feelings—quite the contrary. Emotivism turns a nurse's attention into herself and away from her patient. It replaces her professional responsibility with an obsession onto her ever-changing emotional moods. It makes ethical interaction between a professional and her patient entirely illusory.

"Knowledge" of all these theories is gained by cultural osmosis and expressed in largely unverbalized feelings. None of these theories produces a concern for the person in one's care. Close attention to the appropriate context, and careful analysis based on the nature and purposes of nursing, is what defines nursing.

A Rational Form of Bioethical Decision Making

The intrinsic ethic of a profession is structured by a process of discovering facts, causes, and motives. The contemporary theories demand that a nurse evade her objective, contextual awareness, and the discovery and recognition of immediately given facts relevant to her patient's individual situation. The theories project discovery and recognition away from a patient's values onto her first emotional responses, or onto the sentiments, opinions, and desires of others. For a practice-based ethic, an answer to a dilemma that a nurse and patient share is one that is independent of out-of-context beliefs and attitudes. Ideas based on one or more of these theories strengthen views such as the following:

- Ethics constitutes from issues—euthanasia, harvesting organs from anencephalic infants, research on the incompetent, cloning, medical use of marijuana, and so on.
- Unanalyzed and largely irrelevant individual or cultural opinions are ethical facts.
- Ethical action in certain circumstances is important, but the circumstances requiring ethical action are unimportant.
- What is true or false in a single circumstance is true or false in every similar circumstance.

- Rights are alienable. I would not let you decide for me, but I will decide for you.
- It is the role of a professional to make ethical decisions for her patients, but these roles are not reversible.

MORAL COURAGE AND MORAL DISTRESS

Nurses are obligated to practice in a way that seeks benefit and avoids harm for the patient. Accordingly, the practice of nursing must be moral. Because of economic, political, and social influences the APN role has expanded and evolved to include more direct and autonomous practice. This progression has brought an increase in responsibility for APNs that demands not only expert practice, but also an increased understanding and commitment to ethical practice (Benner, Tanner, & Chesla, 2009; Buerhaus, 2011). To meet this demand, APNs must possess strong moral courage.

Moral courage is the ability to do what is right or moral despite elements that would influence a person to act in another way (Lachman, 2011). It is the resolute commitment to ethical principles despite threat or risk (Murray, 2011). Ethical competence is essential for moral courage and consists of the ability to analyze and respond to moral problems uninhibited by routine, emotional, or dogmatic tenets (Lachman, 2011). Thus, moral courage precludes moral elitism and allows no claims of ethical superiority. The patient within the context is the basis for decision making and action.

Moral courage develops because of repeated experiences that move the practitioner beyond competent practice to one in which there is persistent integration of ethical principles (Miller, 2005; Murray, 2011). Threats to moral courage arise as individuals may face risks such as loss of employment, professional reputation, future advancement, or other negative outcomes. This can lead to moral distress. Moral distress results when the nurse knows the ethical action best suited for the patient in context, but is unable to act because of such considerations as inadequate staffing, institutional requirements, health policy constraints, or cost containment (Repenshek, 2007).

The relationship between moral courage and moral distress is not straightforward. It is tempting to say that if nurses have sufficient moral courage they need not experience moral distress. . . . However, given that organizations are not always supportive and do not always react appropriately, but rather may act defensively to concerns about standards of care raised by conscientious practitioners, even the most morally courageous staff may fear to speak up.

—(Gallagher, 2010, para. 15)

"As nurses advance into leadership positions, the complexity of the decisions they need to make increases, as does the potential for moral distress" (Edmonson, 2010). Unfortunately, "nurse educators . . . have tended to focus [when teaching ethics] simply on the ethical principles . . . [not] on their work environment [as] an ethical context" (Corley, 2002, p. 637). Although moral courage is not sufficient to avoid moral distress (Gallagher, 2010), the practice of APNs, based on the symphonological ethical model, dealing with individuals within the context of their professional practice will support and advance moral courage. Each experience will be a patient-centered, ethical event. In addition, it will enable APNs to be able to justify their decisions and actions. The accumulation of these events will prepare the APN with a strong foundation that will promote ethically driven patient care (Sekerka & Bagozzi, 2007).

THE IMPORTANCE OF CONTEXT

Ethics is concerned with the good of the individual. The good of an individual can only be discovered in a context. A professional ethic assumes that a professional's strength of character is appropriate to produce the flourishing of her patients. So do her patients (Guido, 2006). "Ethics provides structure for placing conduct into action" (Guido, 2010, p. 3). This is basic and the defining end of a professional ethic.

A professional ethic aims at a single end—the end that is the reason for being of the profession. This reason for being establishes and structures the APN's professional context. It relates an APN and a patient internally within this context.

Gastmans (1998) states, "The nurse functions both as a professional and as a human being within a variety of contexts. These contexts influence directly or indirectly the way in which the nurse performs caring tasks" (p. 126).

When a nurse, as an ethical agent, learns how to identify the various parts of an ethical context and their interrelations, she has developed a significant practical skill. When she is able to understand the individual human values that make each context what it is, she has developed an advanced practice competency. The ancient Greek philosophers described this ability as "practical wisdom." The great Chinese thinkers (whose benign influence in the West, although largely unacknowledged, was enormous) called it the *Way*—acting in harmony with the nature of things.

"Context is complex and comprehensive, dynamic, and interactive. Despite how tempting and how much easier it is to resort to the general, the abstract, and the theoretical, any form of bioethics that does not put moral [ethical] problems in their myriad contexts is, in many senses of the word, unreal" (Hoffmaster, 2006, p. 40).

There are three elements of every context that guide objective awareness and action. See **Table 30.3.** First is the *context of the situation.* This context is comprised of the interwoven aspects of a situation that are fundamental to understanding the situation and to acting effectively in it. These are the facts that are necessary to act on to bring about a desirable result.

The second is the *context of knowledge.* This is the agent's understanding of the aspects of the situation that are necessary to its understanding and to acting effectively in it. In other words, this is the knowledge one has of how to deal with these facts most effectively. These resources of knowledge enable a nurse to identify and interweave the two sides of the context into a coherent plan of action.

The third is the *context of awareness.* This is a bridge between the agent's present awareness of the relevant aspects of the situation and of her present knowledge.

An agent's context of awareness includes her awareness of those aspects of the situation that invite action. Every decision that an agent makes, if she acts in (or according to) the context, must be made according to:

- Her knowledge
- That which is appropriate to the situation
- Her present awareness of what she knows, and of what is relevant in the situation (Husted & Husted, 2015, p. 79; also see Table 30.3)

A person's context is the interweaving of these three elements, which provides the resources for making a justifiable decision. Reigle (1996) states, "Knowledge of facts is insufficient if not tempered with the contextual features of each case. Only after the unique conditions of the case are considered can an ethically acceptable solution be identified" (p. 275).

Everything relevant to a context is contained within the context. A multitude of factors that surround that context are irrelevant. These are the factors that play no part in the nature of the dilemma. They neither cause the dilemma nor can they help to resolve it. The resources of the context are resources because they provide *relevant* criteria for ethical decision making.

Here is a simple example: A nurse discovers that a patient is allergic to a certain medicine and acts accordingly. The fact that he is allergic is one part of the context of the situation. Her discovery of this fact, made by virtue of her past experience and her present thinking processes, becomes one part of her context of knowledge. Her purpose is to protect him. This is made possible by her context of awareness.

A context always forms itself around a purpose. One discovers a change to be made or a goal to be achieved and

TABLE 30.3	
The Three Elements of the Context	
Of the situation	The interwoven aspects of the situation that are fundamental to understanding and to acting effectively in it
Of knowledge	The relevant knowledge that a health-care professional brings to the situation
Of awareness	The bridge between an agent's present awareness of the relevant aspects of the situation and of her present knowledge

sets about to learn how, in the circumstances, this is to be done. The key to this is to be able to know the difference between the relevant and the irrelevant. The relevant is any factor in the context that will enable a profession to bring about a change in the context and facilitate the achievement of a purpose. The irrelevant is that which does neither—as in the case of futile care—that which threatens to frustrate the purpose is the inappropriate.

Wurzbach (1999) states that although persons seek certainty in their decisions, "ethical certainty can provide [unwarranted] comfort for the ethical decision maker . . . and stifle dialogue and in-depth discussion of the [situation]" (p. 287). All the certainty that one has in any given context is the certainty that the context allows. One can have contextual and contingent certainty but never final and immutable certainty.

The Levels of a Context

Every context has several levels. The first level is the split second, immediate present—the sensory level of awareness. Observations are taken of all the objective factors comprising the situation at any given moment taken in isolation from one another but without the awareness of their vital influence and relationship. This is the level of the contemporary ethical systems.

The second level is brought into being by a cognitive level of awareness. This level is provided by one's grasp of the nature and relationship of the objective factors as they exist in the present. This is the level of a nurse whose overriding concern is the well-being of her patient.

The third level is produced by foresight. Foresight provides the awareness of relationships, events, and causal sequences as they have evolved out of the past into the present and how they are relevant to the future. This is, or ought to be, an APN's bioethic.

The higher the level of a context and the more an APN relates herself internally to the context, the more appropriate her decisions and the more effective her actions will be. A nurse is "the agent of a patient doing for a patient what he would do for himself if he were able" (Husted & Husted, 2015, p. 17). Her patient is the center of the context. She is acting internally to the context when the values and motivations that produce decisions and actions on her part are her patient's values and motivations. Values and motivations that are not her patient's, but demanded

by the contemporary ethical theories, are external and irrelevant, and often inappropriate, to the context. They produce externally related, out-of-context actions, and very often tragic examples of injustice.

That which is relevant to a practice-based professional ethic is not a matter of tradition or social convention. In the health-care setting, ethical decisions and actions begin with a grasp of those things that are crucially important in the life of a human individual. An APN is a human individual and is capable of understanding and dealing with this.

THE FLOURISHING OF AN ADVANCED PRACTICE NURSE

> Decision-making is that which most characterizes advanced practice. . . . Underlying decision-making are clinical judgments, scholarly inquiry, and leadership. . . . The work of the APN is practice, the product is patient care; therefore, leadership in the advanced practice role supports the scientific process by:
>
> • Interpreting the context of practice
> • Demonstrating influences on care
> • Leading changes in practice
> —(Erickson & Sheehy, 1998, p. 244)

That ethical decision-making skills are part of the core competencies of all APNs is a basic tenet and central to the definition of advanced nursing practice (Reigle, 1996). Ideally, the ethical aspects of practice have developed along with the clinical aspects.

A practice-based ethic aims to relate professionals and patients internally, to bring them into the same ethical context, to make human values its purpose, and to make the health-care setting maximally purposeful and mutually intelligible. An APN can master the art and science of ethical decision making and interacting with what is important in her patient's life. In doing so, she increases her patient's well-being, strengthens the profession of nursing, keeps the practice of nursing contextually intelligible, and establishes for herself the conditions of pride in herself and her profession.

Only by following the definition of her profession can a nurse make her profession intelligible to her patient and to herself. Being the agent of her patient defines her profession. She takes actions for a patient—a person who has been formed by a lifetime of unique experiences and unique reactions to these experiences. In doing this, she develops pride in herself and in her practice. To allow a relatively helpless but competent person to decide for himself is the highpoint of a nurse's pride in her profession and her self-esteem.

The nurse takes actions that a patient cannot take for himself. Yet, although she takes these actions, they are his actions. In coming under her care, he does not give up his right to self-determination—his right to think, decide, and act for himself. He is in a health-care setting to gain the power of expressing himself in action. He is there so that health-care professionals can take the actions that he would take if he were able. These are actions that he has lost the power—but not the *right*—to take.

Every action of an APN is an interaction, whether the action is a cause that results in an immediate effect or a cause whose intended effect occurs farther on down a chain of causal sequences. All cooperation requires interaction.

The noblest action a nurse can take, without which no justifiable action is possible, is her act of accepting her patient as a human being as real as she is. Without this, the context is unintelligible and no real interaction is possible. For the APN, "the importance of developing skills of critical thinking, self-exploration, and the ability to sift through contextually relevant elements of ethical situations" (Doane, Pauly, Brown, & McPherson, 2004) cannot be overlooked.

THE NURSE–PATIENT AGREEMENT

Interaction requires intelligibility. Interaction is possible only when all parties to the interaction know what they are doing, why they are doing it, and what they intend to accomplish. All this requires a prior agreement. An agreement is a shared state of awareness on the basis of which interaction occurs (Husted & Husted, 2015).

A nurse agrees that, for a time, she will be part of a patient's world. Her skills make her a vital part. Decisions can be made and actions can be taken based on an ethical agreement between a professional and her patient. The nature of these decisions and actions is limited by the terms of their agreement. Non–practice-based ethical theories demand that in her ethical decisions and actions she abandon her patient and his world. Her patient is protected by

nothing. He cannot rely on his nurse's dedication. To a greater or lesser extent, his rights and human dignity—his very reality—have been dispensed with.

An APN has the resources for appropriately meeting the demands of the context. An effective health-care setting encourages her in discernment and discovery. Hardt (2001) states: "The . . . [APN] cannot practice successfully in an environment that does not foster context-driven decision making. If [caring nurses] . . . are not able to apply the knowledge they have gained from patients, related to their patient's preferences, then the patient's context is not honored" (p. 45).

A professional, through her open declaration that she is a professional, takes on various obligations as part of the nurse–patient agreement. Through these obligations a patient can rightfully expect the nurse to act ethically and conscientiously within the context. These obligations and these expectations are an integral part of the agreement between a nurse and her patient (Husted & Husted, 2008b).

If a patient's context is not honored, the APN's agreement, in whatever form it takes, is not honored. If the APN–patient agreement is not honored, then the professional is not practicing a profession, but a sham.

Professional practice is sufficient to establish a health-care professional–patient agreement. One human recognizes another. "Seeing each as human, diverse, equal, and worthy were all part of the view of the meaning of human dignity" (Kalb & O'Conner, 2007, p. 200). They recognize the human values that are the basis of their interaction and the attitudes appropriate to guiding these interactions. Because of this, the agreement between them can be formed spontaneously and on an implicit level—the level implied by their relationship. Under the circumstances, the human nature of each guides their awareness, the forming of an implicit agreement to interact, and their interaction. Even with an incompetent, comatose, or very young patient, the nurse's responsibility remains the same. There is a professional agreement in place. She does not have an explicit agreement with this patient, but she does have an implicit, professional agreement.

Even APNs, who are not practicing in the arena of direct patient care, still have the nurse–patient agreement in place. Educators, administrators, and researchers are all ultimately responsible for patients and their well-being. The role of the educator is for the benefit of the patient.

There is a teacher–student–patient agreement. A nurse administrator is ultimately responsible for patients and their well-being. There is an administrator–staff–patient agreement. A researcher must have the well-being of her subjects uppermost in mind, and thus there is a researcher–subject agreement. The research cannot come before the welfare of persons.

THE AGREEMENT ONE HAS WITH ONESELF

Socrates, the first systematic ethicist of the Western world (470–399 BC), is known to have observed that the unexamined life is not worth living.

> Every nurse, [every APN], ought to examine her life, at least to the point at which she comes to an agreement with herself that she will be a nurse. To the extent that a nurse has not made this agreement with herself—a commitment to be a nurse—she resembles a patient more than she resembles what she would be if she were a nurse.
> —(Husted & Husted, 2015, p. 43)

A nurse who directs her actions guided by her awareness of what is needed for her to keep that agreement embraces her profession. A nurse who is inspired by it, and who is dedicated to it, is far less likely to experience burnout. She experiences joy in taking action . . . and pride and confidence in acting as she does.

> A nurse [who] tries to avoid taking those long-term actions that constitute her professional life breaks the agreement she made with herself to be a professional. She becomes indifferent. She undermines herself as a professional and as a person. If she has replaced her confidence and pride with indifference, she has done this because she abandoned herself when she abandoned her profession.
>
> If one is a nurse and is likely to continue to be a nurse, one ought to take the actions [nursing] calls for. At worst, this will make life far less boring. At best, it may restore her to the confident expectations and the pride that she began with at the beginning of her career.
>
> Dedication to what one professes—acting on that which one affirms and believes—is sometimes difficult to do. Adversities and frustrations arise. And these attack one's desire and one's sense of self.
> —(Husted & Husted, 1999, p. 17)

Overcoming adversities through dedication produces pride in oneself as a professional. A patient could not reasonably ask for more and should not find less. He needs a rational agent to do for him what he would do for himself simply because his well-being depends on acting on the basis of reason.

THE ADVANCED PRACTICE NURSE AND THE ETHICAL AGREEMENT

To the extent that an APN acts without regard for her patient's needs and values, she assumes that his decisions and actions have no ethical standing. To the extent that an APN acts for a patient—according to his rational motivations—she shares her patient's rightful authority over himself. His rightful authority over himself is absolute.

Many agreements require detailed, explicit discussion. For obvious reasons, the agreement between an APN, or any nurse and patient, cannot require this. A nurse's interventions, quite often, must begin immediately. What will be discovered during the course of treatment is unpredictable.

An implicit agreement can be formed immediately. This is made possible by the fact that the role of nurse and patient are firmly settled in rational human expectations. Reflection on herself and on her needs gives a nurse a clear idea of a patient's needs and values. Although it is not possible for any person to know fully and completely the lived reality of another, it is the nature of human understanding to draw on common experiences and images to form agreements.

BIOETHICAL STANDARDS

The bioethical standards of autonomy, freedom, objectivity, beneficence, and fidelity signify properties inherent in the nature of every human person. See **Table 30.4.** They are the innate and defining properties of a human life. As guidelines they prevent "contradictions," actions or interactions that conflict with a patient's power to act—his agency.

There are certain individualized characteristics that every patient brings into the health-care setting and retains by right. Any human characteristic—any virtue—that is

TABLE 30.4	
The Bioethical Standards	
Autonomy	Uniqueness, independence, and ethical equality
Freedom	Right to direct the course of one's life
Objectivity	Ability to deal with the reality of one's situation
Beneficence	Right to judge benefit and harm for one's self
Fidelity	Faithfulness to the terms of an agreement

necessary to his successful interaction, first as a human and then as a patient, is a resource that cannot, in any way, be justifiably violated.

It greatly increases an APN's efficiency if she understands the functions of these characteristics to exercise and to interact with them. The bioethical standards signify these characteristics. They are the resources without which any interpersonal agreement or interaction would be impossible, without which a patient's recovery would be inconceivable, and without which a nurse could not function. These are the characteristics of a nurse and patient:

- *Autonomy*—The individual uniqueness of each patient. This uniqueness is the structure of his individual nature, the liaison of his character structures.

His autonomy is structured by the way he uses his mind, the decisions he has formed, his view of his life, his purposes, and the powers and disabilities of his agency. His autonomy includes his power of reason and his animal nature. As a consequence of his rational animal nature, his ethical equality with all other rational agents is established.

Primarily, however, autonomy refers to a person's uniqueness. No two people develop identically. There is no alternative to a human person being unique. Therefore, his uniqueness is a person's innate right. It is a nurse's guidepost to her professional actions.

There is no possibility of one sustaining the excellence of the person he is unless he sustains who he is. Thus, autonomy is a basic virtue.

- *Freedom*—Self-directedness. An agent's capacity, and consequent right, to take independent actions based on his own evaluation of his present situation.

It is the responsibility of a nurse to enable a patient to exercise his freedom. The ability to plan and act effectively in the present with an eye to the future is a value to, and an excellence of, any human being as a human being.

- *Objectivity*—The ability to focus one's attention onto an objective context.

Objectivity is a person's need and right to achieve and sustain his exercise of objective awareness. This standard calls for a nurse to sustain this in her patient and in herself.

To the extent one fails to exercise objectivity, he cannot act to enhance his life. The complete absence of this would destroy the ability to sustain his life. Objectivity is a necessary element of human excellence.

- *Beneficence*—The natural inclination of a person to act to achieve that which is beneficial and to avoid that which is harmful. This implies rational self-interest as the basis of the nurse–patient interaction.

A nurse's actions assist this effort. This standard establishes the right of a patient (or professional acting as the agent of a patient) to act for his benefit. It is the self-interest processes that define life. Rushton (1992) points out that nurses have an obligation to themselves as well as to their patients and others. This is in keeping with rational self-interest as discussed by Husted and Husted (2015). And following on this, "respect for one's own dignity . . . [is] a prerequisite to respecting the dignity of patients, colleagues, and others" (Gallagher, 2004, p. 220).

It is established by the necessity he faces to act, insofar as possible, to acquire the benefits the patient desires and the needs his life requires.

The ability to achieve benefits is what makes life worth living. The ability to avoid harms is a correlate of this.

• *Fidelity*—Adherence to the terms of an agreement. More generally, an individual's faithfulness to his autonomy. And, finally, fidelity to the context.

For a nurse, fidelity is a commitment to the obligations she has accepted as part of her professional role—her professional role being a significant part of her autonomy.

The dedication to continue on courses of action that are appropriate to enhancing life and well-being—this is fidelity. This is essential to human excellence. It is a most desirable virtue.

A nurse ought to recognize these virtues not as obstacles to be overcome but as character resources to be nurtured. She ought to recognize these virtues as her own. A person's life would be a woebegone affair without them. See **Figure 30.1.**

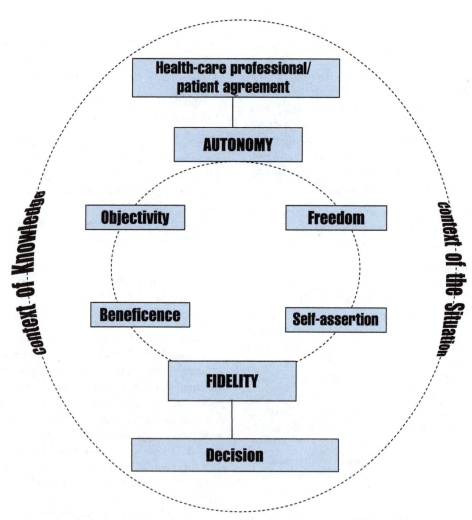

FIGURE 30.1   Husteds' symphonological bioethical decision-making guide.   (Source: Husted, J. H., & Husted, G. L. (2015). *Ethical decision making in nursing and health care: The symphonological approach* (4th ed.). New York, NY: Springer. Used with permission of Springer Publishing Company.)

THE NECESSITY OF THE AGREEMENT

Every APN is at least implicitly aware of a patient's possession of these virtues. She cannot escape awareness of them. Without these virtues, their agreement would not be possible. Without agreement, their interaction would not be possible. If their interaction is not possible, professional actions are not possible. If the virtues are violated, the nurse–patient agreement cannot be sustained. If the agreement is not sustained, interaction is impossible. If interaction is not possible, the practice of a profession is not possible. This is the source of the importance of the bioethical standards to professional practice. Their irreplaceable importance arises in the very first moment.

The Virtues of an Advanced Practice Nurse

Here we are using virtue in its original Greek and Chinese sense: the excellence of a person in performing his role as a person. Thus, the virtue of a farmer is to farm well, of a tailor is to make excellent clothing, and of a nurse is to nurse well. The virtue of every human being is to *live* well, to sustain and enhance his life. Thus, virtue is the excellence of a human being in being human.

Aristotle states, "Now fine and just actions . . . admit of much variety and fluctuation of opinion, so that they may be thought to exist only by convention, and not by nature" (as cited in McKeon, 1941, p. 936). However, fine and just actions follow from characteristics that are fundamental aspects of human nature and the virtues of a human person.

The standard of autonomy includes the inescapable fact (that is too often evaded) that every member of the human species—every rational animal—derives his ethical dignity from his nature as a member of the human species. This produces the fundamental ethical reality. Every ethical agent is the ethical equal of every other. No ethical agent can rightfully aggress against another for the benefit of that second ethical agent (Mill, 1988). Infidelity to, and aggression against, another can never arise from the virtues.

An APN is much more able to take direction from her patient's *autonomy*—his uniqueness—because she is not as engrossed in her own uniqueness as she would be if she were relatively new to the profession. If she is new to the profession, she is more focused on herself because she is, quite rightly, unsure of the requirements and techniques of her profession.

An APN is much more capable of allowing and fostering the *freedom* of her patient because she, herself, has mastered the skills that an advanced beginner must still acquire. Therefore, she is free to act within her patient's entire context. Every APN has taken independent actions to become an APN. Now she can assist her patient to take the independent actions that will restore him to a state of agency. Here, her experience is her best teacher.

An APN has a much greater ability to observe a context and to form *objective,* meaningful patterns of action because her body of knowledge is greater. She has had to exercise objective awareness to acquire the skills of an APN.

An APN has exercised a greater-than-average *beneficence* (rational self-interest) toward herself in achieving the benefit of becoming an APN. She has also made herself better able to assist her patient in pursuing his values. She sees the patient as the beneficiary of her actions and has, hopefully, automatized this in her practice. This is the ethical foundation of her practice.

An APN has had the opportunity to develop a personal and professional integrity to the point that she understands that fidelity to her patient is *fidelity to herself,* to her professional practice, and to her life. As a nurse, she does not see this fidelity as separate from herself.

Because an APN does not have to think solely about the technical aspects of her professional practice, she is free to see the agreement as reciprocal (given the differences in their roles) and necessary.

An APN's knowledge is comprehensive and elaborately organized so that information storage and retrieval is easy. Her clinical knowledge is linked into networks of concepts and relationships, which are then compiled into a higher order knowledge structure that links intricate mental networks into a scheme of relationships and interaction.

Through experience, an APN has become capable of discovering much that a less experienced nurse is incapable of discovering. Progress in an APN's development will move through, and be structured by, her experience to the extent that she has capitalized on her experience. Retaining her experience of ethical situations will increase her context of knowledge. It will enable her to structure and integrate it. As her context of knowledge becomes greater, the context of every situation can become clearer to her. If she deliberates about the meanings of her experiences, this produces a relationship between her context of knowledge, the context of each individual situation that leads to an increase in her professional skill, and her context of awareness. This is also true of her ethical skill generally.

The big picture, and its meaningful details, will become evident through an increase in her knowledge and its attendant power to increase her awareness of present facts and future conditions. The increased acuity of her awareness will form an ever-greater body of knowledge with its power to clarify and sharpen her awareness of her patient's context. This is the source of her ethical competence.

This process of an APN's discovery and learning can never be complete. Learning that makes further learning seem impossible or unimportant has destroyed itself as a biological instrument in human life. The nature of every new situation must be learned. It can only be learned through contextual analysis of each situation.

Ethical efficiency requires that every situation be approached without one's mind being enclosed in a handful of out-of-context-assumptions. Out-of-context truths work *against* ethical judgment.

Even the knowledge that character and motivations are produced by the dynamic complex of relationships among one's virtues (the bioethical standards) is a dead-end to practice if knowledge stops there. This knowledge of the bioethical standards is not sufficient to ethical decision making. It is not knowledge of self-sufficient rules. Through analysis, the bioethical standards are simply sufficient to guide the awareness that they can produce practice-based resolutions to every *individual* dilemma. *The standards must always be applied in the context.*

If there is any reason why nursing diagnosis and treatment is centered on her patient, there is no reason why her ethical decisions and actions should not be. Each serves the same values. To be faithful to the context, an APN cannot turn her back on anything in the context, most especially on her patient. If her patient cannot "call out" to her, then nothing in the context can.

A context-based model actualizes the concept of treating persons as individuals and therefore selecting individualized interactions based on a unique patient's needs and circumstances. It is a nurse's awareness of the patient's perceptions of his situation that assists her in understanding her patient's needs and desires. Symphonological theory is not just another compilation of traditional cultural platitudes. Symphonology presents a method of helping the nurse determine what is practical and justifiable regarding those aspects of her practice. Further, the theory of symphonology recognizes that the context guides what is possible and desirable in the agreement (Scotto, 2008).

ABOUT CASE STUDY ANALYSIS

When ethically analyzing a case study, a difficulty arises in that, in practice, one would request more information—more pieces of data, answers to a greater number of questions—but the nurse can only work with what she has. And so, in a case study, the dilemma must occur entirely within the given context. Now consider the case presented in **Box 30.1.**

Notice that in analyzing this case we did not once use the term *ethics* nor did we name the bioethical standards. Nonetheless, our process was one of ethical decision making from a practice-based perspective. Similarly, a study by Irwin (2004) showed that when patients had an ethical decision to make, they used all the bioethical standards (albeit not the words) in arriving at their conclusions when talking about the decision. In a more complex case, analysis through each standard would be desirable to arrive at the most appropriate decision within the context. (For examples of more complex cases in which analysis is done through bioethical standards, see Husted & Husted [2015].)

As we have demonstrated through the contemporary ethical theories, ethics means different things to different people. By concentrating on decision making and speaking in human terms that everyone can understand, you can probably avoid the chaos that results when, for instance, the head of a societal expectation bumps into the head of a scheme for the greatest good for the greatest number. Or either bumps into the head of an irreconcilable rule.

MUSINGS

Each patient entering the health-care system hopes to derive some benefit. He hopes to regain his competence to perform his normal functions and to live his life as he chooses. He wishes to enter again into the pursuit of

Box 30.1

Case Study

Lois Ott, a 58-year-old, is suffering from end-stage renal disease. She can no longer do anything that gives her pleasure and she is exhausted all the time. She has decided to forego dialysis and let the disease take its course. She has given this decision careful thought. Her family disagrees with her decision and has tried to talk her out of it. They are even thinking about trying to have her declared incompetent on the basis that the toxins in her blood system are making her thought process erratic. Roger, a family nurse practitioner, has been seeing Lois in the dialysis clinic for years. Lois has discussed her plans with Roger. Her family has tried to elicit Roger's help in getting her declared incompetent.

With the dialysis, Lois could probably live another 6 to 9 months. In supporting Lois, Roger can argue as follows:

Lois has had a lifetime of experiences. She has made a lifetime of choices and decisions and formed her life and *herself* according to her experiences and choices. If we, as professionals, have a right to ignore this, then her rights in the health-care system are displaced by habit and force. What we have become through our experiences and choices does not entitle us to erase the person that Lois is and treat her as one object among other objects in the health-care system. There is nothing in this situation that would, objectively, justify our stripping Lois of the right to determine her own life. On the surface, it seems that Lois's family is acting in her place and trying to think and decide with her. However, what Lois needs most is help in convincing her family that they are abandoning her and leaving her all alone in the experience of dying. Lois should not be all alone.

The course of action that Lois has chosen will injure no one and violate no one's rights. If we join her family in making her the instrument of what they desire, we will be harming her and violating her rights. However we go about the business of violating Lois's rights, we cannot make our actions right. We cannot make our actions appropriate and justifiable. It is not appropriate that Lois spend another 6 or 9 months alone, abandoned by the health-care system and her family and suffering during this time.

If we take control of her life and actions, her life will not belong to her. It will belong to us. We will act as though she is not the one living her life. We would not be content for someone else to choose the level of suffering we should endure and the way we should end our life. By the same token, *we* should not choose for *her.*

Lois has expressed her individual desires. Many people would not desire this, but many would, and Lois does. If, in every difficult decision, we were determined that those who disagree with us must accept our perspective, we would simply be acting as terrorists. These arguments can be offered in support of Lois. No comparable arguments can be made against Lois's position.

We made an agreement with Lois that we would act as her agent. Now we are entertaining the justifiability of breaking that agreement. This will make us unfaithful to Lois and unfaithful to our profession. There is no logical way we can justify this.

his happiness. At the very least, he expects to come out better able to live than when he went into the health-care system. Each of the bioethical standards is appropriate to these purposes.

The *standard of autonomy* enables a patient to maintain his way of understanding himself and his world. (In a psychiatric setting, objectivity often replaces autonomy as a goal. Objectivity—an awareness of the facts of the external world—is a necessary precondition of autonomy. An autonomous being is autonomous in his relation to the external world.)

Sara is a timorous 82-year-old lady. Roseanne, her nurse practitioner, relates to her in a manner that implies that it is all right to be a timorous 82-year-old lady. When Sara leaves the health-care setting she will have a sense of her autonomy as strong as, or stronger than, when she entered.

The *standard of freedom* supports a patient's right to function as an independent being. It is the freedom to make the ethical decisions that affect his life.

> Billy is a curious 6-year-old boy. Jane, his pediatric nurse practitioner, talks to him. She explains things to him. She asks his opinion. She allows him to make appropriate choices. Billy leaves the hospital as independent and self-confident as he was when he entered, or more so. In relation to his sense of freedom, Billy's hospital stay has had a positive effect.

The *standard of objectivity* is a patient's ability to function as a reasoning being. To do this, he must have access to the understanding of his situation.

> Jeff has been put on a low-salt, low-fat diet. Robert, his nurse practitioner, takes the time to explain to Jeff why he ought to stay on the diet. He motivates Jeff to stay on his diet by appealing to his understanding (his reason). He makes Jeff an active participant in his plan of care. He does not depend only on a passive emotional motivation that, in a few weeks, will probably fade away.

As Oscar Wilde (1989), tongue in cheek, remarked: "The only difference between a caprice and a life-long passion is that the caprice lasts a little longer" (p. 27).

The *standard of beneficence* protects a patient's reasonable expectation that he will derive some benefit from the health-care system. It is also recognition of a person's right *not* to be harmed, and this includes the right to avoid futile care.

> A patient is dying of metastatic cancer. His family believes that he is going to recover and has made him a full code, despite the evidence of his suffering. While he was conscious he had expressed not wanting to live. He is now semiconscious and cannot make his wants known. The only thing he has to look forward to is avoidance of suffering. Barbara, his nurse, arranges to discuss the situation with the family. If she is unsuccessful, she will request an ethics consult.

The *standard of fidelity*—faithfulness to the nurse–patient agreement—is to establish assurance that purpose of action is not abandoned.

> A child has wet the bed. He begs his nurse not to tell his parents. She promises that she will not. Fidelity establishes a predictable universe for the nurse and for her patient.

The agreement, with the bioethical standards as preconditions, is designed to enable a patient to bring his virtues into a biomedical setting, retain them while he is there, and have them intact when he leaves.

Bioethical analysis and interaction guided by the standards is not possible, in any objective sense, apart from the patient's purposes and attitudes. A patient is passive. His entire ethical purpose is to recover his agency, to act, to once again take charge of his life. The best thing that can happen to him is to encounter a nurse whose purpose is the same.

Through her progress as a nurse, an APN has, if only potentially, come to a greater understanding and experience of herself, of who she is, and hopefully she has come to appreciate the importance of this. Through her experience, she has come to understand the difference in the uniqueness in individuals and has gained a clearer insight into the meaning of this to an individual's progress toward a better life.

Through her experience, she has developed a greater-than-average skill at pursuing long-term goals guided by her objective awareness and an understanding of the importance and joy of this. Because of this, she is able to lead her patient down a version of the same path she has taken.

Index

Page numbers followed by "f" indicate figures, those followed by "t" indicate tables, and those followed by "b" indicate boxes.